ALLE · ZEIT · WACH · 1842

W. Janssen

Forensic Histopathology

Translated by S. Forster

With 162 Figures

Springer-Verlag
Berlin Heidelberg New York Tokyo 1984

Professor Dr. Werner Janssen
Direktor des Instituts für Rechtsmedizin
der Universität
Butenfeld 34, 2000 Hamburg 54
Federal Republic of Germany

Translator: Stephen Forster, BSc,
Furtwänglerstraße 27, 6900 Heidelberg, Fed. Rep. of Germany

Translated and revised from:
Forensische Histologie. Schmidt-Römhild Verlag 1977

ISBN-13:978-3-642-69144-7 e-ISBN-13:978-3-642-69142-3
DOI: 10.1007/978-3-642-69142-3

Library of Congress Cataloging in Publication Data. Janssen, Werner, 1924 – Forensic histopathology. Translation and revision of: Forensische Histologie. Includes bibliographies and index. 1. Forensic pathology. 2. Histology, Pathological. I. Title. [DNLM: 1. Forensic Medicine. 2. Histology.
W 755 J35f] RA1063.4.J3613 1984 614'.1 84-14155
ISBN-13:978-3-642-69144-7 (U.S.)

Softcover reprint of the hardcover 1st edition 1984

2119/3140-543210

Preface

In the literature, there is no comprehensive survey and assessment of the histology of natural and unnatural injuries to humans that has been scientifically researched and practically examined from the point of view of forensic medicine. Even today, an analysis of the international literature shows that the significance of histology in medicolegal examinations has not hitherto been systematically presented in the English language. Above all, there is a lack of a critical appraisal of the evidence value of histology and its significance within the scope of concrete forensic determinations. In the present volume, I have attempted to rectify this situation and thus bridge the prevailing gap in the literature. It is not, however, intended that a new area of histology be established as an independent discipline within forensic medicine. Rather, those facilities of histology will be emphasized that should be considered by scientists in forensic practice.

There are of course older and more recent studies on branches of the subject (Kasianow 1954; Gerin 1965; Raekallio 1965, 1970; Pioch 1966; Berg 1972; Benecke 1972; Perper and Wecht 1980). Otherwise, isolated histological examination findings on organ and tissue damage have been dealt with in old and new standard works on forensic medicine (Hofmann and Haberda, von Neureiter, Walcher, Ponsold, Mueller, Popielski and Kobiela, Prokop, Poulsen, Tedeschi et al., Uotila, Gresham). Finally, the majority of pathoanatomical textbooks and manuals also contain details on the appearance of the corpse, vital reactions, hemorrhages, hypoxidosis, intoxication, etc., which are of interest to the medical examiner.

This book is not only a compilation of generally established findings; it also broaches problems, relates personal experience, and considers basic principles that are of scientific rather than practical significance. As a result, it is unavoidable that ideas are also presented that are perhaps not universally accepted. Many areas could only be touched upon and mentioned with reference to the literature. Various questions had to be left open or excluded because of the inevitable limitation of the large subject area. During the writing of this book, I have endeavored to make forensic histology accessible to as large a circle of interested readers as possible. However, an understanding of the material would be facilitated by an awareness of histopathology and a general feel for the forensic approach to questions. This book is primarily intended for physicians who take the trouble to adopt the methods and findings of histopathology in the solution of forensic problems.

The German edition of this book was completed in December 1976 and published in 1977. Prior to translation into English, the contents were revised and the references updated to the middle of 1981. The pictorial material has been supplemented and in some cases replaced.

I am grateful for the extensive technical assistance of many of my fellow workers at the institute. Similarly, I thank my wife who has helped me as a colleague and I thank all those who assisted me in the preparation of the manuscript. I am grateful to numerous colleagues at home and abroad for their assistance with organic and pictorial material.

Finally, I acknowledge the tremendous work of Stephen Forster with the English translation; he performed this task promptly and with great care.

Hamburg, January 1984 W. JANSSEN

Table of Contents

A. Introduction

I. Subject-matter and Functions of Forensic Histology

In its subject-matter, histology, as the science of cellular structures and their combined functions, results from the findings of morphological examinations and working methods. It is concerned with the study of minute tissue structures and their associated chemicophysical character. Through a direct approach with the direct recording of cellular data, histology – unlike almost any other medical discipline – has promoted the recognition and understanding of natural, pathological, and unnatural changes to the human body. Histopathology, as the study of pathologically altered tissues, and forensic medicine have made use of this knowledge. The inquiry into unnatural death and the tracking down of the causes of injury necessitate that certain fields and specially developed principles of histological investigation require particular consideration. These are the elements of forensic histology, which is not just a branch of patho-anatomical examination but should be understood in the light of its own forensic approach to the problems. Proceeding from the knowledge of diseases and postmortem alterations of human tissue, all histological findings are pertinent which enable forensically relevant facts to be established and the causes of injury recognized from the cellular status (status ex post).

Due to the varied nature of the different kinds of lesion on the one hand and the incidence of similar histological findings with different etiologies on the other, it seems logical to divide the material into two main sections. In the first part, "General Section," those changes and findings will be dealt with that are regarded as basic phenomena. They frequently exhibit regular development and at the same time can lead to injury in several systems of the human organism. These comprise the findings from necroses, postmortem changes, vital reactions, hemorrhages, mechanically induced tissue damage, aspirations, embolisms, hypoxidosis, morphological findings associated with shock, including allergies, and the histological contribution toward identification. In accordance with the classification in morphological pathology – general pathology, special pathology – the first part of the book embraces the tissue changes that can occur largely independent of any specific eliciting cause. In the second part, those topics are presented that involve a special kind of injury with particular subsequent impairment. Among others, these include some diagnostic problems of sudden death from natural causes, "legal obstetrics", including abortion and aborticide, strangulation, drowning, burns and cold, radiation and starvation injuries, and histological findings in poisoning. A comprehensive presentation of the enzyme-histochemical age determination of mechanically inflicted skin wounds, histochemical investigations of thermal skin injuries, gunshot wounds, and nuclear morphological sex determination has been dispensed with. With reference to the relevant books by Raekallio, Pioch, Hellmer and Schwinger we will here restrict ourselves to a brief informatory review.

II. Histological Investigatory Findings as Forensic Evidence

In the evaluation of medical findings in the administration of justice, a particularly high degree of reliability of the evidence has to be observed. It does not suffice, for instance, for a cause of injury or a causal connection to be merely statistically or empirically established; concurrently, evidence must be procured to exclude other, even exceptional, causes. If the evidence is based on the results of histological investigations then the consultant can define its significance in as concrete a form as possible. Moreover, he should ensure that other doctors can verify his assertions with the aid of his investigatory material, for instance, the sections assessed by him.

Statements concerning the value of forensic evidence in the results of histological investigations could be substantially simplified and freed from the risk of false estimation if rigid standards could be set out which would be applicable in practice to as many cases as possible. Despite all efforts toward a scientific standardization of the evaluation of medical findings, such a systematic arrangement is only possible within very narrow limits. The reasons lie in the individual diversity of tissue reactions and in the uniformity of tissue reactions from different causes. Further, in histology, the determination of quantitative properties is only of little use. Of the data relating to quantitative differences, for example, intensive or less intensive staining, many or few leukocytes, there are on the whole no features that have a distinguishing character. Quantitative evaluation is especially difficult in histochemistry (Lake and Ellis 1976). Moreover, it should be borne in mind that histological findings in tissues without organic structures or in badly damaged zones are not precisely measurable and, hence, are inappropriate for quantitative evaluation, even utilizing modern histometric or physicochemical methods. Conversely, the recognition of true qualitative distinctive features is of significance. They can provide information independent of a subjective "many" or "few" and independent of the personal interpretation of the investigator as to the presence or absence of histological criteria.

The value and significance of histological data can be considered from different aspects. First, according to the evidential value of the tissue data itself; second, according to its position within the framework of evaluation which results from the facts of the case that have come to light in combination with other findings. Accordingly, a *principle of classification* can be formulated which results from the relationship between the proven findings and the forensic approach to the problems. We believe that from these basic ideas all the test results of forensic histology can be arranged into three graded groups of different evidential value.

Group 1: This comprises histological findings where identification of their cause, character, and chronological pathogenesis is definite. Findings which are partly or wholly in accordance with these high requirements comprise a class of their own. Specificity and significance of the histological picture here permit, independent of all further data, the assessment of the causal connections between the condition and etiology. Certain stages of tuberculosis and several foreign-body granulomas can serve as examples. The existence and cause of these injuries can be determined on the basis of specific histological findings, even with a certainty to meet forensic requirements. A further example concerns abortion, the evidence for which is regarded as definite with the identification of chorionic villi or other such embryonic components. If this highly critical approach is extended to all histological investigations then the first group is demarcated, where the findings are independent of any knowledge of inferences drawn from additional circumstances.

Group 2: Here, those findings are classified that only have a forensically provable significance in association with further premises. The presence of additional facts is, therefore, prerequisite for the conclusiveness of such evidence. If, for example, the suspicion of homicide by means of an assault on the neck is being investigated, isolated fresh hemorrhages in the deep soft parts of the victim's neck can only be judged as evidence of strangulation if they are in combination with corresponding injuries of the overlying skin and larynx and further indications of asphyxiation and vascular congestion. In themselves, such hemorrhages in the soft parts of the neck are not unequivocal; they are still very much to be taken into account but in the final analysis are not of conclusive significance.

Group 3: This concerns histological findings which neither singly nor in combination with other facts represent evidence that excludes all other possibilities of causal explanation. This group includes many unspecific findings, for example, acute vascular congestion, pulmonary emphysema, petechial serous hemorrhages, cerebral edema, the majority of all parenchymal necroses. As evidence, these findings are basically ambiguous with regard to what can clearly be stated in their evaluation. These findings are either inappropriate or only of limited use as forensic-histological proof. In conjunction with other findings, they can attain informative significance. For example, in the case of pulmonary emphysema and vacuolar cell degeneration in the liver and myocardium, petechial serous hemorrhages can make a subacute death by asphyxiation seem probable.

The foregoing division of histological findings into three groups is a synthesis of medical evidence and forensic methodology; in a given case, it should provide information about the *evidential value* of a histological investigation. The basic requirement is as comprehensive as possible an awareness of histopathology and forensic medicine. In connection with the preceding histological rules of evidence, the practical application is largely oriented to the following questions:

a) Vital or postmortem-induced finding?
b) Cause of the finding?
c) What chronological connections can be established?

The *indication for histological examination* in the sphere of forensic medicine cannot be delimited and defined by universally valid guiding principles (Preda et al. 1965). It was stressed by Pioch (1966), with good reason: "Nothing is so trivial and small that it cannot become the decisive factor in legal proceedings." A hasty curtailment of the histological investigation is frequently a relinquishment of knowledge and evidential possibilities which cannot later be recovered. Investigations and competent opinions on the causes of death and the causal relations of human injuries that demand the minimum requirement of scientific method cannot dispense with histological evidence. Nevertheless, there are varying conceptions as to the necessity of histological examinations, and unfortunately investigations into the cause of death are still being concluded without the use of histology. The reasons are diverse: An enquiry into a case appears sufficiently "clear" from the macroscopic findings alone; mandators and doctors conducting the examination are only interested in a quick "settlement" of a case – especially when no extra fee is involved; specialized knowledge and understanding of the necessity of a histological examination are absent.

Of course, the experienced medical examiner in many cases will be able to appraise, just on the basis of macroscopic autopsy findings, whether further examination is necessary. He knows where and to what extent histological examination is required. However, even the experienced are not beyond being taken unawares, especially when in the postmortem examination there are no particular problems under consideration and it is only later that the etiology and chronological pathogenesis of certain tissue findings require clarification. Here, there is doubtlessly a superiority of the histological examination over the macroscopic observation (Carvalho 1964). It is not only of importance to the novice that as a matter of principle he includes a histological investigation in every case in which tissue findings are to be assessed. He should at least ensure that the organs or organ sections in question are preserved. It is in compliance not only with a general requirement for methodological completeness but also with the necessity for a comprehensive diagnosis of the entire human being that in the final evaluation of an autopsy the histological evidence be presented in the form of an overall status. In many, particularly Anglo-Saxon, countries it is judged an error and a lapse if morphological changes in operation specimens or postmortem findings are not clarified and supplemented by histological examination. It is obvious that the histological finding is important in the clinical and autopsy records.

III. Collection of Data and Examination Technique

The functions of forensic medicine entail that in the assessment of histological findings particular criteria have to be considered and checks made. The results of the investigation are evaluated on the strength of whether those premises and arguments are found that are necessary for offering evidence. The histological finding is, therefore, the basis and origin for all further considerations. Its quality and applicability are, however, dependent on the course of the examination and the methods of data collection. This is in principle also true for clinicopathological examinations – though here it is a question of providing evidence upon which the juridicial consequences of a verdict of guilty or not guilty on other people may be dependent. For this reason, a forensic evaluation of findings must to a particular degree pursue an approach that considers the entire human subject under examination. Despite all specialization, this holistic working method is still firmly established in scientific medicine. The method should nevertheless be a means toward understanding and not an end in itself.

Without going into details, only a few basic principles need be presented, the observance of which is to some extent self-evident.

A statement on histological changes should always be based on a complete postmortem examination. To this end, it is expedient that as far as possible the autopsy and histological examination be in the hands of one doctor or at least performed by the same institution. The advantages of such procedure are already evident in the *removal* and *processing* of the material. The medical examiner knows the macroscopic postmortem findings from his own investigation. In the interests of expediency, he also removes tissue samples himself for further examination. In this connection, the removal of the material, as fresh as possible, should be done with a drawing cut of a sharp knife and not with scissors. The piece of tissue removed, irrespective of the surface area, should not be thicker than 5 mm and must be protected from subsequent damage by immediate transfer into the fixation fluid or by deep freezing. Simple freezing of tissue specimens at temperatures of 0° –10 °C can lead to unwanted damage and cavity formation in liquid-rich organs. In the case of soft organs that are difficult to cut, larger pieces are first immersed and then further cut after about an hour when they have been fixed. The planar parts of organs, e. g., from the gastrointestinal tract, skin, and dura mater, are stretched out on pieces of cork or thick cardboard and thus protected from deformation during the fixation. Of course, taking the appropriate steps, samples for bacteriological or virological tests have to be removed during the obduction and, above all, before fixation of the tissue.

If the topography in a case under examination requires particular consideration or if several findings, e.g., wound sections or parts of the brain, are to be histologically tested then a schematic drawing of the sites of removal, marking of the tissue specimens, and separate preservation of the samples in labeled containers is recommended. Identification is also simple by means of careful threading of white cotton thread (Debarge et al. 1966); in Masson's trichrome stain, this can be selectively stained in the section with saffron. Occasionally, where there is an indistinct overall finding, fixation of the whole organ is necessary; incisions ensure that the fixative fluid also comes into contact with the central parts of the organ. Further, it is important to observe, even during the autopsy and in the removal of samples for the histological examination, that the organs do not unnecessarily come into contact with water, that they do not dry out, and that they do not have contact with other body fluids, such as bile, blood, or stomach contents. Finally, special care should be taken in the removal of small tissue samples, this is also true for biopsy specimens from living subjects, that they do not become contused or otherwise damaged. Orsós (1935) previously emphasized this point. If care is not taken, the histomorphology and quality of the stains suffer heavily.

Unfortunately, there are still setups in which the histological examination and assessment are not conducted by the medical examiner himself. Occasionally, even the tissue samples taken during the autopsy are sent off to other institutes. There, the histological expertise for a further appraisal is available to the forensic medical examiner. In this manner, histological findings are evaluated by forensic medical experts who are in no position to make appropriate judgements for themselves. For a consultant the advantage is thereby lost in knowing from a personal examination of the corpse the connections between the individual findings and the sampling sites of the tissue specimens. This situation applies, for example, in the examination of variously formed wounds, hemorrhages in the scalp and underlying damage to the brain, uncertain strangulation marks, and findings in several lung and brain sections. It must be stressed on this account that first-hand knowledge of the macroscopic postmortem findings facilitates a correlated assessment of the histological data. Personal removal of the tissue samples serves the same purpose; it simplifies orientation in the overall impression of histological sections and encourages the maintenance of topographic coherence in the analysis. The failure to observe these requirements and the omission or incomplete execution of the histological examination are, in the experience of the author, a frequent cause of disputed analyses in foro. For those involved in legal proceedings it is then easy to draw up contrary interpretations and contentions, which are difficult to refute without satisfactory and reproducible examination findings. In many countries in which high value is set on the correct administration of justice, material evidence, as opposed to the testimony of witnesses, is increasingly coming to the fore in legal proceedings. It is therefore to be expected that, likewise, histological material evidence in cases of corporal injury and homicide will gain in importance.

In the further treatment of the removed tissue samples, the choice of the *fixation* method is a science in itself, especially since the nature of the fixing process is still not fully known today. Many factors play a part – type of tissue, diffusive capacity of the fixative fluid, shrinking and hardening of the tissue, precipitation of protein particles, duration, temperature, isotonicity, concentration and pH of the solution,

Table 1. Commonly used fixation and staining methods. (After Romeis 1968)

	Fixation	Stain
General	Formalin 1:4 (Helly, Bovin, Heidenhain, Stieve)	H and E, iron hematoxylin method according to Weigert, trinitrophenol – thiazin red
For special purposes Nucleus (chromatin)	Carnoy, mercuric chloride – glacial acetic acid, Bovin, Allen	Hemalum, iron hematoxylin, gallocyanin, gallamine blue
Mitochondria	Regaud, Champy	Iron hematoxylin
Fat	Formalin – calcium	Sudan, nuclei with hemalum
Glycogen	Carnoy, Rossmann	Best (celloid in embedding) or according to H. Bauer
Blood cells	Helly	Dominici or Pappenheim
Connective tissue (collagenous, argyrophilic, elastic)	Heidenhain with formalin, Helly or Stieve	Azan, Bielschowsky, Gomori or with orcein or resorcinol fuchsin
Bony tissue	Formalin 1:4	With or without decalcification, Becher, galleinaluminium chloride solution
Muscular tissue	"Susa"	Iron hematoxylin, Azan, or Goldner
Nervous tissue	Formalin 1:4 or 1:8 or formalin-alcohol	Gallocyanin, Weigert-Kultschitzky, Bielschowsky, or Feyrter

etc. A great many possibilities, difficult to appreciate fully, are available, which have been expanded in recent years through the development of freezing technology and lyophilization. The selection is governed by the examination material at hand and by the proposed stain and mode of visualization. In routine practice, it should be taken into account that it is frequently not until during the course of the examination that forensically significant questions appear. It is, therefore, preferable to use a fixing agent that guarantees as great a latitude as possible for further treatment, e.g., formol in strong solution with one part 40% stock solution to as many as four parts water for short fixing times up to 24 h – or in weak solution with a dilution of 1:9 for longer periods. A good tabulated survey of commonly used fixing agents with their fields of application which is still fully effective is given by Romeis (1968) (Table 1). The subsequent treatment of the fixed material, the making of sections, and the techniques of staining can only be discussed briefly in the particular subject chapters. Otherwise, the pertinent text books must be referred to, e.g., Roulet (1948), Romeis (1968), Fasske (1964). Moreover, for information on new methods, which are constantly being developed, it is necessary to be aware of the current literature. The fields of electron microscopy, histochemistry, autoradiography, fluorescence microscopy, and immunohistology, which emerged together with histological research, have especially in the last 10–20 years undergone a rapidly increasing specialization that has given these subjects particular importance. The methods and results have already been introduced or comprehensively set out, e.g., Handbuch der Histochemie, Lison (1960), Pearse (1968), Reimer (1967), Lojda et al. (1976). For consideration of the skin in special forensic problems, the books by Raekallio (1965, 1970) and Pioch (1966) examine and summarize numerous histological methods and their applicability.

The successful application of histology with all the modern auxiliary sciences that go with it requires trained assistants and adequately equipped laboratories. These conditions must be similarly fulfilled in forensic medicine through the necessary acquisitions and expenditure. The establishment of large institutes covering all the special disciplines would be suitable (Prokop 1967). At such institutes, the investigation of forensic medical evidence and daily routine practice could be carried out jointly. As a result, corresponding demands would be made on the public institutions responsible for research in the service of justice.

B. General Section

I. Postmortem Changes (Histothanatology)

Preliminary Note. The boundary between life and death cannot be defined in the sense of a sharp dividing line with scientific precision either for the individual as a whole or for particular organs and tissues. It is much more a question of a zone whose time limits are illdefined, in which functional and structural changes occur at various expiry rates. The medical examiner working with histomorphology must proceed from this fact if he wants to tackle the problems of histothanatology (Gerin 1965). From the diagnostic possibilities of morphology, including ultramicroscopic methods, alone, he cannot decide whether a cell or an individual is living or dead. Likewise, he cannot in this manner precisely ascertain at what time death occurred – a fact that already emerged from the basic work by Merkel (1937), Walcher (1927), and Orsós (1935). The decisive criterion is, as Virchow has previously said, the assessment of a function. "Non-irritability and basal metabolism are states that cannot be registered through an analysis of form, for that reason the diagnosis 'death' persists in the range of the functional" (Letterer 1959).

Histomorphologically, the clues toward establishing the occurrence of death can only be provided if there are discernible changes that were produced subsequent to the time of death. These include all *postmortem changes or symptoms* (Merkel 1937; B. Mueller 1975). Histologically, such chances are not always specific for a postmortem origin since they can also arise in similar form in the most diverse toxic and degenerative injuries (Martines 1964). By way of contrast, *supravital reactions* signify those processes that occur after the death of the individual in separate organs or systems in the sense of a "survival reaction". They are due to the fact that the various organs and tissues in an individual do not die simultaneously. From numerous experiments, predominantly carried out on animals, it is known that whole cell systems, e.g., sperm cells in the seminal vesicles, can show mobility for up to several days postmortem. From this relatively long survival time for cells on the one hand to great sensitivity with early functional breakdown on the other, e.g., in nervous tissue, a timegraded *order of death* of the individual tissue types can be derived (B. Mueller 1975). A further breakdown of the zone between life and death with incorporation of agonal changes, such as those analyzed by Orsós (1935), Laves (1931), and Berg (1972), seems to us inappropriate owing to the intricate demarcation of the vital reactions.

In the following section, those histological findings will be presented that are suitable in reliably indicating the occurrence of death in cells and tissue. The *early postmortem signs through autolysis* are of primary importance, since in differential diagnosis they accompany the vital reactions and perhaps present a limited possibility of determining the time of death. A more summarized report requires the histology of putrefying tissues and organs, chiefly with the objective of indicating the border areas of diagnostic possibility. Decomposition, mummification, adipocere, etc. should as far as necessary be specified in the presentation of the particular organ findings. Walcher (1927) has already referred to the difficulties in a precise demarcation of autolysis and putrefaction in practice. Generally, autolysis and putrefaction proceed concurrently for a time.

1. Autolysis and Putrefaction

General

According to the definition by Strassmann (1924), autolysis signifies those postmortem fermentative processes that essentially operate without the participation of bacteria. In the histomorphological sense, autolysis implies the intravital or postmortem disintegration of living structures. Biochemically, autolysis corresponds to a loss in ordered metabolic equilibrium. As opposed to metabolism, metabolic breakdown with degradation of the metabolic substances results in a loss of energy and material. However, a sharp distinction between functional breakdown and decomposition of the structure is not possible, neither can a definite morphological and biochemical delimitation be made between reversible and irreversible processes, which were designated pathobiosis and necrobiosis, respectively, by Koslowski (1959). Autolysis, in the view of many authors, coincides with the activity of certain enzymes, so-called autolytic enzymes, which are already present in the living cell and after death lead to the lysis of the cell's own components (Neubauer 1928; E. Müller 1955; Letterer 1959). The living cell is probably kept from destruction by antienzymes (Merkel 1937; Specht 1937). Unlike autolysis, *heterolysis* depends on the action of enzymes that enter the cell from outside (Letterer 1959).

During the autolytic process, a hydrolytic splitting of proteins, nucleic acids, carbohydrates, and fats occurs. As a result, the postmortem activation of the cell's own enzymes is promoted by acidosis. Even during agony, a displacement of the pH to the acidic side can arise through an inadequate removal of metabolic waste and through the weakening buffering capacity of the blood (Letterer 1959). Decisive in the onset of autolysis is the cessation of the regular oxygen supply (Rössle 1933). According to the investigations of Lorke (1953), a rapid drop in the pH value to 4.7 occurs in the heart, liver, and kidneys during the first 30 h postmortem (HPM) (cf. Severinghaus et al. 1923).

According to Bradley (1922) and Goebel (1955), the acidification of the tissues is due to proteolysis with accumulation of amino acids, which owing to the deficiency of basic valences can no longer be neutralized. In this environment, cathepsin, the optimum activity of which occurs at pH 4–5, comes into effect.

Through the disappearance of the oxidative processes, substances with SH-groups, such as cysteine, glutathione, (Bradley 1938; Glanzmann 1941), which also have an enzyme-activating effect, become concentrated. Schmidt et al. (1959) found that postmortem autolysis occurs in two phases. First, through the continuation of glycometabolic processes, a concentration of lactic acid occurs with a sinking of the pH value. In the second phase, about 48 HPM, proteolysis increasingly occurs, which under aerobic conditions leads to an oxidative protein breakdown with the formation of CO_2 and NH_3, whereby the pH value rises into the alkaline. In this environment, tryptase can come into operation (Letterer 1959). Gallagher et al. (1956) and Richterich (1958) view the nature of autolysis as a disturbance of the metabolic balance, in contrast to postmortem enzymatic activation. Through cytolysis the synthetic capacity becomes suspended and as a result only enzymatically controlled breakdown processes continue which finally lead to a self-disintegration of the cell components (Braun-Falco and Winter 1964). According to the comparative investigations of Gössner (1960) on liver implants, the onset of the autolytic process is explained by the release of hydrolytic enzymes from lysosomes.

The autolytic process is dependent on various factors – temperature, air humidity, and environmental influences (Mackie 1929; Müller 1955; Greuer 1956; Krejci and Hradil 1962; Fukita 1966). Frank (1971) reports the preservative effect of metallic objects. The strongest autolysis occurs at temperatures between 37° and 40 °C. With a rise or fall in temperature autolysis can be inhibited. Autolysis is accelerated after freezing and thawing (Jannoni-Sebastianini 1930). Diseases and disturbed metabolic states also have an accelerating influence (Merkel 1937; Letterer 1959; Braun-Falco and Winter 1964), e.g., in the case of liver atrophy, postmortem cell disintegration proceeds faster and in a modified form (Beek and Haex 1943). From experience, certain tumor cells, especially carcinomas sometimes prove to be particularly resistant to autolysis.

Autolysis experiments of Arnoldt (1937) showed that in alkaline solution the glandula submaxillaris autolyses more rapidly than the glandula sublingualis; in an acidic environment, the reverse was true. Contrary to general expectation, large autolytic resistance was detected in the pancreas; after 24–48 h at pH 8 the nuclei were still comparatively well stained; the islets of Langerhans survived the longest. The suprarenal glands are among the most susceptible organs. The highest resistance was possessed by the sperm cells of the testes. The different reactions of the organs are explained by Arnoldt (1937) as being due to: (1) the different material arrangement of the individual cells, (2) their enzyme content, and (3) the prevailing pH conditions. The occurence of only small differences between a 24- and 48-h autolysis can thus be explained by new substances that emerge in the disintegration which inhibit the progress of autolysis.

Histochemical and Biochemical Findings. In the numerous attempts at an explanation and objective consideration of the autolytic phenomena, histochemical methods have been to the fore. The investigations have largely resulted from the problems of the utilization of histochemical techniques on autolytic or decayed tissue material, however, experimental studies have also ensued in the research into postmortem and autolytic influences on the characteristics of enzymes in the tissues. The results were just as variable in fundamental histochemistry as in enzyme histochemistry.

Generally, the claim is made that as far as possible only fresh living or well-preserved postmortem material should be used for histochemical investigations. However, it can basically be said that most enzymes and histochemically recordable elements remain traceable until, as with the traditional histological stains, autolytic changes become evident (Gössner 1955). The capacity to detect monoamine oxidase decreases relatively early, about 3–5 HPM. Succinodehydrogenase remains sufficiently demonstrable for approximately 6–8 HPM (Eder 1959). The ability to trace diaphorase, ATPase, and 5-nucleotidase is reduced relatively early, whereas esterases and phosphatases are preserved for a long time. In addition, the reduction in the capacity to detect enzymes can be influenced by technically induced fermentation inhibitors and by the different intensity of the compounds that are finally visualized.

Investigations of phosphatases and esterases by Gössner (1966) revealed no substantial changes in their activity and localization up to 12 HPM. Subsequently, a progressive reduction in the reaction and signs of diffusion occurred parallel with histologically detectable structural damage. Autolysis experiments with various temperatures in the livers and kidneys of rats by Holzner and Kaufmann (1962) showed the first impairment of ATPase activity after 12–24 HPM at 4 °C. At room temperature of 18°–22 °C this occurred after 2 HPM in the kidneys and after 4 HPM in the liver. In various vascular walls and in the renal glomeruli, there were still signs of diminished activity for up to 240 HPM. Serial comparative experiments on rat organs by Rozsa and Sotonyi (1964) to examine the various evidence for enzymes at 37 °C revealed after 4–6 HPM substantial structural changes in the cell plasma and, after 6–12 HPM, in the cell nucleus. Two phases could thereby be observed – in the first, granulation and swelling; in the second, homogenization and disintegration. The second phase of disintegration takes place at 37 °C after 24 HPM and at 2 °C after 72 HPM. Moreover, these experiments showed that the changes were often organ-specific. The Gomori-Takamatsu reaction for the detection of alkaline phosphatase only gave useful results directly after death; subsequently, unspecific changes appeared, which can be explained by increased calcium or calcium phosphate bonding of the autolytic tissue. After 6 HPM, therefore, demonstration of alkaline phosphatase with azo-dyes is favored.

In the heart muscle, kidneys, liver, and skeletal musculature of rats and rabbits, as well as in several muscle groups in man, the first decreases in succinodehydrogenase (SDH) activity in the form of localized translucencies are recognizable after 24–48 h with storage at 20 °C, and after 7 days at 0 °C. The activity in ferment-rich organs such as heart muscle and kidneys survived the longest. The SDH activity in the leukocytes of man and rabbits behaved similarly (Nanikawa and Janssen 1964). Quantitative SDH measurements by Nanikawa and Tawa (1960) on 72 mouse hearts showed a clear reduction of activity after 1 day at 25 °C; at temperatures of 0 °C and 5°–10 °C, the activity only decreased negligibly and substantially survived for up to 30 days postmortem. Autolysis investigations by Andersen (1960) on the skin, cartilaginous tissue, and skeletal musculature of human fetuses showed that for up to 6 HPM at room temperature and at 4 °C no loss of metachromasia or polysaccharide and sulfhydryl groups occured. These results are contrary to those of other authors.

Zimmermann and Platt (1962) noticed the influences of oxidative enzymes in anesthesia. With ether anesthesia, the reduction in SDH and isocitrate dehydrogenase activity in liver, heart, and kidneys was clearly more pronounced than after thiogenal anesthesia. At the same time, there was a mitochondrial swelling, which was evident directly after 2-h ether anesthesia or 5–14 h after 2-h thiogenal anesthesia. Short periods of anesthesia of only 15–45 min resulted in an initial increase in enzymatic activity.

With experimental thermal skin lesions and a subsequent autolytic period of 24 h, there was no clear difference in the fine glycogen distribution between intravitally and postmortem burned animals (Pioch 1966); after this time, glycogen was only sporadically demonstrable in the vital and postmortem preparations. However, unspecific esterase was invariably detectable after a 48-h autolytic period at room temperature, which is why this enzyme is particularly recommended for the forensic assessment of burning. Biochemical DNA measurements on bull hearts under extensive exclusion of autolysis showed no reduction in the values for up to 72 HPM. Histochemical preparations of catecholamine and 5-hydroxytryptamine by Penttilä (1971) in various rat organs showed a relatively uniform character with respect to the time of death. The formaldehyde-induced fluorescence of catecholamine completely disappeared within 24 h at room temperature; the autolytic propensities of the particular organs and the original concentration of the amine were here of influence.

General Comments on Putrefaction Histology. Putrefaction signifies the bacterially induced reduction and liquefaction of the organs. With time, autolysis and putrefaction pass one into the other. Normally, putrefaction is initiated by autolytic processes. A histomorphological differentiation of the two processes is only possible within certain limits. In the following section, some features will be emphasized toward a general outline.

Histologically, evidence of relatively large rod-shaped bacteria that can be bacterioscopically differentiated from pathogens characterizes putrefaction in progress. The bacteria reproduce relatively fast in the corpse according to the initial conditions and environment in which the corpse is lying; they tend to spread to the blood and lymph vessels (Fig. 1). The bacteria chiefly appear in those organs rich in capillaries and lymph clefts, especially, therefore, in the liver, lungs, musculature, and in the otherwise relatively putrefaction-resistant myocardium. In the case of corpses found in water, it is not unusual for bacteria and fungi to proliferate in the integumentary appendages (Fig. 2). Bacterial reproduction within the blood vessels can be so considerable as to give the impression of so-called bacterial embolism. Certain boundaries to the bacterial spreading can be set by cell membrane fibers and organ capsules.

According to the investigations of Walcher (1927), Strassmann (1924), and Merkel (1937), which even today hardly require supplementation, intact cell and nuclear membranes can be an obstruction to the penetration of putrefying bacteria for a relatively long time, as can the marginal lamellae of heart muscle fibers. Epithelial cells are usually destroyed by the effects of putrefaction before connective tissue elements. In many cells, e.g., of the adrenal medulla, decay of the cytoplasm is occasionally observed before the occurrence of large changes in the nucleus. Rapidly developing autolysis and putrefaction predominantly lead to diffuse chromatolysis with nuclear and cell wall hyperchromatism. With slow development of the whole process, on the other hand, karyorrhexis and nuclear evagination are observed. Putrefaction studies on animals by Zink and Reinhardt (1978) showed initially a contraction of the cells with an increase in the intercellular gaps and later a swelling with disintegration of the gaps and homogenisation of the organic pattern. Following total loss of chromatin, the nuclear membrane is often preserved, especially in

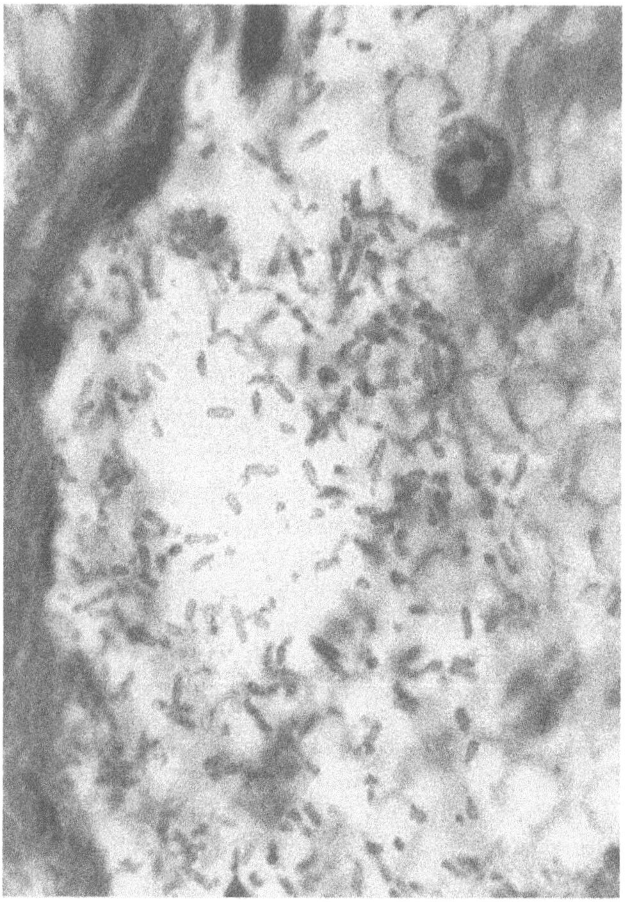

Fig. 1. Putrefactive bacteria in pulmonary interstitium spread intravascularly; 7 days postmortem (PM). H and E stain, 1:250

an earth grave, for as long as 4 months and in isolated cases it can remain over a year and longer. The cell membrane can behave similarly, even when the cytoplasm has already been fully reduced to detritus. Sudanophilic drops within the cytoplasm often outlast the cellular disintegration for a long time. Glia cells and leukocytes outside the foci of infection appear to be the most resistant cells to putrefaction in the human body; the cells of the epidermis follow closely behind. A positive oxidase reaction with decreasing strength and exactness is likewise found in myeloid cells after a long period of putrefaction, e.g., after months in an earth grave.

In the case of strong, rapidly developing putrefaction, a basic change in the neutral fats of the pulmonary vessels can occur leading to the symptoms of so-called postmortem fat embolism. This can, according to Walcher (1927), attain a considerable degree. Sometimes, the differential diagnosis of a vitally developed fat embolism can be difficult (cf. Chap. C II 3 a). In one particular case, the origin of a postmortem fat embolism of the lungs was accounted for by strong putrefaction with

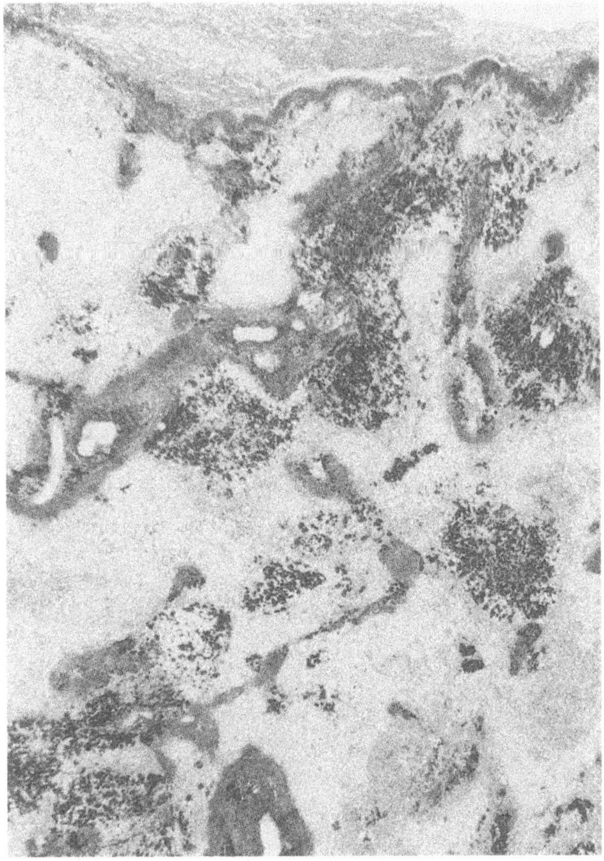

Fig. 2. Skin of the upper arm showing bacterial and fungal invasion of the integumentary appendages; 8 days PM. H and E, 1:40

solution of fat from an intense adiposis hepatica and displacement of the fat by gas being forced into the lungs.

Varied resistance to putrefaction is also seen in connective tissue. Tissues with ample collagen fibers are more durable to putrefaction than elastic fibers and lamellae. The collagen fibers do not disintegrate until the later stages, in which they are penetrated by "filamentary bacilli". Whereupon, a gradual diminution of the fiber substance as complete atrophy follows. A piecemeal decay has, however, not been observed.

Hematogenic and autochthonous pigments have, likewise, proved to be resistant to putrefaction. The postmortem pigment, sometimes very extensive, that frequently appears in the lungs does not contain any ionized iron, for which reason the usual tests for iron appear negative. The pigment shows affinity to the cytoplasm of many cells, particularly to the epithelia of the tubuli renales contorti, leukocytes, and alveolar macrophages. It can, however, also happen that unequivocal, intravitally derived and stored, iron-containing hematogenic pigments are no longer detec-

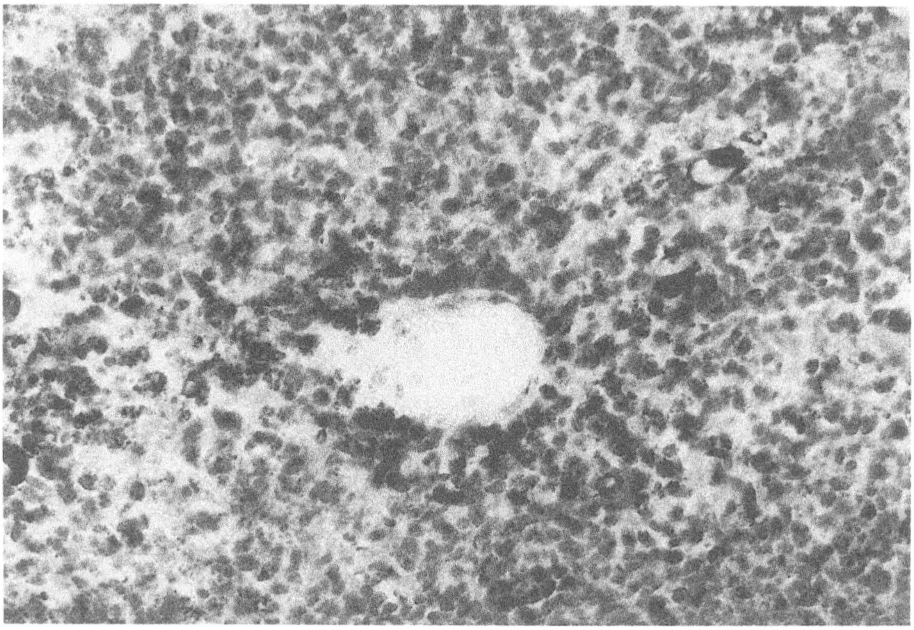

Fig. 3. Hemochromatosis of the liver after 8 month's putrefaction (in vitro). No lixiviation of the hemosiderin. Berlin blue, 1:180

table at a relatively early stage through lixiviation during putrefaction (Mueller 1975). In certain putrefaction experiments on isolated liver specimens with hemochromatosis, no lixiviation of hemosiderins ensued for up to 8 months (Fig. 3). An organic breakdown in the corpse is probably required for this, so that with the postmortem movement of the putrefactive fluid, removal of pigments that are no longer structurally bound is effected (Klages and Wilhelmi 1974).

The studies by Walcher (1927) were concerned with the behavior of pathological soft-tissue alterations during putrefaction. Hyalin-assimilating parts of organs, e. g., glomeruli of the kidneys, central arteries, and centers of infection in the spleen or infarct scars, can still be detected for a relatively long time despite advanced putrefaction. Urinary casts in the collecting tubules of the kidneys (Fig. 4), cicatricial changes in the serous coats, and cardiac callosity can behave in a like manner. In one case of peritonitis post abortum with pneumonia and pleurisy after 6 weeks' burial in late winter, the fibrin with its centers of coagulation was preserved. In concurrence with earlier authors, Walcher (1927) was able to establish that pneumonia can be detected for a long time through fibrin and the increased intra-alveolar cell content. In putrefaction, fibrin is altered to "very soluble globulin" and coagulum, thrombi, and embolisms are believed to be dissolved in the same way.

The macroscopic and histological evidence of gas bubbles within the tissue, as long as there is no presence of gas gangrene infection or other intravital infections with aerogenic bacteria, can practically always be classified as signs of putrefaction. Of course, in the differential diagnosis, care should be taken that traumatic emphysema is not overlooked. From case reports, Borra (1966) pointed out special tissue

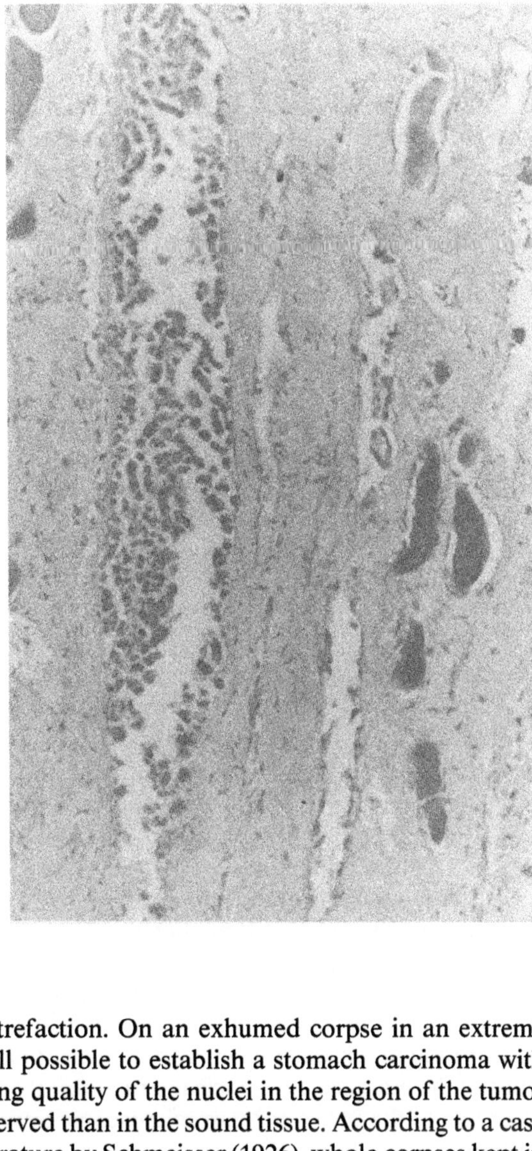

Fig. 4. Lower nephron nephrosis with hyaline and granular casts in the collecting tubules; 11 months' burial. H and E, 1:150

characteristics with regard to putrefaction. On an exhumed corpse in an extreme state of decomposition, it was still possible to establish a stomach carcinoma with metastases in the liver. The staining quality of the nuclei in the region of the tumor tissue was remarkably better preserved than in the sound tissue. According to a case report, evaluation of the older literature by Schmeisser (1926), whole corpses kept in identical conditions can react to putrefaction and decomposition in very different ways.

Mackie (1929) arrived at similar results to those of Walcher (1927) with putrefaction experiments on the organs of apes that had been killed by chloroform. According to a case report by Kimura (1961) on unusually well-preserved remains of the brain following 10-year burial, it is possible that putrefaction was hindered by sporiferous bacteria. Investigations by Wagner (1960) on the state of preservation of human corpses after antibiotic or sulfonamide therapy that had been carried out just prior to death revealed that these medicaments had the effect of restricting putrefaction of the corpse for several months. The most striking reduction in putrefaction of the corpse was obtained with tetracycline preparations. Gantrisin and Leukomycin had a similar though weaker effect.

During the course of putrefaction, liquefaction of the fat with conversion to fatty acids also comes about. The liquefied components of fat carry through into the adjacent organs following hypostasis. It is possible to speak of a regular "fat migration," which begins roughly 2–3 days after death. After 2–3 weeks, deposition of fatty acid nodules in the liver, peritoneum, and on the inner side of the pericardium can occur. Microscopically, this involves crystalline shapes that are composed of "bunches of needles" in a sheaf-like arrangement (Mueller 1975). Marozzi and Lodi (1961) carried out paper chromatographic examinations on organ extracts of the brain, cerebellum, lung, liver, kidneys, and blood during putrefaction. The chromatograms, obtained at different time intervals, can be easily differentiated from those of intoxication.

According to the generally familiar rule of Casper, the ratio of the time taken to reach the same degree of putrefaction by burial in the earth, being in water, or exposed to the air is 8:2:1 (days, weeks, or months). The validity of this rule was decidedly called into question by Walcher (1927). His challenging critique is based not only on the macroscopic but predominantly on the microscopically discernible condition of the tissues and organs.

Specific Cell and Organ Findings

Isolated Cells. A consideration of the extent of morphological variation among living cells is prerequisite (Gropp 1963). The changes to the nucleus and cytoplasm are characteristic in the morphology of autolysis among isolated cells. The light-microscopic findings of the nucleus can according to Müller (1955) and Letterer (1959) be used as a measure of autolysis. Pyknosis, hyperchromatosis, liquid loss and clumping of chromatin, nuclear membrane hyperchromatosis, chromatolysis, karyolysis, and karyorrhexis can be differentiated. All grades occur from pyknosis to total loss of the nucleus, in which the nuclear components display a diverse binding capacity to histological dyes (Laves 1931, 1932). The protein components of nucleoproteins are probably separated during autolysis by activated proteinases and the remaining nuclear protein is broken down by polynucleotidases (Letterer 1959). The nucleolus is one of the most sensitive nuclear structures; it adopts a "luminous" quality, which according to the phase-contrast microscopic investigation of Zollinger (1948) is an early sign of autolysis.

The autolysic changes to the cytoplasm are influenced by the cell type and particular chemical composition. First of all, by the agency of acidification in the dead cell, an opaque swelling or "cadaverous opacity" results with swelling and water uptake in the mitochondria. A clumping and "myelinic degeneration" follow, which ultimately lead to total disintegration of the cell (Mönnighoff 1939; Schümmelfeder 1949; Altmann 1955; Letterer 1959). In the cytoplasm, autolysis can also lead to the appearance of lipoids, e.g., phosphatides and cerebrosides. The signs that emerge resemble fatty degeneration (Dietrich 1904). With the staining method of Smith-Dietrich (Wolff 1924), nowadays better with Baker's "acid hematein test" (Romeis 1968), the cells that have been thus changed, e.g., in the liver, show fine and coarse plaquelike precipitation. Lipoproteins, and not neutral fats, are involved; the former swell through water uptake and lead to myelin forms. These show double refraction in polarized light and can be visualized because of their fatty acid content with neutral red or by the inclusion staining method of Feyrter (Letterer 1969). Occasionally, these substances may also be stained with Sudan or scarlet red (Aschoff 1925); the desired shade is, however, light brown so as to permit the distinction from intravital fatty infiltration (Mueller 1975). More recent investigations by Sinapius (1962, 1963) have shown that in the case of spontaneous and artificial autolysis, histochemically traceable free fatty acid particles and, through the conjunction of finely dispersed fats, so-called *autolysis lipids* (myelins) arise. These changes are dependent on the activity of lipolytic enzymes. Thus, there is histotopographic and quantitative concordance in the localization of unspecific esterases. Previously, Monacelli (1928) discovered in autolysis experiments in vitro fine droplets of monoaminophosphatide precipitation of the cephalin type in the cytoplasm of the epithelia of the stratum basale epidermidis and he spoke of "lipophanerosis". In investigations on putrefactive processes in soil, Minovici et al. (1930) established that saponification-derived fatty acids appear earlier than those derived from protein. From this, it was concluded that fatty acids in putrefaction are formed by protein hydrolysis. Enzyme histochemical and thin-layer chromatographic studies by Lindlar (1962) proved that during autolysis in the pancreas lipoidolytic enzymes of the esterase and lipase type are operative. As a result, higher fatty acids composed of glycerides and phosphatides are released. In advanced autolysis, lysolecithin and lysocephalin are formed from lecithin, plasmalogen, and colamin-cephalin in the pancreas and liver. It is, however, important to bear in mind that vitally induced fat droplets located intracellularly are also preserved after long autolysis and putrefaction and are not to be confused with postmortem "fat phanerosis" (Walcher 1937).

Necrosis occupies a special position as it is involved in intravital cell death. Origin and breakdown can be differentiated from autolysis through the circulation maintained in the surrounding tissue. This ensures a permeation of fluid – a kind of "rinsing effect" – in the mortified tissue area (Eder 1959; Letterer 1959). In necrosis, the autolytic processes are affected by heterolytic enzyme processes from the environment. In centers of large necroses closed off from the circulation of fluids and oxygen supply, changes may nevertheless take place that cannot be structurally distinguished from autolysis (Letterer 1959; R. Müller 1938). Histochemical investigations into the differential diagnosis of autolysis and necrosis showed qualitative and quantitative differences. In necroses, the still traceable enzymes are diffusely localized and a "leak" can be distinguished that is connected with the permeation of fluids from the surrounding tissue. A delayed intravital mortification of cells is designated *necrobiosis*.

According to Letterer (1959), it is possible to distinguish coagulation necroses with increasing tissue consistency from colliquative necrosis with liquefaction of the tissue affected. The capacity to coagulate soon disappears with the death of the whole organism (Koslowski 1959). A necrosis with fatty degeneration, as, e.g., in tuberculosis, is referred to as cheesy necrosis. Trophoneurotic, vascular, chemical, physical, and traumatic necroses can be distinguished according to the causes.

There are a great many efforts that can be made toward identifying, as early as possible, the postmortem changes that can definitely confirm cytolysis. They are not just confined to histological methods. Caesar (1962) in *electron-microscopic* studies discovered a distinct nuclear membrane hyperchromatosis in liver cells after 2-h autolysis. After 6 h, he found a loss of the central matrix in the mitochondria and a tubular distention of the cristae mitochondriales. In the cytoplasm after 6–12-h autolysis, a strong swelling of the ergastoplasmic components and the mitochondria occurred, while the nuclei showed pyknosis and nuclear membrane hyperchromatosis. However, definite regularities in the incidence of the isolated findings could not be established since, e.g., in a great many liver cells there was still no damage that could be assessed with certainty after 12-h autolysis. Further electron-microscopic autolysis studies were performed by Latta (1965), Winkelmann et al. (1965), and Cook et al. (1965) on kidneys and brain tissue with similar results. Combined histochemical, fluorescence-microscopic, and electron-microscopic investigations by Hecht et al. (1962) on experimental heart muscle necroses showed fiber edema, vacuolar changes in the sarcoplasmic reticulum, and the beginnings of distintegration in the structure of individual mitochondria after 15 min. Büchner (1959) arrived at similar results.

After staining adipose necroses with acridine orange (concentration 1:10000 at pH 5.0 and 6.2 – Michaelis buffer), distinct red fluorescence has been observed (Harraszti and Korb 1964; cf. Fahr 1943 and Strugger 1947). Previously, Hadjiolof (1929) noticed signs of fluorescence in Wood's light on autolytic and putrid human and animal organs. The fluorescent phenomena appeared to be connected with the presence of organic substances which had been previously released by oxidation, autolysis, and putrefaction. To visualize strongly decomposed parenchyma, Bernardi and Gatti (1963) suggested treating the material with phosphine solution and subsequent embedding in nonfluorescent oil.

The numerous histological and histochemical investigations hitherto performed on particular organs had the aim of either performing basic research or determining the criteria that would allow a decision to be made as to the time of death. Generally speaking, it appears that different functional states at the time of death, previously existing degenerative and inflammatory lesions, and the conditions in which the corpse is lying exert a very variable influence. These variations affect the chronological development and qualitative and quantitative determinations. They enormously hamper the possibilities for making forensically utilizable conclusions, which only turn out to be sufficiently reliable under laboratory conditions. In the following sections, the essential findings will be briefly be set out that concern particular organs.

Skin. The skin is generally held to be relatively autolysis and putrefaction resistant, probably favored by the rapid cooling after death and the compact lamellar or reticular structure of the epidermis and stratum reticulae cutis. However, with an external source of heat or intravital lesions from thermal and chemical affects, irradiation burns, etc., decay can proceed faster than in the inner organs. In human skin, autolysis acts in a similar manner as in the skin of full-grown mammals. Proteolytic enzymes could be demonstrated at an early stage in skin; the proteases, therefore, were included among the autolytic enzymes. The proteolytically effective enzymes trypsin, cathepsin, glycyl leucine peptidase, and leucine amino peptidase have also been demonstrated in living skin in recent years (Braun-Falco and Winter 1961 –

here further references). With intravital light irradiation of the skin, the postmortem autolysis could be distinctly reduced. Comparisons of pigmented and nonpigmented animal skin showed a more rapid autolyzability associated with pigmentation, with more than 100% increase in the nitrogen values, than with white skin. Studies on the skin of 55 Chinese corpses showed a fall in glycogen within 5 days from threefold positive to zero in the exocrine sweat glands of abdominal skin. In the secretory gland tubes of the surface skin of the hand and foot, the glycogen test remained threefold positive for up to 30 days; in isolated cases a single positive glycogen reaction was still found 55 days postmortem. Generally, however, the intracellular glycogen depots in the skin are broken down early (Braun-Falco and Winter 1964).

The mitochondria-bound cytochrome oxidase and succinic acid dehydrogenase activity also decrease early, from which a structural breaking down of the mitochondria can be concluded. DNA and RNA are broken down later, indicated by a loss of pyroniophilia in the nucleolus and cytoplasm. This would be the first registerable sign of cytolysis in the skin. Unspecific esterases and acidic and alkaline phosphatases survive for a relatively long time. During autolysis, even increased activity in unspecific esterase can appear in the epithelia of the stratum basale. With azo-dye coupling methods, traceable enzymes can show diffusion phenomena. In the detachment of the epidermis during autolysis, the PAS-positive border at the upper corium is often preserved. According to the precipitate in the Hale PAS reaction, decomposing processes with phanerosis of acidic mucopolysaccharides do not seem to occur during autolysis, as is often typical for many pathological processes. On the other hand, depolymerizing processes appear to prevail.

Further investigations into the character of SDH, glucose 6-phosphate dehydrogenase, and reduced nicotinamide adenine dinucleotide phosphate (NADPH) tetrazolium reductase in the early postmortem period by Goffin and Beeckmans (1973) produced no conclusions in the determination of the time of death. Berg (1972) with excised operation wounds established that various enzyme activities are normally detectable longer than the stainability of the nucleus – up to 192 h. Biochemical enzyme determinations of the dehydrogenase group by Miam and Palagi (1968) showed a uniform postmortem decrease, which, however, was not statistically confirmed. With acridine orange secondary fluorescence (SFL), Winter and Braun-Falco (1965) were able to detect a distinct green SFL in the upper portions of the epidermis after a 3-h autolytic period at pH 6.5. At the same time, a dwindling of the SFL in the nucleoli occurred. Soon afterward, intensely orange-red granules, which were coarse and ribonuclease-sensitive, appeared. After 36 h, a yellow-green SFL in the keratohyalin granules was found only sporadically in the stratum granulosum of the epidermis. Simultaneously, a negligible pale green SFL was present in the remaining epidermal layers; in the region of the pyknotic cell nuclei, cytoplasmic vacuoles were found which were occasionally surrounded by orange-red granules. After 72–120 h, the epidermis was extensively broken up.

Postmortem formation of nodules occasionally occurs in the skin of corpses found in water. These are explained by Klauer and Walcher (1937) by the conjunction of calcium ions from the water and phosphate ions from the putrescent gases on the skin surface. Macroscopically, these resemble the shapes of lime soap nodules (Nippe 1913). The histological comparison of skin blisters in putrefaction and after the effects of electricity by Strassmann and Schmidt (1928) revealed that in the case of the action of electricity, peeling of the upper epidermal layers within the germ layer occurs, whereas in putrefaction the whole epidermis is always lifted from the corium.

In conclusion, it should be stressed that, as is well known, the postmortem histological diagnosis of skin diseases is considerably impeded through drying up and hypostasis; even with minimal autolytic effects it is often impossible.

Postmortem Lividity. This is only partly explicable by the action of autolysis. However, as an important sign of the onset of death in an individual it will be discussed here within the framework of postmortem changes. Hypostasis of the blood appears shortly after death and manifests itself histologically in the inner organs and skin by plethora and extension of the blood vessels (Fig. 5). Care should be taken to establish whether in these areas inflammatory changes or thromboses are present. Such findings can also testify to a vital reactive hyperemia. It is also difficult to define a hyperemia occurring directly prior to death, e.g., through a stroke of lightning (personal observation). In the short survival time, histomorphologically or histochemically detectable signs of reaction cannot develop; in otherwise undamaged skin, an intravital hyperemia cannot be distinguished from a postmortem hypostasis. In the region of very pronounced hypostatic livor mortis, normal hemorrhages are often incurred, which can be explained by dehiscence in the walls of overstretched vessels (Figs. 6, 7). These hemorrhages (vibices) do not show any reactive changes in their peripheral areas nor, according to our observations – any fibrin precipitation. It is very difficult to discriminate these hemorrhages from congestive or asphyxial hem-

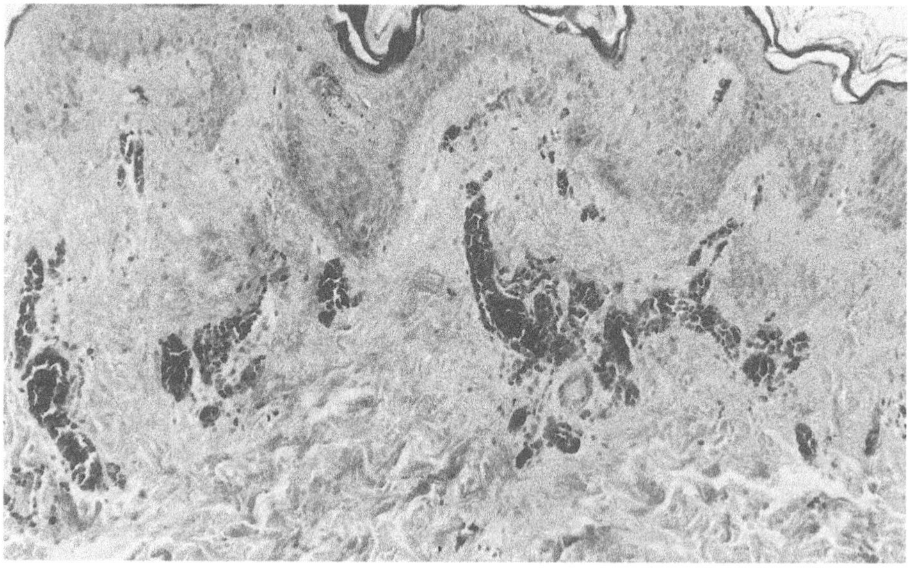

Fig. 5. Livor mortis with hypostasis of the blood vessels in the corium; 26 hours postmortem (H PM). Goldner's, 1:150

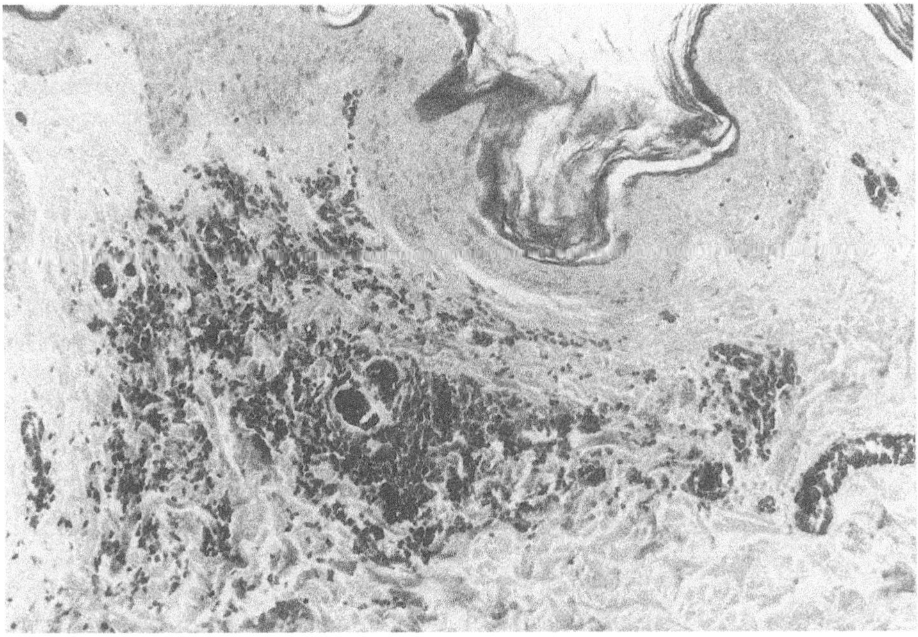

Fig. 6. Discrete livor mortis hemorrhage in the upper layers of the corium; 26 HPM. Goldner's, 1:150

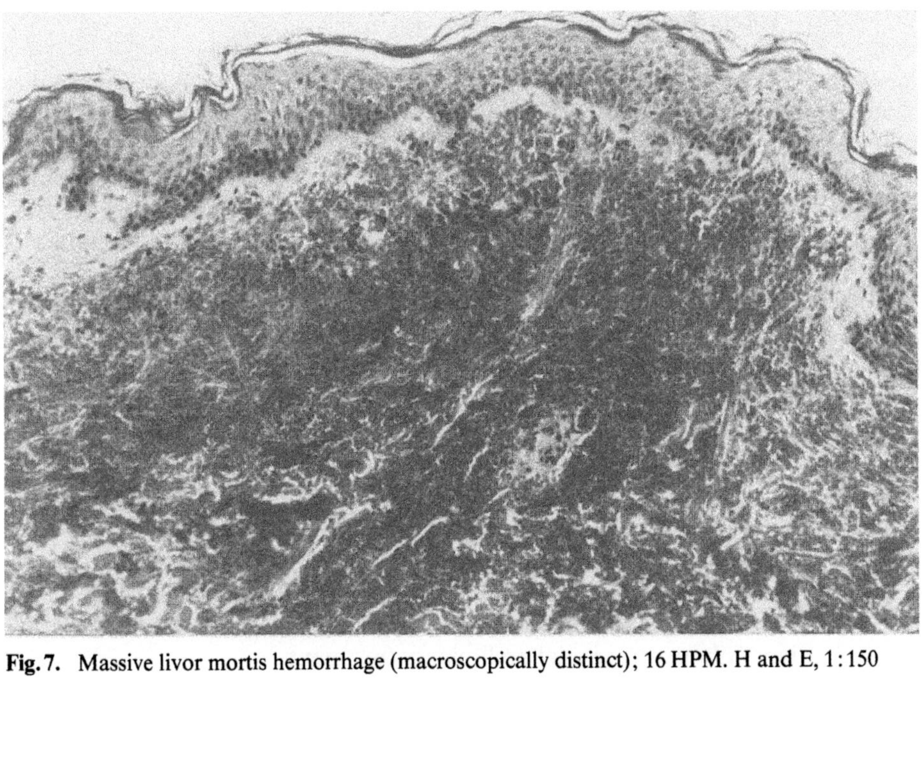

Fig. 7. Massive livor mortis hemorrhage (macroscopically distinct); 16 HPM. H and E, 1:150

orrhages that were caused shortly before death. With histomorphological methods alone it is not possible to make a real differential diagnosis. Basically, the histological identification of intravital hemorrhages is considerably impeded or rendered impossible when these hemorrhages are superimposed by postmortem hypostatic effects. The diagnosis is further complicated in such areas through successive autolytic changes.

The various types of livor mortis development and their transformation in the skin were systematically investigated by Mueller (1951) and Hilgermann (1971). The transition between displaceable or "moveable" and fixed postmortem lividity is, as might be expected – fluid. To begin with, there is intravascularly a disproportionate pallor and lixiviation of the erythrocytes, more rarely true hemolysis with destruction of the erythrocyte membrane occurs. Subsequently, the escaped hemoglobin diffuses through the vascular walls into the surrounding tissue. Occasionally, this can here be histologically determined with Lepehne's stain in the form of a cloud-like confluent precipitation. In the area around the blood vessels, the filamentary components of the interstitium can be imbibed with hemoglobin. Epithelial and muscle cells are also often more highly stained; adipose tissue alone is unaffected. The extension of the hemoglobin in the tissue often follows the flow of the liquid directed to the skin surface, which is caused by dessication (Janssen 1967).

The histological findings in livor mortis have also been evaluated in connection with their macroscopically recognizable displaceability. The first distinct reduction in the displaceability was observed by B. Mueller (1951) when the extravascular hemoglobin "clouds" were confluent. This was usually the case for the time 8–10 HPM. Conversely, Bakulev (1966) took the view that the nondisplaceability of livor mortis is primarily explained not by hemolysis but by inspissation of the blood as a result of seral diffusion out of the vessels ("hemoconcentration") (Hilgermann 1971, 1973 – comprehensive references).

Blood. The postmortem changes in the blood corpuscles and hematopoietic tissues have already been systematically explored several times (Rudnew and Schurpe 1931; Fitting 1950; Werner 1954; Schleyer 1958; Penttilä and Ohman 1977; Penttilä and Laiho 1981). The results are dependent to a high degree on the investigative technique applied. Postmortem hematological smears after 2–3 h are held to present such strong autolytic changes, predominantly in the neutrophilic granulocytes, that it is no longer possible to differentiate the cells. According to these authors, the cells have as good as completely disappeared within 24 h. In histological section, however, blood corpuscles and hematopoietic tissue after suitable fixing and staining can be distinguished for substantially longer (Fitting 1950; Lennert 1952 – description of technique).

The modified method of Moloney et al. (1960) by Leder (1964) has proven useful in the selective enzyme-histochemical preparation of neutrophilic myeloid cells and mast cells in paraffin section. It will be explained in greater detail below. With this method, the histological demonstration of granular inflammatory cells, including their unsegmented preliminary stages, can be performed with material that has been kept for some time and with routinely prepared paraffin sections. The reaction is also positive in tissues that are already clearly autolytic, after formalin or Maximow's fixative, without any special preliminary treatment.

Naphthol ASD Chloracetate Reaction According to Leder (1964): One drop of 4% pararosaniline in 2N HCl and one drop of 4% sodium nitrite solution are mixed and after the hexazotizing has occurred (after 30–60 s) diluted with 30 ml Michaelis buffer (0.1 *M*, pH 6.8–7.6). The pH value is adjusted to 6.3 with HCL, checked by pH meter. Then, 10 mg naphthol ASD chloracetate is dissolved in 1 ml dimethyl formamide. Both solutions are mixed by vigorous stirring, in the course of which a milky, light red, flocculent precipitate appears. At room temperature, deparaffinated sections (as thin as possible and adhering well to the slide) are put into the clear and slightly red-tinged filtrate in the usual way. The incubation time is 30 min. After incubation, the sections are well rinsed under tap water, counterstained in acidic hemalum according to the method of Mayer for 5 min, dyed blue, and covered in gelatinol. The hexazotized pararosaniline combines with the cleavage product of naphthol ASD chloracetate to form a water-insoluble brilliant red dye and guarantees a very precise localization of enzyme activity in the region of the intracytoplasmic granules.

It should be noted that, generally speaking, blood cells in histological section usually appear one-third smaller than in hematological smear. They are, however, better to assess with regard to their spatial interrelationships in section. The signs of postmortem autolysis and decomposition in the cells of the peripheral blood, bone marrow, and lymphatic tissue are only subject to a definite chronological ordering along very general lines. According to circumstances, they begin with varying rapidity after the onset of death . It should also be noted that in many, e.g., septic, states of disease even intravital changes to the leukocytes in the form of clumping, swelling, and vacuolar degeneration occur which are scarcely distinguishable from postmortem changes. According to personal experience (Janssen 1958), postmortem signs of decomposition in the bone marrow and lymphatic tissue commence at quite different times after death with different diseases. Decomposition also proceeds at different rates within the individual types of blood cells. In isolated cases, e.g., in reticulosis, in which an autopsy was performed as early as 25 min postmortem (PM), fine differentiation was no longer possible owing to intense cell changes. In the case of other corpses, e.g., with dedifferentiated lymphoid leukosis, where the autopsy was not carried out until 4 days PM, a good blood cell analysis could be performed without any impediment.

The postmortem morphology of blood cells is predominantly characterized by swellings that appear in the nuclei of neutrophilic leukocytes, with a rounding off of the nuclear shape and dissaggregation of the chromatin network (Werner 1954). Ricci (1957) found complete atrophy of the lymphocyte structure in 15 corpses within a period of 96–108 HPM. During this time, the lymphocytes, baso- and eosinophils, and erythrocytes survived the longest, whereas the mono- and thrombocytes survived the shortest. With the relatively rapid disintegration of the finer nuclear structures, the granulocycytes come to resemble lymphocytes. Schmidt (1965) was able to establish a different postmortem criterion in the mast cells of rat tongues. With the trypaflavine-p-dimethylaminobenzaldehyde technique, sulfuric acid esters could here be detected that corresponded to the heparin. After 10-h autolysis, this reaction became abruptly negative although the granules in the mast cells were still recognizable unstained. An interpretation of this phenomenon has not as yet been possible.

An investigation into SDH activity according to the method of Morrison and Kronheim was performed on human and rabbit lymphocytes from blood smears. The first recognizable reduction in activity was seen after 24–48 HPM when maintained at 20 °C, but not until after 7 days when maintained at 0 °C (Nanikawa and Janssen 1965). According to the studies of Bernardi and Gatti (1963) on 100 corpses, the blood cells of the white series lost their ability to differentiate as late as 24 HPM; the monocytes were the quickest to lose this ability. Similar results were also obtained by Satoh (1955) and Schneider (1953).

According to Schleyer (1958), the fragility of the erythrocytes is considerably increased even shortly after death. A definite dependence of the weakening erythrocyte resistance on the age of the corpse or on the vascular region investigated could, however, not be established. Penttilä and Ohman (1977), on the other hand, believe that postmortem erythrocytic changes occur in a regular fashion and that they can be drawn upon for a forensic determination of the time of death. Under standardized laboratory conditions, they found "peripheral tumefactions" after 4 h, a spherical form to the cell with pointed processes after 24 h, disappearance of the points leaving smooth surfaces after 2–3 days, and variable ruptures in the erythrocyte membranes after 4 days. Under in vitro conditions, these changes developed more slowly. Similar investigations were concerned with the behavior of leukocyte resistance to hypotonic solutions (references in Schröder 1959). This resistance test is suitable for detecting the primary features present in the cells (Schröder 1971). The chronological determination of secondary, i.e., postmortem autolytic changes with reference to the time of death will perhaps be possible when the results of serial investigations with the corpse under different conditions are obtained.

Investigations on the number and function of thrombocytes in the blood of corpses by Harms (1972) showed a decrease in the number of blood platelets in the first 12 HPM to, on average, 10% of the normal value among living subjects. Thereafter, with increasing postmortem time, a further almost linear decrease in the thrombocytes could be observed. Despite early alterations and structural changes, the thrombocytes were still capable of certain functional cell performance after death.

Liver. One peculiarity of liver tissue concerns the expression of the beginning of autolysis, which frequently varies from case to case. Sometimes, the autolytic changes in the individual liver epithelia are prominent, in other cases an early established dissociation of the liver cell texture within the lobuli is more apparent. Laves (1931 a, b, 1932) was particularly concerned with the histological detection of postmortem physicochemical early changes in liver cells using variously buffered staining solutions. He was able to show that the first structural changes appeared in those liver cell regions in which the pH had changed toward the alkaline side. This phenomenon can be interpreted by fine chemical and colloid-chemical reactions preceding the changes in the nucleus and plasma. In our experience, the periodic acid-Schiff (PAS) stain is well suited for the visualization of autolytic structural changes in the liver epithelia.

Considerable difficulties in differential diagnosis arise in distinguishing autolysis from toxic degenerative epithelial damage and changes such as hepatosis or acute liver dystrophy (Magee 1966). Histomorphologically, both processes are able to develop in such a similar fashion that they cannot be differentiated from one another. Likewise, histotopographic criteria, for instance, the localization of liver cell necroses – centrilobular, peripheral, or diffuse – are not sufficiently reliable in defining localized autolytic processes. Intravital, morphologically latent cell impairment favors the expression of postmortem autolysis. Thus, autolytic cell decomposition proceeds essentially more rapidly in dystrophically damaged regions of the liver than in those parts of the organ unaffected by the disease (Beek and Haex 1943). The critical assessment of the quality and extent of intravital liver cell damage can be impaired and even falsified by autolysis. This experience forcibly emphasizes the requirement for the autopsy and fixing of the organs under investigation to be performed as early as possible.

The histomorphology of liver autolysis was studied in particular detail in animal experiments by the working group of Mueller et al. (1965). Their investigations on guinea pig livers kept under different conditions and employing various stains gave the following results. After 2 HPM, there were plasmatic changes and swelling of the mitochondria; at 4 HPM, the mitochondria were indistinct and reduced in number; at 6 HPM, the first breaks in the reticulin fibers occurred – the elastic fibers, on the other hand, survived appreciably longer. At the same time, distention of the nuclei and rupture of the cytoplasmic membrane took place. After 48 HPM, in contrast to the above-mentioned findings, no essential changes occurred. After 4 days, the cell margins were no longer visible and the nuclei, with to some extent still recognizable nucleoli, had almost disintegrated. Reticulin fibers were no longer detectable; the nuclei of Kupffer's cells were pyknotically condensed. After 8 days, only cell shadows could still discerned, and after 15 days only the collagenous and elastic connective tissue framework was still recognizable. A summary of these animal experimental investigations only permits a rough schematic inference to be made with regard to assessing the time of death: Disintegration of the mitochondria and changes in the reticulin correspond to an autolytic time of several hours. The changes in the cytoplasm and cell margins make an autolytic development of 2–4 days appear probable, and destruction of the nucleus with fading of the whole cell morphology testify to a postmortem time of more than 4 days.

The structural changes to liver cells in colliquative and coagulation necrosis, i.e., during intravital cell destruction, have been extensively investigated. The significance of various factors that can counteract necrotic formation – thus, in particular, the mitochondria, lysosomes, nucleolus, membrane permeability, ionic displacement, and the influence of drugs – was presented by Magee (1966, references). From electron-microscopic investigations, Cossel (1966) discovered an increase and swelling in the mitochondria, vacuolar clarification of the cytoplasmic matrix, and clumped homogenization and reinforced development of the predominantly endoplasmic reticulum. These are all changes that resemble the findings in opaque swellings and vacuolar disintegration. The autolytic processes leading to colliquation are retarded by coagulation necrosis. Subsequent to acridine orange fluorochroming on unfixed freezing microtome sections, Harraszti and Korb (1964) discovered green fluorescence of the cytoplasm with matt yellow secondary fluorescence of the nuclei in non-fatty-infiltrated liver necroses from autopsies. Fatty-infiltrated necroses and necroses in autolysis appeared red, and the nuclei could no longer be defined. Here, the green fluorescence can be explained by the loss of the cytoplasmic ribonucleic acids, and the red fluorescence by the binding of the acridine orange reaction to the hydrolytically released fatty acids.

The influence of autolysis on histochemical reactions in liver tissue has thus far been chiefly studied with animal test material under artificial conditions (Holzner and Kaufmann 1962; Lancker and Holtzer 1959; Griffin et al. 1965; Melnikov 1969). Glycogen decreased rapidly after death, especially with material kept at 37 °C. Succinic acid dehydrogenase activity and DNA content showed a distinct reduction 12 HPM at 37 °C; at 4 °C, they only showed negligible changes even after 144 HPM. Alkaline phosphatase level was only slightly lowered after 48 HPM at 37 °C. In the cytoplasmic granules of mouse livers, the bound acid phosphatase and glucuronidase were released very quickly. After 1–2-h autolysis at room temperature, the cytochrome oxidase and glucose 6-phosphate were reduced by 20%. The ATPase activity in rat livers at 18°–22 °C had decreased after 4 h; in vascular walls, traces could be detected for up to 240 h. In experimental mouse liver necroses, succinooxidase and succinate dehydrogenase were appreciably decreased 2–4 HPM and 4–8 HPM, respectively. Here, there is chronological agreement with the electron-microscopically detectable changes to the mitochondrial membranes. Postmortem, the glutamate dehydrogenase showed first of all a modest increase and then a slow reduction in activity. The nuclear enzyme nicotinamide-adenine dinucleotide (NAD) pyrophosphorylase showed, in contrast to the ultrastructural nuclear changes, no alteration in activity. The uricase activity, on the other hand, rose perceptibly postmortem.

The liver fats of corpses were systematically investigated by Sinapius (1962, 1963) in spontaneous and artificial autolysis with regard to esterase activity. He was able to demonstrate, even in formalin-fixed material, that the basophilia of fat drops, which occurs a few hours postmortem, is due to fatty acids, as well as admixtures of phospholipids, released by lipase or unspecific esterase activity. The lipid particles thus caused by the conjunction of easily extractable fats ("autolytic lipids") are diffusely located – intracellular, pericapillary, or irregularly focal, and less peribiliary. With regard to quantity and distribution, there are considerable individual differences, which are dependent on the lipase activity, the amount of finely dispersed lipids, and therefore also on the physiological fat content of the liver cells.

Kidneys. It has already been pointed out by Merkel (1937) that autolytic processes in the kidney cause considerable difficulties in the assessment of microscopic findings. Routine experience reveals a variable onset of autolysis; the secretory epithelia tend to be affected first (Fig. 8). In addition to this, there is the occurrence of lipoid substances and substances detectable with oil-soluble dyes, just as in the liver (Sinapius 1963), which has already been described by Aschoff (1925). The distinction of intravital cell damage, particularly nephrotic tubular changes, is thus sometimes complicated or rendered impossible. Likewise, in the area of clinicopathology, the view is held that many pathological organ injuries, especially in their initial stages, can only be evaluated in an optimal manner from material acquired in biopsies.

The light-microscopically detectable histomorphology of autolysis with regard to the postmortem time-course has been systematically investigated by, among others, Martines (1964) and Osvaldo et al. (1965) under various experimental conditions (Susa and OsO_4 fixing, paraffin and plastic embedding, hematoxylin-eosin

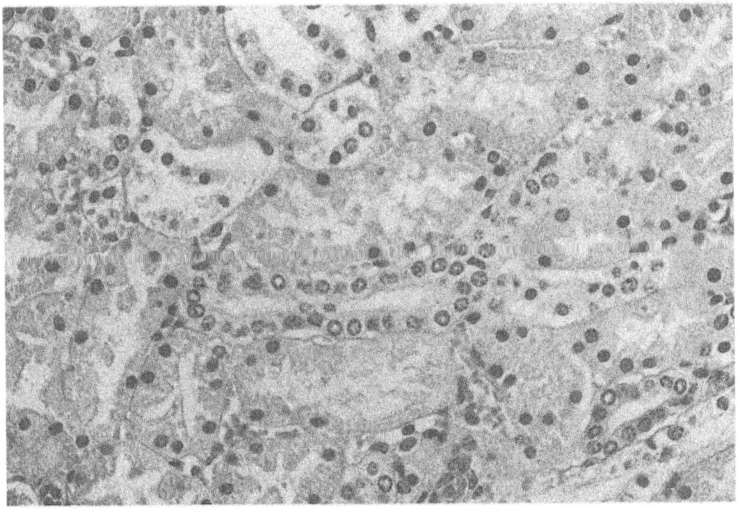

Fig. 8. Autolysis of epithelium of the renal tubule ("postmortem nephrosis"); 3 days PM. H and E, 1:220

and PAS stain). Their essential results are as follows. At the glomerulus, the endothelia and mesangial cells show more rapid autolytic changes than the surface cells, especially in the form of cytoplasmic tumefaction. In the collecting tubule, the first signs of autolysis appear after 8 HPM. In the epithelium of the proximal tubules, there are signs of swelling and contraction of the lumina within minutes. In the distal convolution, there is no considerable autolysis before 2 HPM. In the tubuli contorti at 6 HPM, the epithelial nuclei are not impaired, likewise the cytoplasm of the proximal tubules; the first disaggregation and destruction of the cuticular border occurs. At 12 HPM, there is total destruction of the cuticular border and plaquelike granular plasma transformation, as well as the first chromatin concentration in the nuclei. An increase in nuclear pyknosis and filling of the lumina with cellular debris occurs 24 HPM; at the same time, vesicular changes in sections of the distal tubule and departure of the nuclei from the basal membrane are seen. At 48 HPM, the enlarged lumina of the proximal tubules are filled with amorphous acidophilic material; in the nuclei morular structures appear; in the often discontinuous basal membranes, precipitation of PAS-positive substances occurs (cf. Fig. 9).

Electron-microscopic investigations of autolytic influences on the glomeruli and cortical tubules were made by the working group around Cook and Latta (Cook et al. 1965). They studied in vitro autolysis in rat kidneys after 5, 20, and 30 min, 1, 2, 4, 8, and 24 h in physiological NaCl solution. The results were as follows. There was a very rapid tumefaction of the mesangial cells. Nuclear pyknosis in the endothelium and mesangial cells was more rapid than in the surface cells. At 1 HPM, extensive filling of the capsular space through swollen surface cells and invagination of the tubular epithelia into the capsular space occurred. At 24 HPM, swelling of the basal membrane was seen. In the epithelia of the tubuli contorti, signs of tumefaction and myelin forms appeared very rapidly through the apposition of cytoplasmic mem-

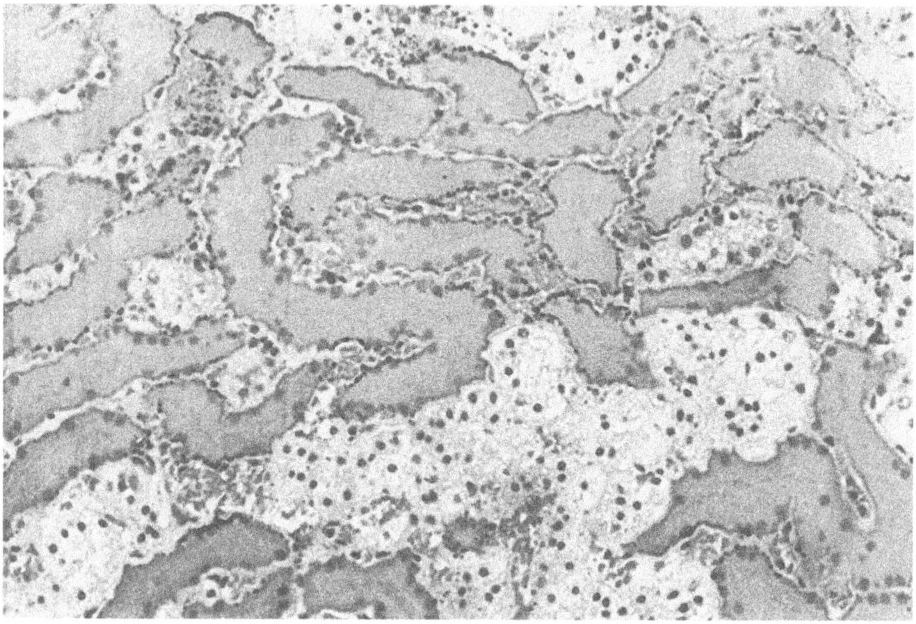

Fig. 9. Advanced autolysis and putrefaction of the kidney; 1 month PM, H and E

branes. In the first 24 HPM, no lysosomal alterations were observed, though there was hyperchromatosis of the nuclear membrane, karyolysis, and karyorrhexis.

Histochemical autolysis investigations by Holzner and Kaufmann (1962) and Kent (1957) on the kidneys of rats and dogs showed, just as in the liver, a fall in ATPase activity in the tubuli, detectable 2 HPM. In the glomeruli, the enzyme was evident for up to 240 HPM. SDH and DNA were clearly diminished 12 HPM. Alkaline phosphatase at 48 HPM had only decreased a little, whereas diffusion of the enzyme could be observed at 12 HPM.

Heart. Among the inner organs, the heart is regarded as relatively resistant to autolysis and decomposition (Fig. 10). It is possible that this is connected with its cytoplasmically dense myofibrillar structure. In the assessment of pathological findings, however, various postmortem changes have to be observed. Holczabek (1970) observed a cyanochrome lipoid granulation in the myofibrils in 11.5% of the corpses he examined, which he interpreted as a postmortem autolysis-dependent myelinic demixture. He assumed that this phenomenon was caused or at least favored by vital disturbances in lipoid metabolism. Occasionally, edema of the mycardium can present difficulties in differential diagnosis.

Comparative investigations on fresh and preserved human hearts showed in the case of real edemas of the myocardium a dissociation of the heart muscle fibers that had survived and were not homogenized or fragmented, usually with isolated eosinophilic leukocytes in the interstitial tissue. With postmortem liquid absorption, the fibrils on the other hand were forced apart, homogenized, and had poorly defined

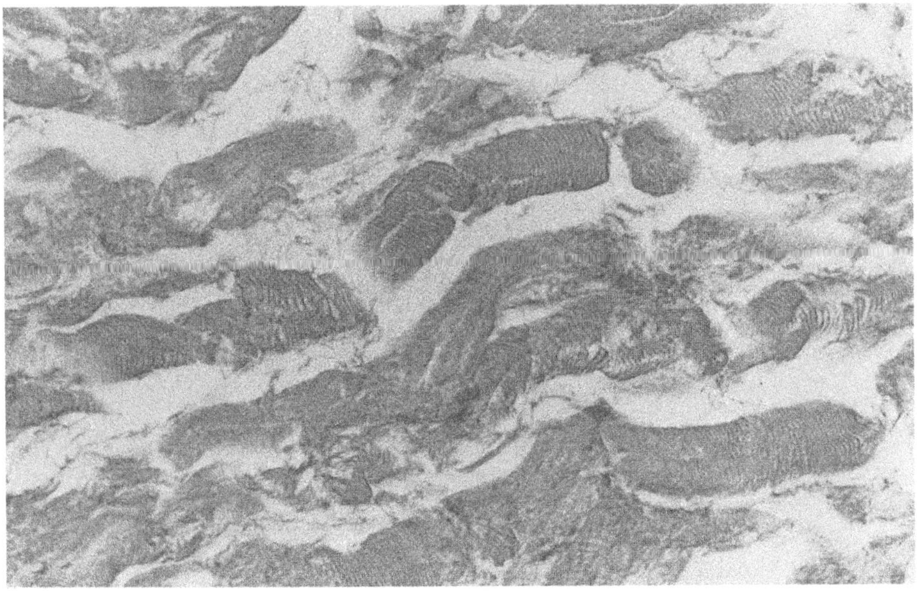

Fig. 10. Myocardium after 5 months' burial. Transverse striation partially preserved. H and E, 1:280

borders. After 72 HPM, a distinction between vital and postmortem myocardial edema was no longer possible.

Systematic autolysis investigations and electron-microscopic observations on human and rat hearts by Nicolas et al. (1969) showed comparable findings. In the first 6 HPM, no light-microscopic changes were detectable. At 6–12 HPM, there were the beginnings of pyknosis and hyperchromatism in the nuclei of muscle cells. At 12–18 HPM, the onset of fragmentation of heart muscle fibers occurred, easy to recognize in longitudinal cell sections. At 18–24 HPM, intensification of nuclear pyknosis and fragmentation of the fibers were seen. At 24–48 HPM, there was a diffuse increase in the fragmentation. After 3 days PM, lysis of the muscle fibers with homogenization, loss of transverse and longitudinal striation, and rounded or oval deformation were observed (cf. Fig. 11). On about the 6th day, there was complete dissociation of the homogenized and deformed fiber fragments. On the 15th day, the tissue was only held together by the coronary vessels; the cell nuclei and myofibrils had entirely disintegrated. Under the electron microscope, distension and deformation of the sarcosomes, impairment of the cristae mitochondriales, and vesicular degeneration of the granules could be observed in two cases in tissue samples taken from heart muscle 15 and 20 min PM. Moreover, the nuclear chromatin was fragmented and deposited along the nuclear membrane. Later examination of preserved material showed a decrease in glycogen and an "empty" quality to the sarcosomes 1 h later. After 3 h, the glycogen had completely disappeared. In rat hearts, the electron-microscopic investigations showed alterations in the mitochondria and nuclei and a loss of glycogen 15 min PM.

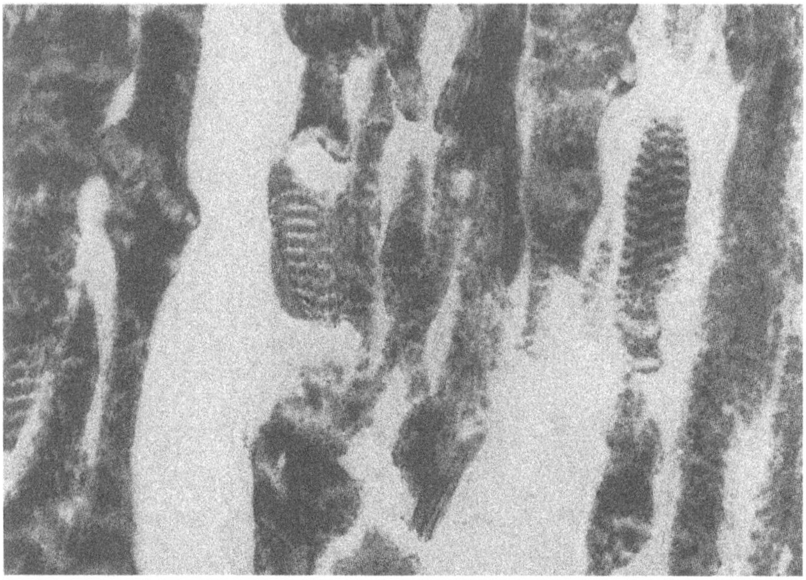

Fig. 11. Myocardium 3 days PM; partial loss of myofibrillar transverse and longitudinal striation. PTAH, 1:280

The rapid postmortem decrease in glycogen could also be histochemically attested (Kent 1957). DNA and alkaline phosphatase behave similarly to the way they do in the liver and kidneys. Qualitative and quantitative investigations on myocardial SDH, which is very stable to autolytic influences, in humans and white mice by Nanikawa and Janssen (1964) showed that it was only possible under standardized conditions to make any assertion as to the definite temperature-dependent postmortem decline in this enzyme activity. After 24–48 HPM at 20 °C, the first reductions in the form of localized clarifications were observed; at 0 °C this did not occur before 7 days (Figs. 12, 13). Quantitative SDH investigations on mouse hearts according to the method of Nanikawa and Tawa (1960) resulted in a distinct fall in activity after 1 day at 25 °C. At 5° or 10 °C, however, the enzyme activity in the main survived for up to 30 days.

Histological investigations on rigor mortis in ox and rabbit hearts for up to 16 HPM revealed generally circumscribed, narrow closing together of the muscle compartments such that the A and I bands could no longer be differentiated (Gallos 1960). From this, a varying ATP concentration of the myocardium during the period is inferred. Even poisoning the animals with γ-hexane could not alter these findings. The histochemistry of heart muscle infarctions has shown in postmortem autolysis in animal experiments a more rapid loss of activity for SDH and alkaline phosphatase (AP) than in comparable undamaged muscle regions (Hecht 1962). Buss (1970) found a strong decrease in the PAS reaction for glycogen, 5-nucleotidase, lactate dehydrogenase, and cytochrome oxidase in rats following coronary ligature and 4-h survival time as a result of autolysis. Among human subjects with myocardial infarctions of varying age, the enzymes of energy transportation, the transami-

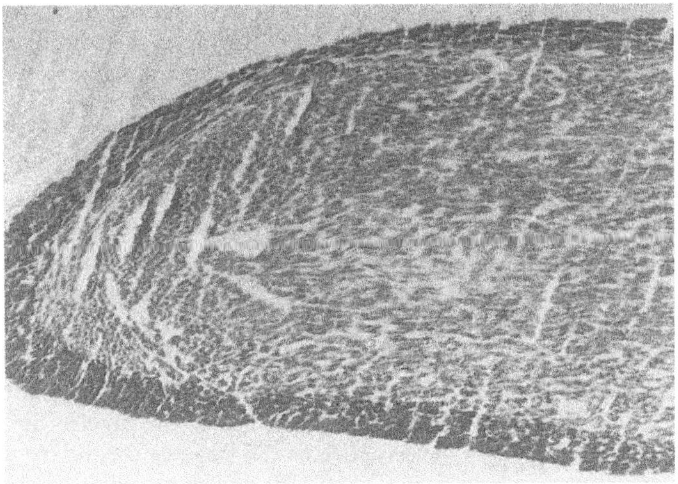

Fig. 12. Papillary muscle infarction (ca. 3–4 h old). Positive SDH reaction of the subendocardial muscular tissue; 3 days PM

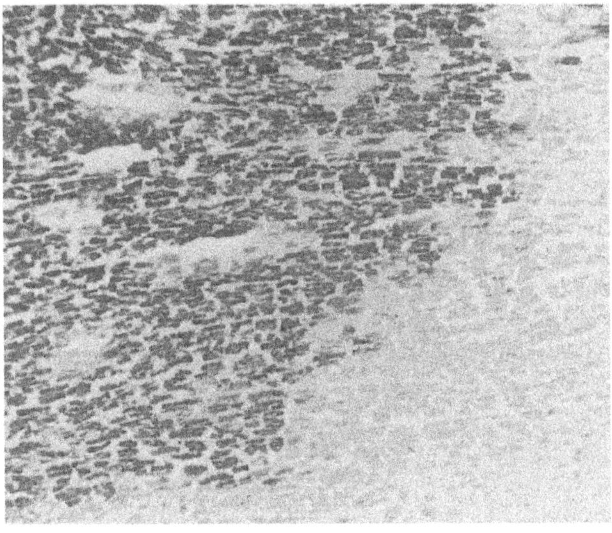

Fig. 13. SDH reaction in the periphery of a ca. 2- to 4-h-old myocardial infarction; 3 days PM at a temperature of ca. 6 °C

nases, the dehydrogenases, and the enzymes of glycolysis showed basically a similar behavior though with quantitative differences (v. Smekal et al. 1973). The reduction of enzyme activities was clearest in the center of the infarction and the decrease was generally more strongly expressed in the left ventricle than in the right.

By way of contrast, the activity of the enzymes that activate the pentose phosphate shunt (6-PGDH and G-6-PDH) was increased in the infarction center. The activity of G-6-PDH was also raised in the marginal zone, while both enzymes were slightly lowered in the right ventricle. Owing to the complicated interrelationships, no conclusions can be drawn from these investigation results in the diagnosis of fresh myocardial infarction in forensic practice.

Musculature. The few existing investigations to date have exclusively confined themselves to skeletal musculature, which like the myocardium has a relatively high autolytic resistance. Comparative studies on the biceps and triceps musculature of humans, rabbits, and guinea pigs were carried out by Kitaev (1962). Here, the appearance and progress of rigor mortis was evident in uneven increasing interruption of the bright ionophragma bands and thinning of the isotropic and anisotropic plates, with subsequent cell destruction. In the musculus gastrocnemius of mice 3–6 HPM, with increasing rigor mortis, numerous fine granules are evident under the electron microscope on the filaments of the myofibrils in the region of the A bands (Suzuki 1976, references). In the stage of secondary muscle atony, granular decay and disintegration of the fibrils occur. Autolysis experiments on guinea pigs by Debarge et al. (1966) showed dissociation of the connective tissue and myofibrils and opaqueness of the nucleus after 6 HPM. Two weeks PM, the muscle parenchyma had disintegrated, leaving just remnants of the connective tissue. Light- and electron-microscopic parallel investigations by the same study group (Bernheim et al. 1966) have confirmed these results. According to them, N bands appear to be the first to be affected by autolysis. The Z bands were detectable for up to 10 days.

Lungs. The majority of autolysis and putrefaction investigations of lung tissue have largely been aimed, even in advanced organ decay, at establishing histomorphological findings, e.g., the determination of whether newborns had lived, the diagnosis of death by drowning, aspirations, pneumonia (Fig. 14). After autolysis and putrefaction of several weeks' duration, usually only parts of the connective tissue framework, vascular walls, bronchial cartilage, and anthracotic pigments can be recognized (Strassmann 1924; Fornari and Pierucci 1965). The alveoli of putrefied lungs frequently contain large cell-like structures, which include poorly defined brownish pigment granules. These do not show any positive reactions in the usual iron preparations. They are not, therefore, heart-failure cells. Also, the pigments cannot be removed with the technique of Kadasewitsch. In our experience, Lepehne's stain is sometimes weakly positive. We may therefore assume like Strassmann that alveolar cells into which hemoglobin has diffused, are probably involved, and altered postmortem. The alveoli of autolytic or putrescent lungs also contain a more or less prominent accumulation of liquid, which is explained by the postmortem penetration of tissue and blood fluid in consequence of the breakdown of all membrane functions. The differentiation between this and a vitally developed pulmonary edema can be difficult, especially when signs of putrefaction, such as gas bubbles and bacteria, are sparse or completely absent. The detection of protein in the alveolar fluid by yellow-green fluorescence on unstained paraffin sections (Bernardi and Tappero 1964) is not reliable enough in our opinion. With an unequivocally positive result, an edema can of course be proven; with a negative result, it is not, however, out of the question since the protein content can be very slight and the existing protein may be broken down by postmortem disintegration.

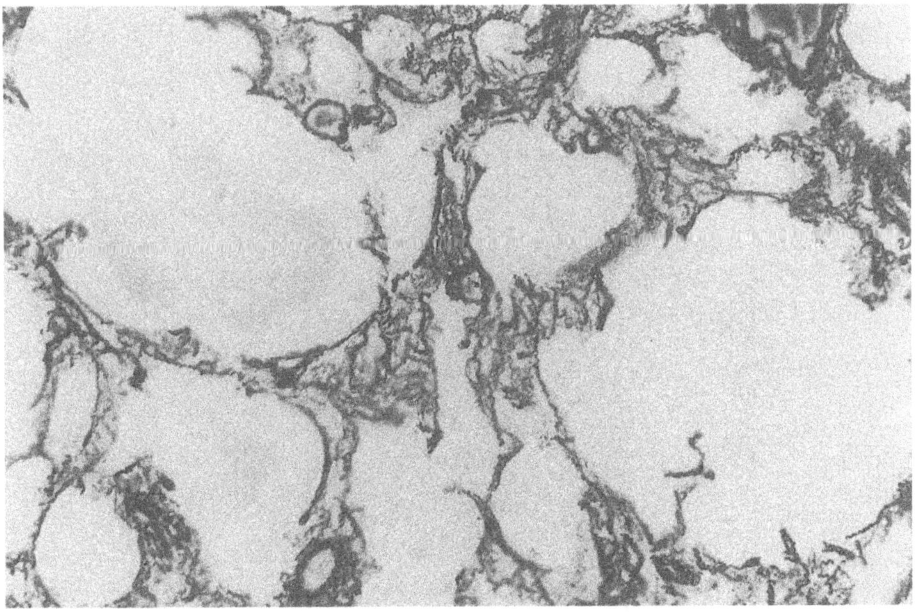

Fig. 14. Reticular fiber structure of the pulmonary parenchyma; 5 months PM (exhumation). Acute emphysema. Subject: 66 years old, ♂, coronary thrombosis. Gomori's

The lungs of neonates are thought to decompose at different rates according to whether or not they have inspired oxygen – a distinction which deserves special mention (see p. 201). This may have something to do with the rapid propagation of putrescent germs from the unfolded alveoli (older references in Strassmann, cf. Bryc et al. 1972). In our experience, such a distinction cannot be substantiated; it was refuted by Schleyer (1952). The forensically important question of what postmortem time has elapsed in the neonatal lung cannot be morphologically answered with certainty. This is based on systemic observations on the lungs of mature and immature neonates. First of all, in the lung epithelium, there is a reduction and pyknosis of the nuclei with coarsening and crumbling of the nuclear structure. Subsequently, vesicular swelling ensues, leading to complete cytolysis and rarefaction of the lung parenchyma.

The changes in the pneumocytes and alveolar macrophages can under certain conditions be dependent on supravital changes and thereby also on the postmortem time of examination. Through oxygen deficiency in protracted death from asphyxia, swelling and proliferation of the very reactive macrophages especially in the region of edemas can persist long after the death of the individual. In combination with autolytic cell tumefaction through absorption of fluid, these processes can affect the histological picture of the lungs (Janssen 1963; Janssen and Bärtschi 1964; De Bernardi and Tappero 1965). Quantitative differences in macrophage reproduction can, therefore, be simulated in such cases depending on the time of examination.

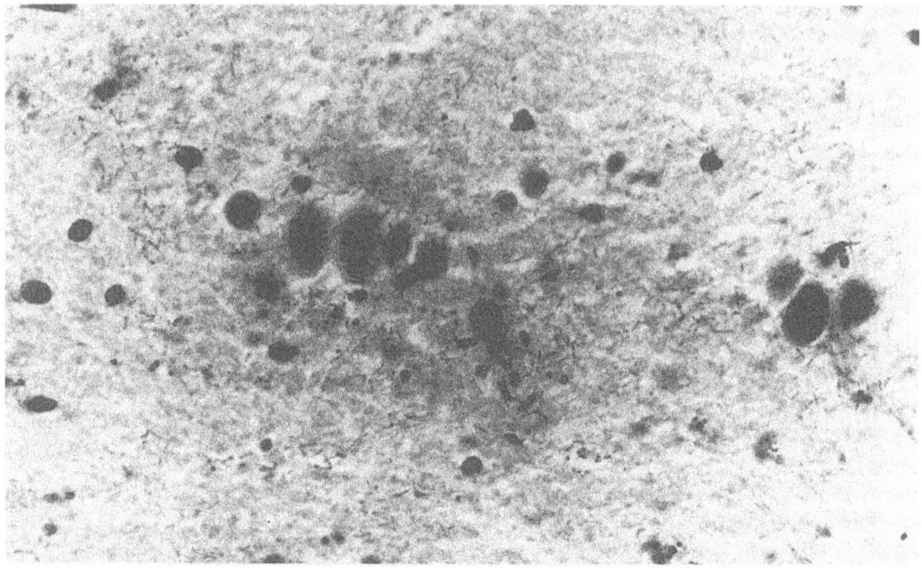

Fig. 15. Autolysis of the brain. Globular myelin decomposition. Subject: 15 years old, ♀, soporific intoxication, 4 days PM. H and E, 1:280

Central Nervous System (Fig. 15). Experimental investigations by Ardenne et al. (1970), with measurements of the pH trend upon death in the cerebrum of rats, revealed rapid hyperacidity to be a particular feature of cerebral tissue. This pH behavior, which is also significant in histochemical investigations, could be observed as soon as the oxygen supply or oxygen utilization was impaired in the experimental setup (prussic acid administration, hyperglycemia, or anesthetic overdose). The acute change in pH would seem to be responsible for the rapid irreversible damage to cerebral tissue, as well as, e.g., the short resuscitation time. Also dependent on the postmortem time is the diffusion of the intravascular plasma albumin in the perivascular, periventricular, and subpial neuropil, where it can be detected with Evans blue fluorescence (Oehmichen and Gencic 1980).

The first morphological changes in the vermis of the cerebellum of white rats could be observed under the electron microscope by Winkelmann et al. (1965) 10 min PM in the mossy fiber membranes. These changes could not be continuously tracked for any longer than this. After 1 HPM, electron-dense particles, (possibly pigments), strong swellings, and break-up of the cristae of glia cell mitochondria appeared in the dense cytoplasm of nerve cells. After 2-h autolysis, the cell membranes were destroyed and the synaptic formations could no longer be distinguished. The glia cells were then strongly swollen in the cerebral edema. Basically similar findings were recorded by David et al. (1970) in various areas of the brains of guinea pigs.

Specific studies have also been carried out on the granular layer of the cerebellum (Marcinkowski 1963; cf. Henn 1971). This cell layer is, on the one hand, held to be markedly autolysis-resistant, on the other hand it is here that circumscribed necroses without reactive changes occur, which are difficult to interpret (Fig. 16). Are

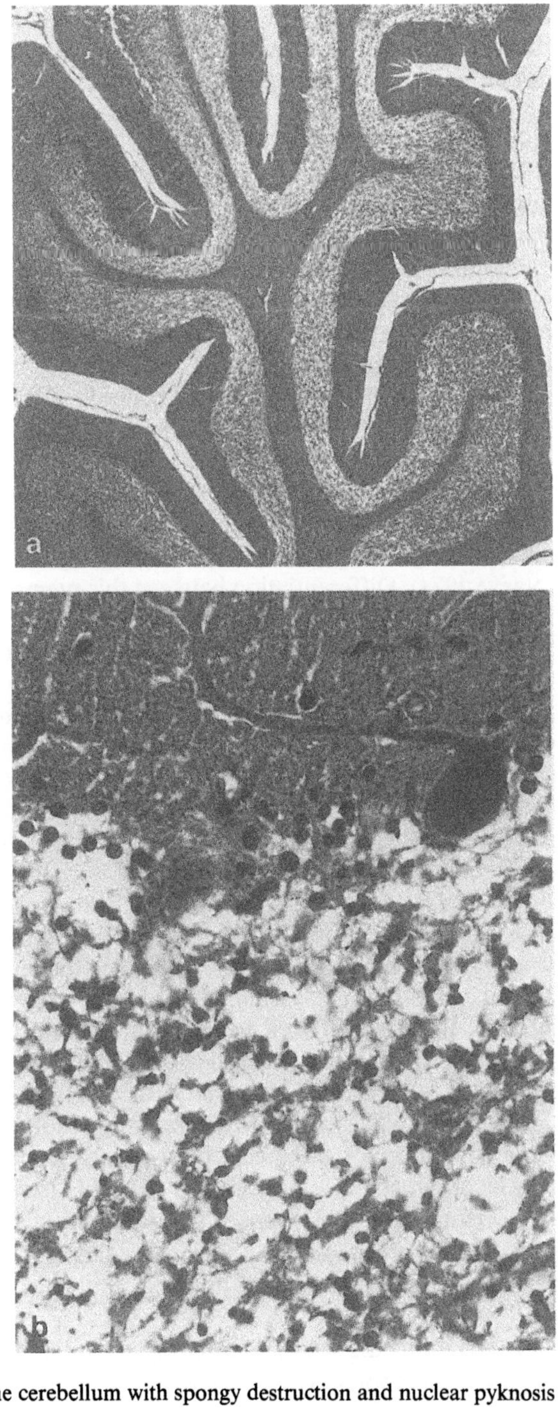

Fig. 16 a, b. Granule cell necrosis of the cerebellum with spongy destruction and nuclear pyknosis (autolysis). H and E, 1:180, 1:350

these granule cell necroses a purely postmortem manifestation of autolysis or are they intravital lesions that appear in this form early postmortem? This question cannot be satisfactorily answered in many cases. According to Ikute et al. (1963), granule cell necrosis can be artificially generated by incubation in liquor cerebrospinalis at 37°–45 °C within 48 h. Older experimental investigations by Lambertini (1930) on the fetal spinal cord of humans and other mammals revealed long-term autolysis resistance, especially using Donaggio's method (molybdenum fixation), in the neurofibril network. It was only after 70 HPM that the mesh of the network began to disaggregate. Exceptional cases should be noted in which in localized areas of the brain the coarser cell structures survived even long periods of autolysis and putrefaction. In the case of one exhumation, Strassmann (1924) still found histologically well-recognizable glia cells and solitary pyramid cells 9 months PM.

Experimental investigations by Schrader (1924) on the brains of paralyzed individuals revealed that even in advanced putrefaction with dissolution of the macroscopic brain structures, demonstration of the characteristic perivascular iron pigment absorption with the method of Spatz was possible in crush preparations. The same is true for malarial pigment, which in the erythrocytes of brain capillaries even after disintegration of the glia cells and ganglia was still detectable for a long time (Naeve 1971). Differentiation between this pigment and hemosiderin in old hemorrhages is not difficult owing to the unusual extravascular localization of the former.

Problems can occur in differentiating postmortem cerebral changes from intravital tissue reactions. Thorough investigations on this subject were carried out by Petersohn (1962, 1963) and involved the postmortem effects of water, pressure, punctures, and cuts on rat brains. Results showed that if the nuclei do not show impaired structure, cell forms that deviate from the norm are not due to intravital damage. Petersohn also showed that a closely circumscribed compacted form of the ganglia points to a postmortem event. Vital ganglion necroses evoked by ischemia can resemble postmortem changes in the initial phase, with the appearance of tigrolysis, nuclear opacity, and fluid intake. With a survival time of several hours, however, signs of regression, such as plasmolysis, hyperchromasis, vesicular nuclei, incrustations, diminished or reactively intensified enzyme activities, and hematogenic or glial cell reactions (Colmant 1965), occur which mostly cannot be observed postmortem. It is also difficult to appraise cerebral injury in the case of vita reducta, since even with prolonged clinical survival all reactions around areas of the brain that are already necrotic can be lacking (Adebahr 1963). According to Grohme et al. (1969), the displacement of prolapsed and autolytic cerebellar tissue into the spinal subarachnoid space and the accompanying meningeal cellular reactions, which can only be observed in some cases, are proof of "intravital brain death". In a recent review, Oehmichen (1980) makes the observation that in the first 6–8 HPM no substantial structural changes visible under the light microscope or biochemically detectable alterations in enzyme activities can be expected in cerebral tissue.

In the following section, those organs and tissues will be presented about which only isolated reports exist in the available literature.

Pituitary Gland. The first postmortem changes are observed in the anterior lobe of the pituitary gland. Here, endolysis begins in the γ-cells after 30 min, in the α-cells after 36-h autolysis. The early changes in autolysis are thought to be connected with an unrestrained postmortem hyaluronidase effect (Latka and Adam 1953).

Pancreas. Mukai (1955) examined the degree of autolysis in 181 pancreases from humans and 57 from rabbits with regard to inferring the time of death. Form and structure of the nuclei, zymogen granules, interrelationships of acidic and basic dyes, coherance of the tissue, cell outlines, and the character of the elastic fibers between the individual lobules were recorded. His criteria, graded in six phases and set out in tabular form, certainly provide a useful classification of the postmortem state of the organ. However, in our experience, the pancreas is not at all suitable for a histological assessment of the time of death owing to the very variable postmortem cooling in this region and the variable vital and agonal conditions of circulation and function even under laboratory conditions.

Spleen. Histological studies by Tappero (1969) on the postmortem structural changes in 20 exhumed corpses with periods of burial between 5 days and 4 months gave the following results. After 15 days, there was dyschromia of the erythrocytes, good nuclear stainability in the follicles but less so in the red pulpa; the staining of connective tissue was good. After 30 days, there were only phantom corpuscles; the nuclear staining was unchanged; staining of the connective tissue was better with Mallory's stain than with van Gieson's. After 60 days, there was deterioration in the nuclear staining, differentiation of the lymphoplasmic cells with the Unna-Pappenheim stain was, however, still possible; the red pulpa had degraded to granules. After 120 days, only sporadic traces of nuclear staining in the follicles were still present; the staining of collagen according to the method of Mallory was still satisfactory.

Small Intestine. Loehry and Creamer (1969) provide methodological indications that despite the frequent early autolytic decomposition of the mucous membrane, a satisfactory evaluation of the villous structure is still possible. After treatment with formalin and alcohol and staining with 5% alcoholic eosin, pictures can be taken under the dissecting microscope in 8 × magnification that permit an adequate diagnosis with only slight qualitative variations due to different postmortem times (Fig. 17). In a general assessment, it is the structure of the mucous membrane and not the mucosal epithelium that is important.

Vascular Endothelium. According to the investigations by Sinapius (1958), after 6 HPM the most frequent early signs of death are dissociation and detachment of endothelial cells, whereas nuclear changes are absent or only present to a negligible extent. Under favorable conditions, the endothelium can be unaltered for longer than 48 HPM. Granular transformation and increased stainability of the cytoplasm can be commonly recognized in the detached endothelia (Fig. 18). Temperature decrease and blood content exert great effect.

Epididymis. Liebhardt and Spann (1968) attempted to infer the time of death by determining the numerical proportion of living to dead spermatozoa in the epididymis. For the cell differentiation, vital staining with eosin was employed, which en-

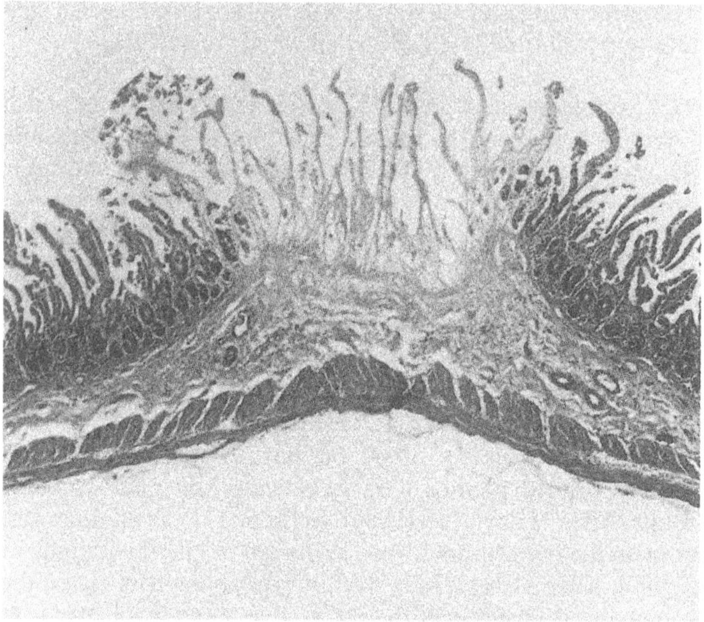

Fig. 17. Autolysis of the small intestine with circumscribed destruction of the mucosal folds. Subject: 22 years old, ♀, automobile accident, 3 days PM. H and E, 1:40

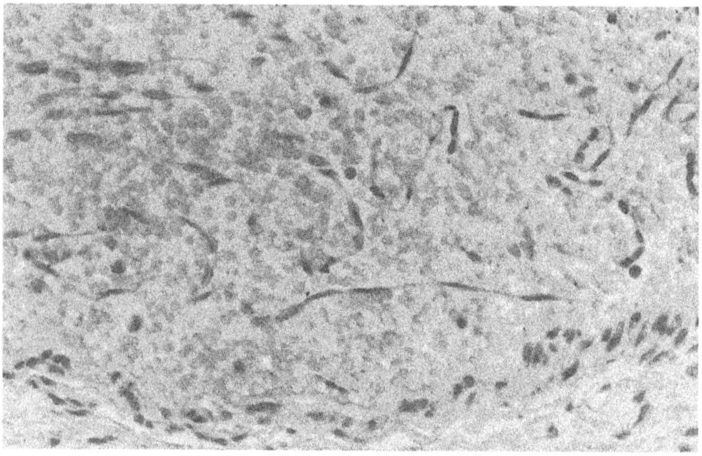

Fig. 18. Detachment of the vascular epithelium; 2 days PM. H and E, 1:220

ables a simple distinction to be made. This method has proven to be better than stimulation with Baker's solution and the assessment "motile" or "nonmotile". Provided that living spermatozoa are actually found, it appears that within particular time limits a certain inference is possible as to the time of death.

Bones. For the determination of the postmortem time, the reader is referred to the relevant material in the textbooks and manuals. Here, note should be made of the differences in autolysis which were found by Remagen and Stolpmann (1962) following decalcification of rat femoral epiphyses with acid according to the method of Plank and with neutralized buffered Titriplex III. Autolysis ensued for up to 24 h at 37 °C in physiological saline. With acidic decalcification, the cell structures were badly damaged; after Titriplex III decalcification, the mucopolysaccharides, as evidenced by the toluidine blue reaction, survived longer and better in bone and cartilage. The very thorough histomorphological investigations by Berg (1963, 1964) and Berg and Specht (1958) into the detection and evaluation of the degree of decomposition revealed the onset of decay in the bone tissue to occur after about 20 years in the region of the outer and inner ground lamellae. Depending on the type of soil, different forms of decomposition can be distinguished histologically: breakdown of the bone substance spreading from the Haversian canals, with faveolate disintegration of the osteon centers, or the onset of decomposition occurs in the region of the intermediate lamellar areas, whereby the osteon centers survive the longest. The fibrillar systems that remain intact can be best recognized in polarized light in the typical sectorial anisotrophy of the osteons; they can still be detectable even after the first thousand years postmortem.

Hair. The possibilities for diagnosis and postmortem investigation have already been presented in numerous reports (e.g., Lochte 1938; B. Mueller 1975; Berg 1957; Prokop 1966). After a long postmortem time, hair, which is very resistant to autolysis and putrefaction, mostly shows a sorrel-red discoloration. In a series of tests on variously pigmented hair samples from humans and animals, Krefft (1969) was able to obtain the same shade by treatment with nitric acid and ammonia. The discoloration would seem to be analogous to the oxidative and reducing processes in putrefaction and decomposition and occur by means of chemical transformation of the keratin building block tyrosin and its breakdown products (Volk 1970).

Adipocere. The nature and chemistry of adipoceratous formation will not be discussed here in any great detail (for references see Berg 1970). According to the relevant sources (Mueller 1975; Prokop 1966), the corpse needs to lie for, on average, 2–4 months under favorable conditions, i.e., damp, anaerobic, before adipocere can occur. Under certain circumstances, e.g., in oxygen-poor water and with loss of the outer skin, a considerable acceleration of the adipoceratous formation must be expected (Mueller 1961). From a personal examination of the corpse of a 3-year-old child who had been concealed by her mother in a cabinet under damp garbage and clothes, we were able to detect circumscribed adipoceratous foci that contained crystals and were partly confluent. The foci were found at 8 weeks PM in the cutis and subcutis of the bend of one elbow (Fig. 19). Exhaustive histological investigations by Mitsuki (1962) using all the common stains on an adipoceratous corpse that had been lying for tens of years revealed among other findings that bones, the brain, and kidneys were the most resistant; connective-tissue fibers survived longer than the musculature. According to Prokop (1966), a combination of adipocere and mummification can occur in adipose corpses: the skin dries up and hinders the flow of putrefactive fluid, whereby adipoceratous formation is favored in the interior of

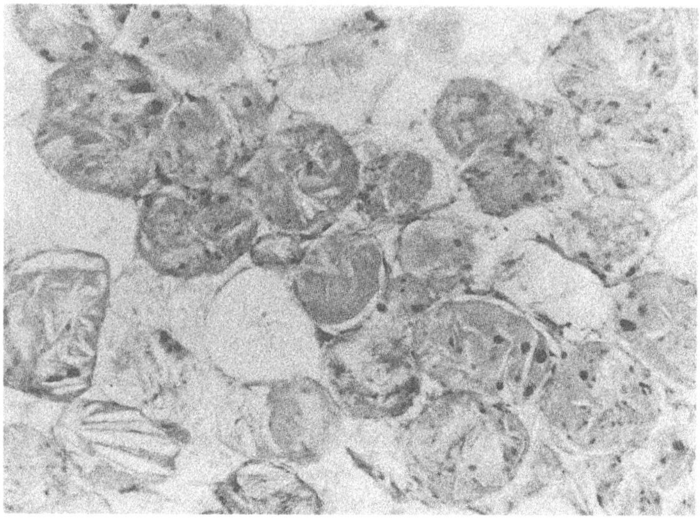

Fig. 19. Adipocere (cubital skin). Infiltration of the subcutis with confluent round crystalline adipoceratous foci. Subject: 3 years old, ♀, 8 weeks PM. H and E, 1:220

the corpse. Histologically, the soft parts still partly contain collagenous and elastic fibers, sometimes also muscle cells with transverse striation (Born 1959; Evans 1962 – here further references).

2. Histological Determination of the Time of Death

A comprehensive evaluation of all histologically, histochemically, and electron-microscopically detectable postmortem changes shows that human tissues and organs are decomposed and broken down in a certain sequence. Theoretically, it can be assumed that there is a fixed "autolytic regularity." Basically, the necrotic order of organs and tissues postulated by Mueller (1975) can be confirmed. In practice, however, in a given case, this order may only be recognized with difficulty or not be seen at all. In laboratory experiments, it is possible with artificial autolysis under precise conditions to establish histologically and histochemically the course of the first 48 HPM of this process. Under laboratory conditions, therefore, after a suitable series of tests and controls, the postmortem time could be determined from the degree of decomposition found in an organism. The numerous experiments carried out thus far have proven, however, that even with standardized animal material comparatively negligible changes in temperature and evironment entail accelerated or retarded autolysis, sometimes even producing autolysis of a qualitatively different kind. In this regard, experience in the area of clinical pathology has shown that early autolysis in human organs is already established in the course of dying or shortly after the death of the individual. For a scientific and clinical assessment of morphologically distinguishable organic lesions, especially in the incipience of a disease, biopsy material is therefore preferable. In forensic practice, the influencing factors are extremely diverse and cannot be taken into account. This applies, e.g., to the time-course and manner of death as well as to the postmortem cooling of the inner organs, which, with the difference in subcutaneous adipose tissue formation especially in the trunk region, cannot be exactly determined by measuring the temperature of the corpse. The same is true for the effect of previous injuries, the different functional states of the organism as a whole, ingestion, digestion at the time of death, different circulatory conditions, etc. For forensic purposes, a determination of histological-histochemical autolysis and of the time of death can, therefore, only be attempted when all possible influential factors are known. Valid findings indicating the time of death can perhaps be taken from the cardiac musculature, skeletal muscles, kidneys, and liver. On no account do such findings have proof value. An attempt to estimate the time of death without knowledge of the environmental conditions is entirely futile and forensically unjustifiable. This observation also applies for the combined utilization of histological, histochemical, and biochemical methods (ct. Daldrup 1979).

3. Histological Examination of Exhumed Corpses

Sometimes, the expediency of an exhumation is judged differently, particularly when the corpse has been buried for some time. Even experienced doctors tend to decline, if they are in a consultative capacity and are confronted with specialist problems, e.g., whether another soft-tissue injury or hepatitis, encephalitis, etc. could be identified. From the forensic point of view in this matter, however, there should be unanimity that an exhumation is virtually always to be recommended in the clarification of the cause of death or the establishment of other legally relevant facts of the case. In advising public authorities and insurance companies, it should be pointed out that in most cases an exhumation following a general line can lead to the clarification of particular questions (Mueller 1975). The practical experience that has been made with exhumations has been particularly good (Schmeisser 1926; Althoff 1974). Familiarity with technical practice in exhumations must here be assumed; this also includes making the preparations for a histological examination. This should be attempted in every case, even where there is heavy decomposition of the corpse. Unfortunately, sometimes in the case of advanced decay, the histology is rashly dispensed with.

The material for histological examinations must be removed as early as possible, during the exhumation and autopsy, and immediately preserved in fixing solutions. In higher grade decomposition with dissolving organ remains, e.g., brain, spleen, or hemorrhages, pretreatment with induration of the whole organ is recommended. For example, with the brain, preservation of the whole head with fenestration of the dome of the cranium and gradual fixation or cold-hardening may become necessary. In our experience, alcoholic or 3% formalin solutions have proven best for the fixation of heavily decomposed exhumed corpse material. Care must here be taken with the common occurrence of so-called autolytic pigments, which are mainly the products of blood decomposition and are difficult to differentiate from formalin precipitates. Subsequent treatment to remove the formalin precipitates in autolyzed material using the method of Kadasewitsch leads to further impairment of the existing tissue structures. Particular care must, therefore, be taken with the degree of purity of the formalin. With extensively decomposed dissolved organ material, e.g., brain, increased use should also be made of the possibilities for making teased-out or crush preparations.

In the histological assessment of preparations, the investigator must understand precisely the processes in corpse decomposition and consider them in detail (B. Mueller 1975). To obtain the practical experience required, taking part in a routine histological examination of autolyzed or putrefied corpse material, even where there are no particular problems concerned, is recommended for junior medical doctors in this special field. Further, the histological examination of exhumed corpses should not be carried out on a restricted selection of organs but in the form of a comprehensive status of the whole available material. In this way, the investigator has a general impression of the autolytic and putrefactive condition of all the organs. A relative assessment of the intravitally derived changes, e.g., from necroses, is thus facilitated.

The positive approach to the histological examination of exhumed corpses advocated here is supported by a great many reports of forensically utilizable findings that were made after a surprisingly long time postmortem (Strassmann 1924; Schmeisser 1926; Merkel 1936; Mueller 1975; Prokop 1966; Evans 1962; Althoff 1974 – here further references). Such communications cannot be dismissed by the argument that exceptionally long preservation of the tissue structures was responsible. The majority of isolated findings demonstrate very strikingly just what histological diagnoses are still possible in exhumations. This source of knowledge should not be dispensed with. Of particular interest is, for example, the evidence from the following partly wellpreserved tissues that Evans (1962) was able to provide histologically from 33 corpses which had been put into coffins under natural conditions and been buried in dry soil for 103–127 years: vascular wall structures; musculature, partly with transverse striation; pulmonary alveoli; anthracotic and silicotic foci; connective tissue structures of cardiac valves, liver, gallbladder, and kidneys; tissue structures of the uterus, testes, and cutis; cartilaginous and nervous tissue. The adipocere copiously present stained reddish-brown with Sudan IV. The entire iron stains were, however, negative. In other investigations, the cellular components of soft-tissue hematomas and hemorrhages into the body cavities could still be detected 7 months after death. Intravitally developed products of blood decomposition, such as hemosiderin, can survive even longer. Attention should be paid to postmortem lixiviation of the ferriferous parts of stains and a displacement, or migration, of the iron (Klages and Wilhelmi 1974). Inflammatory cell infiltrates in the region of soft-tissue injuries and in the aryepiglottic folds have still been detectable for up to 4 months after death.

The following pathological findings might be histologically detected in exhumed corpses even after long periods of burial, from months up to several years: Scars in the outer skin which cannot be macroscopically discerned, deposits of metal (e.g., argyra), and foreign bodies. The brain and its membranes may show older inflammatory changes with accompanying cicatrization, hemorrhages with signs of decomposition (epi- and subdural hematomas, hemorrhagic internal pachymeningitis), paralysis-iron, malaria, degenerative and inflammatory vascular processes, and Wer-

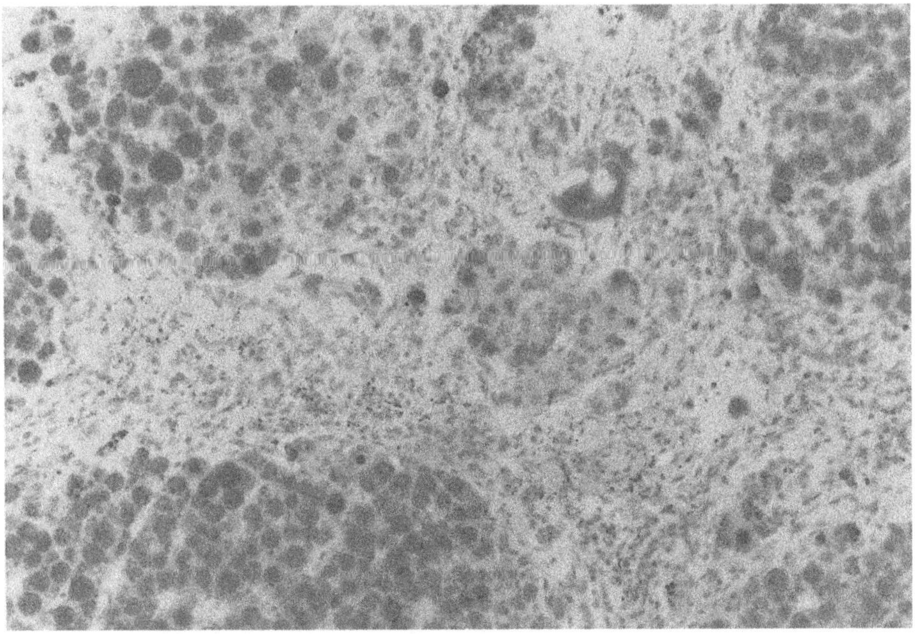

Fig. 20. So-called fatty cirrhosis of the liver; exhumation 3 months PM. Sudan, 1:150

nicke's encephalopathy (polioencephalitis acuta hemorrhagica). The granular layer of the cerebellum deserves particular attention in that it is occasionally preserved for a long time, it can also, however, be an early indicator of intravital lesions (Henn 1971). In the liver, advanced stages of cirrhosis with heavy cicatrization (Fig. 20), hemochromatosis, lipofuscinosis (Fig. 21), scar formation in the region of the capsule, Glisson's triangles, and in the region of the efferent biliary tracts and gallbladder wall can be found. In the lungs, there may be evidence of inorganic matter, e.g., in heavy anthracosis or advanced silicosis; pneumonia, aspiration material, especially of putrefaction-resistant foreign bodies, and granulomatosis with heavy cicatrization may be identifiable (Fig. 22). In the myocardium, the structure of which according to experience is well-preserved for a long time, callosity and degenerative parenchymatous changes can be recognized years after death; inflammatory changes, on the other hand, rarely survive (Fig. 23). After a long period of burial, shrinking of the muscular parenchyma must be taken into consideration, whereby an increase in the interstitial connective tissue may be simulated. In the kidneys, changes in the glomeruli from chronic nephritis or vascular lesions with hyalinization can be seen as well as hyaline casts and pigments and calcification in metabolic disturbances. In the spleen, which commonly decomposes very rapidly, pigments, e.g., in malaria or general hemosiderosis, can occasionally be detected. In the mucous membranes of the gastrointestinal tract, buccal cavity, and urinogenital tracts, scars, e.g., following gastric ulcers, can be histologically substantiated. In the uterus, the mucous membrane of which according to experience decomposes relatively quickly, fetal components can survive for a long time. In the whole of the arterial

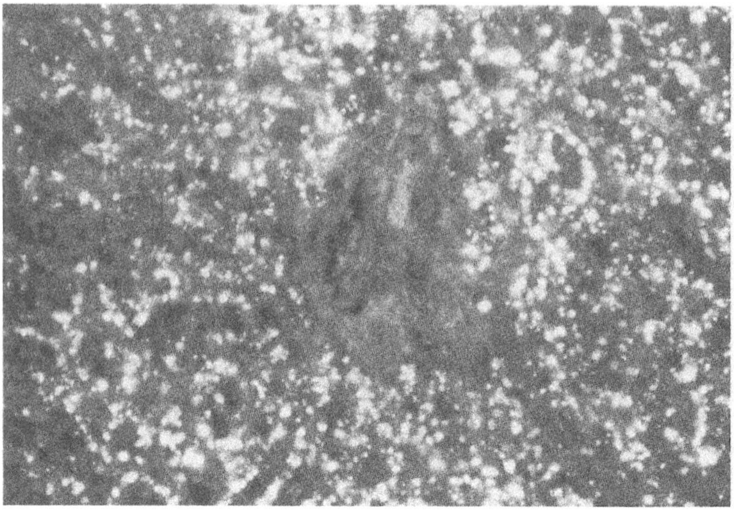

Fig. 21. Pronounced centrolobular lipofuscinosis of the liver; exhumation 3 months PM. Primary fluorescence, 1:150

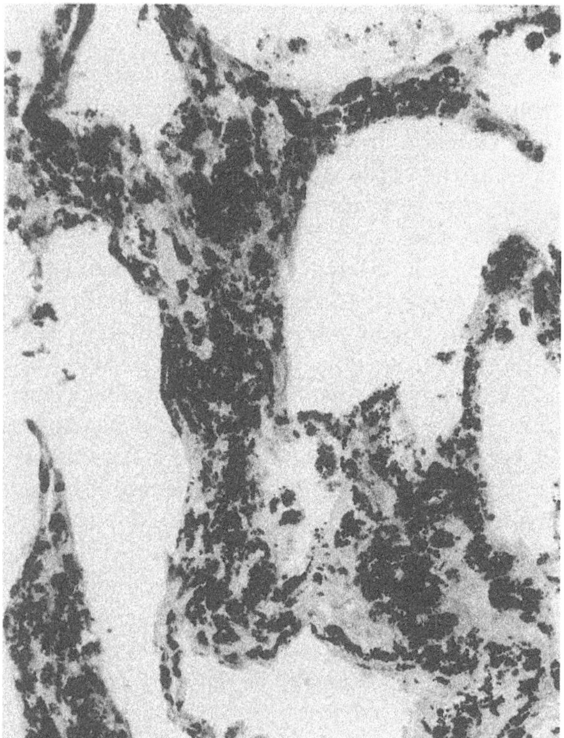

Fig. 22. Asbestosis and anthracosis of the lung; exhumation 14 months PM. H and E, 1:150

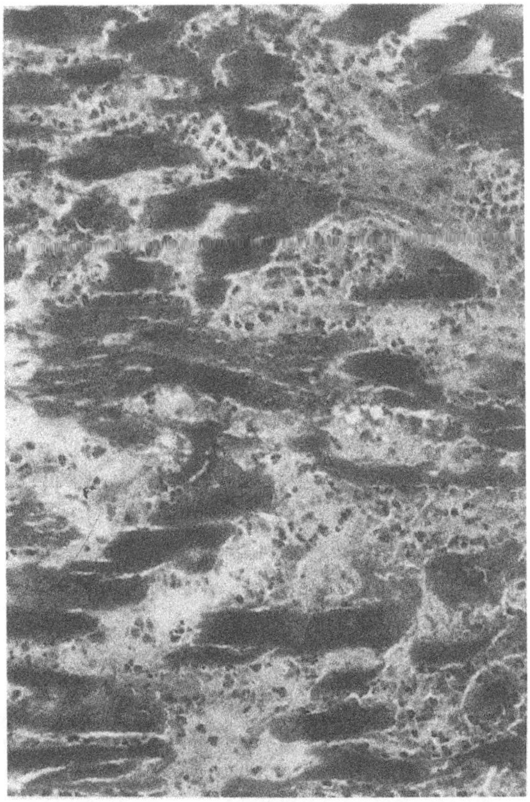

Fig. 23. Myocarditis purulenta; exhumation 2 months PM. PTAH, 1:220

Fig. 24. Coronary artery with atherosclerosis and calcareous deposits; exhumation 14 months PM. H and E, 1:60 ▽

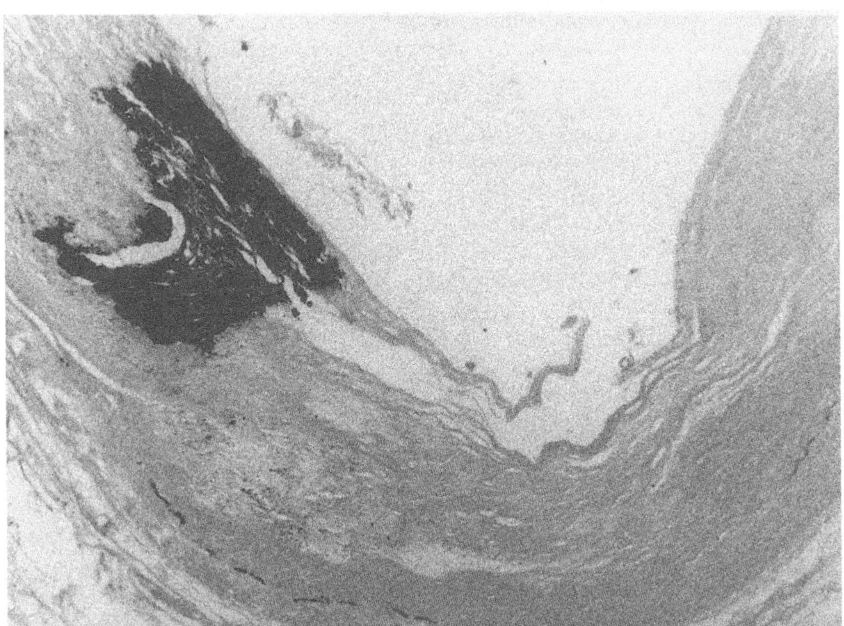

Table 2. Macroscopic and histological findings in exhumed corpses, time after death (author's findings, reports in the literature)

Organ	Finding	Own findings		Literature
		Macroscopic	Histological	
Brain	Cerebral hemorrhage	73 days	73 days	549 days
	Meningeal hemorrhage	34 days	–	84 days
	Epidural hematoma	63 days	–	84 days
	Metastases	23 days	23 days	44 days
	Leukemic infiltration	–	40 days	–
	Cerebral contusion	–	63 days	–
Trachea, bronchi	Bronchiectasis	60 days	–	24 months
	Bronchial carcinoma	56 days	–	1–2 years
Lungs	Embolism	189 days	189 days	13 months
	Fat embolism	–	38 days	4–½ months
	Bronchopneumonia	–	73 days	2 years
	Blood aspiration	34 days	53 days	–
	Tuberculosis	28 days	60 days	12 months
	Emphysema	547 days	–	2 years
	Metastases	23 days	23 days	–
	Bronchitis	–	52 days	–
	Edema	–	189 days	–
	Heart-failure cells	–	78 days	–
	Leukemic infiltration	–	40 days	–
	Asbestosis	–	288 days	–
Heart	Hypertrophy	68 days	60 days	95 days
	Myocardial calluses	145 days	145 days	2 years
	Fresh myocardial infarction	12 days	–	1 month
	Metastases	23 days	23 days	–
	Myofibrosis	–	93 days	–
	Leukemic infiltration	–	40 days	–
	Myocarditis	–	189 days	–
Coronary arteries, aorta, vessels	Coronary and aortic atheromatosis	288 days	145 days	–
	Medionecrosis of aorta	–	42 days	–
	Coronary and vascular	547 days	145 days	12 months
Liver	Metastases	263 days	263 days	44 days
	Liver cell fatty infiltration	–	189 days	59 days
	Liver cell necrosis	–	46 days	–
	Fibrosis	–	46 days	–
Kidney	Cortical scars	145 days	–	–
	Hyaline glomeruli	–	60 days	13 months
	Arteriosclerosis	–	69 days	–
	Leukemic infiltration	–	40 days	–
	Suppurative nephritis	–	19 days	27 days
	Pyelitis	–	19 days	27 days
	Hypernephroid carcinoma	–	23 days	–
Bladder, genitalia	Prostatic hypertrophy	–	23 days	95 days
	Interstitial prostatitis	–	19 days	–
	Prostatic adenomatosis	–	19 days	–
Pancreas	Tumor	263 days	263 days	–
	Leukemic infiltration	–	40 days	–
Stomach	Pyloric scar	41 days	–	24 months

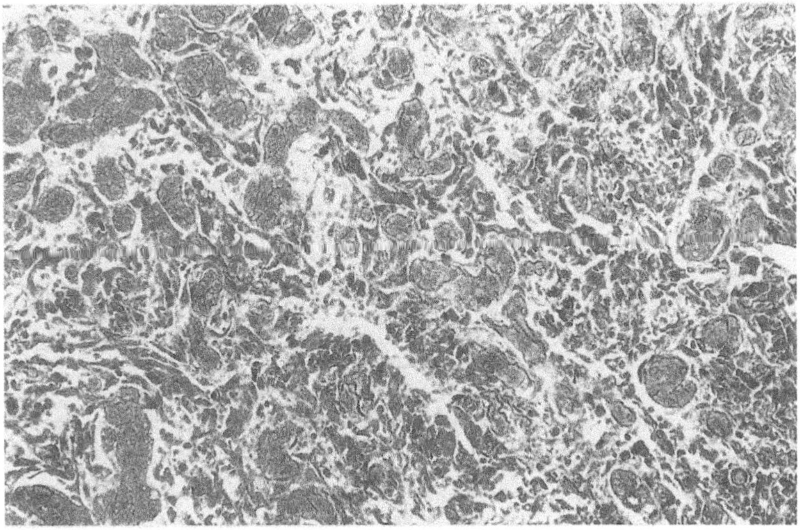

Fig. 25. Angiosarcomatosis of the liver; exhumation 10 weeks PM. H and E, 1:180

system, particularly in the region of the coronary and renal arteries, it is not unusual for arteriosclerotic alterations with heavy cicatrization and calcification to be preserved for years (Fig. 24).

It is only seldom that generalized and local illnesses with tumors, granulomatosis, tuberculosis, leukemia, etc. offer the possibility of histological verification (Fig. 25). Exceptions can exist when, for example, in the region of tumor metastases or foci of tubercolosis calcareous deposits occur. As a general principle, bone sections from the skeletons of exhumed corpses should also be macroscopically examined for such processes.

From the nature of the subject, it is inevitable that the assertions of individual authors as to the longest postmortem time after which pathological findings can still be established turn out to be different. An ad hoc examination on the indicative value of the material that we obtained working on behalf of professional organizations is summarized in Table 2. These results are compared with the statements of other investigators, in particular with the very thorough presentations of Althoff (1974) and Bandmann (1977). In the histological examination of exhumed corpses, the same basically applies as in the examination of fresh corpses. Along with a general histological status examination, every suspect macroscopic finding should also be histologically checked.

II. Vital Reactions

The vital reactions are of central importance in the forensic medical examination and assessment of changes to tissues and organs. The significant findings with regard to the chronological order of the established data are related to these reactions. Hitherto, it has been customary for vital reactions to signify predominantly those changes that arise during the life time of an individual as a result of external or internal injury; their study was mainly confined to local reactions by Walcher (1936). Forensic medical practice, however, necessitates a comprehensive approach. Reactions and organic changes also occur that are largely or wholly independent of tissue damage or external trauma, the finding of such reactions and changes is nevertheless proof of a vital origin. The histology of thromboses, embolisms, and aspirations is therefore discussed in the General Section of this book. These remarks are supplemented in the Special Section among the individual types of injury and damage with regard to the application in practice.

The existing literature on vital reactions is so voluminous that it cannot be completely covered here. Reference is made to the following broader summaries: Orsós (1935, 1940); Walcher (1935, 1936); B. Mueller (1953); Lindner (1967, 1971); Berg (1972); Beneke (1972); and Raekallio (1965, 1970, 1980). Generally speaking, it is necessary that the findings with regard to the vital reactions are sufficiently described and understood. On the other hand, the significance and conclusiveness of the individual finding and the definition of postmortem changes are frequently problematic mainly due to the necessary reference to the clinical time of death. However, such an approach is at odds with the fact that clinical death does not occur at a fixed point in view of the gradual death of the individual tissues; clinical death is indistinctly marked by a smooth transition (Berg 1972). The difficulties with a forensic assessment oriented to a specific time of death become particularly apparent when disturbances connected with central nervous regulation are under consideration. Orsós (1935) has already pointed out with reference to older observations by various pathologists that in subjects with severe commotio cerebri the vital reactions can be almost completely absent. Earlier, such observations were only sporadic but nowadays they can be expected much more frequently due to the increased possibilities of resuscitation and intensive care. In this connection, it should also be borne in mind that in the case of organ transplantation the necessary measures for the assessment of death demand a longer period of time.

Hitherto, the following classification and demarcation of the vital reactions, though sometimes only theoretically possible, was customary: Vital reactions – agonal reactions – intermediate reactions – supravital reactions – transition to postmortem changes.

However, with a rigorous forensic approach making use of all available scientific findings, the following classification appears to be more justifiable: *Definite vital reactions – organ findings that could have occurred at the time of death – postmortem changes.*

1. Hemorrhages

Hemorrhages will here be discussed under general considerations. Even today, hemorrhages are of great significance as signs of vital reactions in very different kinds of injury. However, they warrant a particularly critical evaluation.

Origin, Histomorphology, and Degradation

With regard to the cause and origin of hemorrhages, it is generally understood that hemorrhages from diapedesis need to be differentiated from hemorrhages through rhexis. The etiology of diapedetic hemorrhages extends from the various blood coagulation diseases to hemorrhages resulting from disturbed circulation or disturbances of the vascular wall through toxic influences and oxygen deficiency. The cause of these hemorrhages will be discussed under the particular form of injury concerned. Their histology has not hitherto been the subject of specific and systematic investigation.

The cause of hemorrhage per rhexin is easier to detect than that of diapedetic hemorrhages. Splitting of the vascular wall occurs through mechanical action and blood escapes into the surrounding tissue. The mechanical action may involve a blunt force, with contusion and rupture of the tissues including the blood vessels, or a sharp or semi-sharp force, with direct severance of the blood vessels. The continuity of a vascular wall can also be partly or completely interrupted by stretching. A further possibility for the origin of hemorrhages per rhexin occurs in the vicinity of inflammatory, liquefactive, or tumorous lesions, which lead to erosion or displacement and trophopathy of the vascular wall. The histological finding of a diapedetic hemorrhage or hemorrhage per rhexin can be simply characterized when corpuscular components of the blood are detectable outside a vessel. This criterion is, however, limited in the region of the pulpa lienis where there is essentially an open connection between the sinus and the extrasinuous space.

The corpuscular components of blood, erythrocytes, leukocytes, and thrombocytes, are found in the region of a hemorrhage between the cellular and fibrillar elements of the particular organ or soft-tissue sections affected. In the case of injuries associated with natural cavities in the human organism, e.g., abdominal and thoracic cavities, pericardium, gastrointestinal tract, or subdural space, there is of course no connection between tissue and blood corpuscles.

Hemorrhages within the tissue can present a great diversity of form. They can occur with or without displacement of the tissue concerned (Fig. 26a); they can continue spreading in the fissures of the connective tissue. Extravasation is usually found in the hypodermis under excoriations, even if this is not macroscopically evident from the outside. Adjacent to deeper incised wounds, the extravasation fre-

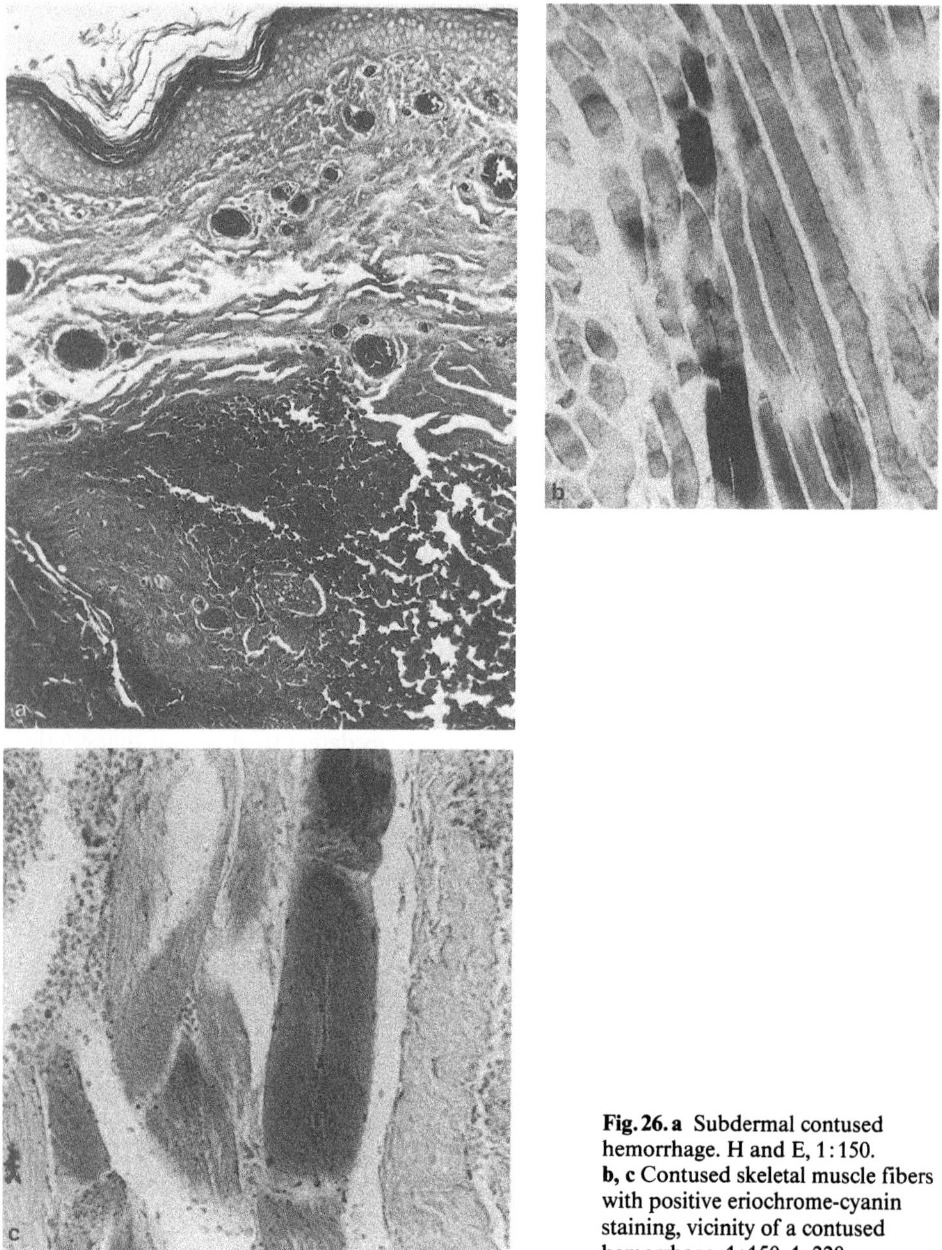

Fig. 26. a Subdermal contused hemorrhage. H and E, 1:150. **b, c** Contused skeletal muscle fibers with positive eriochrome-cyanin staining, vicinity of a contused hemorrhage. 1:150, 1:220

quently occurs between the muscular fascicles. In the case of laceration or contused wounds, lesser extravasation is occasionally seen at some distance from the main hemorrhage and should not to be construed as an independent process. It is caused by blood at the periphery of the primary extravasation extending along the muscle bundles, becoming more pronounced at particular sites, and appearing there as independent hemorrhages. The connection between primary and secondary extravasation can be established by serial sections.

A histological distinction between hemorrhages per rhexin and diapedetic hemorrhages is often not possible unless the splitting of the vascular wall or parts of the adjacent tissue can be found in histological section. In investigating hemorrhages due to pressure and passive hyperemia, we attempted to visualize the vicinity of the vessels concerned, e.g., in the region of skeletal musculature, using special techniques to stain compressed though not destroyed musculature. Using eriochrome cyanin stain, which is normally utilized in visualizing metals, an increased stain-binding ability could be detected in the muscle parenchyma damaged by pressure (Fig. 26b, c). This is thus an indirect means of differentiating the cause of hemorrhage. However, even with this method, there is no certainty of establishing the mechanism of origin in every case.

Caution should be taken with artefacts in the course of histologically processing the examination material. It is possible for blood components to be washed out of intact vessels as a result of the incision. Sections of capillary wall can also be torn, which then gives the impression of so-called capillary wall ruptures. A certain degree of experience is necessary in being able to recognize such artefacts in histological section. Blood corpuscles that have been washed out can be detected by the fact that they do not occur between pre-existing tissue components, rather, they tend to overlie them. Hemorrhages in the medulla and medulla-cortex boundary of the adrenal glands (Janssen 1962; Dohm 1965; Adebahr 1971) have to be assessed with particular care in the case of neonates and young children. Regressions of the inner cortical layer caused during development or large congestive hyperemia can here be deceptive (Fig. 27). One particular area that has been repeatedly investigated is left ventricular subendocardial hemorrhages, which can be elicited by various causes, such as trauma, intoxication, cessation of breathing, intracranial processes. Histologically, these subendocardial hemorrhages accompany necroses of the muscle cells, inflammatory reactions, and vascular lesions in the area of the entire myocardium, especially in the papillary muscles (Rajs 1977).

For the visualization of discrete hemorrhages, the use of Goldner's or Lepehne's stain is recommended.

Very special demands are made in the diagnosis and assessment of hemorrhages in view of the fact that they can also occur spontaneously or be caused in the tissues and organs of humans after death. Even in the older literature (Haberda 1898; Lesser 1912; references in Werkgartner 1926 and Janssen 1968), numerous causes of such postmortem hemorrhages were specified: ecchymosis and vibices in the skin, particularly where the corpse is in the prone position; postmortem vascular ruptures; hemorrhages in the region of hypostases and livor mortis (cf. p. 26); postmortem fractures of the cervical spine; postmortem or agonal hemorrhages in artificial respiration; extravasation caused during burning of the corpse; formation of hemorrhages in the soft parts of the neck during the anatomical examination, etc. Further, care should be taken with sanguineous colliquation and cavity formation incurred postmortem in the medulla of the adrenal glands (Fig. 28), which are sometimes difficult to distinguish from intravital hemorrhages of the adrenal medulla (Janssen 1962). In his review of the work of Christeller (1920), Werkgartner (1926) stated that hemorrhages in the soft parts of the neck in the case of sudden

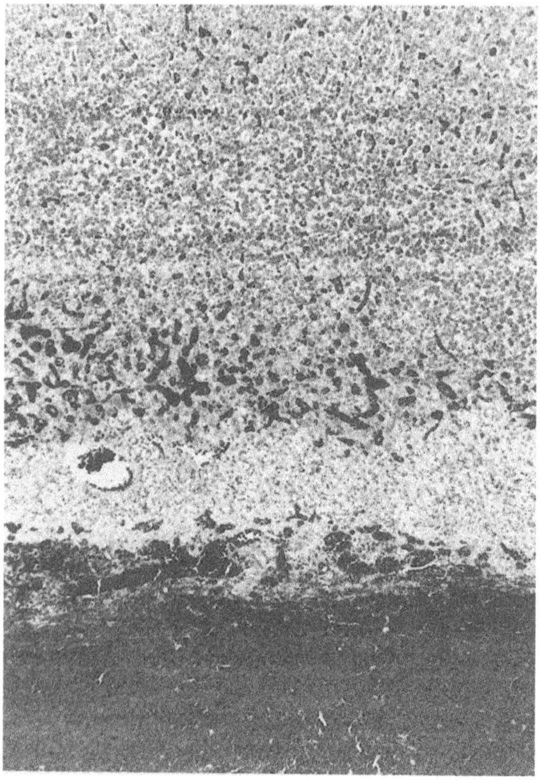

Fig. 27. Hemorrhage in the adrenal medulla through birth trauma; physiological hyperemia of the cortex. Goldner's, 1:80

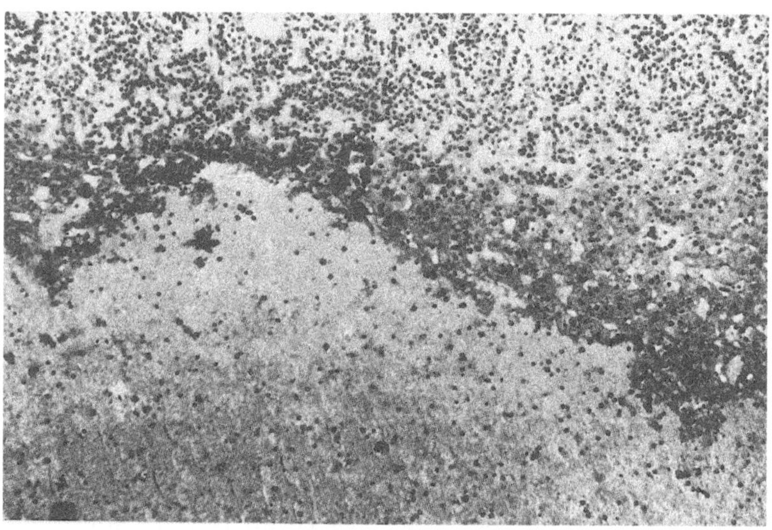

Fig. 28. Postmortem sanguineous softening of the adrenal medulla (autolysis with subsequent postmortem infiltrative hemorrhage). Hemoglobin imbibation of the marginal regions. Subject: 6 months old, ♀, autopsy 3 days PM. H and E

death from natural causes are extremely rare and that on no account can the suddenness of death and the speed of heart failure be inferred from such findings. He considers the hemorrhages observed by Christeller to be postmortem artefacts that developed during the preparation.

It has to be generally acknowledged nowadays that almost every manner and form of hemorrhage can be artificially manufactured by postmortem trauma. In our own investigations studying the effects of blunt force on the skull, cerebral findings could still be produced several hours after death that macroscopically and histologically could not be distinguished from typical contusion foci (Naeve and Bause 1974). In the cervical region, Schulz (1896a, b) and later Prokop (1968) produced hemorrhages that had the appearance of vital hemorrhages in the first hours after death. We have arrived at similar results.

According to the investigations of Gordon and Mansfield (1955), petechial hemorrhages of the pericardium may arise postmortem. They are caused by venous ruptures during rigor mortis. Haberda (1898) described the development of pericardial hemorrhages in connection with observations of postmortem lividity. As a result of the non-uniform development of rigor mortis in the musculature of arteries and veins, associated with differences in pressure in the arterioles, variable blood distribution occurs in the smallest branches of the veins, which eventually brings about postmortem ecchymosis. The diverse causes of conjunctival hemorrhages among living and dead subjects have been investigated and summarized by Prokop and Wabnitz (1970).

A histological comparison of hemorrhages that occurred just prior to the death of an individual with those produced not long after death does not reveal any conclusive histomorphological features. This particularly applies to the quality and distribution of the corpuscular components of blood. The evidence of fibrin as an indication of a vital origin of hemorrhage has diminished in importance: with hemorrhages that are definitely of vital origin, a histological test for fibrin can appear negative; conversely, fibrin can be present in hemorrhages of postmortem origin (B. Mueller 1953, 1964; Dotzauer and Tamaska 1968). Also, with immunohistochemical methods using fluorescent antibodies (Laiho 1967 and literature; cf. Geiler 1965), a reliable distinction between fibrin of vital and postmortem origin is not possible. The macroscopic test on the ability of a hemorrhage to be eluated is evidently still better than the histological examination (B. Mueller 1964). One restriction emerges from the investigations of Hinz and Tamaska (1971), who produced postmortem hemorrhages in the anterior spinal ligaments of the cervix which could only be partly eluated. The erythrocytes in this firm and fiber-rich tissue are probably held fast even without fibrin.

Although the presence of fibrin nowadays no longer has decisive bearing in the investigation of vital and postmortem hemorrhages and wounds, it should nevertheless still be taken into account in all appropriate examinations of hemorrhages. If a distinct fibrin network is present, particularly in the marginal regions of hemorrhages, this points to the hemorrhage having occurred during the lifetime of the individual, provided further vital indications are at hand. The histological visualization of fibrin should be checked on unequivocally positive material; the PAS stain, the staining method according to Weigert-Schueninoff, and phosphotungstic acid hematoxylin (PTAH) are recommended. Finally, the presence of elastic fibers in the

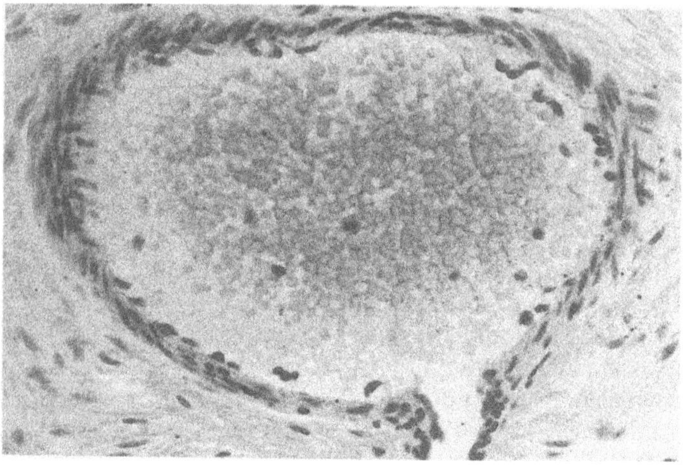

Fig. 29. Postmortem lixiviation of erythrocytes in the periphery of a vein. H and E, 1:180

region of the hemorrhage, especially in the center of larger hematomas, should also be considered. The fibers, which can be detected by means of specific elastica stains, have a certain degree of diagnostic significance for a vital origin of a hemorrhage according to Kernbach et al. (1937).

In the case of death from exsanguination, Adebahr and Weiler (1976) investigated the blood distribution in the kidney using the benzidine stain according to the method of Pickworth on 30 to 50-µm thick sections. In acute exsanguination, the cortical vascular system and both serially connected capillary regions were devoid of blood; in protracted exsanguination, on the other hand, the capillary network of the glomeruli located between the arterioles was filled. In forensic practice, inferences can be made from this as to the exsanguination time and assertions are possible regarding hemorrhages occurring at two different times. In the fractional bleeding of guinea pigs, Berg et al. (1974) found a reduction in the histamine level and number of mast cells in the lungs. Similarly, they found in the case of death by exsanguination in humans, a lower concentration of mast cells in the perivascular connective tissue of the lungs than in other forms of death involving shorter agony.

The changes in hemorrhages during the lifetime of an individual have particular importance in assessing when such hemorrhages occurred. Lixiviation has been regarded as the first indication of vital change in the erythrocytes. This is seen as a pallor of the erythrocytes chiefly in the marginal areas of the hemorrhage, whereas in the central sections the hemoglobin loss proceeds more slowly. Within the scope of postmortem hemorrhagic changes, however, it has to be emphasized that lixiviation and pallor of the erythrocytes can also occur after death, e.g., in the peripheral sections of thin-walled vessels filled with blood (Fig. 29). The pallor or lixiviation of erythrocytes should, therefore, no longer be utilized in the chronological assessment of hemorrhages (Janssen 1967b).

There is in principle no difference between the examination of open and covered wounds. The changes in covered suffusions develop somewhat more slowly. At the outset, the course is characterized by a more or less heavy exudation, with disaggregation and permeation of fluids in the immediate vicinity of the hemorrhagic focus. Histologically, widening of the fibrous septa is seen; sometimes, there is also a swelling of the ground substance and a slight PAS-positive reaction even before the appearance of cell infiltrates. This early, noncellular, exudative phase passes over into the beginning of the leukocytic reaction. Numerous investigations have dealt with the cytology, histomorphology, and time-course of this process. It should be noted that not only the white blood cells extravasated with the hemorrhage are detected, but also the granulocytes that migrate out of the neighboring blood vessels. The disputed interpretation of autochthonous granulocyte genesis is not discussed here.

A conglomeration of leukocytes in the marginal regions of the hemorrhagic focus occasionally causes some confusion; this should not be evaluated as a leukocyte reaction but as a distribution phenomenon of the cellular hemorrhagic components. Care should be taken that an actual infiltration of the neighboring tissue is present; the interstitial connective tissue and marginal areas of the damaged tissue are the vehicles of the infiltration. A swelling and enlargement of the local immobile connective tissue cells, occasionally coupled with an altered stain-binding ability, only has indicative value for a vital, reactive event, since such changes can also occur postmortem. The same is true for the margination of vascular leukocytes, described by Tannenberg, and also for so-called leukostasis. It remains to be seen whether the general vascular leukocytosis described by Schulz (1968), e.g., of the myocardium in the case of violent death, will gain recognition as a diagnostic principle.

The beginning of a leukocytic reaction as a tissue response to a hemorrhage has been variously described. It was rightly pointed out by Berg (1972) that many details are not compatible. The term "leukocytic reaction" has been variously interpreted. Histotopographic differences have not been taken into consideration and, on the whole, there has been a lack of systematic investigation into the influence of the tissue affected. In addition, practice shows that with covered dermatorrhagia in the form of "bruises", the subcutaneous tissue is affected far more than the epidermis and corium. With the effects of blunt force in the region of the scalp, in our experience, usually only the connective tissue layers lying directly above the periosteum present hemorrhages; the layers on top of these are free. Correspondingly, the intensity of the leukocytic reaction is affected by the vascularization of the tissue concerned.

The earliest recorded leukocytic reaction of 20–30 min observed by Walcher (1930) in vital excoriations is often cited. Assertions as to the time of the first appearance of leukocytes in the vicinity of a hemorrhage or wound vary between 1 and 24 h after occurrence of the lesion (Ojala et al. 1969; Raekallio 1965; Lindner 1967; Ross and Benditt 1961; Smith 1945). In specific investigations concerning the age determination of subcutaneous hemorrhages, Berg and Ebel (1969) detected the first influx of polymorphonuclear leukocytes after about 4 h. In animal experiments, the reactions proceeded substantially quicker. After 30 min, there were the beginnings of an edema of the connective tissue mesh in the region of the hemorrhage; after 1.5 h, a distinct infiltration of leukocytes on the edge of the hematoma was present. These studies performed on rats can be contrasted with guinea pig experiments adopting a different approach (Janssen et al. 1968). Following contusion of the quadriceps musculature and generation of massive hemorrhages, distinct leukocytic infiltrates were seen in the marginal areas of the damaged tissue region after 20–30 min.

The leukocytic reaction to a hemorrhage is gradually superseded by an increasing mononuclear cell reaction. However, it should be observed that isolated mononuclear cells can appear relatively early, frequently at the beginning of the leukocytic reaction. The first leukocytes to migrate become increasingly necrotic after about 15–30 h and are superseded by mononuclear wandering cells or phagocytes, which are probably derived from hematogenic monocytic cell elements. Origin of the pericytes of the vessels adjacent to the adventitia has also been discussed (Zollinger 1962). Further changes lead either to complete dissimilation of the hemorrhage without scarring or to the development of granular tissue through mobilization of the histogenous wandering cells, which can take place after about the 2nd day (Berg and Ebel). In the case of bland resorption without scar formation, the components of the hemorrhage are evidently broken down by fibrinolysis and erythrocytolysis and removed humorally. Further histological evidence of a vital reaction to hemorrhage is seen in hemostasis caused by thrombosis in vessels damaged by rhexis. The formation of blood clots, which are composed of balloonlike blood platelets and closely packed fibrinous fibers, has been systematically investigated by Jorgensen and Borch-Grevink (1963) (cf. Böhm 1974b; Laiho 1975) with different periods of capillary hemostasis. Care should be taken in the identification of postmortem-hemolyzed, intravascular components of blood, which when they have a homogenous and hyaline quality are sometimes misinterpreted as fibrin thrombi.

The breakdown of hemoglobin is important in the chronological assessment of hemorrhages. The data concerning the first appearance of iron-containing pigments in the region of a hemorrhage are very variable; the pigments have been sporadically observed in phagocytes after 24–48 h. The first evidence of hemosiderin is probably also substantially affected by the method applied. Comprehensive reports on the histochemistry of detecting iron and on the formation of the iron pigment are found in Timm (1960), Gedigk and Strauss (1954), Bessis (1962), Richter and Bessis (1965), and Wille et al. (1969). Hemosiderin is histologically and light-microscopically evident as intracellular granules with a positive Berlin blue reaction (Fig. 30). Chemically, it is a very non-uniform substance; its protein, iron, fat, carbohydrate, copper, and calcium content is very variable. Electronmicroscopically, hemosiderin can be evident in different forms: (1) as crystalline ferritin; (2) as ferritin surrounded by a protein membrane; (3) as a substance with a definite structure, composed of various substances such as fats, PAS-positive material, and membranous formations containing ferritin; (4) as a hybrid; and (5) as an accumulation of ferritin molecules without crystalline form.

According to Timm (1960), who provides a critical survey of all the possibilities for histochemically detecting iron, Turnbull's blue is the best means of tracing hemosiderin. There is, however, a considerable disproportion between the histochemically detectable and the chemically analyzable tissue iron. This phenomenon can be explained either by a very fine distribution or by a special binding of the iron in the tissue. Kellner (1964) indicates a means of detecting iron which is supposed to be highly sensitive and easily regulated. The reaction is performed on paraffin or celloidin sections and involves ascorbic acid solution, iron II chloride stock solution, iron II chloride carrier solution, potassium ferrocyanide solution, and hydrochloric

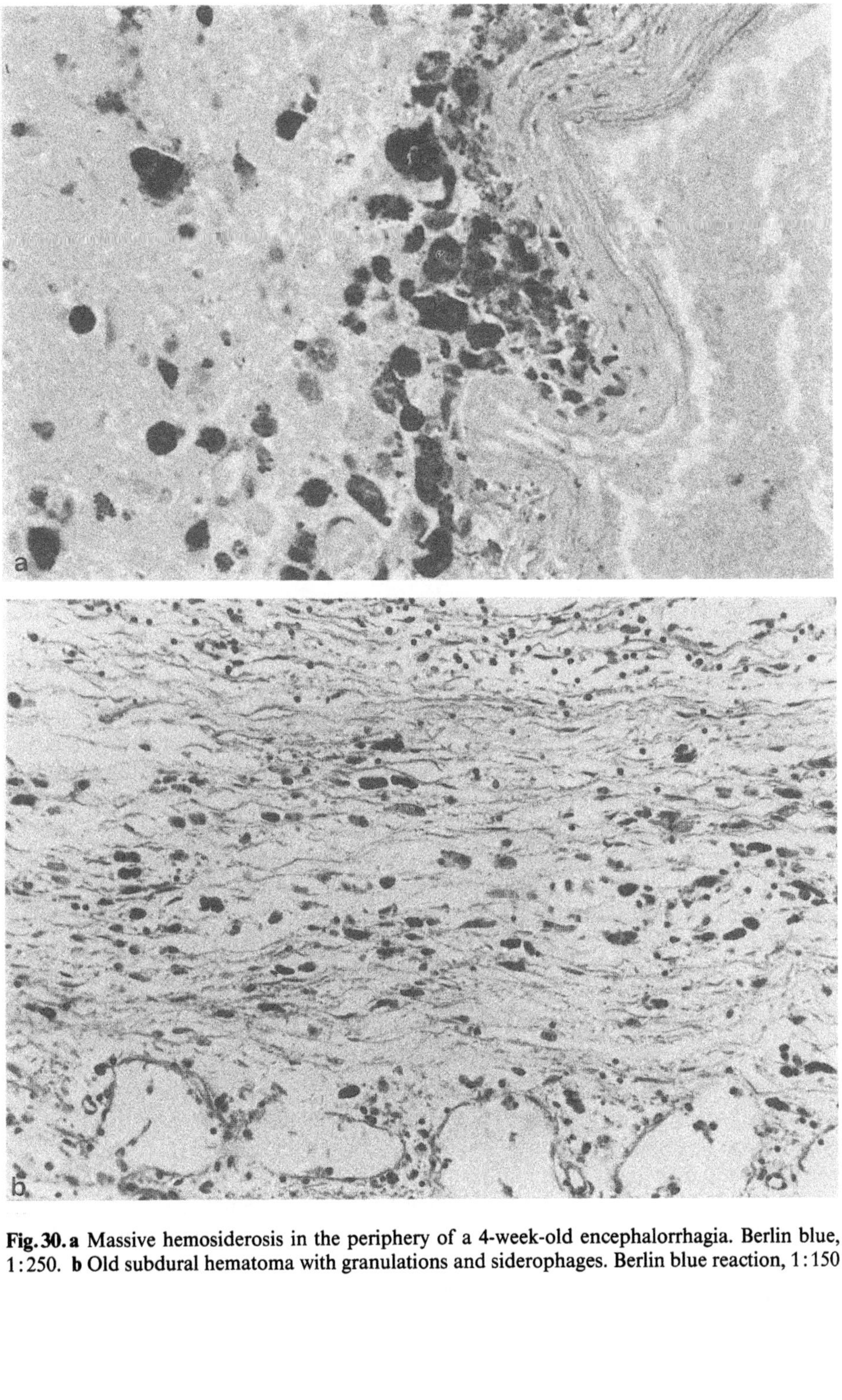

Fig. 30. a Massive hemosiderosis in the periphery of a 4-week-old encephalorrhagia. Berlin blue, 1:250. **b** Old subdural hematoma with granulations and siderophages. Berlin blue reaction, 1:150

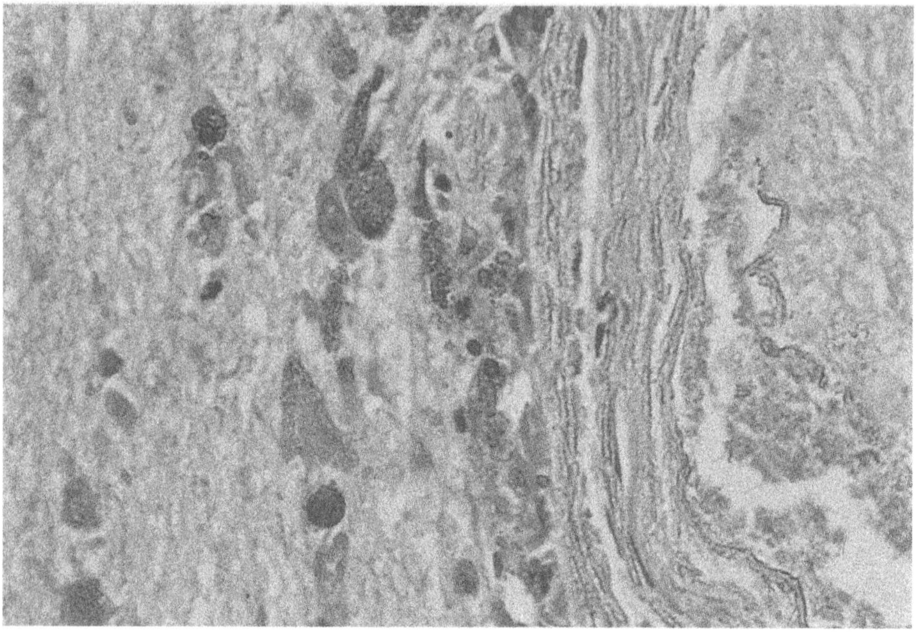

Fig. 31. Nonsiderous pigment (hemotoidin) intra- and extracellularly evident in the periphery of a 19-day-old cerebral hemorrhage. Berlin blue, 1:250

acid. Ferrous and ferric iron are detected in the reaction. With the tannic acid – phosphomolybdic acid – phloxine B method (according to Puchtler and Sweat), Wille was able to obtain positive reactions 4 h after hemorrhage formation (Wille et al. 1969). In a normal case, however, it should be assumed that with the Berlin blue or Turnbull's blue reaction, hemosiderin cannot really be detected in the vicinity of a subcutaneous hemorrhage before 2–3 days have elapsed; some authors cite the 3rd–4th day (B. Mueller 1953) or the 9th day (Walcher 1930, 1936) after hemorrhage formation. The development of iron-free pigments can normally be expected after 1 week according to Gedigk (1958), according to Walcher (1930) this does not occur until after 9 or 11 days (Fig. 31). Extensive reviews of the iron-containing pigments and the breakdown of hemoglobin are found in Hueck (1912, 1921), M. B. Schmidt (1940), Masshoff (1946), Schwerd (1962), and Merker (1968).

Of more theoretical interest is the identification of further pigments such as melanin, paralysis-iron, and malarial pigment. Mention should also be made of the iron-free, brownish inner pigmentation of impacted fetuses due to hemoglobin breakdown, so-called Lobstein's cirrhonosis (M. B. Schmidt 1934). Histochemical investigations have gained increasing significance in recent years in the scientific study of early tissue reactions to hemorrhages and lesions. Histochemical examination methods were also established to a broader extent in forensic practice by Raekallio (1965, 1972) and Pioch (1966a). This will be comprehensively discussed in the age determination of wounds and hemorrhages.

Covered hemorrhages in the subcutis were first subjected to a systematic enzyme-histochemical investigation by Berg and Ebel (1969). In 25 cases from routine autopsy material, they found the first definite reaction in the form of an increase in ATPase activity in the vascular walls 2.5 h after hemorrhage formation. At the same time, there was an increase in the activity of aminopeptidase, especially in the connective tissue mesh and vessels of the panniculus adiposis in the vicinity of the hematoma margin. These reactions were identifiable in many previous cases in the appearance of leukocytes. The authors stress that in forensic practice the presence of the reactions only permits the age of the hemorrhage to be tentatively concluded, since retardation may be possible. Negative findings on the other hand are to be assessed with caution.

Postmortem Changes

In the histological assessment of hemorrhages, the findings relating to postmortem changes also have to be examined. The most important findings capable of giving rise to deception and limiting the histological evidence value will be briefly mentioned here.

Shortly after formation of a hemorrhage, probably after 10–20 min, extracellular hemoglobin can be observed in the vicinity of the hemorrhagic focus even when the subject is still alive. In such cases, the hemoglobin probably originates from traumatically damaged erythrocytes. After death, hemoglobin can be traced in the immediate surroundings of hemorrhages, both of vital and postmortem origin. With the comparatively sensitive Lepehne's stain, the hemoglobin takes on a distinct yellow-brown shade. The occurrence of hemoglobin quantitatively increases apparently uninfluenced by the onset of death. Hemoglobin diffusion out of the erythrocytes in the region of the hemorrhage leads relatively rapidly to the surrounding tissue becoming imbibed. Diffusion of hemoglobin into the area around hemorrhages could be detected by serial tests on hemorrhages of diverse vital and postmortem traumatic origins and on hematomas produced postmortem by the injection of blood (Janssen 1967b). This postmortem hemoglobin diffusion can reach the skin surface from the deeper areas within 1 HPM in loose tissue regions (Fig. 32), e.g., under the eyelids; it thus occurs considerably earlier than the formation of diffusive livor mortis. Histologically, there is as a rule no displacement or migration of cellular parts out ot the hemorrhagic focus connected with the diffusion. A consequence of this diffusive phenomenon that is macroscopically perceptible from the outside is an apparent enlargement and displacement of the hemorrhage. Such postmortem changes have been occasionally misinterpreted as vital indications. These misconceptions have also led to a doctor being reproached for failure to help after having carried out the first examination of a person killed in an accident. The postmortem hemoglobin diffusion is probably affected by the fluid content of the tissue concerned and by the postmortem movement of fluid toward the body surface as a result of desiccation.

There is no regularity in the development of postmortem hemoglobin diffusion: It can sometimes be entirely absent; in some cases it can already be distinct after a few hours; occasionally, it only becomes conspicuous on the body surface after a matter of days. Pallor of the erythrocytes accompanies this diffusion, especially in the peripheral areas of the hemorrhage. If the hemorrhage is located within adipose

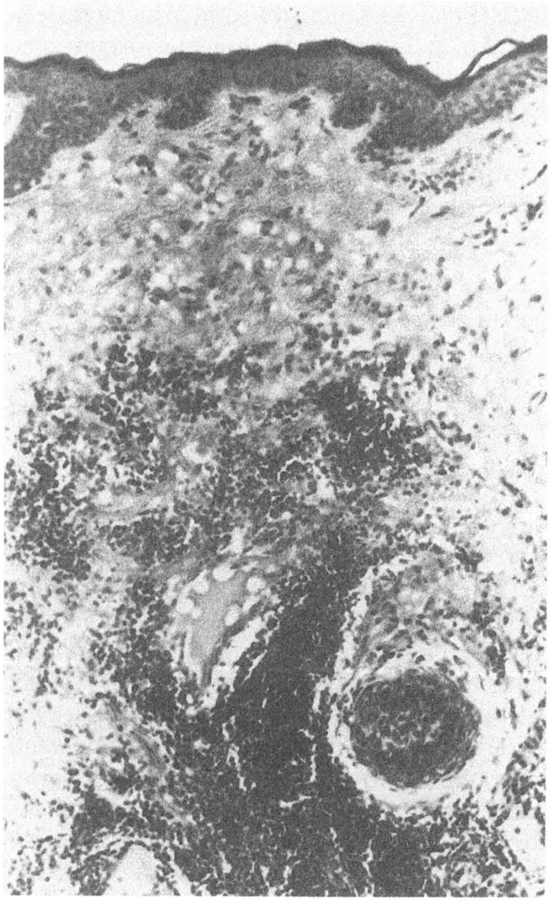

Fig. 32. Intravitally developed subcutaneous hemorrhage with postmortem hemoglobin diffusion to the skin surface. Lepehne's, 1:120

tissue, the hemoglobin diffusion may only be minimal. Imbibation of the adipose tissue, particularly of the adipose tissue cells themselves, is evidently not possible.

The postmortem occurrence of fairly large, poorly defined impregnations, sometimes also circumscribed and red, should be taken into account, e.g., in the pectoral and cervical musculature. These findings, which can be macroscopically confused with hemorrhages, are created by rapidly commencing autolysis and putrefaction and may be identified in an otherwise well-preserved corpse. Histologically, these changes are seen as a very intensive hemoglobin imbibation. In differential diagnosis, such findings can give rise to problems if the erythrocytes are already homogenized or lysed postmortem. Identification of traumatically dependent hemorrhages of vital origin then becomes difficult. Conversely, the presence of a vital hemorrhage cannot be demonstrated with the necessary reliability in such areas.

In older hemorrhages, the iron may be washed out of the hemosiderin comparatively soon after death (B. Mueller 1953). Precise chronological data on this phenomenon are not as yet available. Klages and Wilhelmi (1974) carried out a putrefaction experiment for almost 2 years on a liver containing a large amount of hemosiderin. They discovered a rearrangement of the hemosiderin test reaction with a high concentration on the free surfaces and in the crevices and vessels of the decaying liver after about 7–9 months. At the same time, a conversion of ferric to ferrous iron probably took place. The iron-containing incrustations partly receded again with the hydration of the organ, and a more diffuse finely dispersed accumulation of iron-containing pigments became dominant in the surviving organ structures. A positive hemosiderin test was detectable at the end of the 2-year experiment.

The age determination of hemorrhages is made in connection with the assessment of mechanically caused tissue damage.

2. Mechanically Caused Tissue Damage

Mode of Origin and Histomorphology

Every kind of mechanical trauma comes into consideration as a possible cause. This concerns in particular contused trauma with the formation of laceration, bruising, and dehiscence in the region of the skin, including the hypodermis and, in severe cases, the underlying soft parts down as far as the bone; partial detachment of the skin (décollement); abrasions; excoriation; incised wounds; puncture wounds; blows, including all associated forms of internal injury; and special kinds of contused trauma (e.g., gunshot wounds, explosions, hydrostatic explosive effects). All mechanically caused tissue damage, therefore, comes into consideration that is characterized by deformation or interruptions in the tissue continuity. The histomorphology of mechanically caused tissue damage does not, with few exceptions, include any characteristic features that are indicative of the cause. The main function of histomorphological investigation is age determination and the establishment of whether damage is of vital or postmortem origin.

Some histological findings of more general significance, however, require a brief description.

Excoriation, Desiccation. As is generally known, this concerns skin changes in the corpse caused shortly before or after death by the effects of contused trauma. These changes can be brought about up to several days after death by blunt force. Very shortly after the trauma, discoloration from light yellow increasing gradually to dark reddish brown occurs in the cutaneous area affected. Histologically, these cutaneous areas are characterized by compression usually of all layers of the epidermis with simultaneous detachment of the stratum corneum and strong compression of the upper layers of the corium. In the case of older excoriation, stratification within the epidermis can no longer be discerned. The papillary body is in most cases more extremely flattened. Hyalinization and clumping can occur in the region of the stratum basale (B. Mueller 1934, 1953). Flattening of the cell nuclei of the stratum germinativum takes place in the area around skin desiccation and it is independent of the developmental mechanism. These flattenings of the epithelium can occur in skin desiccation produced with or without considerable effects of blunt force; they have, therefore, no practical forensic medical significance. Our own attempts

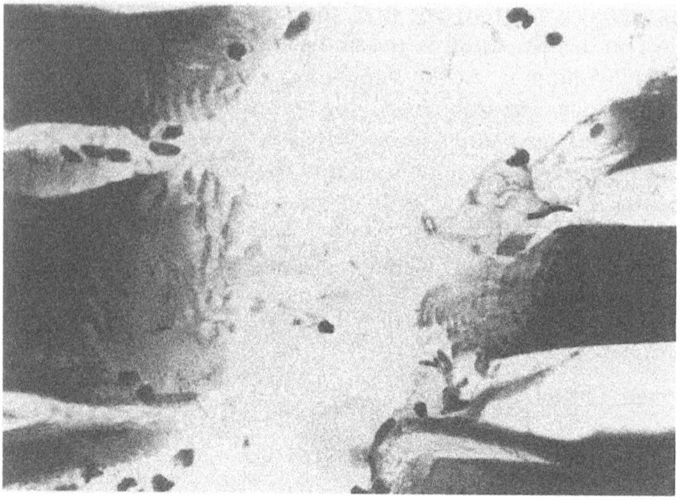

Fig. 33. Contusion with separation of the skeletal muscle fibers. Divergence in the transverse striation. Eriochrome-cyanin, 1:350

at visualizing the histochemical characteristics were without success. Broadly speaking, only one slightly elevated stain-binding ability compared with normal staining was found.

Lacerated, Contused, and Incised Wounds. Histologically, there is a possibility of differentiating contused and incised wounds. Careful fixation with protection of the tissue topography is essential, best done by mounting the excised piece of tissue. In addition, the use of serial sections is recommended. In this way, a smooth division of the tissue elements concerned, especially of bundles of fibers and vessels, can be seen histologically in clearly cut incised wounds. Retraction of separated fibers resulting directly after the trauma must be taken into account. This might lead to an irregular margin to the incision appearing in the histological picture. With lacerated and contused wounds, a divergence in the transverse striation is detectable in the region of skeletal and cardiac musculature near the sites of division (Fig. 33).

Metachromasia, Fluorescence, and Adipose Tissue. In the histological assessment of vital reactions, particular value was seen by Orsós (1935) in the stained visualization of so-called metachromasia in damaged connective tissue. Using Mallory's stain, he saw an alteration in the normal blue color of the collagen fibers; they stained red in the region of various mechanical, chemical, and thermal lesions. This finding can also be observed in postmortem lesions (Blum 1937). In experiments on bites carried out on volunteers, Millington (1974) observed a changed staining character toward Masson's reagent in the collagen after circumscribed compressive application; the change was restricted to the directly affected areas and persisted for at least 5 days. For the differentiation of pre- and postmortem lesions of the cardiac musculature, Ökrös (1961) developed an impregnation method: Embedding in paraffin, cauterization in potassium bichromate solution, aqueous safranine solution, toluidine blue solution, silver nitrate solution, and ammonium silver nitrate solution. The vitally damaged myofibrils of the heart bind the metal salts much more intensely than the undamaged fibrils. This involves, to some extent, metallophilia of the traumatically damaged fibrils and an affinity for chrome and silver salts that does not occur in postmortem lesions of the cardiac musculature.

The phenomenon of metachromasia is also evident in the area of desiccation. Orsós (1935) was thus able to distinguish a lesion metachromasia from a desiccation metachromasia. The latter is supposed to be reversible with prolonged hydration, but this was not confirmed by Lindner (1971). Orsós (1935) assumes that a displacement of the albumin fraction to the globulin side is the cause of metachromasia in the protein substance of the affected connective tissue fibers. In fluorescence-microscopic investigations on wounds and abrasions, Krauland (1955a) could detect no change in the primary fluorescence of the various tissues. Only with heavy desiccation of the wound margins and with abrasions could a negligible increase in fluorescence be found. This obviously developed as a consequence of the greater density of these tissue sections. After fluorochromatization with acridine orange (phosphate buffer mixture pH 2-11.5), the circumstances were more difficult to assess due to the different shades involved. No reliable differences could be determined between wounds of vital and postmortem origin, just as in unstained sections. In contusion of the hypodermis, the fat droplets in the lipocytes may be finely dispersed and emulsified. This phenomenon is thought not to occur in adipose tissue in the vicinity of rope marks in postmortem strangulation (Blum 1937). Fat emulsion could not be produced in animal experiments (Hubalbeck 1951).

Special Organ Findings. In the brain, the effects of mechanically caused injuries are predominantly manifest in the form of cortical contusions, cerebral medullary hemorrhages and vascular lesions with intracerebral hemorrhages, and subdural and epidural hematomas. The histomorphology has been exhaustively investigated and described (Krauland 1950, 1963; Peters 1969; Unterharnscheidt 1972a, b; Jellinger 1977). Injuries to cerebral tissue involve some special features not common to other organs. Even without any demonstrable interruption in the continuity of cerebral tissue, rhectic hemorrhages suddenly occur at the moment of trauma. The vessels show a perivascular border of blood corpuscles and later lymphocytes appear; the surrounding cerebral tissue becomes displaced. Hemorrhages tend to be found in the cupulas of the convolution gyri; smaller hemorrhages are confined to the cortex of the brain, whereas larger hemorrhages extend as far as the subcortical cerebral medulla. The tissue continuity in the region of cortical contusion foci may initially be preserved in the early stages following trauma. By means of careful serial sectioning, circumscribed lacerations can be demonstrated in the vessels in areas affected by trauma. These are probably the cause of the hemorrhages, which tend to be perivascular and appear as annular hemorrhages in section.

The nerve cells in the area of cerebral hemorrhages are reduced in size and deformed; the cell body is shrunken and elongated. The nucleus is similarly deformed and tends to stain diffusely (Fig. 34). In assessing ganglion cells, care should be taken with postmortem effects, e..g., "dark neurons;" these have a round pale nucleus with dark cytoplasm and cell processes that can be traced a long way into the periphery. These cells are regarded as a consequence of postmortem traumatization in

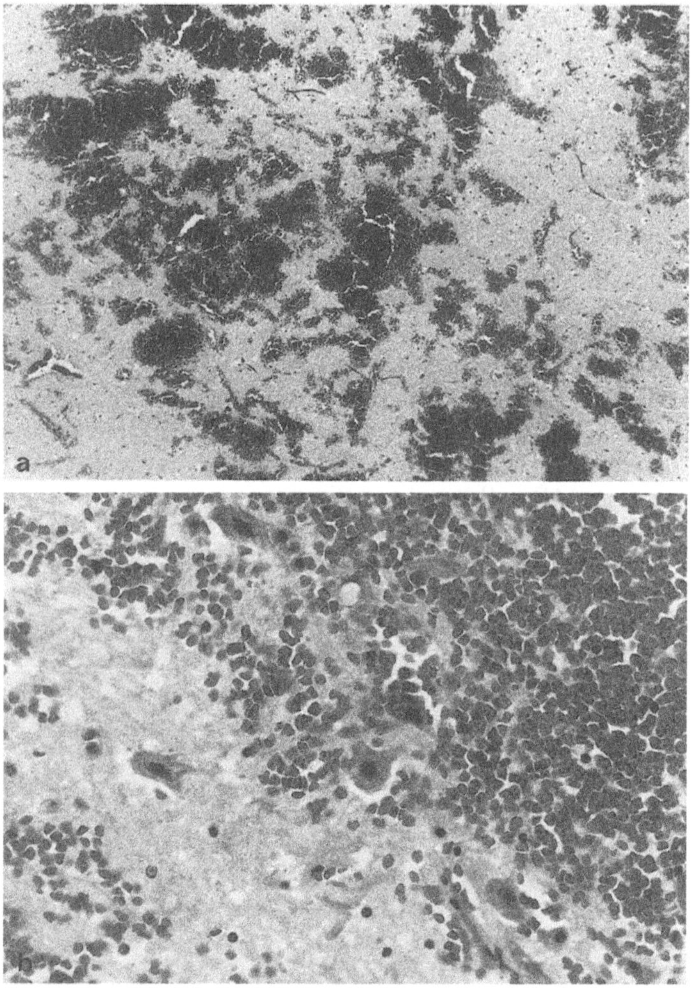

Fig. 34. a–c

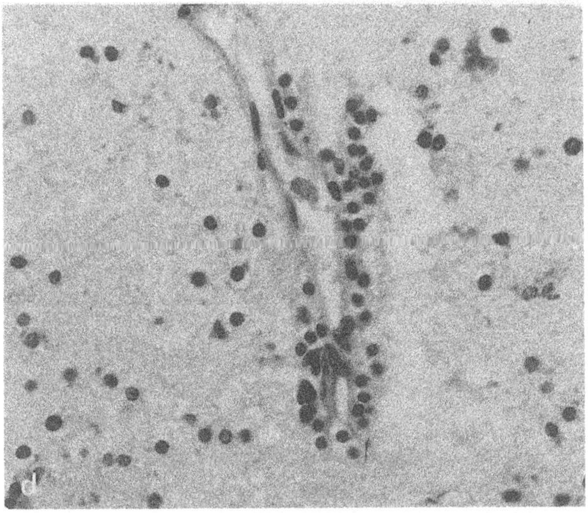

Fig. 34. a Cerebral contusion with fine-maculate cerebral medullary hemorrhages. H and E, 1:80. **b** Contused hemorrhage of the brain with alteration of the ganglion cells. H and E, 1:250. **c** Perivascular cerebral hemorrhage in the vicinity of a contusion focus. H and E, 1:180. **d** Perivascular round-cell infiltrations of the brain, 4 days after contusio cerebri. H and E, 1:200. **e** Cerebrum with "neuronophagia" of ganglion cells in the region of a contusion focus. H and E, 1:250

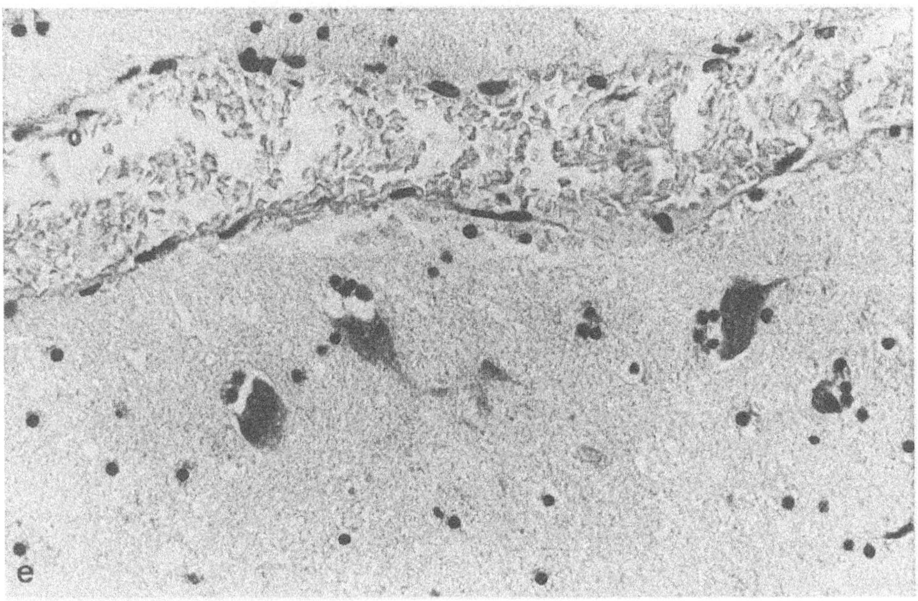

unindurated brains. It is believed that in removing the brain, the deformations induce a substantial strain in the transitional zone between the gray and white matter, with the result that the unfixed neurons can be damaged (Cammermeyer 1978; cf. Oehmichen and Gencic 1980).

In an area of hemorrhage, the cerebral tissue is poorly stained with Nissl's method and the zone appears altogether lighter. In cerebral tissue damage with and without a break in tissue continuity, the early tendency toward necrotic formation is characteristic. This is probably due to early edematization and the resulting poor nutritional supply. Central brain injuries deserve special attention since they are sometimes difficult to distinguish from spontaneous cerebral hemorrhages; the histomorphology and traumatic origin were thoroughly investigated by Krauland and his followers (Bratzke 1979). According to them, isolated vascular ruptures and "cerebral ruptures" are responsible, brought about by short violent blows from the front and side or by violent rotation of the head.

In 52 fatal craniocerebral traumas, Weiler (1979) was able to demonstrate histologically 36 pituitary hemorrhages, which were combined with primary and secondary traumatic chiasmatic changes in ten cases. Following acceleration stress on albino rats, Roudier et al. (1965) found a removal of Gomori-positive material in the hypothalamus-pituitary system. The changes in the central nervous system in epilepsy and trauma were histologically and histochemically examined in rats by Wegman et al. (1970). In these extensive experiments, spasms were produced by electric shocks and cardiazol; with other animals, cerebral necrotic foci were caused by hot needles. The results are predominantly of significance to basic research.

The histological assessment of mechanically incurred cerebral injuries becomes problematic when no breaks in continuity, contusions, or other morphologically detectable destruction exist. Here, one can speak of an area of concussion in the broadest sense, including the regions marginal to the tissue contusion. In the case of commotio cerebri, the extraordinary difficulty in correlating mechanically caused dysfunctions of an organ with morphological, particularly histological, features is apparent. Numerous efforts have been made in trying to detect the tissue effects of cerebral commotio with disturbance of the state of consciousness. To bring about a concussion syndrome, it appears necessary for there to be mechanically conditioned irritation of a particular extent and intensity in a localized part of the cerebrum (Unterharnscheidt 1972a, b; cf. Jellinger 1976). It is still not known which cellular structures are affected by the mechanical irritation. A kind of reversible paralytic mechanism in the cells produced by mechanical traumatic means would be a possibility. The symptoms of cerebral concussion cannot be explained by a reaction of the circulatory system in the affected tissue since they do not become immediately effective. The damage to the brain cannot be detected by the light-microscopic methods of investigation currently used. The small hemorrhages frequently referred to in the region of the brain stem have thus far not been established as related morphological features.

The same difficulties with regard to the histological evidence of concussive damage also apply to other organs, for example, the heart. After contusion of the thorax with distinct clinical functional disorders of the heart, it is possible that despite the most painstaking histological investigations on the heart and its tunica, no traumatically dependent changes can be detected. Further problems arise in the diagnostic examination if older pathological changes are present, if a long interval between trauma and death is involved, or if early microtraces are evident in the region of the conductive system (Rosenkranz 1971; Walther 1972; Geppert 1978; Vesterby and Gregersen 1980). In the case of blunt trauma without interruptions in tissue continuity and without evident contusion, the only histological indications of the preceding trauma are occasional disturbances in the blood distribution. The vessels in this area are distended and filled with blood. Sometimes, leukostasis is also seen, though its diagnostic value is disputed. On no account are such findings a definite sign for the onset of an inflammation. So-called traumatic myocarditis generally

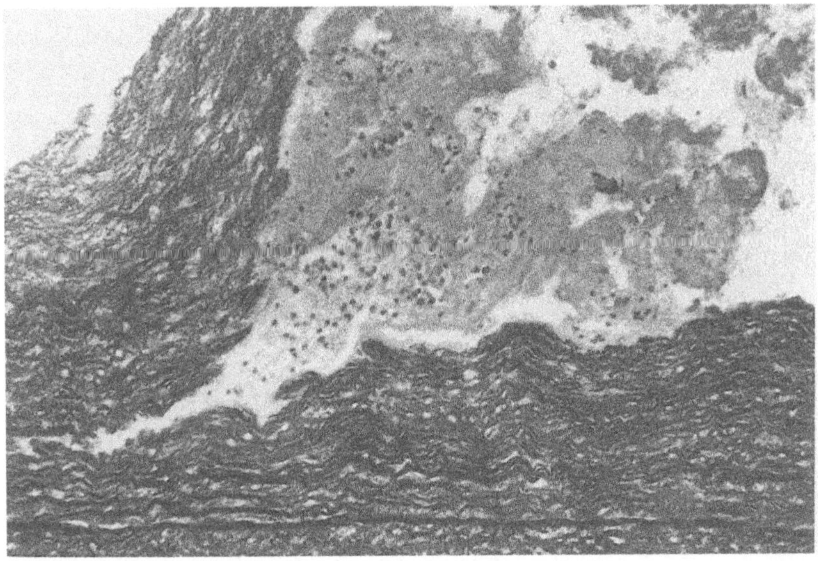

Fig. 35. Intimal laceration of the aorta with fibrin thrombus. Subject: 30 years old, ♂, automobile accident, survived 5 h. Elastica-van Gieson, 1:150

gives rise to a lot of problems (Plueckhahn and Cameron 1968). An inflammation alone is normally not a morphological feature indicative of trauma.

Histological investigations and critical examinations of traumatically caused damage to the larger arteries and veins require particular discussion. The histological inspection of fresh traumatic intimal lacerations or complete or partial breaks in the tissue continuity in previously healthy vascular branches does not give rise to any difficulties (Fig. 35). Serial sections parallel to the vascular axis with various cell and fiber stains (elastica van Gieson, H and E, PTAH, silver staining) are recommended for the investigation. However, traumatic lesions in blood vessels that only later, sometimes after development of aneurysm, lead to rupture are difficult to assess (Figs. 36–38). The investigation and assessment of such cases is further impeded if in the area of traumatic vascular wall lesions previous inflammatory or degenerative vascular diseases, such as arteriosclerosis, arteritis, medionecrosis, lues, are present. Even the diagnosis of vascular disease is not easy if advanced stages, healed defective states, or combinations of several vascular diseases exist. Vascular or aneurysmal ruptures produced spontaneously or by incidental causes can thus for the most part not be excluded with certainty. Under such circumstances, it is also difficult to differentiate between aneurysms of congenital and traumatic origins.

On the whole, critical reserve and restraint are necessary in histologically determining the quality and extent of traumatic or morbid vascular damage. Generally, exhaustive histological investigation and evaluation is an indispensable requirement in the appraisal of every kind of vascular lesion. Forensic evaluations without verifiable histological evidence are fragmentary: The pathologist submitting such evidence runs the risk of its not being accepted. For specific questions concerning different traumatic and morbid vascular lesions, the examples in the following

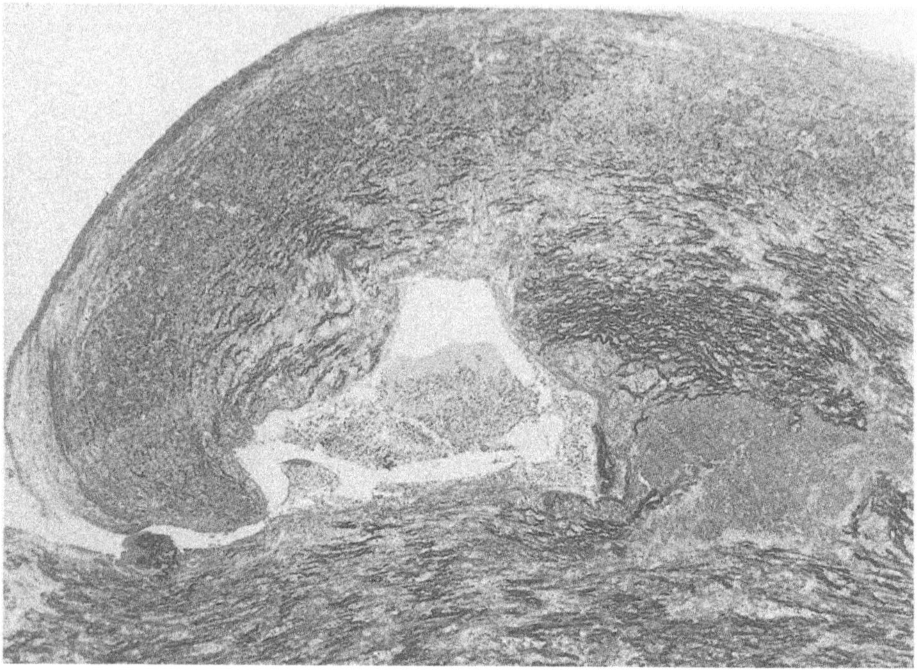

Fig. 36. Intimal laceration of the aorta with dissociated hemorrhage and degeneration of fibers. Subject survived 5 days. Elastica-van Gieson, 1:60

studies are referred to: Krauland (1955b, 1961 – references), Klages (1970), Naeve and Brinkmann (1971), Brinkmann (1975), Hirst and Gore (1976), Schlatmann and Becker (1977), Plamenac et al. (1977), and Weiler et al. (1980).

A clinical condition due to traumatic lesions of the vessels and bile ducts in the liver was summarized by Illichmann-Christ (1952) under the term "metatraumatic hepatopathy." Histologically, this involves disturbances in the permeability of the capillaries and the formation of a protein-rich perivascular edema with a subsequent adverse effect on the adjoining parenchyma. Disaggregation occurs in the fibrous framework along with desmolysis, histolysis, and tissue necrosis with increasing exudation. Very similar changes are found in hyperthyroidism, burns, heavy infections, intoxications as well as in connection with other causes; according to Roessle (1944) these changes represent an acellular "serous inflammation." The hepatic cells become surrounded by exudate, dissociate out of the tissue structure, are cut off from the natural nutrient and oxygen supply, and finally fall to necrobiosis and cytoclasis. Metatraumatic hemobilia can also develop as a result of a traumatic liver lesion (Fig. 39); this is thought to occur by the flow of blood out of the hepatic arteries or veins and into the bile ducts. In ruptures of the liver, traumatic anastomosis can come about through a central blood-filled rupture cavity in the liver with a valvelike outflow mechanism, or it can be the result of transmitted angionecroses. Central and deep ruptures of the liver and subsequent tissue necroses, in rare cases also tumors, intra- and extrahepatic aneurysms, and cholecystopathy, can also give

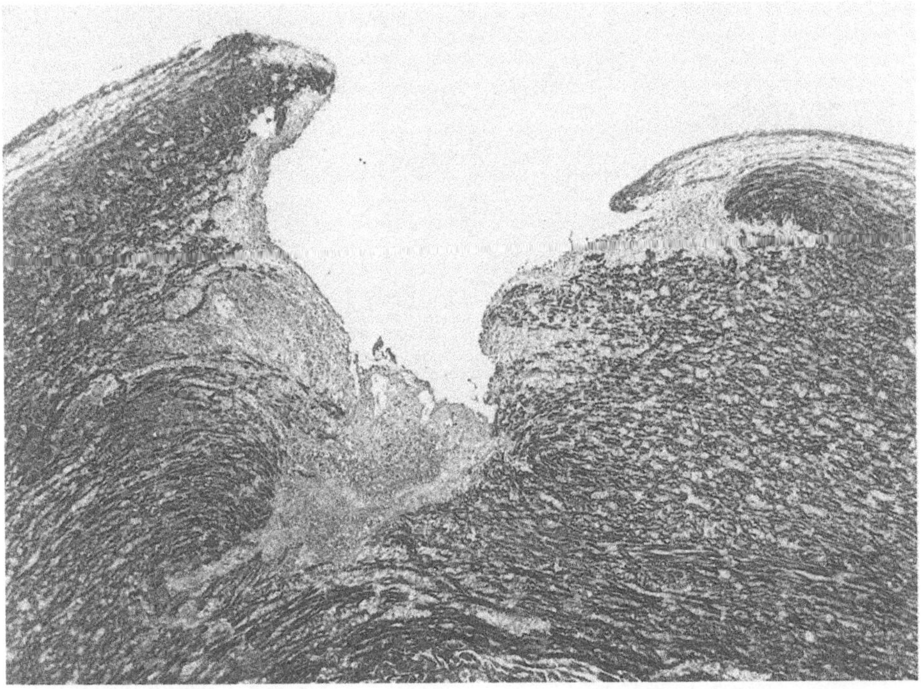

Fig. 37. Intimal-medial laceration of the aorta with granulations. Subject survived 12 days. Elastica–van Gieson, 1:60

rise to the clinical symptoms of hemobilia. These symptoms are characterized by spasms in the right epigastric region, intermittent obstructive jaundice, hematemesis, melena, and subsequent severe anemia (Bässler 1959 – references). Very occasionally, complications arise from the traumatically incurred communication between the larger bile ducts and hepatic veins with the penetration of bile into the blood and extremely high bilirubin levels (Kleiber and Bause 1976).

Another incidence of organ involvement concerns the kidneys following mechanical injuries with hemorrhages and muscular damage, incorrect blood transfusion, and in connection with a number of other causes. As a result of hemolysis, myolysis, or both, often accompanied by cardiovascular disorders and shock, the histologically very striking picture of hemolytic nephrosis (i. e., lower nephron nephrosis) results (Zollinger 1966, references). The swollen kidneys, which stain a brownish color on the cut surface, are seen histologically to contain numerous casts largely in the distal and collecting tubules (Fig. 40). The casts stain brown-red; some are granular, whereas others are more bandlike. The granular components of the stained protein casts are very variable in form and size and individually very much smaller than erythrocytes. Hemoglobin- or myoglobin-containing protein precipitation is probably involved; therefore histochemical differentiation between hemoglobin and myoglobin is not possible here. In the middle of the plaquelike chromoprotein casts, calcium oxalate crystals can also occasionally be detected. Necrobiotic epithelial changes develop in the distal portions of the main parts of the widened tu-

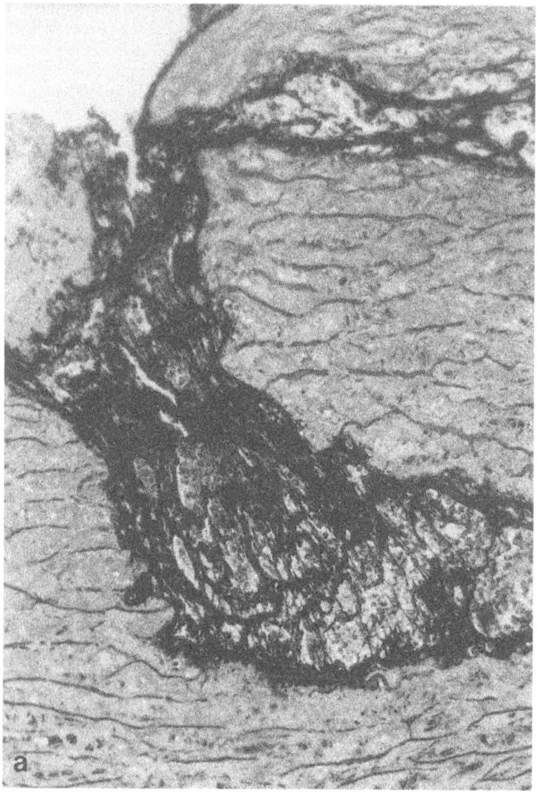

Fig. 38. a Traumatic rupture of the artery occurring at two different times with fibrin and blood in the crevice of the rupture. Subject survived 12 h. PTAH, 1:150

bulus and in Henle's loops. Regenerative budding in the epithelium of these sections and in the collecting tubules occurs in later phases.

In the case of traumatic rhabdomyolysis, renal changes occur which are histologically similar and are also often accompanied by anuria (Weitbrecht et al. 1976 – references). This acute syndrome does not receive a great deal of clinical attention. It is attributed to completely different causes, such as intoxication, infection, and other muscular lesions; histologically, the skeletal musculature shows ceraceous plaquelike and vacuolar degeneration of almost all muscle fibers, between which are found isolated empty sarcolemmic tubes.

A particular histological finding was detected by Meinel et al. (1977) in the area around ruptures of various tendons. This involves fibrillary structural disturbances in the form of crack deformation, which can also be found in experimentally overstretched and relaxed collagenous fibers. Ruptures of the Achilles tendon are normally due to degenerative alterations of the tendinous tissue. A traumatic disruption caused by an accident can only be verified if normal tendinous tissue is histologically traceable and the accident itself is judged to have been capable of bringing about a rupture (Keyl 1979).

Foreign Bodies. In the histological examination of wounds, particularly of deep soft-tissue and organ injuries, foreign bodies are also occasionally found sur-

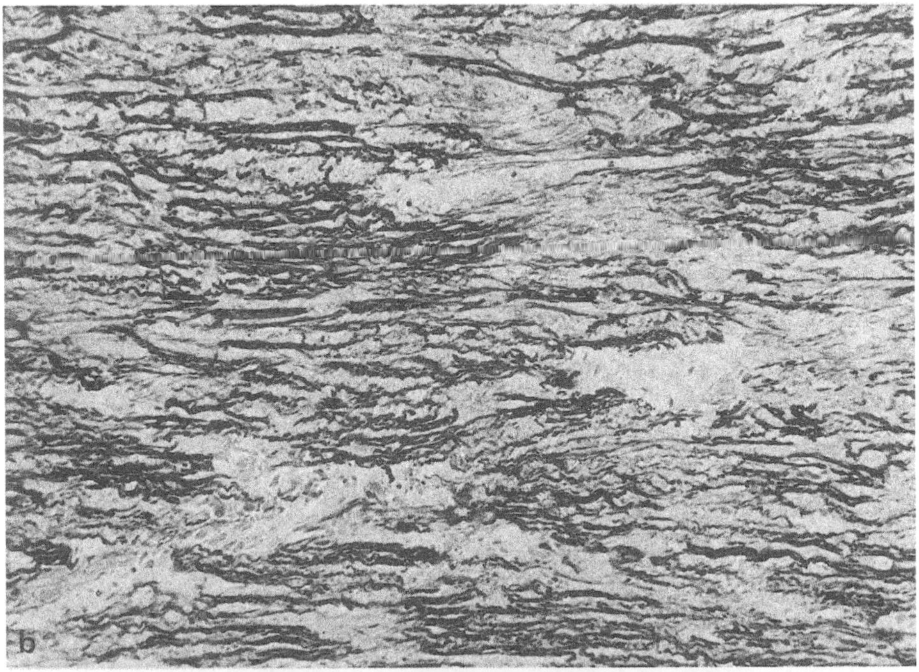

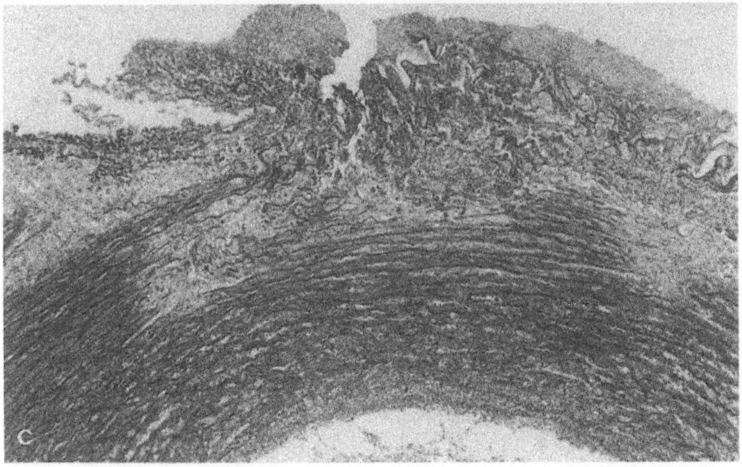

Fig. 38. b Edema and fibrous degeneration of the aortic media in the vicinity of a rupture occurring at two different times. Elastica-van Gieson, 1:180. **c** Aorta: traumatic laceration of the adventitia and media with incomplete repair of the connective tissue. PTAH, 1:60

rounded by granular tissue and foreign-body giant cells, containing multiple, mainly centrally located nuclei (Figs. 41, 42). These foreign bodies can be composed of all kinds of material, mainly, particles of clothing, particles of dirt, metal and glass splinters, cellulose-containing fragments, and powdery components. The investigation of foreign bodies in histological section aims at describing their topography with regard to the injury and identifying them as precisely as possible. From this, in-

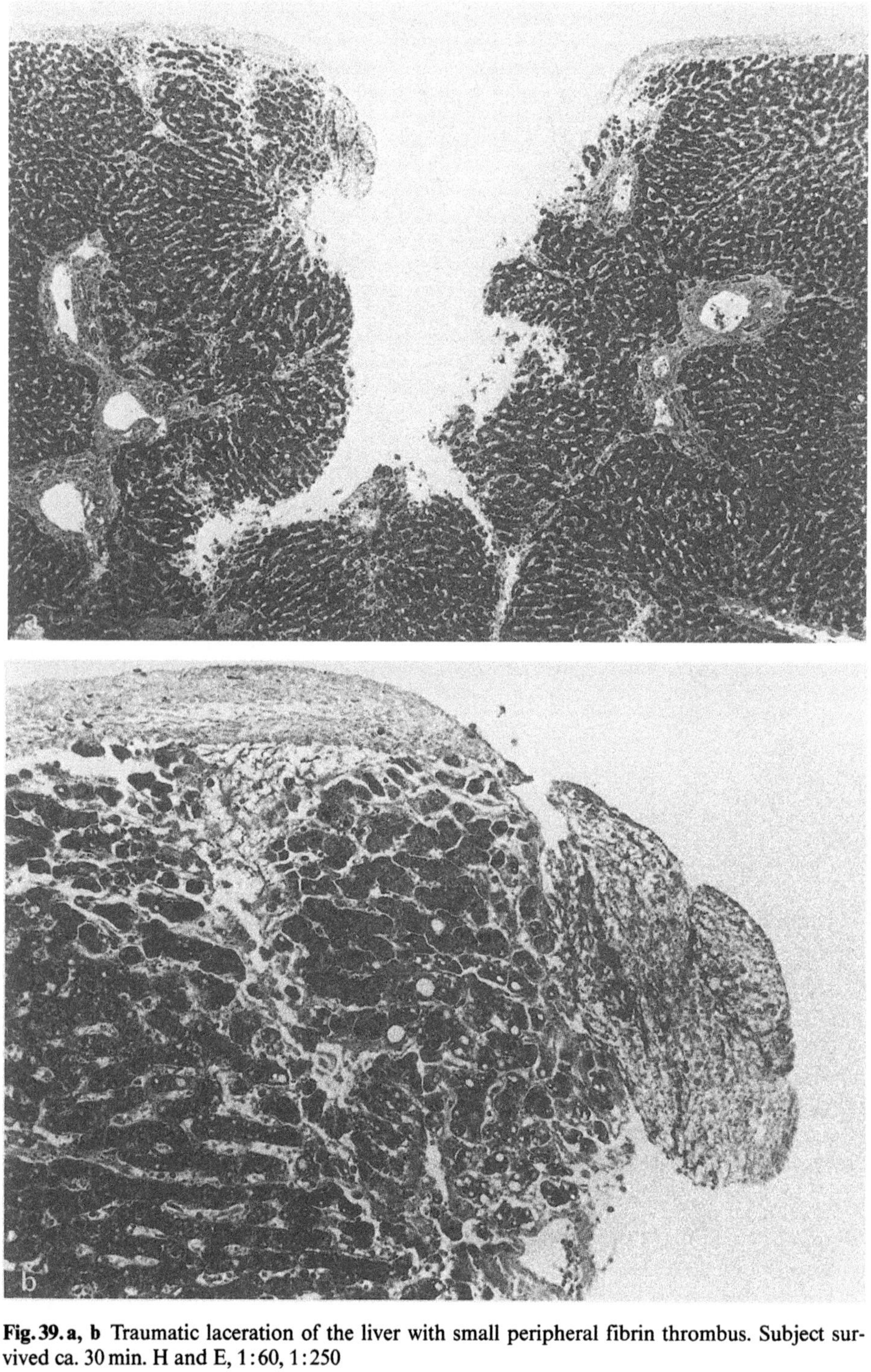

Fig. 39. a, b Traumatic laceration of the liver with small peripheral fibrin thrombus. Subject survived ca. 30 min. H and E, 1:60, 1:250

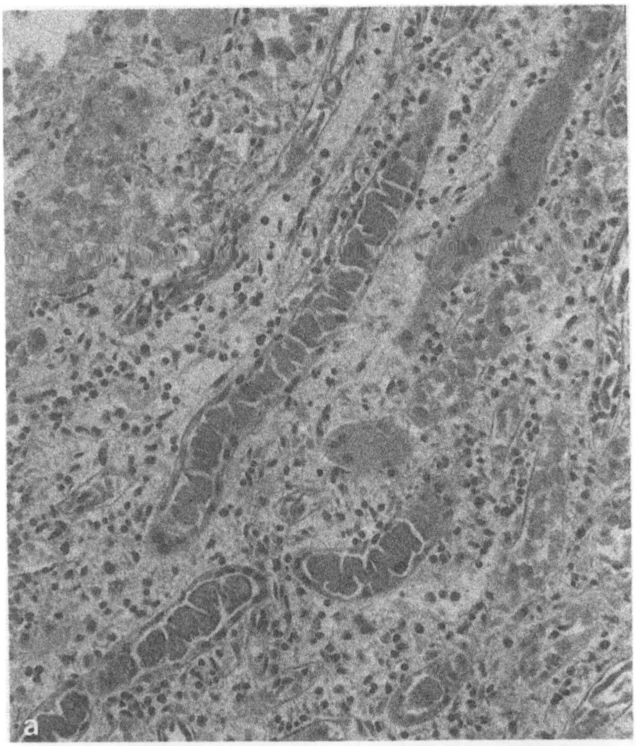

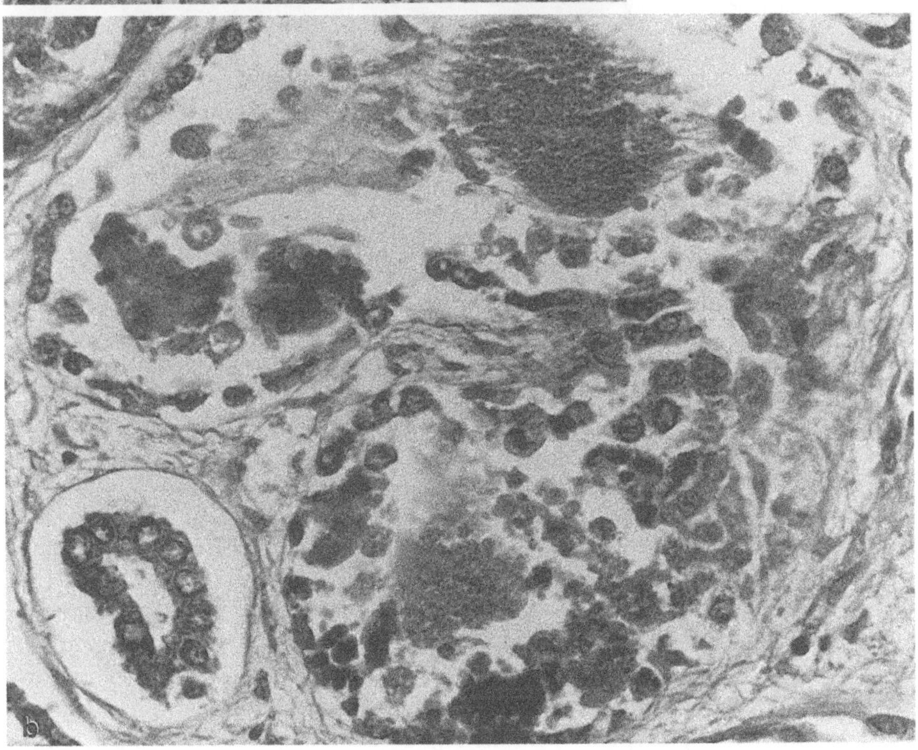

Fig. 40. a Kidney with granular casts in the collecting tubules (lower nephron nephrosis). Subject: 35 years old, ♀, transfusion accident. Lepehne's, 1:150. **b** Lower nephron nephrosis with fine-granular casts (hemoglobin and myoglobin). Multiple crush injuries to the soft tissue. Subject: 24 years old, ♂, Lepehne's, 1:250

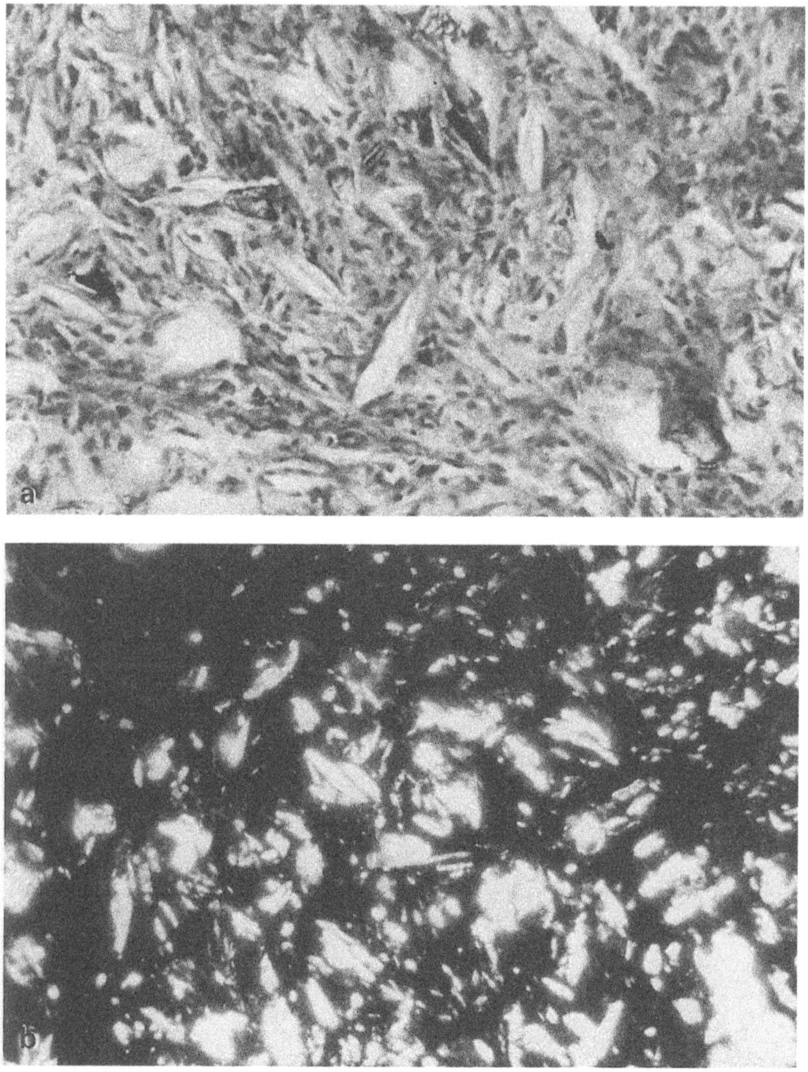

Fig. 41.a Foreign-body granulation tissue with crystalline inclusions and giant cells. H and E, 1:200. **b** Same findings as in **a** in polarized light

ferences can be made as to their origin and significance in causing the wound. Histological evidence of foreign bodies in the region of soft-tissue injuries can, therefore, contribute to the clarification of mechanically induced lesions. A histological investigation should always, therefore, be carried out.

Endogenous particles that reach deeper tissue layers or the intracorporal region should also be included among the foreign bodies in these circumstances. Parts of the epidermis, integumentary appendages, and all other specifically structural tissues, e.g., bone and musculature, come under consideration here. In the region of the abdominal cavity, the post-traumatic implantation of parenchymatous compo-

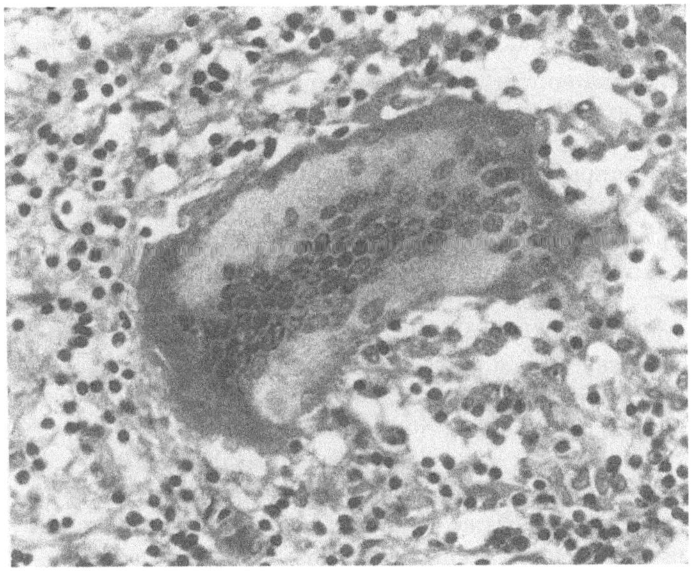

Fig. 42. Giant cell with multiple central nuclei. H and E, 1:280

nents in the wrong position has occurred in isolated instances. Klein (1951) found several tubercles up to the size of cherry stones in the serous membrane of the small intestine of a 40-year-old man who died 23 days after a road accident suffering from severe contused abdominal trauma. In the well-preserved marginal areas with central necrotic zones, these tubercles were identified histologically as liver tissue. A personal observation concerns a 27-year-old man killed within a few minutes in a road accident. The autopsy and histological investigation revealed multiple, well-preserved splenic tubercles up to the size of peas in the serosa, especially of the lower small intestine. Owing to the locality and pattern, accessory spleens did not come into question. This man, whose case history was not known until the time of the forensic autopsy, had had a splenectomy 3 years previously because of traumatic splenic rupture. Autopsy and histology here had indicated the case history from the finding of post-traumatically implanted splenic tissue (traumatic splenosis, Böhm and Wybitul 1980).

In the identification of foreign bodies, all available methods should be employed, for example, tests in polarized light, evidence of metals (Timm 1958; Voigt 1971), botanical and zoological comparative investigations, tests on unstained sections, and the use of phase-contrast microscopy.

Wound Healing

To be able to understand a presentation of histological findings concerning mechanically caused tissue damage in humans, it is necessary to have a certain basic knowledge of the character and development of inflammations and tissue repair.

Numerous surveys and classifications exist in which histomorphological findings and criteria toward the determination of age and the differentiation between vital and postmortem injuries are summarized with regard to forensic considerations. Just as in the critical examination of hemorrhages, all such classifications must be used with caution and critical reserve, particularly in the presentation of findings concerning age determination. The reason for such an attitude is that theoretically the natural wound healing process proceeds in phases which permit inferences to be made as to the time of infliction of tissue damage. Practically, however, these individual phases are not histologically demarcated by sharp boundaries, but to some extent develop concurrently. Moreover, in the question of supravital reactions, reference to the time of death (by which is meant the death of the individual) cannot be made precisely, since death does not occur at a single point in time but over a period which cannot be exactly defined.

According to the principles of general pathology, the essential histological features that occur when tissue is mechanically damaged in living humans are as follows (for the present without precisely considering the chronological development): Interruption in tissue continuity with breaks in the parenchymatous or connective tissue structures; contusion and destruction of the affected tissue; lesion and disruption of capillaries or larger blood vessels; escape of blood in the region of the tissue damage, into preformed cavities, or to the outside; exudation, with the escape of blood plasma and edematization of the damaged and surrounding tissue; thrombosis, particularly in the area of the affected blood vessels; hemostasis and blood coagulation; formation of fibrin; migration of granulocytic leukocytes from the neighboring blood vessels; migration of mononuclear cells; formation of inflammatory halos; necrosis of the directly or indirectly damaged tissue sections; purulent liquefaction with or without infection; migration of histogenous cells; budding of capillaries; formation of granular tissue; formation of collagenous fibers; gradual regression of the resorptive inflammatory process, subsequent retrogression of the granular tissue; increase in the fibrous portion until termination of the tissue repair in the form of a scar.

Breakdown of the hemorrhages with the formation of hematoidin and hemosiderin occurs parallel to the wound healing process. The healing of covered hemorrhages can also occur without granular tissue in the form of "bland resorption" (Berg and Ebel 1969). The preceding, rather summary enumeration of histological criteria makes it clear that the healing of mechanically produced wounds should be seen as a particular form of inflammation. In this context, some tissue characteristics and influential factors deserve mention. The earliest signs of necrosis in interposed soft parts, especially musculature, in the region of fractures have been observed after a survival time of 2 h 20 min. In animal experiments, myonecroses have been found in the case of a 65-min-old fracture (Panning 1940). In the deep periosteal layers, Haversian canals, and in the medullary cavity, the proliferation of cells did not begin until after 20 h. Experiments by Pierucci and Gherson (1970) revealed medullary tissue, especially marrow cells, in the region of rib fractures in 17 of 28 cases, even where there were agonal and early postmortem fractures from extrathoracic cardiac massage. The histological and cytological differentiation of such findings is important in distinguishing them from vital leukocytic reactions. In primary healing of bone, the size of the fracture line is a significant factor. The limit of tolerance is about 0.5 mm for a primary osseous bridging-over (Schenk and Willenegger 1977); with greater damage, intermediary connective tissue is formed. For the duration of the healing, an osseous apposition rate of about 1 μ/day may be assumed.

The healing of skin lesions can present certain differences according to the age of the individual. In serial tests on surgical wounds, fibroblastic proliferation in the corium was predominant in infants; in adults, the rapid regeneration of the epidermis was more apparent (Bednár 1976). Investigations into wound healing in secondary and tertiary wounds by Seitz et al. (1978) revealed differences in the resistance to rupture which were attributable to a rapid collagenous fiber formation in secondary and tertiary wounds. The resistance of the wound can be negatively influenced by antibiotics (Struck 1976). Experiments on the behavior of mast cells in wound healing in the skin of rats showed an initial disappearance of these cells (Miller and Whitting 1965). Not until after 3–7 days did the mast cells once again become evident, mainly without granules. After about 14 days, a pattern of mast cell distribution could be identified corresponding to that in normal uninjured skin. It is supposed that the mast cells play a part in the stimulation of connective tissue cell division. In mechanical damage to skeletal musculature, regeneration with partial fibrous hyperplasia occurs after temporary fibrous atrophy (Schmalbruch 1976). Glycogen-free mitotic myoblasts form very rapidly following thermal necrosis; after about 2 weeks, new muscle fibers are present. In animal experiments, in all, four types of muscle fiber regeneration can be distinguished.

Experiments specifically concerned with the behavior of elastic fibers within lesions revealed, using Weigert's stain, fine, broken, contracted elastic fibers with an irregular inner structure between the erythrocytes. In the case of injuries caused shortly before or after death, this finding was only slightly expressed (Lomenzo 1962). Investigations on wound contraction in guinea pigs suggest that the source of contractile force is located more within the wound rather than in the wound margins or surrounding tissue (Zahir 1964). According to older experiments by Krause (1927), the elastic fibers have a particular significance in the histological age determination of wound healing processes. They first appear after the termination of cellular regenerative and resorptive processes and after the development of collagenous fibers. This late differentiation permits a histological age determination at a time when there is no overlapping with other tissue elements.

The structure of granular tissue has been extensively studied in numerous experiments with various methods (Fuchs 1965; Kischer 1979). It has been electron-microscopically established that the erythrocytes are moved passively through the vascular walls. In this way, small quantities of fluid can also be transported. The perivascular tissue pressure increasing in this manner can ultimately prevent further diapedesis, whereby the hemorrhage stops by itself. The capillary endothelium can facilitate or aggravate this process by strong constrictions or tumefactions.

Histological analyses of punctures and incised wounds have revealed distinct cutlike alterations around the site where the blade of the instrument used was inserted into the tissue, and in the area where the blunt back of the knife had been there were changes characteristic of pressure (Zagryadskaya 1965). In carrying out the examinations, the investigator is recommended to take sections with a thickness of 20–30 μm parallel to the skin surface. The author was unable to detect any deep spreading of parts of the epidermis in scissor wounds. Rauschke (1956), on the other hand, reported invaginations of the epidermis where the outer edges of the scissors had been inserted. Similar observations have also been communicated by Bosch (1968). With stab wounds, he was also able to determine spreading of parts of the epidermis in the puncture channel, especially where the back of the instrument had been applied. Displacement of the elastic fibers in the region of the back of the knife and their severance on the opposite side can be histologically clarified in the same way.

The occurrence of foreign-body giant cells in connection with mechanically produced lesions is mainly due to the introduction of foreign material or displaced and denatured endogenous substances. The giant cells thus induced are components of granular tissue. The cytomorphology of the giant cells is characterized by multiple nuclei, which are on the whole centrally located, and a relatively dark cytoplasm. The cells are on average 50–80 μm in size. They commonly enclose the foreign bodies that brought about their formation. In the case of foreign bodies that have been incorporated and fully encapsulated, a weakening of the stimulus caused by the foreign bodies occurs and with it a disappearance of the giant cells. The data as to the period of development are variable: Wurm (1956) = 3 weeks, Wohlgemuth (1962) = 6–10 days, Köberle (1956) = 3 h. According to the autoradiographic investigations by Silverman and Shorter (1963), the polynuclear giant cells in foreign-body granulomas produced in animal experiments develop from macrophages. According to other interpretations, the foreign-body giant cells are formed from phagocytes that derive from mononuclear hemocytic elements. Additional pertinent investigations into the histology and histochemistry of foreign-body giant cells come from Letterer (1959), Bassermann (1960), Guseck and Uerlings (1958), Goldstein (1954), Giese (1960), Leder and Nicolas (1965), and Kuske (1965).

There has been no lack of experiments investigating the factors of influence in the process of wound healing (references in Gilsa 1966; Berg 1972). The following factors have inhibitory effects: Irradiation, corticosteroids, scurvy, diabetes, hepatic cirrhosis, uremia, denervation of the wounded area, loss of blood, cold, commotio cerebri, shock, and all other "vitality-reducing conditions." A reduction of inflammatory reactions in prolonged severe lesions of the central nervous system leading to death has often been cited. The apallic syndrome and coma dépassé should here be considered (Ore et al. 1977). The investigations of Berg (1972) argue against inhibition of the inflammation by cranial trauma, blood loss, and cold. After the administration of psychotropic drugs to rats, Seiffert and Friedrich (1965) discovered a lowering of the wound resistance. Following the massive application of psychostatic drugs to guinea pigs, Suppan (1963) found only a negligibly delayed healing of femoral fractures. Delayed wound healing was also observed in rats when the wounds were generated with an electric knife (Hupe and Roeper 1965). There was only a slight impediment of histoid leukocytosis through the influence of acids and lyes on intact and mechanically damaged guinea pig skin; however, a lowered increase of enzyme activity in the wound margins was obtained (Kampmann et al. 1978). In postmortem incised wounds and subsequent cauterization, a distinct rise in the histamine level occurred in the wounded area. This is a finding that deserves particular consideration since it is well established that an excess of free histamine

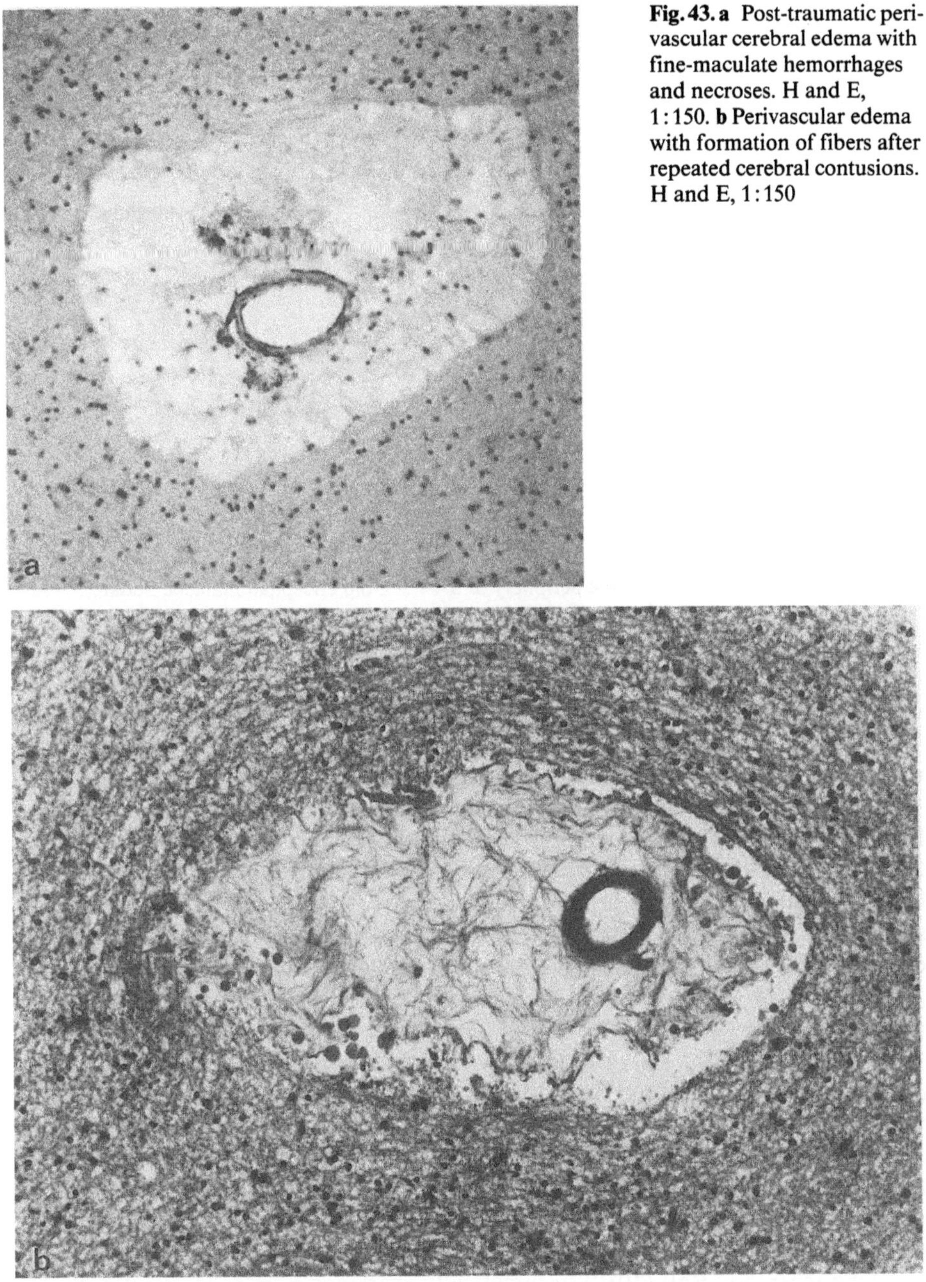

Fig. 43. a Post-traumatic perivascular cerebral edema with fine-maculate hemorrhages and necroses. H and E, 1:150. **b** Perivascular edema with formation of fibers after repeated cerebral contusions. H and E, 1:150

compared with undamaged control skin is to be regarded as a vital reaction. In skin burns, therefore, cautious interpretation of histological and biochemical findings is advisable.

In the examination of wounds that have been altered postmortem by autolysis or putrefaction, the employment of histochemical enzyme tests appears to offer

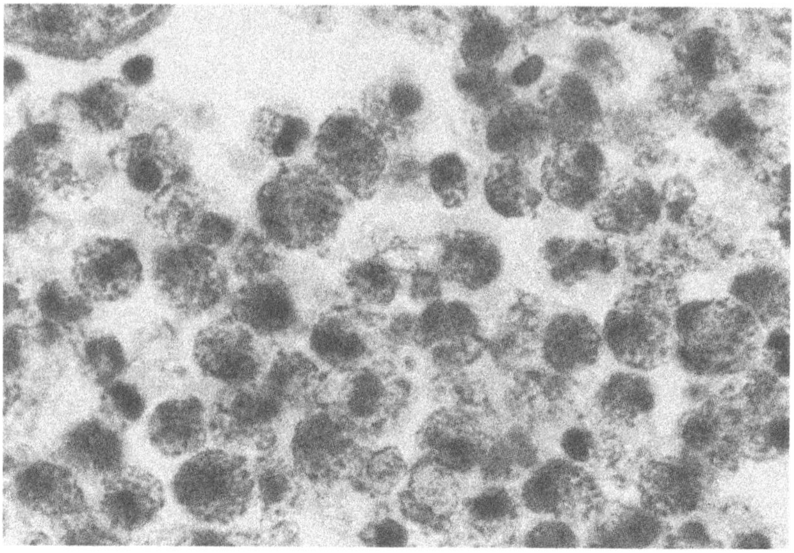

Fig. 44. Fatty granule cells from the periphery of a 4-week-old encephalomalacia. Sudan, 1:350

more promise in diagnostic assessment than the use of the customary cellular and nuclear stains. In systematic putrefaction experiments on excised surgical wounds, Berg (1972) proved that a whole series of enzyme activities regularly survive longer than the nuclear stainability in the cutis and subcutis.

The interesting question of whether there are specific properties in the various tissues which can affect the course of healing in mechanically caused tissue damage has hitherto not been systematically examined. A certain individual character can be distinguished in the healing process in cerebral tissue. According to Unterharnscheidt (1972a, b), passive regressive changes predominantly occur in the first stage of hemorrhages and necroses (Fig. 43). Two kinds of tissue lesion can be distinguished here, those detectable in the case of immediate death and those whose appearance requires a minimum survival time. In the second stage of resorption and organization, intense reactive and proliferative tissue processes take place, in which the cells of the undamaged supporting tissue and vigorous macrophage activity, with degradation of the necrotic histoid material and formation of fat granule cells, are prominent (Fig. 44). In the final stage, fluid-containing cystic defects persist with negligible cicatrization on the surface, mainly without fusion to the dura mater. Occasionally, dystropic calcification of ganglion cells also occurs in the surrounding cerebral tissue (Fig. 45).

Oehmichen and Raff (1980) systematically examined a series of histological parameters toward establishing a chronological order of histomorphological changes in corticocerebral contusion foci among 116 cases with a known post-traumatic interval. They examined when the criteria during the post-traumatic interval were detectable for the first and last time in each case. In an earlier investigation, Oehmichen (1978) described the significance of macrophages in various reactive states in the brain. A great many reference points for the histological assessment of brain in-

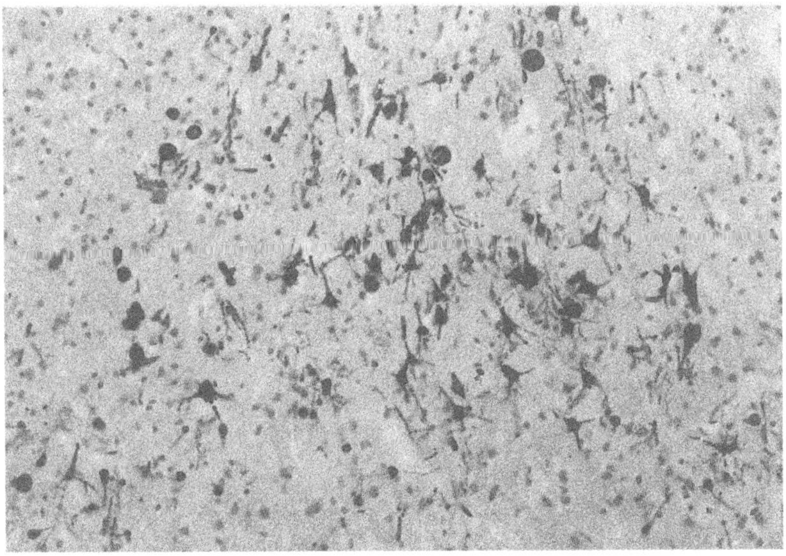

Fig. 45. Margin of a post-traumatic cerebral scar. Calcification of the ganglion cells in the cortex. H and E, 1:180

juries are provided in these large-scale studies. The origin of traumatic necroses in the region of the pallidum, corpus callosum, and medulla and the cerebral changes following post-traumatic unconsciousness lasting for several weeks have been examined and described, particularly by Adebahr (1960b, 1963).

A special form of "wound healing" concerns the degradation of hemorrhages on the interior surface of the dura mater. Closely connected with this is a difficult problem in the examination, namely the distinction between traumatically incurred subdural bleeding and pathological changes of the dura mater with hemorrhage on its inner surface, especially in hemorrhagic internal pachymeningitis. The very comprehensive investigations by Krauland (1954 – references) revealed that a fundamental difference cannot be established from histological evidence between hemorrhagic internal pachymeningitis and a traumatic subdural hemorrhage in resorption. Both processes are histologically characterized by vigorous cell reactions and capillary budding just under the epithelium of the interior surface of the dura mater, resorptive breakdown of the hemorrhages, hemosiderin deposition, capillary cavity formation, secondary hemorrhages and exudation, and fibrous membrane and capsule formation on the outer and inner sides of the hemorrhages. The histological examination is a valuable aid in estimating the age of the changes.

Enzyme-histochemical experiments on traumatic tissue damage in guinea pig and human brains revealed changes in the activity of NAD-diaphorase, malic dehydrogenase, and succinic acid dehydrogenase 3–4 h after causation of trauma. The findings could only be established in those traumatized areas of the brain in which a hemorrhage was present. The enzyme changes are assumed to be connected with a local oxygen deficiency. In investigations on changes in the activities of unspecific esterases in the wound healing process by Bonte and Herrmann (1978), no correlation between enzyme finding and age of the wound could be ascertained that was of use in estimating the time of occurrence. In investigations on dogs following brain injuries, Carvalho (1964) initially found a circumscribed vascular reaction and not until after this did he find a generalized tissue reaction. After 6 h, there was a clear microglial and astrocytic proliferation, connected with giant-cell formation (cf. Wegmann et al. 1970).

Mityaeva (1965) points out one particular feature: In cranial trauma and injuries of the pelvis and lower extremities, a narrowing of the lumen with a high degree of sinuosity of the elastic fibers was found in the pulmonary vessels if death occurred up to 1 h after the severe injury. However, extreme vasodilation was present in the case of longer survival times of 4–15 h.

Age Determination of Lesions and Hemorrhages

The establishment of findings that permit one to infer the time of injury are of prime importance in the forensic medical assessment of lesions and hemorrhages. This involves criteria that indicate in living or dead subjects the time of causation of an injury and from that the survival time. In living human subjects, the examination is almost always confined to a macroscopic investigation. It is only seldom that a specific histological examination by biopsy sampling from the damaged area comes into question for the purposes of determining the age of a wound. Unfortunately, little use is made of the possibility of carrying out a forensic histological examination on excised wound material obtained in the course of clinical treatment of injured subjects.

The forensic medical age determination of injuries and hemorrhages must also be defendable in court. Consequently, the reliability of the diagnosis is of prime importance. Scientifically justifiable certainty, verified by experiment and statistical tests, is often not sufficient for forensic purposes. All factors that cannot be definitely excluded but which could influence the outcome of the age determination must be taken into account in the evaluation of an individual case. Thus, it is generally only possible to specify maximum and minimum limits for the survival time. Some of the more important difficulties that have to be observed in age determination are set out in the following section.

In examinations of corpses for the clarification of the survival time, reference to a clinical time of death signifies unreliability. It has already been pointed out that the process of dying covers a certain period of time and permits no reference to a particular point. Important problems result from this in the distinction of vital and postmortem injuries and hemorrhages. In this regard, the presence of tissue reactions and enzyme activation even after the onset of clinical death in the individual has led to the revision of viewpoints held earlier. The great number of results from studies of wound healing, which are not in complete concordance, makes a forensically utilizable presentation of the age determination of wounds very difficult. Many experiments have been carried out more in the sense of basic research; a forensic significance test was frequently not performed or only done as a subordinate measure. An examination of the results shows it to be necessary to keep a check on the findings with regard to their evidential, indicative, and unspecific value.

The processes at work between causation of tissue damage and cicatrized healing have to be considered as a whole from a general medical point of view. The development in time-graduated phases is the most important reference in determining the survival time. In a given case, however, it is impossible to distinguish the phases exactly from one another. The numerous factors that influence the development of the wound healing processes and which have already been specified in the preceding section are not always known and frequently cannot be recognized. In addition, there are other, more general findings. In the subcutaneous fat, the traumatically released reactions are basically detectable earlier than in the region of the epidermis and corium (Berg 1972; Hirvonen 1968; Ojala et al. 1969). To what extent these findings either empirical or obtained in serial tests, can be regarded as reliable in a given case must remain open for the time being. The same also applies to injuries to the inner organs, where traumatically incurred reactions take longer to be established than in the hypodermis. A comparison of the experimental results from different animal species reveals that the reactions begin substantially earlier and proceed faster in small laboratory animals than in humans (Thomas 1977). The dependence of wound healing on the age of the individual concerned has been demonstrated clinically and in animal experiments (Struck and Engelhardt 1971). In young animals, closure of a wound predominantly comes about by primary healing, whereas in the older animals it is frequently by secondary healing. Histologically, a delayed epithelization and development of granulation tissue was found among older animals. The metabolism of collagen shows a decreased "turnover" and a displacement of equilibrium toward collagen synthesis in older animals. The absolute firmness of the wound increases with age, whereas the relative firmness decreases. The application of such results to the individual case, however, remains problematic.

In the past, the age determination of lesions and hemorrhages relied largely on histological and cytological criteria. In recent years, numerous, and for some time also forensically utilizable, data from histochemistry and biochemistry have been added to these sources. The essential results from research and individual findings are presented in the following books and Monographs: Raekallio (1965, 1980), Raekallio and Mäkinen (1970), Lindner (1967, 1971), Pioch (1966a, b, 1969, 1971), Berg (1972), Beneke (1972), Helpap et al. (1977), Kampman et al. (1980), and Oehmichen and Raff (1980).

For a presentation of the histomorphological and cytological data, the prevailing division into phases of wound healing has proved good despite all critical objections. The classification by Ross (1968) has been frequently cited:

Inflammatory phase:
a) Vascular response
b) Hemostatic response
c) Cellular response – polymorphonuclear cells, lymphocytes, macrophages and monocytes, mast cells

Proliferative phase:
a) Epithelial regeneration
b) Connective tissue regeneration – morphology of fibroblasts, origin of fibroblasts, function of fibroblasts, budding of capillaries

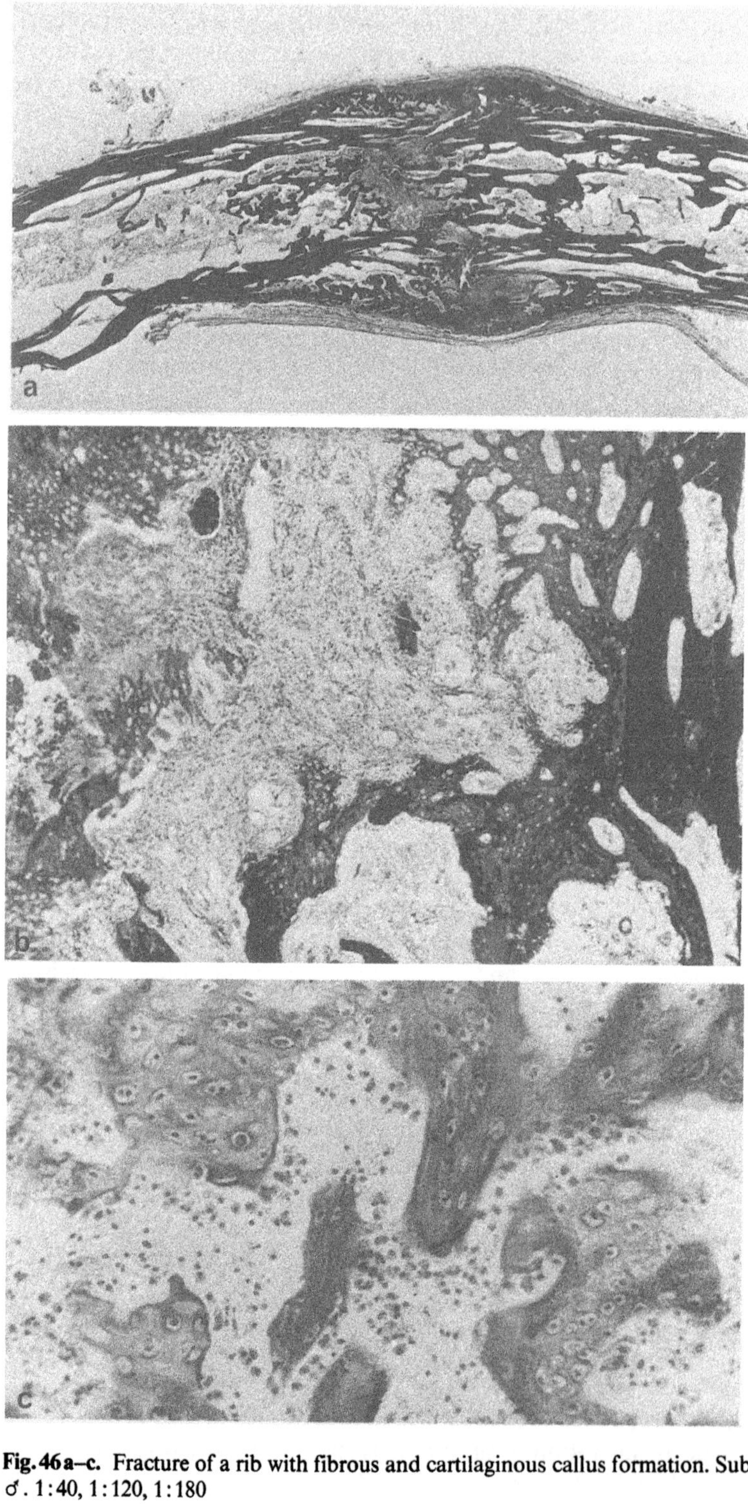

Fig. 46 a–c. Fracture of a rib with fibrous and cartilaginous callus formation. Subject: 65 years old, ♂. 1:40, 1:120, 1:180

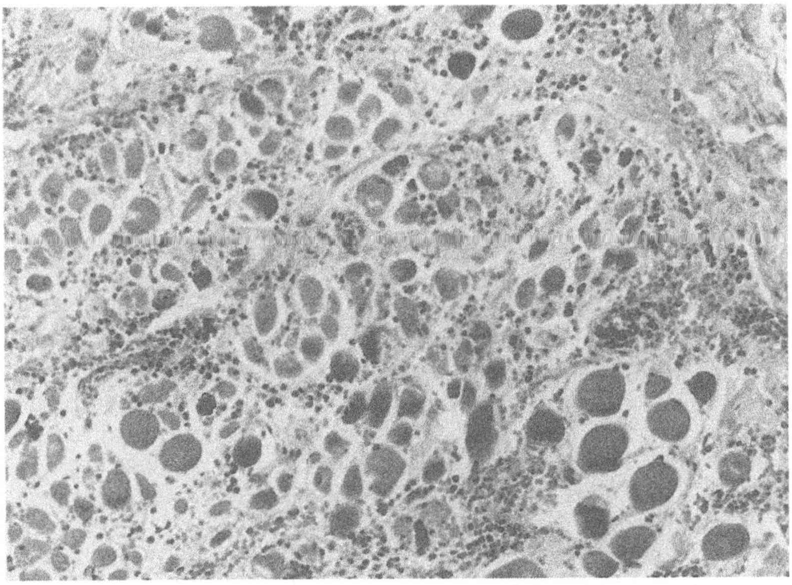

Fig. 47. Three-week-old contusion of the musculature with hemorrhages. Inflammatory and proliferative phase predominantly with monocytes and macrophages. H and E, 1:180

c) Fracture healing (Fig. 46)
d) Muscle healing (Fig. 47)
e) Nerve healing
f) Healing of particular tissues.

Reorganization or transformation phase

Before a synoptic presentation of the essential criteria in the age determination of lesions and hemorrhages at the end of this chapter, some principles and the most important utilizable findings from histochemistry and biochemistry should be discussed. In the presentation of the first cellular reactions, care should be taken that the terms and findings utilized are comparable. Wound leukocytosis has frequently been differently interpreted in humans and animals. A leukocytic reaction should not be considered as such until infiltrates are unequivocally present. At least three to four polymorphonuclear leukocytes per visual field should have permeated the tissue at no less than two different sites in the section outside the vessel. Leukocytes that are located in the middle of hemorrhages cannot be evaluated in terms of a leukocytic reaction. In humans, polymorphonuclear leukocytes have been histologically determined in the marginal areas of laparotomy wounds at the earliest after 20 min. At the same time, white thrombi had formed in the blood vessels (Ojala and Lempinen 1968).

The further course of the cellular reaction is determined by the transition to histiocytic infiltration. This change in the cell picture is of great diagnostic value according to Berg (1972). Here it should be observed that even in the early post-traumatic phase, e.g., in covered skin contusion, mononuclear cell elements can appear (cf. T. Büchner 1971). Postmortem, an escape of leukocytes from undamaged vessels, even with preserved ameboid mobility at the moment of cardiac arrest, is impossible in animal experiments. Once the inflammation has begun, it does not proceed any further in the dead animal or in a detached piece of skin with ligature of the blood circulation (Busse-Grawitz 1964). According to Lindner (1971), on the other hand, the local intravital reactions develop further for a certain time even after the death of the individual. According to Hirvonen (1968), even phagocytosis is possible postmortem. Weak signs of activation can also appear (unspecific esterases in the epidermis and activation of aminopeptidase in mesenchymal cells) in early postmortem damage, according to Pioch (1969). In damaged connective tissue, primary acidosis, which can attain a pH value of 6.0, occurs in the first minutes following stimulation (Lindner 1971). This is caused by an accumulation of acidic metabolites and a change in the normal eucolloids of the tissue concerned. Parallel with this is a release of acidic mucopolysaccharides in the ground substance. This primary ground substance reaction can be produced and detected within 30 min following various types of intravital skin damage. It can also be detected more weakly in lesions of agonal and premortal origin. However, this evidence cannot be applied in forensic practice. The phagocytosis of the traumatically destroyed or phlogistically released parts of tissue and phlogogens leads to the activation and synthesis of enzymes in the fibroblasts. The enzyme patterns in the macrophages and giant cells that emerge are very similar to one another. Impetus has been given to modern connective tissue research by the introduction of radiochemical experimental methods. In this way, it has been shown that fibroblasts in the region of damaged sections of tissue are capable of extremely rapid metabolic reaction and can incorporate a wide range of labeled substances.

Several studies have been concerned with the forensic medical age determination of brain injuries (Krauland 1973; Eisenmenger et al. 1978; Oehmichen 1978; Oehmichen and Raff 1980). From these studies, a greater importance is attached to the mesenchyme and glia than to the nerve cells and fibrous elements. The breakdown of hemorrhages in cerebral tissue and the behavior of fat granule cells as a reaction pattern for the microglial cells are the essential elements for a more precise chronological determination. Light microscopically, hemosiderin is detectable after 3–4 days and the appearance of fat granule cells from day 3 onward. The greatest caution, however, needs to be exercised in the assessment of the findings since these fat granule cells can persist in the tissue for a long time and then be erroneously assigned to other, later events. As in animal experiments in other organs, an effect of the lesion type upon the progress of wound healing can also be demonstrated in the kidney (Helpap et al. 1977b). Comparative tests on local cryopathy and heat injury revealed a retardation of the wound healing by thermal necroses.

The extended application of histochemical and biochemical methods as well as electron-microscopic techniques has obviously also opened up new areas and brought new findings for the forensic medical assessment of lesions and hemorrhages. In the morphological detection of early local vital reactions using combined investigation techniques, Böhm (1979) was particularly concerned with the utilization of normal and scanning electron microscopy. He presented criteria that permitted a distinction to be made between vital and postmortem clot formation. Many histochemical methods have been broadly applied in morphological examinations

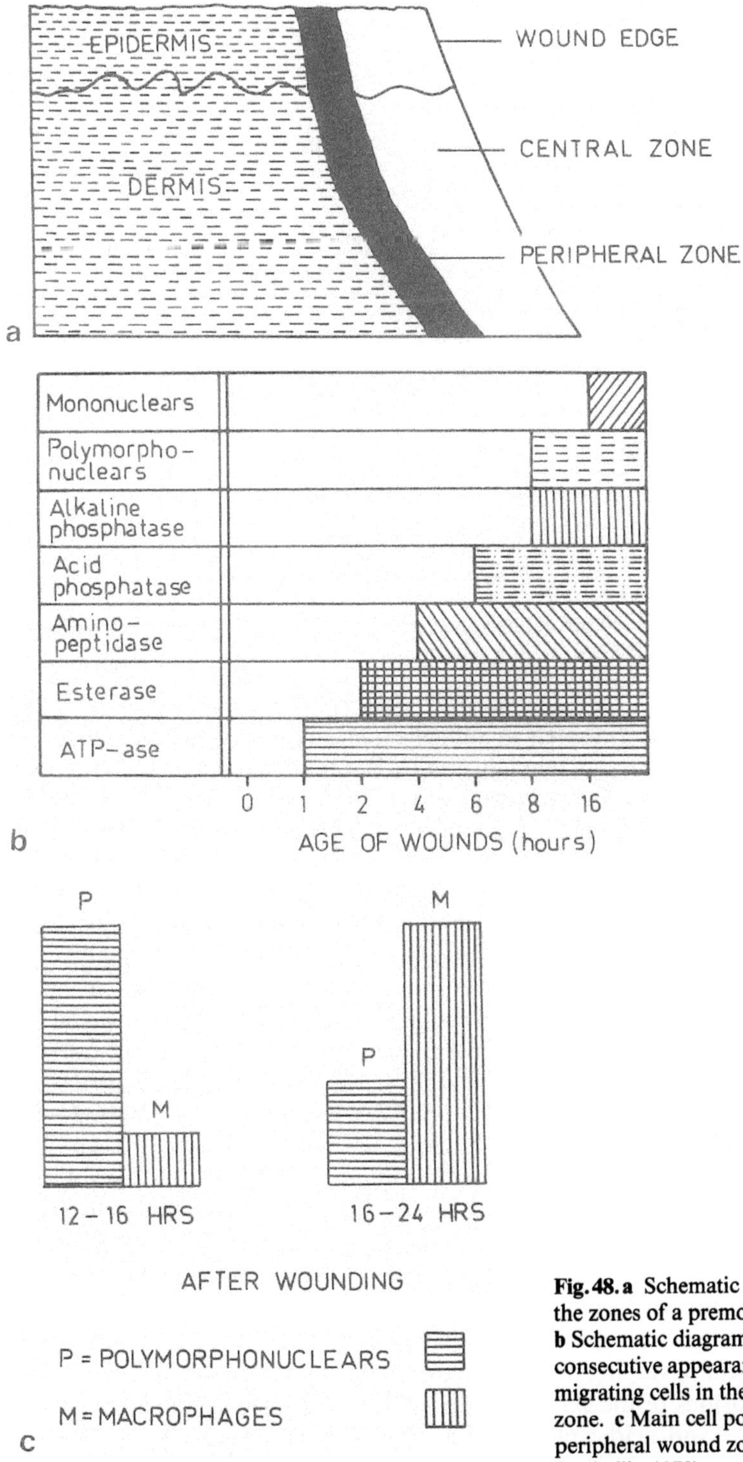

Fig. 48. a Schematic diagram showing the zones of a premortal wound. **b** Schematic diagram showing the consecutive appearance of enzymes and migrating cells in the peripheral wound zone. **c** Main cell populations in the peripheral wound zone. (After Raekallio 1972)

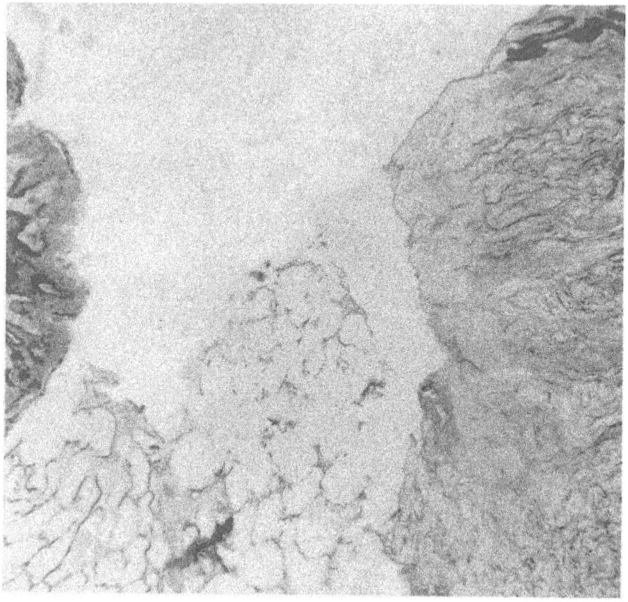

Fig. 49. Puncture channel with peripheral necrotic zone. Invagination of epidermis and displacement of fatty tissue. PTAH, 1:80

in forensic medicine following tests in animal experiments. Routine methods from unrelated fields, summarized in tabular form by Raekallio, are now available. Raekallio (1976) designated the 1st h of lesion survival time as the domain of biochemical analysis, the 2nd–3rd h as the domain of enzyme histochemistry, a central "joint region" in which concurrently histology and histochemistry have the same significance, and the 8th–16th h as the domain of histology (Fig. 48).

It should be observed that in human skin, the histochemical reactions generally commence considerably later than in rats and guinea pigs (references in Berg 1972). The detectable enzyme activities are on the whole structure-linked. They facilitate the cytological differential diagnosis and assignment to individual hematogenic cell series. The majority of routinely detectable enzymes contribute to the activation of fibroblasts. In the peripheral area of sharply defined wounds, the infliction of which was survived by about 1 h, an inner zone can be detected, 200–500 μm wide on average, having diminished enzyme activity. Externally adjacent to this is a zone, 100–300 μm wide on average, with enhanced enzyme activity (Fig. 49). This subdivision into a negative vital reaction in the region of the inner zone and a positive vital reaction in the outer zone, which has been verified in numerous experiments by Raekallio (1965), has won acceptance in principle. It cannot be detected until a later stage using the customary histological stains.

Quantitatively, the enzyme-histochemical reactions of the cutaneous and subcutaneous tissue occur in varying degrees of strength (E. Müller et al. 1971). In incised wounds and abrasions of the skin, ATPase, anilide-acid esterase, unspecific esterases, and alkaline and acidic phosphomonoesterase can essentially be detected more strongly than in contused wounds. The difference is explained by the fact that necroses in contusions are frequently dispersed. Inhibition of aminopeptidase activity in the phase of early wound healing by hydrocortisone could not be seen in animal experiments (Mäkinen and Raekallio 1967). However, it must be taken into account that with clearly nonfatal wounds despite painstaking observation of all procedural requirements, an enzyme-histochemical visualization of vital reactions may not succeed in the peripheral areas of a wound (cf. Berg and Ebel 1969; Raekallio and Mäkinen 1971 a). A negative histochemical finding must, therefore, be evaluated with great caution. Lack of reaction is no proof against a vital origin of the wound. From personal experience, an enzyme-histochemical investigation is usually unsuccessful when strong dehydration of the wound margins has occurred. Around injuries of the subcutis, the cellular reaction can be detected just as quickly (if not more so) as the histochemical reaction according to Berg (1972), Ojala et al. (1969), and Hou-Jensen (1969). From personal investigations, this is also the case in the region of contused musculature in guinea pigs (Janssen et al. 1968). Recently, an increase in ribonucleic acid has also been reported in the region of open wounds (Buris 1978).

In determining the age of lesions of inner organs, there is the disadvantage that, unlike skin injuries, some histochemical methods are not suitable for use with human corpse material. From the results of animal experiments, Beneke (1972) distinguished the following separate processes in injuries to inner organs: (1) cardiovascular changes, (2) degenerative changes of organ-specific cells in the periphery of a lesion, (3) cellular reactions of cells from the bloodstream, and (4) cellular reactions of cells from the vicinity of the lesion (organ-specific cells and fibroblasts). In the liver, kidneys, and adipose tissue, fairly similar phasic histomorphological changes can basically be detected, just as in wound healing in human skin. Histological and histoenzymatic studies on hepatic lesions in humans and animals revealed a discernible reduction in the activity of NAD-diaphorase and β-hydroxybutyric acid dehydrogenase as early as 10 min after trauma (Gherson and Pierucci 1968). In recent animal experiments on the morphology and biochemistry of wound healing in incised wounds to the liver, Kampmann et al. (1980) demonstrated that tissue leukocytosis is less suitable for the age determination of wounds. With short survival times, the liver epithelia showed signs of hypoxidosis and glycogen loss in the vicinity of the incised wound. Proliferation of organ-specific and mesenchymal cells did not appear until after 24 h. The activities of various enzymes (acid phosphatase, glucose 6-phosphatase, and ATPase) were distinctly increased after 1½ h. The proliferative processes occurring later in the traumatically damaged liver were the subject of thorough cellular kinetic investigations by Helpap and Cremer (1970, 1972), Helpap (1973), and Helpap et al. (1977 a).

In experimental fractures on rats, enzyme-histochemical investigations revealed the first reactions after survival times of between 6 and 10 h, especially for unspecific esterases, ATPase, acid phosphatase, and leucine aminopeptidase (Raekallio and Mäkinen 1971 b; Kovacs and Hársanyi 1971). Emission spectrum investigations on the bone marrow of individuals who died directly after mechanical trauma showed a significant rise in the proportion of sodium to copper and a reduction in the proportion of sodium to magnesium compared with bone damage produced postmortem (Filippov and Pashinyan 1971). Age determinations of covered subcutaneous hemorrhages in humans and animals by Berg and Ebel (1969) revealed in particular

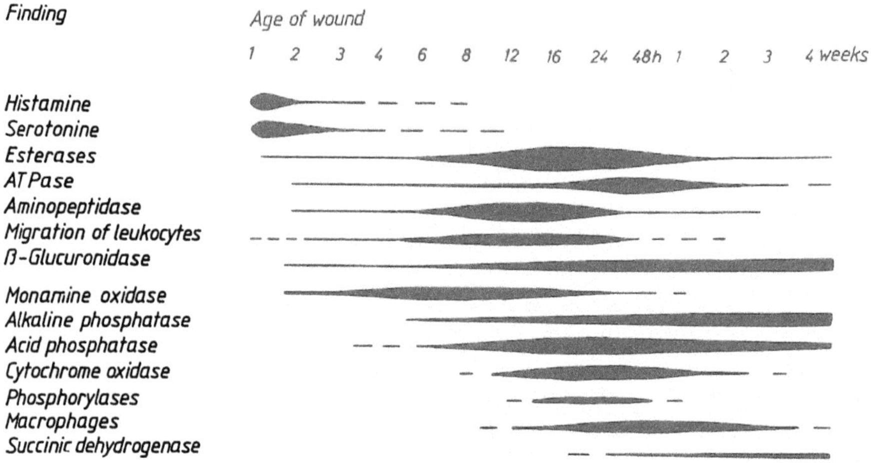

Fig. 50. Chronological graduation of findings in traumatized skin. (After Berg 1972)

the following findings: After 2½ h ATPase reaction in the connective tissue structures adjacent to hematomas; aminopeptidase and unspecific esterase reaction after 4½ h; first migration of polymorphonuclear leukocytes after about 4 h; distinct mononuclear cell reaction after about 9 h; hemosiderin after 90 h; hematoidin after 9 days; granular tissue was only rarely observed in the region of the hemorrhage, however, there was mainly light resorption with only sparse phagocytosis.

In recent years, age determinations of lesions have also been successfully carried out with biochemical methods. These investigations, which can only be briefly mentioned here, are based on the fact that in every healing wound there is a complicated, highly integrated system of efficient, interlocking local and general effects brought about by active substances of a stimulatory and inhibitory nature (Kühnau 1962). Essentially, the following active substances have been quantitatively detected with regard to forensic problems – alkaline phosphatase, aminopeptidase, esterases, histidine decarboxylase, lactate dehydrogenase, histamine, serotonine, and catecholamine. In this connection, studies by the following authors are referred to: Raekallio and Mäkinen (1967, 1969, 1970, 1971 a, b, 1973), Berg et al. (1968), Berg (1969, 1972), Berg and Bonte (1971), Fazekas (1967, 1970, 1971), and Gevers (1975). The most suitable approach appears to be the detection of alpha esterases, serotonine, and histamine in the early post-traumatic phase. According to Berg (1972), there is no doubt as to the basic usefulness of the findings in detecting early vital reactions in forensic practice if the requirements concerning the correct removal of material and methodical precision are fulfilled and postmortem changes are given appropriate consideration. This particularly applies to the detection of reactions within the first hour following damage to the skin, i.e., before morphological or enzyme-histochemical changes become evident. The most prominent findings and processes were summarized by Berg (1972) (Fig. 50). Any attempt at a synopsis of the essential reliable results that are suitable for determining the age of lesions must be largely oriented to the investigations and summaries of Lindner, Raekallio, and Berg (Table 3).

Table 3. Time-course of healing of injuries

Time after injury	Histological, histochemical, and biochemical findings and reactions
1 h	Hemorrhage, exudation, tissue swelling, acidosis, isolated polymorphonuclear leukocytes, ATPase, unspecific esterases, aminopeptidase, increase in histamine, serotonine, and alpha esterases
2 h	Mast cell degranulation, polymorphonuclear leukocyte infiltration, fibrous disintegration, ground substance segregation, extracellular enzymatic activation – glucosidase, monoamine oxidase
2–4 h	Appearance of mononuclear cells, phagocytosis
4–6 h	Increase in hyperemia, fibrin precipitation, formation of a leukocytic wall, increase in mononuclear cells
6–8 h	Cellular and further tissue disintegration, development of inflammatory demarcation, increase in phagocytosis
8–12 h	Further increase in mononuclear cell elements, alkaline phosphatase, cytochromoxidase, phosphorylases, sporadic occurrence of macrophages
12–16 h	General preponderance of mononuclear cells, disintegration and recession of polymorphonuclear leukocytes
16–32 h	Mobilization of macrophagic cell elements, cellular proliferation with increase in fibroblasts, onset of capillary regeneration
32–72 h	Development of granulation tissue complete
3–4 days	Ground substance formation, fiber formation, beginning of wound elasticity, decrease in macrophages, regeneration of mast cells, possibly foreign-body giant cells
4–10 days	Reduction in water content, reduction in histochemical stainability of the ground substance, further fiber formation, gradual regression of the cell contents, onset of scar formation

3. Thromboses and Embolisms

The occurrence of thromboses and embolisms in very dissimilar injuries and diseases would appear to necessitate a summary presentation under general aspects of forensic histopathology. What is more, thromboses and embolisms are, on the whole, to be regarded as vital processes. Certain exceptions occasionally arise in the case of fat and air embolisms in the corpse. Microcirculatory disturbances, microthromboses, and histological findings in consumptive coagulopathy will be dealt with in the chapter on shock (Chap. C IV).

Stratified and Agglutinative Thromboses – Thromboembolism

Thrombogenesis. In the formation of thrombosis, the well-known causative trio of Virchow – vascular change, slowing of the circulation, change in the blood coagulative ability – is generally acknowledged even today. The last factor in particular has undergone comprehensive scientific study in recent years (references in Bang et al. 1971). Blood clotting consists of the two mutually independent processes of coagulation and conglutination (platelet agglutination). Coagulation is a function of the blood enzymes that maintain a dynamic equilibrium between fibrinogenesis and fibrinolysis and thus ensure an intact endothelial seal. If this enzymatic equilibrium is disturbed, the danger of either thrombosis or hemorrhagic diathesis develops. Experimentally, platelet agglutination can be induced by ADP and Ca or Mg. The adenosine of ADP settles on the thrombocytic surface, whereby Ca or Mg establishes the connection between the phosphate groups of ADP. Platelet agglutination can also be effected by thrombin or isolated collagenous fibers. Positive surface charges on damaged vascular endothelia likewise induce the negatively surface-charged thrombocytes to agglutinate (Mason et al. 1977). Simultaneously, thromboplastin formation is set in motion by activation of factor XII on damaged vascular walls. Thromboplastin formation together with platelet factor III regulates the conversion of prothrombin to thrombin. In this way, fibrin is formed from fibrinogen by the splitting of two peptides and acquires strength and retractility from the influence of various factors. Fibrin appears in four forms according to Bergerhof (1954) – reticular, homogeneous, as bundles of fibers, or as single elements. However, no importance can be attached to these forms of fibrin with regard to the age determination of thromboses (Irniger 1963). The "viscous metamorphosis" of thrombocytes is induced by the autocatalytic reactions of thrombin; coagulation-promoting and vasoactive substances, which are released from the thrombocytes, cause an increased agglutinative disposition and adhesive power of the thrombocytes. The blood platelets partly adhere to one another, partly to the vascular endothelium. Apitz (1942) has already shown experimentally that in arterial and venous hemorrhages, vascular occlusion does not occur spasmodically but through the formation of a stratified thrombus. Only in capillary hemorrhages does the obstruction occur through endothelial adhesion.

The electric conductivity of the vascular wall and the blood components is of decisive importance in the onset of blood clotting. The potential difference between the vascular wall layers and the formed and unformed components of blood is the "zeta potential." If the negative intimal charge is changed to positive by a lesion agglutination of the surface-negative thrombocytes, viscous metamorphosis and fibrin precipitation occur. E. Müller (1956), using conductivity measurements, determined that with intimal swelling the zeta potential was reduced, whereas in the region of necroses it was increased. A stratified thrombus should thus tend to form in the region of intimal swelling foci. The intimal edema in the region of the adhesive site of a thrombus observed by many authors, which according to Irninger (1963) takes place after a few hours, is, therefore, probably not the result but the cause of thrombus localization. The level of the zeta potential is affected by the pH of the blood and by the heparin pool.

The reactions of the blood following contact with exogenous surfaces, e.g., in vascular protheses and in extracorporal circulation are an area of special interest. Of causal significance to the plasma and platelet phase of blood clotting are here the molecular interactions that occur between the exogenous material and blood plasma (Scarborough 1971). Investigations based on these findings strive toward the development of compounds whose surface thrombosis resistance is comparable with that of the normal vascular endothelium.

Increased thrombophilia can occur by an increase in the coagulation substances, e.g., factor X, prothrombin, fibrinogen in pregnancy and after operations, and by reduced inhibition of the activation of coagulation factors, e.g., in reduced antithrombin formation in isolated cases of hepatic cirrhosis. In experiments with rats, coronary thromboses and parietal stratified thromboses in the left ventricle could also be generated by a thrombogenic diet (Howard and Gresham 1964). The coronary changes in the rat induced in such a manner are, however, difficult or impossible to compare with the circumstances in humans. Nonetheless, the basic possibility of being able to interfere with the system of blood coagulation through dietetic measures is remarkable. A diminished clearance in the clotting factors by blockade of the reticuloendothelial system is of importance in the Schwartzmann-Sanarelli reaction. A further causal complex concerns the occurrence of thromboses, particularly in the arterial system, after the taking of oral contraceptives (Warniez and Loffredo 1977). According to the results of a large-scale statistically evaluated series of tests, a connection between ovulation inhibitors and thromboses would seem to be demonstrable from a scientific point of view. Forensically, such a connection could be scarcely established with the required level of certainty in a given case (cf. Asbeck et al. 1972; Dalal and Pitney 1972). Virchow's trio mentioned at the beginning has, therefore, in two points – blood composition and vascular wall damage – undergone basic modification and integration without losing its validity. The third component, slowing of the bloodstream, also fits into the mechanism presented above: Segregation of the axis cylinder occurs in the bloodstream, the corpuscular elements of blood come to marginate at the vascular wall, and agglutination is stimulated by turbulence in the area near the intima. More general factors such as age, obesity, time of year, weather, geographical differences, and sex cannot be entered into here. For postmortem blood coagulation see Dettori et al. (1962), Harms (1971), and Schneider (1974).

The Pikro-Mallory method is suitable for the histological visualization of preserved blood platelets within thrombi. A thrombocytic antigen can also be detected by immunofluorescence microscopy. For this, Carstairs (1965) used the indirect method with absorption of the antihuman thrombocyte globulin, obtained from rats, with human renal cortex homogenate and a mixture of pulverized human kidney and guinea pig liver, kidney, and spleen. The influence of platelet concentration, glucose, and calcium chloride on the morphological changes in platelets and fibrin during coagulation and retraction could be demonstrated by special embedding and staining with eosin-phloxine by Gainter et al. (1962). After the experimental generation of multiple thromboses in mice, Hoak (1964) using light and electron microscopy detected large platelet aggregates which were surrounded by erythrocytes and leukocytes (cf. Schulz 1968; Laiho 1975). In the center of the aggregates, the platelets were particularly compact. Unlike the platelets in the center, those on the margins of the aggregates did not contain any mitochondria or granules.

Electronmicroscopic studies on hemostasis in severed vessels of rats and guinea pigs showed the first thrombocyte aggregates, which were surrounded by red blood corpuscles, after 30 s (Johnson et al. 1965). One minute after the onset of hemorrhage, the platelets were in disordered clusters in rosette form. The "thromboplastic cell component" is thought to be involved in the formation of the rosettes. It is further supposed that by degradation of ATP to ADP in the red corpuscles, the ADP released starts the agglomeration of thrombocytes. After 30 s, disolving of the marginal platelets can also be seen to commence. Fibrinous fibers are then present, which penetrate the platelet aggregates and interweave around the erythrocytes. These fibrinous fibers are not plasma fibrin, but develop from the platelets which are located in the center of the aggregates and contain granules. After 7 min, the electron-dense fields, which are completely composed of fibrin, have substantially expanded and sustain the hemostasis.

Tissue lesions of various kinds are of influence in thrombogenesis. Bergström et al. (1959) were able to show experimentally in rabbits that thrombogenesis directly post-trauma is due, on the one hand, to a reduction in the blood volume, on the other, to a release of thromboplastin from the damaged tissue region. The development of thrombin some time after traumatism, however, is thought to be the result of reduced suspensory stability of the blood.

The morphology of fibrinogenesis, its methodical visualization, the protein structure of the fibrinous fibers and fibrils, and the bundle-like closing together of fibrinous filaments were extensively described by Fonio (1964). From a study of the development of fibrinous fibrils, it is seen that in the clotting process first of all the compact amorphous fibrinous mass is precipitated, and subsequently the fibrinous fibrils are formed by the protein structure. By a bundle-like closing together, the fibrinous filaments then emerge and extend through the fibrinous mass. The transverse striation of the fibrinous fibrils is functionally connected with the contractile process and resembles the contraction of myofibrils. The compact amorphous fibrinous mass acts passively in this.

The differentiation of agglutinative and stratified thrombi is important in forensic histology. In practice, pure forms are seldom found, predominantly , stratified thrombi or combination forms, so-called mixed thrombi, are seen (cf. Beneke 1976).

Agglutinative Thromboses. These are induced by hypercoagulability or slowing of the circulation and within a short period of time may suddenly fill large areas of the venous system, especially in the lower half of the body. A change in zeta potential within the cellular and plasmatic blood factors underlies this form of thrombosis. By reduction of the plasmatic potential, coagulation-promoting plasma factors give rise to fibrin precipitation, which can take place within a very short time. Macroscopically, an agglutinative thrombus has a uniform dark red character as a result of the inclusion of numerous erythrocytes. A distinctive structure and stratification as in the stratified thrombus do not as a rule exist. Histologically, the erythrocytes in the fresh stage are not connected with the vascular endothelium but are only loosely associated with it. They have a uniform character in the peripheral and central sections. Stratification is also undetectable microscopically (Fig. 51). The histological evidence of agglutinative thromboses, as autochthonous or embolic thrombosis, is an indication that this thrombosis was caused by generally effective factors. Local genesis, caused directly after trauma or inflammation, is thus out of the question. Unless traumatically dependent, general immobilization, especially in older previously injured people, or more large-scale tissue damage with the release of thromboplastin caused the thrombosis via hypercoagulability.

The fresher and moister an agglutinative thrombus, the more difficult it is to differentiate from a postmortem coagulum (cruor). The certainty sometimes shown here by many investigators cannot be histologically justified (Table 4). The exami-

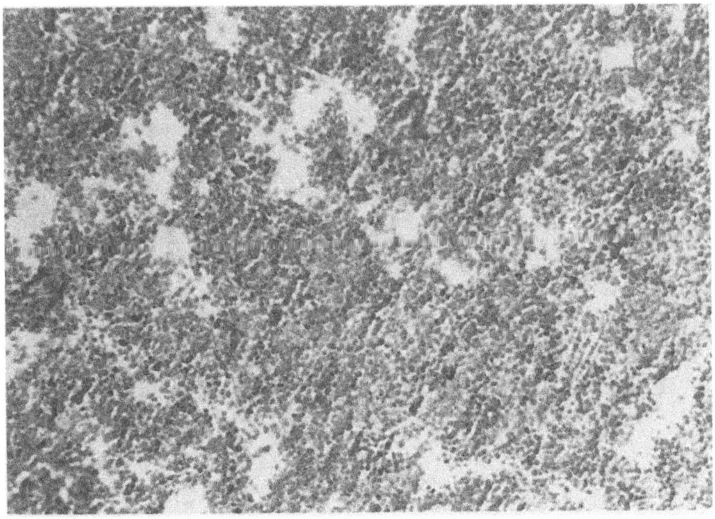

Fig. 51. Fresh agglutinative thrombus with loosely associated erythrocytes. No certain differentiation from postmortem cruor can be made. H and E, 1:150

Table 4. Differential diagnosis between intravital and postmortem thrombi

Intravital thrombus		Postmortem thrombus	
White	Red	Cruor	Buffy coat
Macroscopic			
Dry	Dry-moist	Contain more fluid	
Partially fragile	± elastic	Somewhat elastic	
Fluted surface	Smooth surface	Smooth and reflective surface	
Partially adhesive	Not immediately adhesive	Nonadhesive	
Gray – gray/white – gray/red	Blue-red	Blue-red	Gray-gray/yellow – yellowish
Border between white and red parts unrelated to position of corpse		Border between gray and red parts horizontal with unchanged position of the corpse	
Microscopic			
Compact aggregation of platelets, layered or festoonlike	Predominantly erythrocytes Little fibrin Few platelets (difficult sometimes impossible differential		Loose fibrin fiber network Leukocytes changeable Occasionally platelets
Fibrin ± erythrocytes	diagnosis!)		

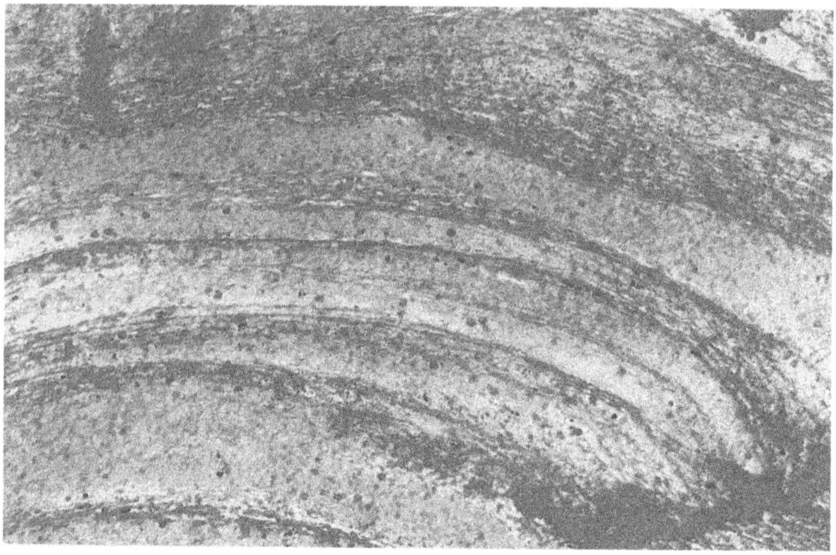

Fig. 52. Stratified thrombus with typical alternating layers of fibrin and blood corpuscular components. Weigert's fibrin stain, 1:80

nation of the microscopic structure and physical and chemical characteristics of buffy coat, white and gray thrombi, cruores, and red thrombi by Jakoby (1930) led to the conclusion that a detectable fundamental difference between fresh and postmortem thrombi does not exist in every case: "The criteria valid for particular clear cases overlap a great many borderline cases." The physicochemical process is basically similar in intravital and postmortem thrombi. In this respect, the opinion of Ribbert (1915), according to whom postmortem thrombi correspond to "agonal thrombi," finds support from Jakoby (1930). Tendeloo (1933) infers that buffy coat thrombi have a vital genesis from the fact that he never came across such a finding in his autopsies in cases of sudden death. A basic point here is the knowledge that in the majority of cases after death a more or less solid coagulation of the corpse blood occurs in the large vessels; the fibrinogen, however, can also disappear without any evident clotting process. In this connection, according to Harms (1971), the blood shows a strong fibrinolytic activity in half of all cases. The postmortem fibrinogen depletion is apparently based on consumption through clotting processes. If blood is made incoagulable by the addition of anticoagulants, the fibrinogen level remains unchanged postmortem (Im Obersteg 1956; Satoh 1955; Satoh et al. 1953). Coagulation and spontaneous decoagulation of postmortem thrombi can be obtained by streptokinase activation (Harms 1972). In a case of rapid death, the fibrinogen is probably transformed into fluid intermediary products, which do not appear as extra gradients in electrophoresis. As profibrin (Apitz 1939) or prefibrin (Satoh 1955), they are broken down so quickly under the effect of plasmin that formation of a fibrinous fiber network can no longer occur. Firm clots can, however, also be wholly or partially dissolved again. Following consumptive coagulopathy, the reduction of microthrombi caused by postmortem fibrinolytic activation can similarly be observed (Harms 1971).

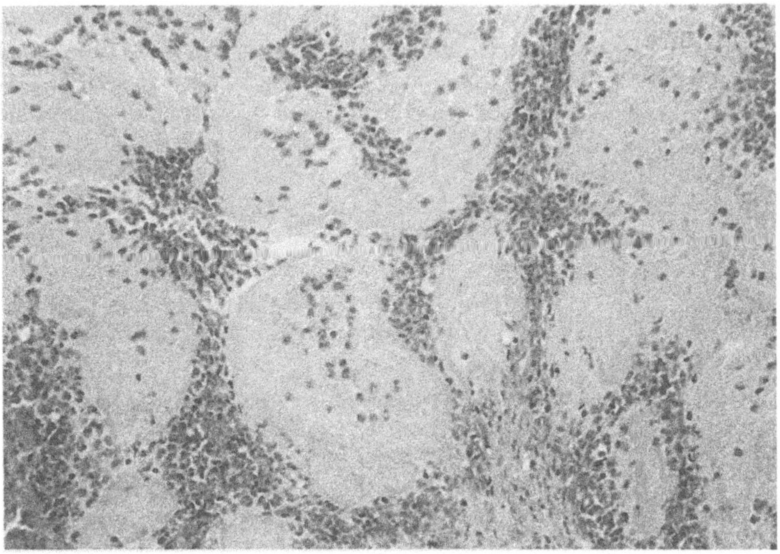

Fig. 53. Mixed thrombus with festoonlike stratification of fibrin and blood corpuscular components. H and E, 1:150

Stratified Thrombosis. Histologically, this macroscopically "white" or "gray" thrombosis is particularly characterized in its incipience by more or less firm contact with the vascular intima and by stratification. The layers are formed by depositions of varying thickness of the corpuscular components of blood, especially leukocytes and fibrins (Fig. 52). The fibrinous portions are soon homogenized and are often lightly undulating. On the surface, particularly in the tail part of the thrombus, regions can develop that resemble an agglutinative thrombus.

Mixed Thromboses. This form of thrombosis is the one most commonly found in forensic medical practice. It is composed either longitudinally or transversely of successive gray and red thrombi. In section, onionskinlike or festoon-like laminations are also found (Fig. 53). The surface is transversely fluted to the direction of flow. The oldest, head part, which is directed against the circulation flow and adheres to the wall, usually corresponds to a mixed thrombus. In the direction of flow, the tail part attaches itself as a red agglutinative thrombus. Retrograde thromboses, i.e., those developing against the direction of circulation flow, are also common. This leads, e.g., in the arterial supply system, to complications if the thrombus grows beyond the vascular ramifications and in so doing occludes a proximal supply area. In isolated forms of thrombus growth, the section between two vein branches is not crossed. The intermediary form crosses various venous segments, and the so-called continuous form is distinguished by multicentric growth.

For the histological examination of thromboses, removal of the whole vessel, if possible without cutting it open, is recommended, followed by fixation in Orth's solution in order to facilitate the preparation of the histological sections of blood components. Parts of the tissue, as large as possible, should be taken from the vicinity of the blood vessel concerned and also be included in the examination. In this way, data can be obtained concerning external damage to the vessel. In serial sections, a check should be made as to whether a lesion of the vascular wall caused by thrombosis had developed from the intima or media or had attacked the vessel from outside. In this manner, the cause and mode of action of lesions can often be easily detected histologically.

In traumatic damage to arteries and veins, longitudinal extension with lacerations of the intima or development of deep vascular wall necroses can also occur. Such partial lesions of the vascular wall, which are easily detectable histologically, can lead to the development of a spurious aneurysm given the appropriate survival time. In the aneurysm, formation of marginal stratified so-called parietal thromboses then directly follows.

It should of course be observed during the histological examination whether previous nontraumatogenic vascular diseases are present. Arteriosclerosis is of major importance here; its course is generally seen intermittently and proceeds with numerous regressive metamorphic variations. The assessment of post-traumatic thromboses can be extremely difficult in such arteriosclerotic areas. Along with the usual criteria in the evaluation, such as the local and chronological links with trauma – which should if possible be histomorphologically detectable – the greatest emphasis should be laid on registering the quality and extent of previous vascular disease. It has to be borne in mind that spontaneous thromboses may be brought about by causes that cannot always be clarified and that not every trauma occurring prior to thrombosis, or at least thought to have occurred prior to thrombosis, can be identified as the cause (B. Mueller 1953). One important area in the overall assessment that gives rise to many problems of correlation concerns the traumatically derived thromboses in the region of the head and neck (Dotzauer and Adebahr 1964; Foedisch and Kloos 1966; Nejmark 1975; Reisner et al. 1976; H. Reisner and T. Reisner 1976). Thromboses of the large carotid arteries in juveniles, the etiology of which is not on the whole satisfactorily clarified, are markedly rare (Vadasz et al. 1973). By means of interesting case reports and experimental studies, Holzer (1965) pointed out the connections between occlusion of the vertebral artery at the atlanto-occipital joint and subsequent thrombosis through lateral rotation of the head. Kaeser (1955) has reported unilateral carotid artery thromboses with hemiplegia and encephalomalacia following strangulation. The vessels concerned were arteriosclerotically altered. Whether thrombotic occlusions are also able to form in healthy vessels following strangulation appears dubious.

The histologically recordable effects and changes in the associated supply area also have to be included in the histological assessment of thromboses. It is generally acknowledged that a coronary thrombosis can develop on an arteriosclerotic patch and thus become the cause of a myocardial infarction. The thrombosis can also, however, develop retrogradely, to a certain extent, out of an area of primary myocardial infarction. Sometimes such questions can only be clarified by histological evidence of primary deposition at the adhesive site of the thrombus (cf. Krauland and Stögbauer 1961). The elucidation of such a question can be significant with respect to a coronary embolism (Oeser 1977) if, for example, an endocarditis recognized as an occupational disease comes into consideration as the focus of the embolism. The inflammatory nature of the embolism can be histologically detected in fresh cases. The differentiation of resorptive organic processes is occasionally difficult in adherent embolisms and thromboses. Inflammatory intimal lesions come into consideration as the cause of a thrombus chiefly in connection with thrombophlebitis in the veins of the lower half of the body. Thromboarteritis (Winiwarter-Buerger) and panarteritis (=periarteritis nodosa) are rare causes mainly of multiple and heterotopic thromboses.

The importance of infection as a cause of thrombosis is nowadays undisputed, however, the pathogenesis is not clear in many cases. Many authors believe that pathogenic organisms or their toxins directly damage the vascular intima, in contrast to the view that abacterial, reactive, and allergic inflammations are involved. With thromboses in the region of the neck and head, the proximity to infective processes doubtlessly plays a decisive role, confirmed in the older literature. Investigations on isolated thromboses of the sinus cavenosus by Uta (1924) revealed that 50% were attributable to an infection of the nasal passages, and 16% to an infection of the aural region. The role of angina as a causative factor was indicated by Juhl (1921) and Reye (1923). Thrombi were found in the vena jugularis with anaerobic streptococci, pneumococci, and staphylococci in postanginal sepsis. Necrotic deposits on the intima and on the thrombi are, according to Juhl (1921), evidence of the affinity of the influenza virus to the vascular walls. Further reports concerning the propagative pathway and sites of precipitation of thromboses in the vicinity of the jugular vein following septic infections in the pharyngeal region and in the area of the smaller cerebral vessels have come from Greifenstein (1931) and Lauterberg (1923).

Clot formation could not be produced in animal experiments by stasis of the intravascular blood alone. Not until after sensitization of the vascular walls by pretreatment with colibacilli injections and reinjection of bacteria did a reaction take place in the form of disaggregation of the endothelium, fibrin deposits, veil-like striations, and transition to thrombosis. In humans, it is thought that these primary changes in the wall are, on the whole, not evident in connection with thromboses.

Iatrogenically caused thrombosis is closely associated with infectious pathogenesis, and for reasons of criminal or civil law, this form of thrombotic origin becomes a matter for forensic investigations. Tissue lesions, even following aseptic operations, create dyscratic changes through histolysis that can cause a distant thrombosis similar to infections. Stöhr and Kazda (1928) found postoperative distant thromboses in 1.16% of over 20000 obductions; the thromboses largely affected the venous region of the pelvis and legs. According to Nordmann (1930), 2.2% of patients undergoing operations suffer a thrombosis after a few days; the figure is as high as 2.8% in patients with conservatively treated fractures. A correlation of thrombosis with acute operative blood loss cannot be established according to Tapfer (1933). Similarly, narcoses have no thrombosis-promoting influence (Kunz 1932). According to recent literature, the extent of histolysis and the susceptibility to infection are decisive in the formation of a thrombosis. Laparotomies are thought to be twice as prone to thromboses as all other operations. According to Axhausen (1930), 51.7% of internally caused thromboses can be attributed to disorders of the organs of circulation. Reduced inhibition of coagulation factor activators has been found in liver cirrhoses. A significant correlation between intravenous injections and thromboses was negated following large-scale statistical investigations by Mayer (1932), Axhausen (1930), and Ratschow (1959). In cases in which a connection between injection and thrombosis formation may be supposed, either through coincidence of time or position, particular attention should be given to the kind of drug administered, since it is possible that this can promote coagulation. Lob (1968) points out that in unsuccessful venipuncture the artery can be damaged, leading to the development of an aneurysm in the region of which a striated thrombus forms. Venous thrombi in the pelvic region and lower extremities were evident in 40% of 1350 random autopsies on adults in the year 1974 (Schwarz et al. 1976).

Thromboembolism, Embolic Thrombosis, Embolism. These are the most important complications of thromboses. In routine practice in forensic and pathoanatomical autopsies, they are significant, in the form of pulmonary embolism, as causes or concomitant causes of death. However, often in cases where the macroscopic evidence appears clear, a histological examination of thromboses and emboli is dispensed with. Occasionally, this omission entails that questions which might later arise concerning place of origin and age of the emboli cannot be answered.

The optimistic attitude that followed the introduction of thrombotic prophylaxis has subsided in favor of a more critical approach (Ziegler 1977). Pulmonary embolism has been reported in diverse communications in the literature as having had a uniform incidence, as having doubled since the pre-war period, or as having considerably increased up until the mid–1950s with subsequent constant levels. The following have been specified as reasons for the increase in pulmonary embolisms – prosperity, nutrition, raising of life expectancy. Close correlation exists between age and frequency of lung embolisms. In childhood, they are rare. Over a period of 20 years, Ziegler (1977) found pulmonary embolisms in 17.4% of approximately 4000 clinical autopsies, more frequently among women. In 11% of cases, it was the sole or main cause of death. Schwarz et al. (1976) found pulmonary embolisms in 23.5% of their postmortem examinations; a fatal fulminant course was evident in 7.8% of all cases. The data concerning hemorrhagic pulmonary infarctions fluctuate between 46% and 65.4% of all pulmonary embolism cases. Recurrent and clinically non-apparent pulmonary embolisms can lead to the development of a chronic cor pulmonale, according to Ziegler (1977) in 5.2% of the total number of all pulmonary embolisms. It is not exceptional for small parietal thrombi of no clinical significance to be detected in the region of vena cava catheters. There is a particular danger of embolisms in the course of intensive therapy. With regard to ovulation inhibitors, Ziegler (1977) was unable to determine an increase in pulmonary embolisms.

In two-thirds of all cases, the deep veins of the leg are the starting point of venous embolisms (Schulte 1932). According to Schmidt (quoted by Lob 1968), 65.7% of pulmonary embolisms originate in the femoral veins, and 14.8% in the deep fibial veins. Brack (1933) and Lob (1968) point out that in hypertonic blood pressure crisis, the danger of thrombolysis is especially high. The embolic complications following kidney damage or kidney operations are thought to be relatively frequent.

The loosening of the thrombus at the adhesive site results from fibrinolysis or retraction (Lob 1968). The results of Sandritter and Bergerhof (1954), however, argue against such an explanation. In their experiments, they were unable to observe a dislodging of the thrombi despite strong enzymatic influence and high flow velocity. They considered the onset of the embolic process to be associated with fibrous or-

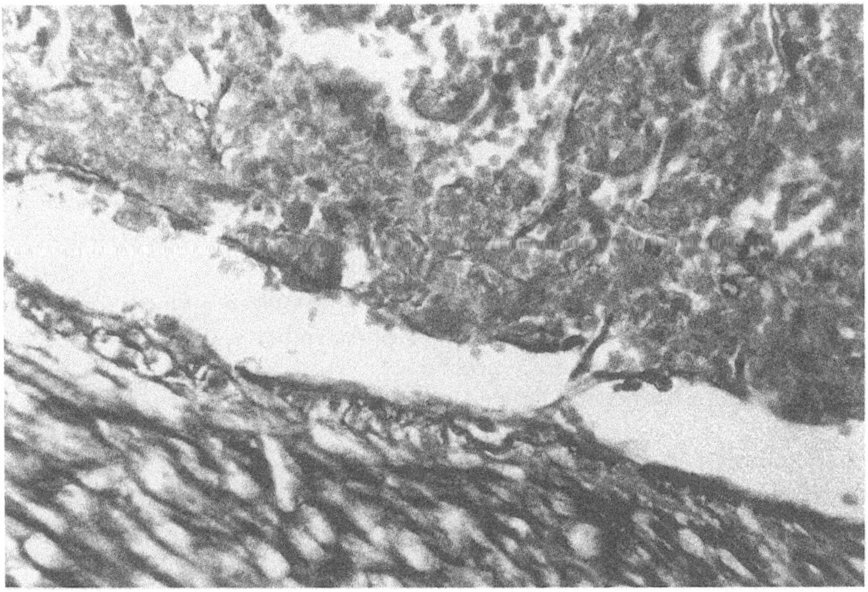

Fig. 54. Splitting between the vascular wall and thrombus with ingrowing fibroblasts. Elastica-van Gieson, 1:220

ganization of the thrombus, especially since, according to the investigations of Barker, 65% of all embolisms arise in the first 5 days following appearance of clinical thrombotic symptoms. According to Irninger (1963), the retraction of the thrombus was so far advanced 3–8 days after the beginning of the thrombus that sinusoids, clefts, and cavities formed. From our own investigations, it emerged that these fissurations predominantly form on the border between the thrombus and vascular wall (Fig. 54). Dissolution of the thrombus in this region appears plausible. This also explains why occasionally following complete thrombolysis, the original thrombus adhesive site can no longer be detected even by histological examination.

Generally, embolic spreading of the thrombi arises in the lower half of the body and proceeds through the lower vena cava, via the right heart, into the pulmonary arteries. From the forensic point of view, an examiner can be faced with the question of whether a blood clot discovered in the pulmonary artery is an embolus or a locally derived earlier thrombosis in which a recognizable vascular wall reaction has not taken place. Even if intimal changes are already present, this does not argue against an embolism. As is generally known, an embolus in a nonfatal pulmonary embolism is organized like a thrombosis in the pulmonary arteries. Winter (1931) reported the partly organic structure of carcinous metastases in the pulmonary arteries, whereby intimal fusion and thromboendoarteritis can occur. Certain diagnosis of an embolism with a superimposed secondary thrombosis is particularly difficult. The possibility of autochthonous thrombogenesis by striation in inflammatory or tumorous conditions of the adjacent lung tissue should be considered. If all differential diagnostic possibilities are taken into account, then an embolism can only be established with a probability verging on certainty by the presence of the following findings:

1) The area of embolic origin is detected and it is possible to indentify a lacuna corresponding to the embolism. However, the simultaneous occurrence of thromboses and blood clots in the pulmonary arteries is sometimes not proof of an embolic process. A general hypercoagulability with multicentric thrombosis could be present.
2) The embolus is typically divided into a head and tail and the white head part is not adjacent to the vascular wall.
3) The embolus or the infarcted lung tissue is colonized by a pathogen which is identical with that in the area of origin of the embolus.
4) A so-called riding embolus is present.
5) The embolus has become tangled up during its migration.

Putnoky (1932) conducted specific investigations concerning the localization of embolisms of the pulmonary arterial system: 18% of all emboli are found in both main branches, 15% in the truncus, 2% exclusively in one main branch, and in 29% the embolisms were found in the peripheral pulmonary arterial branches of the 2nd–4th order.

Arterial thromboses and embolisms cannot as a general principle be distinguished from those of the venous system. The foci are usually inflammatory changes of the cardiac valves and endocardium or inflammatory degenerative and traumatic lesions of the vascular intima. At one time, endocarditis lenta was particularly fatal as a source of embolisms; since the improvement in therapy, this disease appears more rarely and is generally no longer complicated by embolisms.

Occasionally, parietal thrombi can be loosened out of aneurysms by puriform softening and become embolized. Wilhelmi and Hildebrand (1972) observed a rare case: Following a trivial trauma, a large arteriosclerotic aneurysm of the aorta abdominalis broke through into the vena cava inferior and led to a massive pulmonary embolism of thrombotic material from the aneurysm. According to Sandritter and Beneke (1966), thrombotic morbidity of 0.5%–5%, embolic morbidity of 0.1%–2.6% must be expected in clinical patients. Of all venous thromboses, 25%–50% lead to embolism, and 5%–10% of these develop fatally. The frequency of embolisms is given as 8.14% in pathoanatomical autopsy cases; in 2.5%–3% of these, the embolism was the cause of death. Venous thromboses are markedly scarce in infancy (Beau et al. 1963 – references).

The histologically detectable transformations and signs of organic structure and dissolution can have forensic significance as evidence since they provide information regarding the chronological development. In the dissolution of human striated and agglutinative thrombi, puriform softening in the central sections and surface changes by enzymatic effects from the bloodstream have to be taken into account. The various forms in which fibrin occurs must be considered. According to Sandritter and Bergerhof (1954), the following forms can be distinguished: (1) Three-dimensional fibrin network composed of long, fine or coarse threads with strong prominent intersectional sites and pistonlike distensions, staining intensely with azan; (2) fibrin in the form of loose or close parallel fibers with the formation of bands; (3) in the form of homogeneous masses which sometimes appear hyaline.

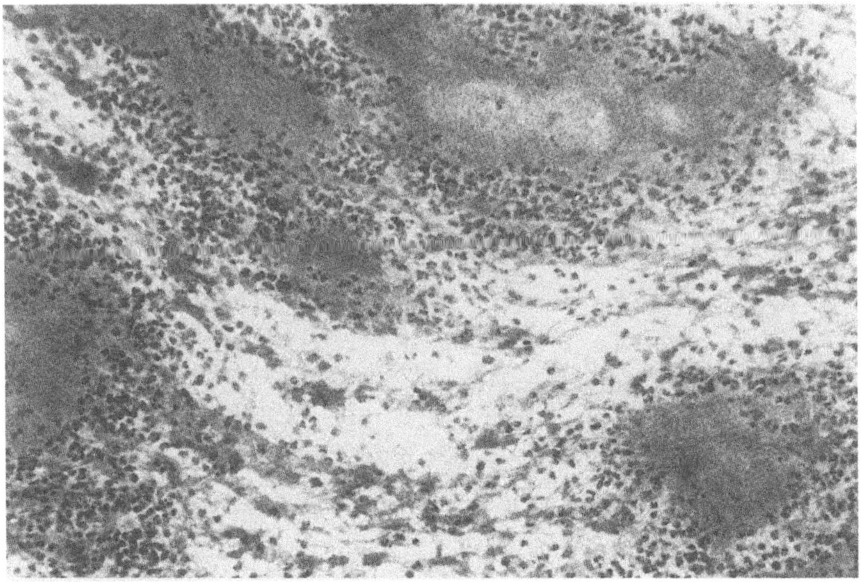

Fig. 55. Stratified thrombus with puriform softening. H and E, 1:180

In the last phase of blood coagulation, contraction of the blood clot appears, in which the serum is pressed out and the clot is consolidated. This process, familiar as a reaction, occurs by contraction of the fibrinous fibers under the influence of an enzyme from the thrombocytes (retractoenzyme) and is already established a few minutes after the onset of coagulation. A measure of the progress of the retraction after 5 min is the increasingly poor lysability of the coagulum with streptokinase, which completely ceases after about 2–3 days. This phenomenon is explained by the squeezing out of the plasminogen, whose transformation to the fibrinolytic enzyme plasmin is activated by streptokinase. After a lapse of over 3 days, even completely retracted thrombi can be lysed by streptokinase. The plasminogen diffuses out of the plasma and into the thrombus again; the fibrinolytic enzymes, which at first are intracellular, are released within the thrombus and older thrombi lose their content of plasmin inhibitors.

In the enzymatic lysis of fibrin, the fibers disintegrate into larger and smaller fragments. Prior fixation with formalin makes all enzymatic proteolysis impossible. With alcohol-fixed fibrin sections, lysis can be achieved by chymotrypsin, trypsin, and plasmin, and less well by pepsin and papain (Beneke and Hey 1965). The outlines of the fibers appear vague. Granules with indistinct outlines occur. With azan stain, a dirty violet shade is produced, which is in distinct contrast to the orange–red-stained unaltered fibrin. The platelet trabeculae initially retain their shape. On the whole, the fibrin is broken down more easily than the platelets. Distended puriform softening occurs in the interior of thrombi through the proteolytic enzymes of leukocytes (Fig. 55). Externally, fibrinolytic enzymes of the blood are active, as a result of which the surface of the thrombus appears macroscopically mucous and filaceous (Fig. 56). The fibrin mantle of the thrombus is broken down from

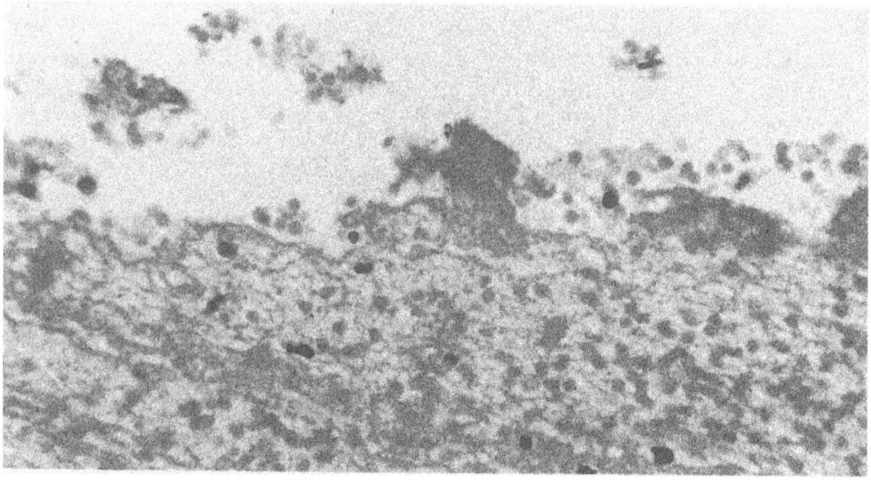

Fig. 56. Enzymatic breaking up of the thrombic surface, which has the appearance of having been "gnawed." H and E, 1:220

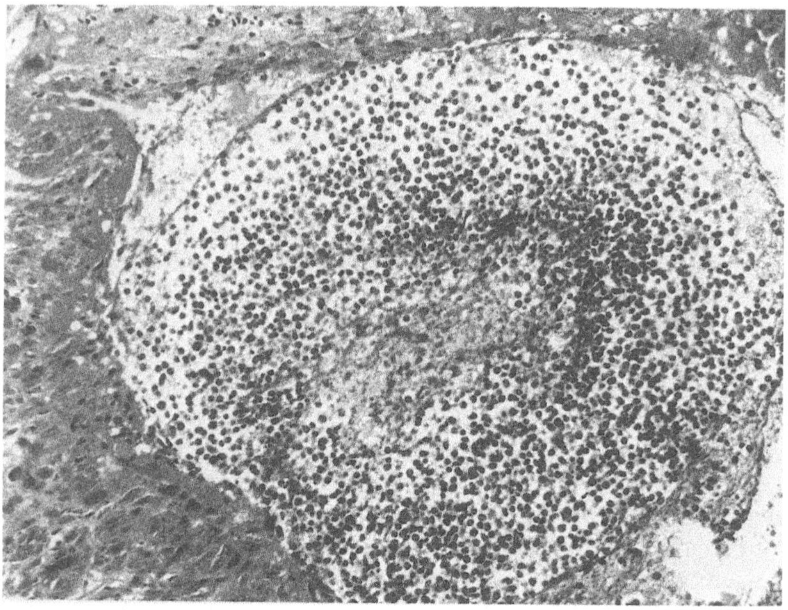

Fig. 57. Inflammatory thrombic liquefaction in a uterine wall vein. H and E, 1:180

the surface and has a gnawed appearance, basically, a similar process as in puriform softening. The agglutinative thrombi are dissolved more quickly, owing to their high fibrin content, than the striated thrombi, in which the lysis-resistant thrombocytes predominate. Along with enzymatic autolytic dissolution, real suppurative liquefaction occurs following infective colonization (Fig. 57).

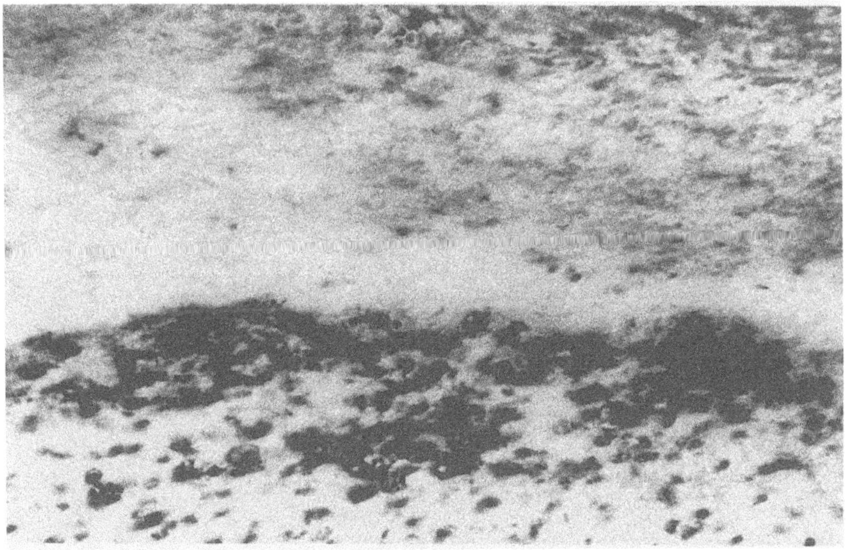

Fig. 58. Thrombus adhesive site with increased activity of unspecific esterase in the fibrocytes of the intima (below). 1:220

The frequently observed transformation of the thrombus by organization is suitable for a forensically utilizable age determination. In this manner, different stages of development can be detected which may be correlated with a particular chronological sequence. At the thrombus adhesive site, increased enzymatic activity initially occurs (Fig. 58). Proliferating granular tissue develops in the dead thrombus masses, starting at the vascular wall, by means of which vascular connective tissue is formed (Fig. 59). The capillaries which rapidly spread within the thrombus masses grow outward into the vascular wall and there connect with the vasa vasorum. Growing toward the vascular interior, the capillaries reach the free surface of the thrombus. This organization process can lead to extensive breakdown and complete recanalization of the thrombus. It can also however, result in deposition of hemosiderin (Fig. 60) in the region of the granular tissue and vascular wall and also result in deposition of calcium salts with the formation of phleboliths (so-called vein stones). A myxomatous transformation can occasionally be observed in large parietal thrombus masses of the cavities of the heart. According to the experimental studies of Jurukova and Knieriem (1970) on carotid thromboses of Wistar rats, the organization of arterial thrombi is brought about by the ingrowing of smooth muscle cells and fibroblastlike muscle cells, which originate in the arterial tunica media. The medial muscle cells situated under the thrombus show increased cellular activity as a result; their mitochondria and free ribosomes are more numerous, the endoplasmic reticulum is enlarged. Moreover, the smooth muscle cells contribute to the phagocytosis of thrombocytes and erythrocytes. The organization of arterial thrombi by smooth muscle cells can be taken as indicative of the general trend of the vascular wall in reacting uniformly with the proliferation of its smooth muscle cells following lesions.

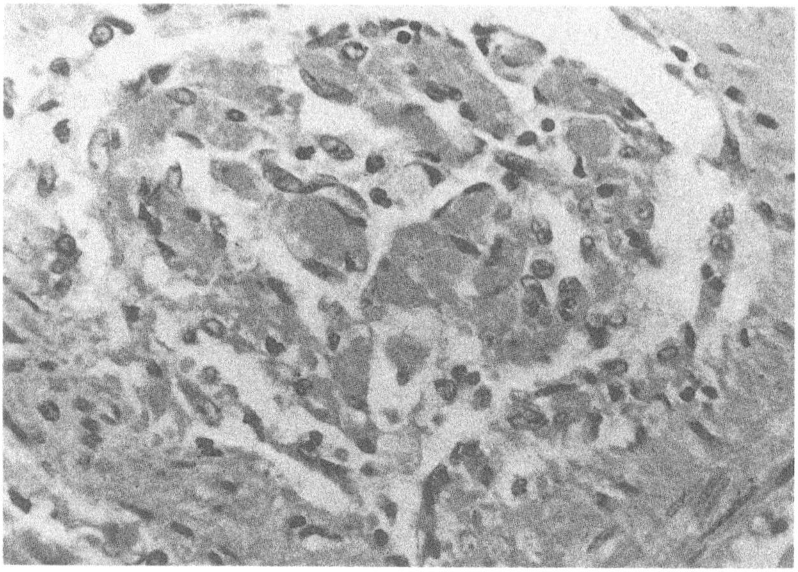

Fig. 59. Thrombus undergoing organization and the spreading of capillaries. H and E, 1:220

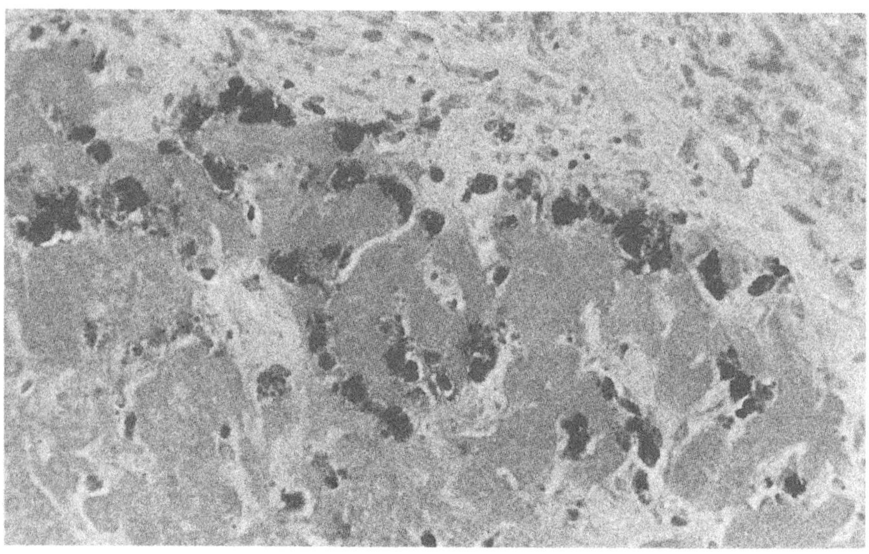

Fig. 60. Organization of thrombus with hemosiderin deposits in the region of the thrombus adhesive site. Berlin blue, 1:280

Specific investigations into the organization of coronary thromboses by Emmrich (1969) have revealed that the speed of the organization process is influenced by the extent of the thrombus, the state of the arterial wall at the adhesive site of the thrombus, and the size of the contact area between the thrombus and the vascular wall. Histological and histochemical investigations of 60 parietal and occlusive coronary thromboses of different sizes and structures by Sinapius (1967) showed intra- and extracellular fat droplets in 63% of the parietal and 46% of the occlusive thromboses. The amount of fat was greatest in 3- to 7-day-old thrombi. The fat droplets almost completely regressed during the organization process. The intracellular fat results from resorption of the extracellular fats with increasing age of the thrombi. The location of the fat droplets, close to the lumen, within the thrombus attests to the infiltrative origin of the fats from the bloodstream and argues against an origin from components of the thrombus or from the vascular wall. Histochemically, cholesterin and phosphatides can be detected as essential fat fractions in coronary thromboses.

Circulatory disorders in the affected areas of the organ are among the regional effects of thromboses. Very diverse clinical symptoms arise as a result of reduction or interruption of the circulation in addition to vascular congestion, edema, hemorrhagic infarcts, gangrene, and the development of collateral circulation. The clinical symptomatology, therapy, and prophylaxis of thromboses and their sequelae have been comprehensively presented in the books by Gross et al. (1977) and Ratschow (1959). The extent of circulatory disorders is dependent on the localization of the thrombus. The proportion of arterial to venous thromboses is 1:3 according to Brack (1928), and 1:5.25 according to Axhausen (1930). The peroneal veins are the most frequently affected by thromboses (Rössle 1937; Neumann 1939; Ratschow 1959). As a result of embolism of the suprarenal arteries, the clinical symptoms of Addison's disease have been observed (Furuta 1924). Similar symptoms have been described following renal vein thromboses (Veit 1922; Schauwecker 1930).

Chronic circulatory disorders in the lower extremties, which develop from a deep thrombosis of the veins of the legs, lead to the post-thrombotic syndrome. It is caused by destruction of the endothelium with irreparable damage to the venous valves. As a result of rigidity of the damaged vessel and incompetence of the valve apparatus, the pump mechanism of the leg musculature fails. Venous pressure increases and a chronic edema develops, which finally leads to interstitial fibrosis. The skin becomes chapped and discolored. Varices appear, which can be distinguished from the idiopathic kind by their diffuse distribution over the whole lower part of the leg. The development of ulcers of the skin (ulcus cruris) is among the further sequelae. Similar symptoms, which are difficult to differentiate, are found in Sudeck-Leriche syndrome. The assessment is obstructed by the fact that, often without intermediary symptoms, the symptoms do not appear until 2–4 years after they were caused.

Thromboses of the portal vein, the splenic vein, or the upper vena cava are relatively rare (Lob 1968).

Histological Age Determination of Thromboses and Embolisms. This is an important task of forensic medicine and requires thorough knowledge of the general and specific pathology of striated and agglutinative thromboses. The histological assessment should, as far as possible, always be performed in conjunction with the surrounding vascular wall of the uncut blood vessel with at least three to six different transverse incisions. With embolisms, the red terminal section should be included in longitudinal section if present. Hematoxylin-Eosin, van Gieson, and iron are recommended for the histological staining. According to Irninger (1963), the following

Table 5. Histological age determination of thromboses and embolisms. (After Irninger 1963)

Phase I 2nd day (1st–3rd day)	No reactions between endothelium and thrombus. White blood cells, fibrinous ribbons with blood platelets unchanged. Erythrocytes mainly densely packed in the center (agglomerated), peripherally looser.
Phase II 5th day (3rd–8th day)	Penetration of fibroblasts and endothelial budding. Free surface of thrombus may already be covered by endothelium. Onset of hyalinization, mainly central. Enclosed white blood cells pyknotic. Monocyte nuclei enlarged and bright. Through shrinking of thrombus, peripheral fissures and "sinuous" cavities can develop in which loosely aggregated erythrocytes are found.
Phase III 10th day (4th–20th day)	First capillaries, fibroblasts, mesenchymal cells, and hemosiderin-accumulating histiocytes, endothelium under thrombus, hyalinized thrombus split into separate large clumps. Scattered nuclear debris of white blood cells. Monocytic swelling still evident
Phase IV 3rd–4th week (8 days to 2 months)	Onset of fibroplasia (argentophilic and collagenous fibers). Numerous capillaries. In hyalinized thrombus shadowlike nuclear debris from white blood cells. After 8th-17th day, no more monocytic swelling.
Phase V 6th month 2nd–th month	Isolated capillaries, argentophilic, collagenous, and isolated elastic fibers in addition to some cellular elements. In the completely hyalinized thrombus occasional groups of fusiform cholesterol crystal cavities. Infrequently, vessels budding in from the adventitia. Central sinuous cavities, occasionally with fresh flowing blood, possibly thrombus remains.
Phase VI older than 6–12 months	Completely recanalized by larger vessels, between which compact, fiber-rich and cell-deficient connective tissue. Absence of thrombus remains.

criteria deserve particular attention in age estimation: changes in the thrombus, such as pyknosis of the nuclei; platelet disintegration; hyalinization, enlargement, and translucence of monocytic nuclei. Further, endothelial proliferation and the appearance of mesenchymal cells, capillaries, collagenous fibers, hemosiderin, and elastic fibers are of importance. The occurrence of these cellular elements and fibers is quantitatively very variable. Their qualitative appearance, on the other hand, is almost always constant. In accordance with the experimental results of Irniger (1963), the most important findings concerning thrombotic changes and thrombotic organization are summed up in Table 5, which are also recommended in the forensic-histological age determination. Even greater variations in time arise if from the point of view of criminal law an expert assessment has to be made of the minimum or maximum age of a thrombosis or embolism. According to Schäfer (1977), only three stages can be distinguished from one another with any degree of certainty – 1–6 days, 5 days to 8 weeks, older than 2 months.

Fat Embolisms

Fat embolism can unreservedly be accepted as a vital reaction if organs of the systemic circulation are affected. However, the finding of a pulmonary fat embolism calls for discriminating and quantitative evaluation with a simultaneous consideration of the other organ findings. Neutral fats histologically evident in the pulmonary vessels should be assessed with particular care if the organism was subjected to burning or scalding either when still alive or after death. The histochemical and paper chromatographic studies of Wagner (1959) were concerned with this difficult problem. With the postmortem action of heat, the intravascular lipoferous compounds in pulmonary tissue were closely restricted to those places where the effects of heat or flames were locally at their most intense. The histological picture then gave the appearance of lipemia. It was very seldom that histological changes with intravascular spherical neutral fats resembled a fat embolism as a general finding. Genuine capillary fat embolisms could not be detected in these experimental postmortem burns. The partly increased predominance of neutral fats is explained by a heat-dependent local fat phanerosis. The experiments and studies by David and Reimann (1960), Schollmeyer (1962, 1965), and Eidlin (1965) gave similar results. According to them, a genuine fat embolism, with histologically detectable, intravascular neutral fatty deposits that are sausage-shaped and coherant, can always be regarded as an intravital finding. In corpses, a subpleural fat compression into the interstices of the lungs and pulmonary vessels and an intravascular finely dispersed de-emulsification of the blood fat occur through the postmortem effects of heat.

Following attempts at resuscitation with fractures of the ribs and strong compression of the soft tissues, a fat embolism of the lungs is no reliable proof of a vital reaction (Wegener and Sack 1967; Szabo 1971; Schneider and Klug 1971). Under these circumstances, a fat embolism of the lungs cannot be so readily accepted as the cause of death. It has, however, also been debated whether death could have been caused by such an artificial, intravital fat embolism. Finally, liquefied fat can be driven into the pulmonary vessels by gas pressure in advanced putrefaction. In such cases, the histological detection of fat proves poor. A differentiation between intravital and postmortem fat embolisms does not, therefore, generally incur any great difficulties (Meixner 1940; B. Mueller 1953, 1975). According to the studies of Henn and Spann (1968) and Schollmeyer (1971), embolized neutral fat can still be determined quite well in the pulmonary vessels for months after death.

The diagnosis of a fat embolism of the lungs and organs of the systemic circulation cannot be substantiated without appropriate histological evidence. Similarly, following blunt traumatic violence, a fat embolism cannot be excluded without histological study. The comprehensive literature will here only be considered with regard to histological findings. On the origin, frequency, and significance of fat embolisms, I refer to the monographs of Sevitt (1962) and Szabo (1971) and to the clinical and statistical studies by Säker (1955), Shapiro (1962), Knoch and Lenser (1963), Greendyke (1964), Palmovic and McCarroll (1965), Böttger and Strik (1970), Motin et al. (1970), Ander and Jung (1976), Huth (1971), and Brinkmann et al. (1976).

Etiology of Fat Embolisms. Even today, the classic view is predominantly taken that the coarse droplets of neutral fats, which appear in the circulation in a fat embolism, derive from traumatized sections of the lipoferous bone marrow or other fatty depots. At the same time, in recent decades the idea has been developed that the coarse droplets of intravascular fats detectable in fat embolism form by separation of the plasmalipids. Accordingly, through the primary traumatically destroyed and infiltrated fatty tissue, following overburdening of the enzymatic defence mechanism, secondary additional fat is released from the fat depots. In addition, a traumatically induced release of lipase increases the amount of fat reaching the circulation by mechanical means and affects the finely dispersed distribution of the plasma lipids in the form of a coarse-droplet de-emulsification. This "enzyme theory of fat embolism" has often been critically examined (references in Bschor 1962; Moylan et al. 1976; Hausberger 1976). The changes in the blood in alimentary fat excess and other symptomatic hyperlipemias should also be considered. Bschor (1962,1963 a–d; 1964) deserves recognition for the detection and demonstration of physiological and pathological forms of fat in the blood, particularly of the chylomicrons and their aggregates. It should be observed that in alcoholic hyperlipemia, intravascular coarse droplets of fat can appear which are of a similar kind to those found in traumatically conditioned fat embolisms. Hyperlipemia (hyperchylomicronemia) probably also occurs through lipometabolic disturbances in the case of chronic abuse of alcohol.

Other studies on the etiology combined with histological findings have been concerned with the occurrence of fat embolisms following: Phosphorus poisoning (Puppe 1896); injections of soapy water in abortion (Weinig and Schwerd 1951); decompression sickness (Fischer 1963); fatty infiltration of the liver (Bschor 1963 a; Stelzig and Kössling 1969); frostbite in both lower extremities (Hardmeier 1963); kidney homotransplants with corticosteroid treatment (Jones et al. 1965); and mycetismus (Schulz and Hildebrand 1977).

Animal experimental, clinical, and pathoanatomical studies have also been occupied with the nature of fat embolisms: On their genesis and pathogenesis (Bergentz 1961; Adkins and Forster 1962; Burkhardt 1970); on morphological findings following parenteral administration of fine-droplet fat emulsions (Schubert and Krüger 1962; Lewis and Pappas 1969); traumatic bone marrow and fat embolism (Büchner 1964); breakdown processes following experimentally induced fat embolism (Solovay et al. 1970); physiological and anatomical studies in animal experimental fat embolism (Jacques and Saini 1962; Herberg et al. 1965; Hegglin 1965; Whitenack and Hausberger 1971); and histological studies combined with electrocardiographic and X-ray examinations (Kaulbach and Benninger 1962; Kraus et al. 1961).

The histomorphological demonstration of a pulmonary fat embolism is relatively simple and does not cause any difficulties (Fig. 61). Frozen sections are used after fixation in 10% formalin or cryostat sections. Sudan III or Ceres B, scarlet red, or Sudan black B come into consideration as stains. Part of the fat can be lost from the section through the staining process due to the effects of alcoholic solutions. Sudan black B can be recommended because it stains even the finest fat particles strong black. Staining the fat with Nile blue sulfate is also advantageous since it can be used in aqueous solution. In this respect, the method of Lorain Smith (Prinz 1958; Romeis 1968) should be observed: in the tissue, the esterized liquid and soft fats are stained pink and the liquid fatty acids are stained blue with this method. This procedure requires the use of fresh or briefly fixed tissue, since with fatty tissues kept in old formalin for a long time a color change of pink to violet and ultimately to blue can be observed. This is caused by formic acid which develops in old formalin. Such a color change also arises, however, when using formalin-free fixative fluids, after 2–3-h lipase digestion, and in fresh tissue. Nile blue sulfate is not only an effi-

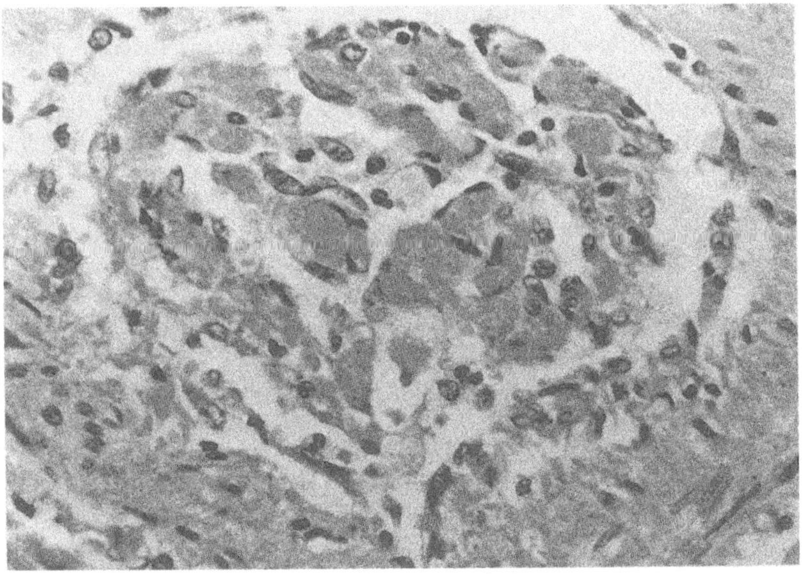

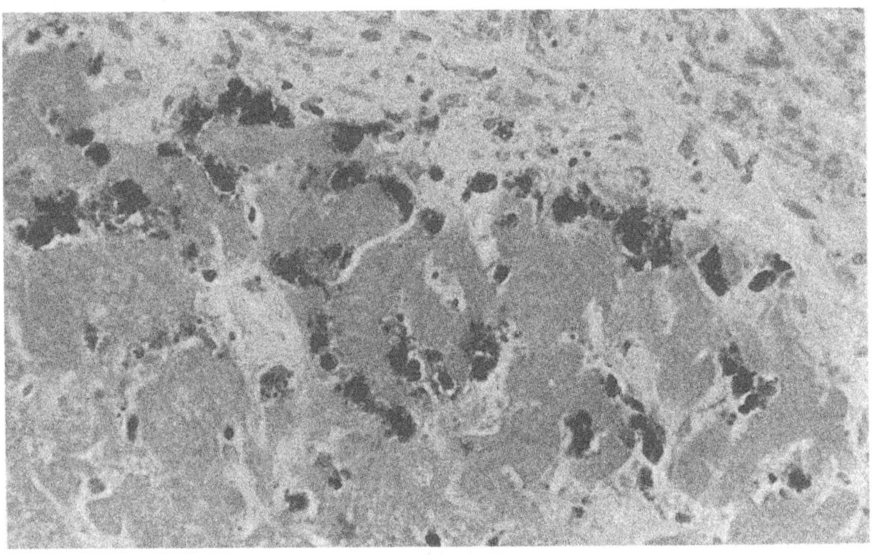

Fig. 61. a Massive pulmonary fat embolism after polytraumatism. Subject survived 5 h, 63 years old, ♀. Sudan red, 1:220. **b** Pulmonary fat embolism of a larger arteriole showing signs of disintegration. Subject survived 5 days: 45 years old, ♂, automobile accident. Sudan black, 1:220

cient diachrome but also a fat fluorochrome. The pink-stained fat droplets show a strong, luminous, gold-yellow fluorescence in UV light, which is stronger with a stain that has been boiled than with one used cold. Bschor (1962, 1964) and Perjès and Kadàs (1968) are referred to for further properties of this stain and its possibilities in the detection of fat embolism. In fixed material, coarse-droplet fat is still evident many months after the autopsy. The Sudan-positive plasma, on the other hand, loses stainability after a few days. The detection of fat embolisms by Popwassilew et al. (1971) using luminescent polycyclic hydrocarbons is recommended with the following method: staining of the tissue sections of fixed pieces of lung with saturated Perylen solution in ethanol, embedding in glycerine, and examination under the luminescence microscope, in which the fat deposition presents a bluish luminescence.

An important methodical contribution to the diagnosis of fat embolism was produced by the studies of Holczabek (1964 a, b, c, 1968 a, b) and Holczabek and Machata (1971) with the introduction of thin-layer chromatographic studies on tissue slurries and sections. To obtain objective data on the percentage distribution of the various lipid fractions (cholesterin, fatty acid, triglyceride, cholesterin ester), the chromatograms are determined by densitometry in reflected light. In the case of sudden natural death without traumatic effects, the triglyceride values came to 12.6%–13.7%, whereas in the case of violent death with pulmonary embolism they were 41.1%–72.1%. Nadvornik and Pavelcova (1968) arrived at similar results. Gas chromatographic comparative tests of the various lipid fractions by Holczabek and Machata (1971) have indicated that the depot triglycerides detectable in the lungs infiltrate from the site of traumatization. Within the lungs, the upper and middle lobes tend to be affected by fat embolic vascular obstructions (Brunner and Schellmann 1979). The organic manifestations of a fat embolism and its functional implications have led to the distinction between a primary (pulmonary fat embolism) and a secondary fat embolism (general fat embolism).

Primary Fat Embolism (Pulmonary Fat Embolism) As Cause of Death. It is not rare for considerable difficulties to arise in deciding whether a histologically detected pulmonary fat embolism could have played a role in causing the death of a person. Special demands are made on the evidence if the primary fat embolism comes into consideration as the sole cause of death. If large parts of the arterioles and capillaries of the pulmonary tissue are filled with neutral fat over long vascular sections, and if this finding is evident in at least four different areas, then the pulmonary fat embolism can be recognized as the cause of death according to B. Mueller (1953). Here, examination using about $\times 100$ magnification is recommended; at least four to six connected neutral fat infiltrations should be visible per microscopic field. However, if only solitary particles are found in every microscopic field and if whole sections are free of fat, the pulmonary fat embolism cannot be accepted as the cause of death (Meixner 1940). In the comparative registration and evaluation of histological pulmonary fat embolism findings, the classification by Falzi et al. (1964) is recommended (Table 6).

An analysis of our material by Brinkmann et al. (1976 – references) was particularly concerned with the significance of pulmonary fat embolism as a cause of death. Their histological examinations and quantitative analysis of fat revealed that evidence of histological grade III according to Falzi et al. (1964) and a pulmonary

Table 6. Graduations of fat embolisms. (Modified after Falzi et al. 1964)

Grade of FE	Form of embolism	Localization
I = light FE	Drop-shaped	Sporadic in every microscopic field[a]
II = distinct FE	Sausage-shaped or rounded	Multiple, disseminated in every microscopic field
III = massive FE	Antler-shaped	Numerous everywhere, in every microscopic field
0 = Not FE	(Punctiform)	(sporadic, not in every microscopic field)

[a] FE, fat embolism; here: enlargement × 25

total fat content of about 20 g in humans without conflicting diseases and organic damage is proof of death through fat embolism. In low histological grades of embolism, a pulmonary fat embolism can only be accepted as a contributory cause of death with the required degree of certainty if other organic damage involved in causing death can be detected. The establishment of death from pulmonary fat embolism is, therefore, to an exceptional degree diagnosis by exclusion, which in any given case has to take into account all the findings from a thorough status examination. In the histological diagnosis, evidence has also to be adduced that the fat embolism led to morphologically detectable effects, e.g., microhemorrhages, capillary damage, perivascular edemas, microthrombi, and other features associated with shock.

Studies have been carried out as to whether connections between the post-traumatic survival time and the intensity of the fat embolism can be established. Of 300 people who died as a result of accidents, 20% of the casualties, who died directly after the accident, had no fat embolisms in their lungs; 80% had minimal or high-grade fat embolisms. Of those who survived the accident for 6 h, 96% had a fat embolism; of those who survived 12 h, 100% had a fat embolism (Palmovic and McCarroll 1965). Generally speaking, positive findings of a pulmonary fat embolism increase with survival times of up to 2 days. On the other hand, bone-marrow embolisms, which appear at the same time as fat embolisms, can subside 2–5 h after their traumatic origin (Mason 1968). The influence of states of shock on the formation and extent of pulmonary fat embolisms has also been confirmed in other connections. In posthemorrhagic cases of death in which trauma was excluded, Bauer and Missliwetz (1978) detected low- to middle-grade pulmonary fat embolisms.

The removal of embolized fat is effected in different ways in cases of survival. Electron-microscopic studies of the blood-respiratory system by Rubia and Schulz (1963) revealed that 1 h after the onset of experimental fat embolism, fat droplets were present in the cytoplasm of the vascular endothelia. The fat droplets had reached the endothelia by mechanically induced membranous defects. Part of the fat was emulsified in the lumen of the capillary and phagocytized by thrombocytes. At the same time, lipids infiltrated the intercellular spaces and reached the alveolar septa. From here, the fat was absorbed by the alveolar macrophages and stored in the cystosomes of these cells. Following transformation into lipoids, they gave rise to reticular structures, myelin figures, and crystalloid precipitation. In the capillaries obstructed with fat, the endothelia showed considerable tumefaction and a distinct increase in the vesiculation processes. The capillary lumen can become constricted in this way in a fissure-like manner. The blood-respiratory system was enlarged ten- or twentyfold mainly by this strong endothelial swelling. David et al. (1967) arrived at similar results. They found, moreover, ruptures of the alveolar septa, probably as a result of increase in pressure, along with escape of fat droplets and erythrocytes into the alveolar lumina, where small leukocytic foci, though no pneumonia, developed. Experiments with iodine-containing contrast media on rats by Kaufmann (1970) led to numerous lung parenchymal hemorrhages with vigorous macrophage activity.

Further propagation toward a secondary fat embolism occurs via the pulmonary capillaries or through an open foramen ovale. The terminal vascular systems in the brain, kidneys, and cardiac muscles are then affected. Holczabek (1968b) has drawn attention to the significance of arteriovenous anastomoses in the lungs. He was able to demonstrate that very shortly after traumatic effects, sudanophilic substances and bone marrow components appear in these shunts. The function of obstructed arteries in hemorrhages and minor hemorrhagic infarctions of human lungs in the case of fat embolism was also studied by Adebahr (1979). He was able to show that by means of these obstructed arteries, fat droplets that had previously passed into the systemic circulation or bonemarrow components are also transported as a fat embolism into the pulmonary region cut off from the functional circulation. A primary fat embolism of the liver is also possible with injuries in the inflowing area of the portal vein.

On the whole, there is no doubt as to the damaging effects of fat embolisms in the brain and cardiac muscle. Systematic investigations by Henn and Spann (1965) on the histological cerebral findings from 140 cases of traumatic death showed that with increasing survival time, the number of cases with cerebral fat embolism similarly increased. Distinct fat infiltrations into the cerebral capillaries were not observed until after an interval of several days, with the exception of one case in which death occurred 30 min after the trauma. With increasing severity of the injuries, the cases of cerebral fat embolism also increased. Altogether, the investigation results revealed that pulmonary fat embolism essentially occurs earlier and more frequently than cerebral fat embolism. Even after a survival time of 30 min, no case was found without pulmonary fat embolism. Factors related to the post-traumatic reaction of the circulation are thought to explain the very diverse occurrence of cerebral fat embolisms.

In cerebral fat embolisms, the histological changes are found preferentially in the cerebral cortex. These predominantly involve spherical or annular hemorrhages with an arteriole or capillary in the center, which may contain infiltrated neutral fat. In older annular hemorrhages, the central regions become necrotic (Fig. 62). There are also cases of multiple necroses without hemorrhages, and similarly of fat-plugged vessels without changes in the surroundings. Positive findings are provided by examining the plexus chorioideus and cerebral tissue in teased-out and unmodified preparations. Occasionally, circumscribed necroses (elective parenchymal necroses), together with reaction and lipopexia of the neighboring microglia, are found in the vicinity of cerebral fat embolisms survived for longer periods of time (Fig. 63). Cases of brain purpura following trauma cause problems when a fat embolism cannot be histologically detected. Spann and Henn (1970) therefore caution

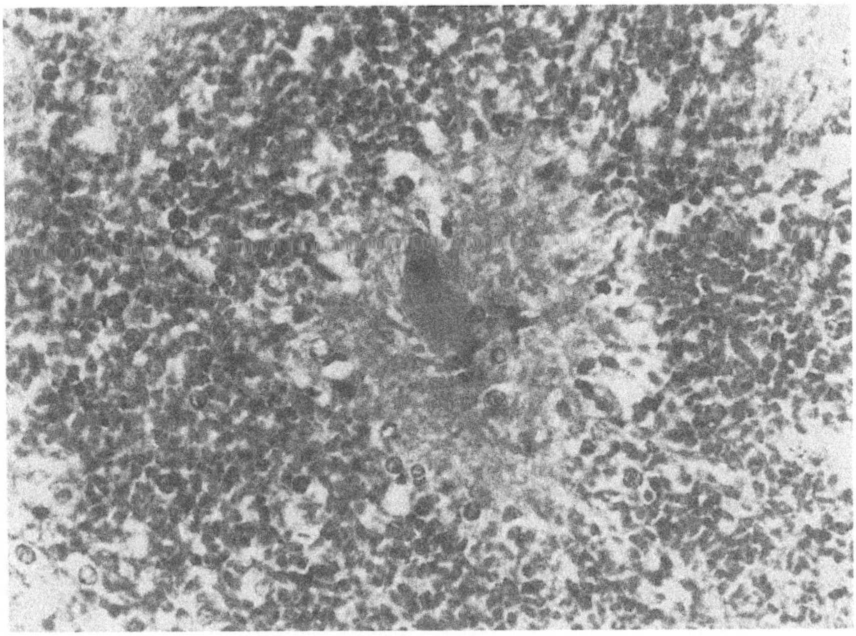

Fig. 62. Fat embolism of the brain with surrounding necrosis and annular hemorrhage. Subject survived 5 days: 45 years old, ♂, automobile accident. Sudan black, 1:220

against a macroscopic diagnosis of "cerebral fat embolism" when there is no histological evidence of medium-grade fat embolism of the brain, but the sequelae of a circulatory disorder in the parenchyma of the brain and clinically the symptoms of a cerebral fat embolism are present. Brain purpura following trauma without infiltration of fat into the capillaries can be attributed to consumption coagulopathy through inflow of tissue thromboplastin into the bloodstream. Vascular occlusion gives rise to the surrounding necrosis, and the simultaneous hypocoagulability of the blood produces the externally adjacent annular hemorrhage. This mechanism for the development of a brain purpura following trauma also makes it clear why clinical symptoms indicating a cerebral fat embolism do not appear until after a few days. The connections between fat embolism, microthrombosis, and consumption coagulopathy or clumping of the erythrocytes in the capillaries (sludging) have already been pointed out (Sessner et al. 1962; Bschor 1963c; Serck-Hanssen 1965). The trichrome staining method according to Goldner is recommended for the demonstration of fibrin precipitation in the microthrombi in the case of fat embolism, particularly since Weigert's fibrin stain often fails in such cases. Further details concerning the mainly unspecific histological changes in the brain and particulars on the pathogenesis of cerebral fat embolism are found in Schmidt (1929), Weimann (1929), and Gee (1967). Schewe (1968) has also drawn attention to the differential diagnosis of purpura cerebri, with its various patterns of distribution.

Marcinkowski (1964) described the peculiar finding of isolated fat embolisms in the capillaries of the brain following complete severing of the head in a railway ac-

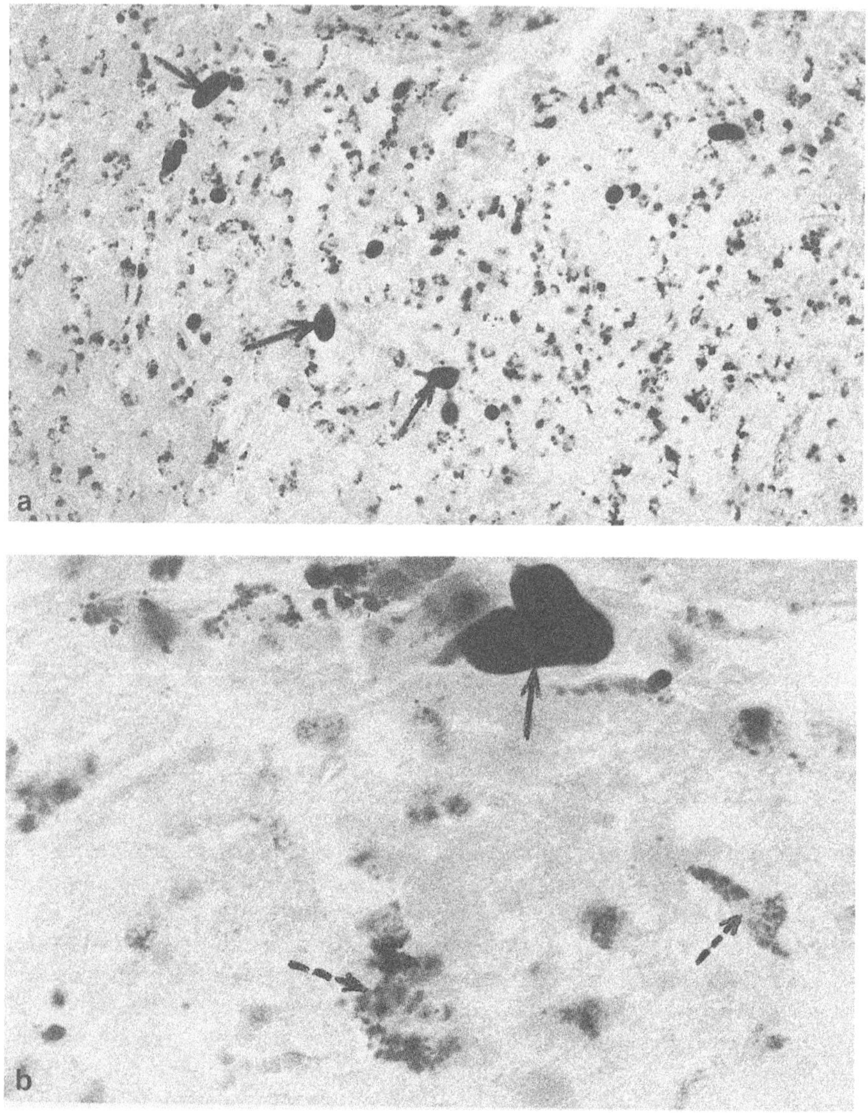

Fig. 63. a, b Fat embolism of the cortex (↑). Selective parenchymal necrosis in the removal stage with lipopectic microglia (↑). Sudan III, 1:180, 1:350

cident; the lungs on the other hand were clear. He explains this finding as being due to contractions of the vessels, whereby fat pressed out of the cervical tissue is conveyed up to the capillaries of the brain. Wojtek (1955), Neugebauer (1959, 1961), Kelemen (1962), Fromm (1962), and Girgen (1966) report on cerebral late sequelae, differential diagnostic investigations, and rare forms.

There have evidently been no systematic studies on the forensic significance of fat embolisms in the kidneys. Histologically, the fat embolism tends to be manifest in the vascular loops of the glomeruli, and to a lesser extent in the cortical capillaries. Escape of the neutral fat with transport as far as to the collecting tubules is possible, according to our own investigations.

The histological findings from the myocardium do not suggest any particular systematic process. Bschor (1963 d) produced very striking findings on chylomicron aggregates in cardiac muscle capillaries. In animal experiments, localized fibrillar necroses with slender hemorrhagic halos could be observed on the myocardium following fat embolisms (Anderson 1971; Harman and Ragaz 1950). In experimental fat embolisms on dogs, small-macular necroses of the myocardium were found much more frequently in the right than in the left ventricle (Hecht and Korb 1960). The occurrence of the necroses is explained by the duration of the mechanically obstructive phase in the pulmonary circulation caused by the fat. The cause of death in the case of fat embolism was right ventricular failure. The lethal dose was 2.0 ml fat/kg body weight in the experiments with dogs. Schmidt et al. (1970) have called attention to the links between fat embolism and idiopathic femur-head necrosis.

Air Embolisms

As with all embolizations of finely dispersed material, the distinction between venous and arterial air embolisms has to be made. For a description of their etiology, pathogenesis, pathophysiology, and macroscopic autopsy findings, the following textbooks, manuals, and reviews are refferred to: Meixner (1940), B. Mueller (1953), Rössle (1944, 1947, 1948), Gormsen (1961), Mallach (1978), and Palzelt et al. (1979). An acquaintance with these studies is essential in the histological examination and assessment of causes of death by air embolisms.

The diagnosis of a venous air embolism, regardless of its cause, relies largely on the macroscopic examination findings. The venous air embolism can be diagnosed much more reliably by an early and thorough autopsy, with the evidence of air bubbles or frothy blood in the right heart, afferent large veins, arteria pulmonalis, and coronary veins, than by histological investigations. Of course, the possibility of deception through postmortem gas formation and errors in the autopsy should here be taken into account. Naturally, just as in every case, the histological status should be examined to see whether other, macroscopically imperceptible agents could have contributed to the cause of death.

Hitherto, there have only been systematic histological studies on venous air embolisms by Adebahr (1949, 1953, 1954, 1960 a, b, 1963), Adebahr und Kupffer (1967), and Adebahr and Staak (1969). Even after a short survival time of a few minutes, Adebahr found, in animal experiments as well as in forensic autopsy material, changes in the venous blood of the heart which he attributed to the foreign-body influence of small air bubbles. These were seen as unstained vesicles in the blood of the right heart and sometimes also the large afferent veins, coronary veins, and arteria pulmonalis. In the immediate surroundings of these vascular formations, which were interpreted as embolized air bubbles, leukocytic infiltrations, platelet aggregations, and solitary fibrinous threads were found (Fig. 64). Further, in experiments on rabbits following venous air embolism by injections into the veins of the ear, and sporadically in humans e.g., after air-filling of the hip joint, platelet aggregations with surrounding leukocytic borders have been observed in the branches of the arte-

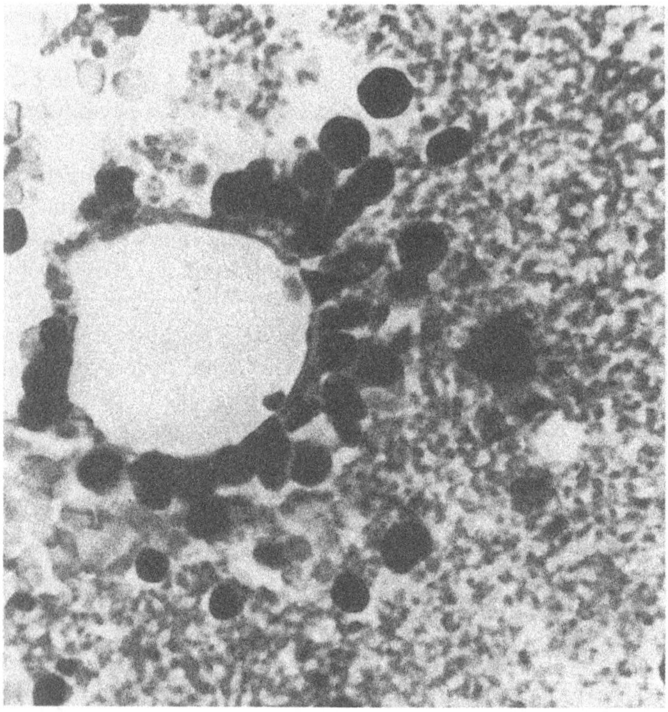

Fig. 64. Venous air embolism with small bubbles of air in the right heart, surrounded by leukocytes and thrombocyte aggregates. (After Adebahr 1966)

ria pulmonalis. Adebahr sees in these changes, particularly in the vesicles of the venous cardiac blood, a histomorphological basis for the venous air embolism. Without the presence of a vital air embolism these finding could not be produced postmortem.

In our own serial-section investigations on blood from the right ventricle, fixed in 5% formalin or in Orth's solution, following death through venous air embolism, we were unable to record similar results in four cases (attempted abortion, transfusion accident, cut wounds on the neck). Of course, in the middle of the blood coagula, there were to some extent quite numerous unstained vacuoles, but in the marginal areas of these recesses the leukocytic infiltrations and thrombocytic aggregations were absent.

Numerous systematic histological investigations have nevertheless been carried out after cases of death through arterial air embolisms. In this area, the histological findings are of prime importance. For proof of an arterial air embolism, that is of forensic use, an assessment is necessary of the clinical findings and histological evidence of vital organ changes that developed as a result of the air embolism. Evidence of the embolized air itself is not easy to detect. After a relatively short survival time of only a few hours, the air disappears out of the vascular areas and organs affected, probably by resorption and exhalation through the lungs (Meixner 1940; B. Mueller 1953). Occasionally, however, it has been possible to demonstrate the

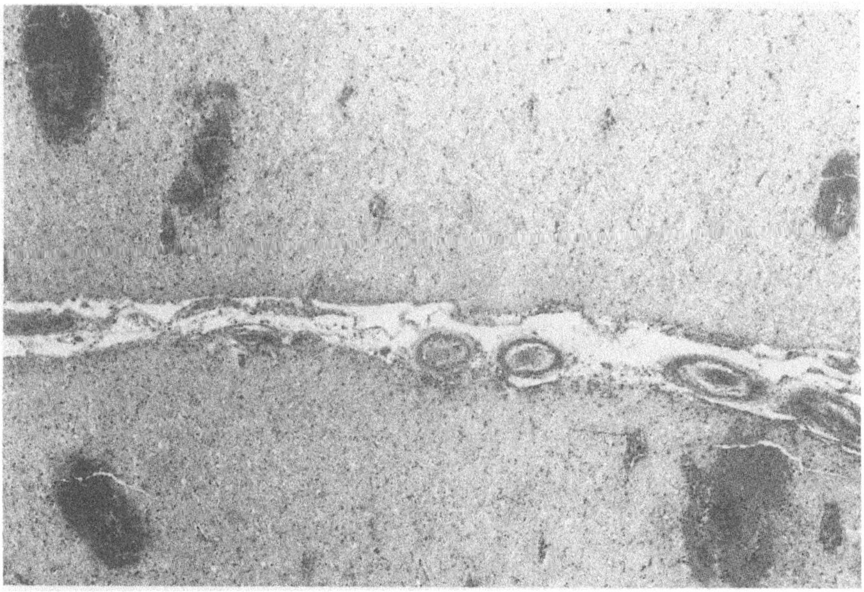

Fig. 65. Air embolism of the brain. Multiple spherical hemorrhages in the cortex. H and E, 1:120

embolized air in histological section, chiefly in the capillaries and arterioles of the brain (references in Rössle 1944, 1947, 1948; B. Mueller 1953). In the cerebral capillaries, irregularities in the columns of erythrocytes were found histologically; the tightly packed erythrocytes were in places interrupted by sharp boundaries. In the small engorged blood vessels, the unstained vesicles could also be observed, which were directly adjacent to the vascular intima. The perivascular Virchow-Robin spaces were in parts irregularly vesicular and unstained. Similar findings with interruptions in the erythrocytic borders were also evident in the capillaries of the myocardium (Hausbrandt 1938; Harter 1947). However, according to the critical studies of Köhn (1952a, b), such findings as proof of an arterial air embolism have to be assessed with great caution since artefacts can sometimes develop a similar appearance.

Tissue lesions to the myocardium and, particularly, to the brain are substantially more important. In combination with clinical data and other organ findings, they can be forensically considered as evidence of arterial air embolism. The survival time after which relevant histological findings were detectable in these organs is variously given; it extends from 30 min to 1 or 2 weeks. In the brain, macroscopically evident purpura is of chief interest. Systematic studies on the frequency of brain purpura in the case of cerebral air embolism have not been published. Histologically, brain purpura involves annular or spherical hemorrhages which are mainly irregularly distributed in the cerebrum (Fig. 65). In several cases, a variable tendency to affect the gray or white matter has been evident (Janssen 1967a). This diverse distribution of the hemorrhages is probably associated with the functional and circulatory condition of the brain. On the whole, the gray matter of the cerebral cortex appears to be less affected by the hemorrhages since there is a more intense vascular

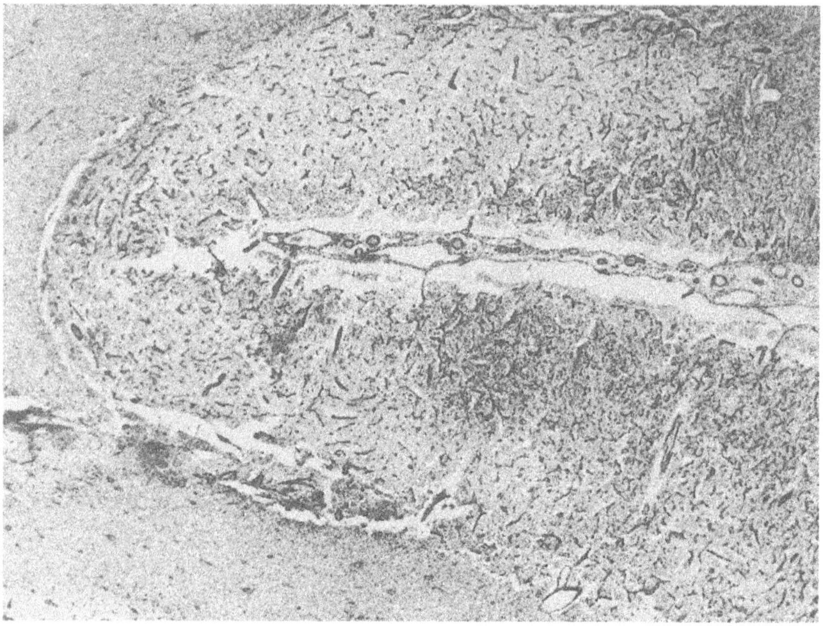

Fig. 66. Air embolism of the brain. Isolated total necrosis of the cortex with vascular reaction (onset of removal stage). H and E, 1:80

supply with better tissue compensatory possibilities in this area (cf. Henn et al. 1970). According to the results of serial-section investigations, the annular hemorrhages are composed of tubular hematomas in the vicinity of capillaries or arterioles. In tangentially cut surfaces, they appear as spherical hemorrhages. With a section perpendicular to the vascular axis, the blood vessel is in the center and is surrounded by a zone of necrotic cerebral tissue. After a survival time of several days, necroses of the wall can be detected in the centrally located vessels. In advanced stages, the structures of these vessels can only be recognized as shadows. Leukocytic reactions in the region of vascular wall necroses occur only seldom. On the other hand, in the case of cerebral air embolisms in humans and in animal experiments, microthrombi have occasionally been detectable in the central vessels of spherical hemorrhages. The fibrin stain according to the methods of Weigert and Goldner as well as with PTAH was positive. Under the fluorescence microscope, the microthrombi showed a distinct primary fluorescence and, following fluorochromization with acridine orange, a strong secondary fluorescence. In other areas of the brain, the capillaries and arterioles contained agglomerated erythrocytes and thrombocytes.

Typical sludging was involved. In the case of cerebral air embolisms survived for longer periods of time, localized total necrosis of the cerebrum sometimes also occurred (Fig. 66).

The remaining regions of the brain, particularly the hypothalamus, contained the ganglion cell changes, with fading in Nissl's stain, destruction of the cytoplasm, and the beginnings of glial proliferation, that have already been exhaustively described in the literature (see Rössle 1944). Usually, a survival time of at least 12–15 h is required for the manifestation of these histologically detectable findings.

The formation of annular and spherical hemorrhages in the brain following air embolism, as well as after cerebral fat embolism or other embolizations of finely dispersed substances, has already been repeatedly investigated and considered. It has been considered that vascular and cerebral tissue necroses with the surrounding hemorrhage are only the consequence of an embolic vascular obstruction with circulatory and nutritive disorders. It is difficult, however, to account for the formation of the microthrombi and the surrounding annular hemorrhage with such an explanation. In personal investigations (Janssen 1967 a), it was concluded that in at least some of the cases, consumption coagulopathy following cerebral air embolism was involved. Through disturbance in the microcirculation in the terminal vascular system with alteration of the local coagulation potential, precipitation of microthrombi occurs along with subsequent hypocoagulability of the blood. At the beginning of the microthrombosed vascular stretches, there is then extravasation of blood, which surrounds the central necrotic zone (cf. Henn et al. 1970). In concurrence with H. G. Lasch (personal communication, 1967), the microthrombi and annular hemorrhages are to be interpreted as histological manifestations of consumption coagulopathy following cerebral air embolism. Disseminated intravascular coagulation and fibrin precipitation in the whole organism are not necessarily involved in consumption coagulopathy. Evidence of this theory is given when a whole organ is affected; there is impairment of the microcirculation in cerebral tissue, which particularly appears with arterial air embolism. According to the studies of Schubert (1963), most organs are accessible to the gas via arteriovenous anastomoses in arterial gas embolisms. The diameter of the gas bubbles is usually 40 µm or more; the primary arterial gas embolism can thus become a venous embolism. The brain deserves particular attention in this regard since it is more vulnerable than other organs owing to its high oxygen consumption. The fine vascular distribution (cf. Pfeifer 1930) functionally corresponds to the system of "last meadows" (Zülch 1955). This anatomical and functional peculiarity makes it clear why in arterial air embolism disorders in the microcirculation with subsequent consumption coagulopathy particularly occur in the brain.

Adebahr and Staak (1969) were unable to detect changes indicative of gas embolism in brains, apart from negligible necrotic vascular changes with leukocytic reactions. However, it should be taken into account that in these experiments venous air embolisms were produced primarily by injection into the ear veins of rabbits. In our own investigations (Janssen 1967 a), we produced primary arterial air embolisms by injecting air into the cavum of the left ventricle of experimental animals. The contractions of the left ventricle in this way gave rise to an air embolism, with the corresponding disturbances, directly in the organs of the systemic circulation, particularly in the brain. This probably explains the differences in the results of the two studies.

No significant dependence of cerebral injuries on the kind of gas applied was evident in experimental cerebral air embolisms on dogs. The greatest amount of gas was tolerated with carbon dioxide. Nitrogen and helium behaved similarly to air. Oxygen had a low mortality, though a high morbidity (La Torre et al. 1962).

The effects of an arterial air embolism on *heart muscle* measured in terms of mortality, are probably more dangerous than in the brain (B. Mueller 1953). Apart from an early detection of intracapillary air, which is occasionally successful, histological demonstration of an air embolism in heart muscle is virtually impossible. This fact is probably explained by a short survival time as a result of early decrease in the performance of the myocardium in the case of air embolism.

Decompression sickness can, provided there is an appropriate survival time, lead to ischemic circulatory disorders and necroses through the incidence of gas bubbles in the vascular system (Rózsahegyi and Soós 1956; Haymaker 1957; Hartmann 1961; Haberer et al. 1972 – and further references in these studies).

From a forensic point of view, a great many histologically detectable organ changes occurring in venous and arterial air embolism do not in themselves have any proof value. The presence of an air embolism cannot be excluded by negative examination findings. In combination with appropriate clinical observations, histological cerebral findings, after the exclusion of other causes of death, may obtain proof significance. This also applies to histological evidence of gas bubbles with cellular reactions in the case of venous air embolisms in the blood of the right heart, according to the investigations and conclusions of Adebahr (1949, 1953, 1954, 1960a, b, 1963), Adebahr and Kupffer (1967), and Adebahr and Staak (1969).

Even without detailed knowledge of circumstances and possible causes, histological findings can occasionally draw attention to death from air embolism. An example from my own practice will serve to demonstrate this: A 38-year-old married woman was found lying unconscious on the floor of her apartment. Upon admission to hospital and for the next few days, persistent tonoclonic spasms were observed. The neurologist diagnosed an etiologically unclear focal cerebral symptom. On the 3rd day in hospital, a 4-month-old fetus was aborted by the woman. Despite intensive symptomatic treatment and circulatory support, the woman died without regaining consciousness on the 8th day in hospital.

The forensic autopsy and histological examination showed a status post abortum, a flaccid dilation of the cavities of the heart on the right side, and a pronounced purpura cerebri, with particular involvement of the cerebral medulla. Numerous cerebral capillaries and arterioles were necrotic in the region of the hemorrhages and partly occluded by fibrinous thrombi (Fig. 67). There had been strong cerebral pressure, which in combination with the multiple cerebral hemorrhages had led to death through central regulatory disorders. In the myocardium of the left ventricle, some localized necrobioses were found histologically (Fig. 68). With this position of the evidence, although the foramen ovale of the heart was closed, an air embolism was conjectured to have taken place following an attempt at abortion, with the entry of air via the pulmonary circulation and subsequent arterial and cerebral air embolism. Such an entry of air is known to be possible (B. Mueller 1953).

This supposition was communicated to the public prosecutor's office as the result of the examination. Thereupon, renewed inquiries were conducted and revealed that the woman had resolved to perform an internal douche upon herself in her apartment in the presence of a witness. About 5 min after the completion of this manipulation, the woman suddenly fainted and collapsed as she was cleaning the instrument. Despite concerted further investigations, the witness could not be proven guilty of complicity. In this example, the primary supposition of death of the

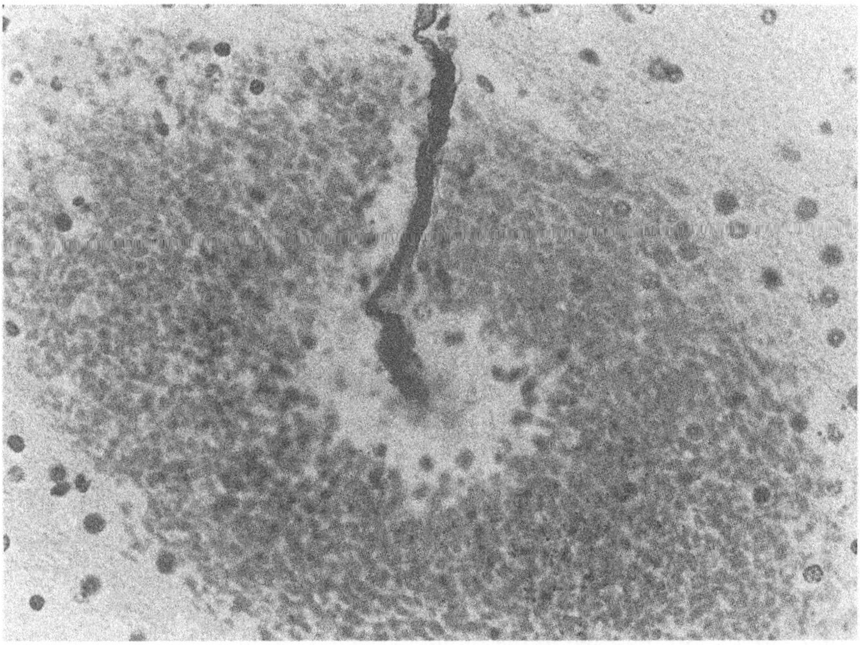

Fig. 67. Air embolism of the brain after expulsion with fibrinous capillary thrombosis, surrounding cerebral necrosis, and annular hemorrhage. Subject survived 8 days, 38 years old. Weigert's fibrin stain, 1:220

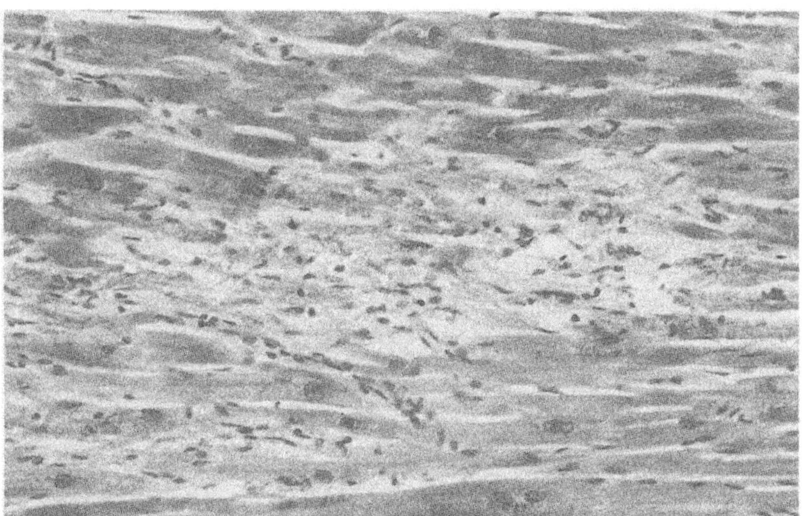

Fig. 68. Air embolism after expulsion with circumscribed necrobioses of the myocardium (direct effect of the embolism?). Subject survived 8 days, 38 years old. H and E, 1:180

woman through air embolism with cerebral involvement, which was at first only histologically based, became a certainty through further inquiries that were suggested on the strength of the histological evidence.

Amniotic Embolisms

The amniotic embolism presents a special form of vital reaction which arises in connection with pregnancy and childbirth. As a cause of sudden, unexpected, and inexplicable death, it demands forensic interest, above all when criminal offences are supposed, e.g., abortion or medical mispractice.

An amniotic embolism is caused by the passage of amniotic fluid and its components into the veins of the uterus. The passage is induced by injuries to the fetal membranes, especially in association with detachment of the placenta. The embolic material comprises amniotic fluid, meconium, lanugo hairs, sebum, epidermal epithelia, mucus, components of the decidua, and, in rare cases, amniotic and chorionic components. Histological evidence of an amniotic embolism can be adduced if these well-formed components of the amniotic fluid are detected intravascularly. They are chiefly found in the small vessels of the pulmonary circulation (Fig. 69). In the case of a closed foramen ovale, they have occasionally been found in the systemic circulation; passage in the pulmonary circulation is thus possible. Amniotic fluid by itself cannot be histologically detected.A survey of acute and subacute amniotic embolisms, their frequency, their paths of propagation, and their consequences is provided in the comprehensive studies of P. Müller (1964) of Jena; older references are found in Slodder and Lock (1952). Among 3500 autopsies, death in 20 women occurred in the course of gravidity, during or following childbirth. Of these, the cause of death was in 12 cases a definite, and in three cases a possible, amniotic embolism. In three cases, the birth was without complications; in nine cases, surgical measures or intrauterine intervention had to be undertaken. In 11 cases, damage to the uterus was evident. Using formalin fixation of the entire pelvic organs and serial-section investigations, the embolic course of the amniotic components could be determined in the maternal venous system. Corpuscular embolic products, with and without thrombi, were found in the intrauterine veins, particularly common in the venae ovaricae and venae uterinae, occasionally in the plexus uterovaginalis and rectalis cranialis and ligamentum rotundum. Other than in the lungs, amniotic components have been observed in the brain, kidneys, and intrahepatic branches of the portal vein and liver sinusoids.

The *effects of the amniotic embolism* have to be judged in relation to their extent, the path of embolization, and the reaction of the body. It is only in a few cases that the cause of death can be traced to damage to one particular organ. Of central importance is death from an acute right ventricular failure, just as with thromboembolisms. The histological assessment of findings in the lungs is carried out according to the same criteria as with fat embolisms. In the material examined by P. Müller (1964), 10 of 15 cases were found to bear indications of a heavy hemorrhagic diathesis, and in two cases there was an eclamptic liver with thromboses spread into branches of the portal vein and parenchymal necroses. In one case, urticarial exanthem occurred. Amniotic allergy is, therefore, debated; it is assumed that an ana-

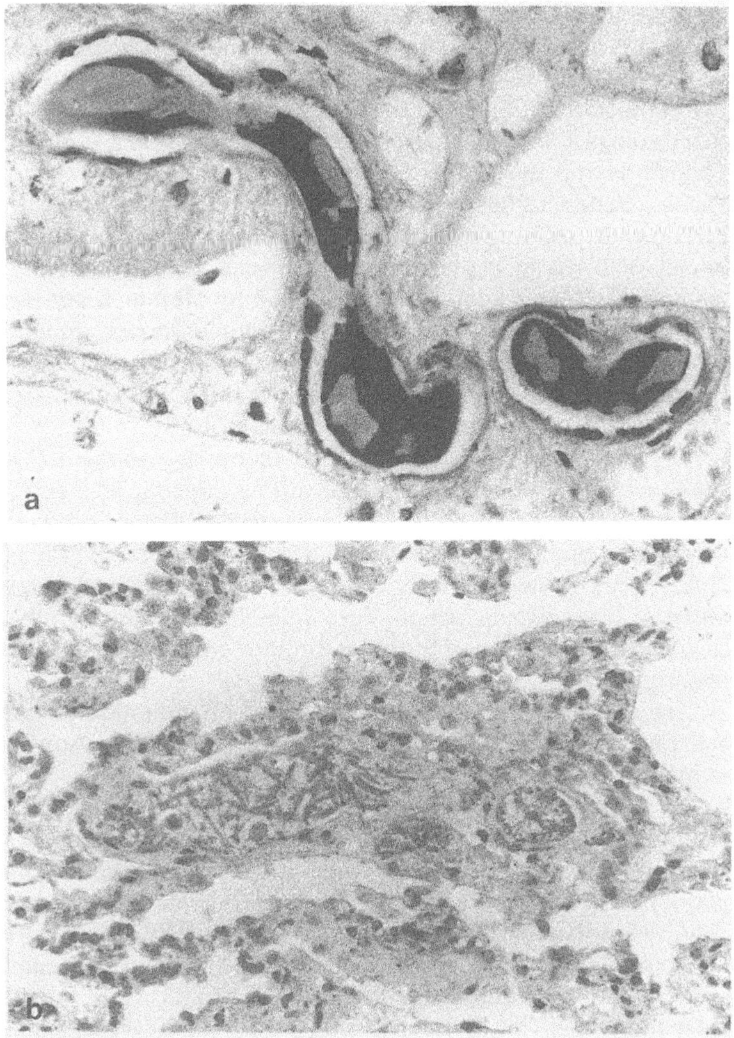

Fig. 69. a Amniotic embolism with deformed chorionic epithelial cells in the pulmonary capillaries. Subject: 30 years old, status post partum. H and E, 1:400. **b** Same subject as in **a**. Fibrin precipitation and shock bodies in the pulmonary capillaries. Mallory-Goldner, 1:220

phylactic shock induced by amniotic fluid is important as an essential contributory factor in the cause of death in certain cases.

From our experience of three fatal amniotic embolisms and numerous investigations into cases of death post partum, histological evidence from the lungs, where it is not massive and unequivocal, has to be examined in many respects from the approach of a differential diagnosis. Not every intravascular giant cell in such cases is derived from the chorion or decidua. Following heavy blood loss, which is known not to be uncommon in partus, acute stimulation of the bone marrow with flooding out of the megakaryocytes occurs; these megakaryocytes can then be detected in large numbers in the pulmonary circulation (cf. shock, p. 165). Recognizing megakaryocytes and differentiating them from giant-cell structures of the uterus is not always simple. The cells are considerably deformed by being pressed into the capillaries of pulmonary tissue and suffer extensive loss of their cytoplasmic borders, such that cytological differentiation, even with specific stains, e.g., Giemsa, modified by Lennert, is impeded. Occasionally, there is spreading of the larger decidual fragments with dimensions up to 580 × 160 μm, which after a long survival time are broken down by resorptive granulation tissue (Cameron and Park 1965). Filtering the blood, followed by staining of the extracted cellular elements according to the method of Papanicolaou is recommended by Möttönen and Isomäki (1971) as a supplement to histological investigation. Moreover, care should be taken with the differentiation of embolized foreign matter, which, e.g., in therapeutic and diagnostic procedures, can enter the bloodstream and thus the pulmonary capillaries by intramuscular or intravenous injection (Brüning 1955).

Experimental studies on dogs and rabbits by Attwood (1964) and P. Müller (1966) with intravenous injections of various amniotic elements revealed the semisolid components of amniotic fluid, in particular mucous substances to be responsible for the acute symptoms collapse, dyspnea, shock, convulsions, right ventricular failure. They acutely obstruct the pulmonary arteries and cannot be quickly disposed of by enzymatic action. Pure amniotic fluid, on the other hand, led more slowly to the formation of fibrinous thrombi, which were then dissolved again relatively quickly.

The embolized corpuscular components of amniotic fluid are apparently broken down very slowly in the lungs. In animal experiments, Attwood (1964) was able to identify histologically epithelial scales for up to 3 weeks and mucin for up to 7 months. Lanugo hairs, the only amniotic components to induce negligible reactive changes in the vascular walls, behave similarly. Arteritis was only found once among 40 experimental animals. It is thus doubtful that human amniotic embolisms play a part in the development of primary pulmonary hypertension.

A very important complication, also histologically detectable, is the incidence of *blood coagulation disorders*. The amniotic fluid and its components consume a large proportion of the thrombocytes and coagulation factors of the blood within a relatively short time. Thus, even after short survival times, an accumulation of thrombocytes and fibrin precipitation occurs around components of vernix caseosa, which then fill the capillaries of the pulmonary circulation at numerous sites. These signs of disseminated intravascular coagulation (Hardaway et al. 1961–1964) are then found in other organs, e.g., the liver sinusoids and capillaries of the renal cortex. This blood coagulation disorder induced by the amniotic fluid with obstruction of the terminal vascular system, further complicated by a subsequent increased hemorrhagic tendency, doubtlessly has fatal consequences in many cases which go beyond the primary effect of inhibiting the circulation in the pulmonary vascular system. Clinically, this process is characterized by a typical pathological course, whereby initial hypercoagulability, which can be verified by coagulation analysis, is followed by afibrinogenemia, thrombopenia, and reduction in the prothrombin complex (Duda and Papilian 1962; Slunsky and Mirejovsky 1963).

Finally, in the forensic assessment of an amniotic embolism, care should be taken in differentiating postpartum shock without anatomical substrates, endotoxin shock in terms of a Schwartzman phenomenon, and an acute circulation crisis with hemorrhagic shock syndrome. Here, the histologically established evidence of amniotic components is of prime importance (Petersohn 1968).

Tissue and Foreign-Body Embolisms

Venous and arterial embolisms of endogenous tissue components and foreign material are to be regarded as vital reactions. It should be borne in mind in this respect that in rapidly established putrefaction with dissociation and detachment of parenchymal cells, e.g., from the liver tissue, isolated cells can be propelled postmortem by putrefactive gases into the veins and even carried into branches of the pulmonary arteries.

The origin of traumatically induced tissue embolisms is usually a severe injury, whereby tissue debris enters the veins by direct traumatically caused communication and then is usually carried into the smaller ramifications of the pulmonary circulation. If parenchymatous organs are affected, the traumatism is normally fatal. The tissue embolism can then usually not be held to have caused death.

Embolisms of organ fragments of the liver, brain, and bone-marrow tissue have been histologically detected and described (Nunes 1966, 1970, 1971; Pioch 1964; Karkola and Möttönen 1971 – further references in these studies). There have also been reports of a fatal cerebral embolism following traumatic rupturing of an echinococcus cyst in the wall of the left ventricle of the heart (Preda et al. 1963) and fibinous embolisms following severe tissue trauma (Remsch 1964). In the latter case, however, it is not altogether certain that a traumatic shock-induced intravascular clot was not present. Brettel and Lutz (1972) reported a cartilage embolism as a special form of vital reaction following stab wounds to the neck involving incision of the larynx and vena jugularis. Following the operation on an atrial septum defect in a 6-year-old child, there was an embolism of cardiac muscle and fatty tissue into the right arteria cerebri media (Buris et al. 1979). The embolism of skin fragments into the pulmonary arteries, e.g., due to functions of the peripheral veins, is distinctly rare (Andrew 1976; Gilbert and Borchard 1980). Arterial embolisms from atheromatous intimal ruptures without the influence of foreign material occur in the case of severe arteriosclerosis of the large vessels with the spreading of cholesteremic material. Occasionally, in advanced anthracosis with heavy involvement of the tracheobronchial lymph nodes, direct malacic incursions into the pulmonary veins result, which lead to arterial embolisms. Carbon-containing particles can then be found histologically in the capillary systems of practically all organs of the systemic circulation, largely without further circulation-induced damage.

In rare cases, it is also possible for foreign material entering the bloodstream via therapeutic and diagnostic procedures or through injuries to lead to embolisms that are transported into the terminal pulmonary circulation (Figs. 70–74) (Brüning 1955a, b). Reports have been made of a metal splinter embolism in the brain following an industrial accident (Althoff 1967) as well as various bullet embolisms (Miner and Handel 1978; Pauwaa et al. 1979; Glass et al. 1980).

In animal experiments on pulmonary detritus embolisms, Voigt (1962) found numerous thrombi in the pulmonary arteries as early as 24 h following the injection

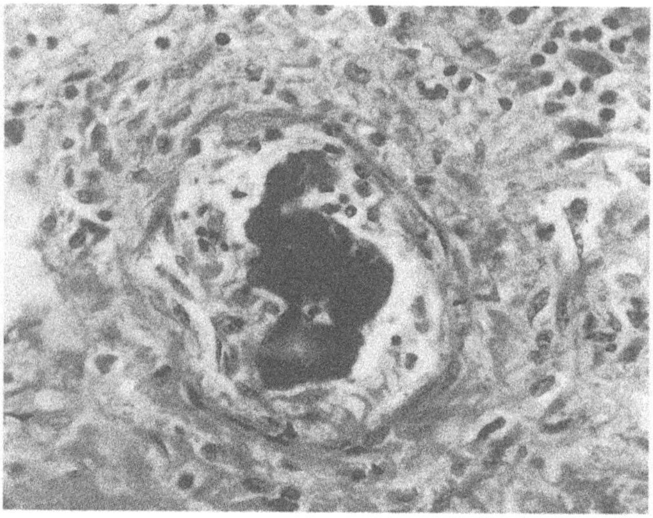

Fig. 70. Particles of bile embolized in the lung following liver biopsy in a case of biliary cirrhosis. Subject: 30 years old, ♂. H and E, 1:220

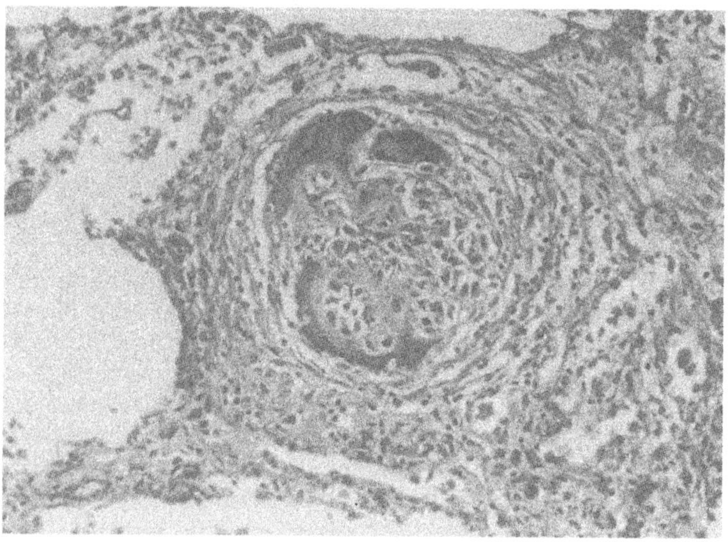

Fig. 71. Pulmonary arteriole with foreign-body granulations; status following repeated injections. H and E, 1:220

of nonlethal doses of subcutaneous tissue and skeletal musculature. The thrombi were organized just as rapidly as the other embolized particles in the pulmonary arteries. Intravenous injections of polyvinylchloride with a particle size of 50–200 μm and polystyrene in rabbits caused pronounced right ventricular hypertrophy after 3–4 months. Histologically, fresh cardiac muscle fiber necroses and numerous ste-

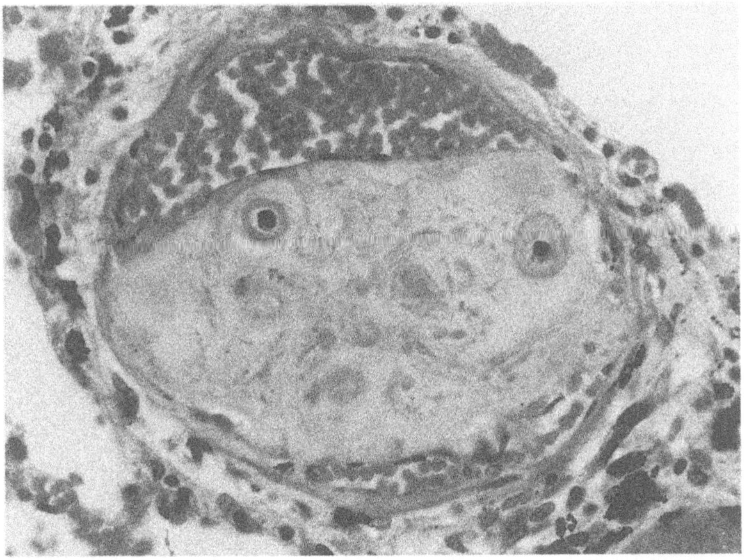

Fig. 72. Pulmonary arteriole with embolized material that is no longer identifiable (animal parasite?). Subject: 48 years old, ♂, soporific intoxication. H and E, 1:280

noses with foreign-body inclusions in the branches of the pulmonary arteries were detected (Köhn and Berg 1965).

Occasionally, embolized substances that cannot be identified are found histologically in the pulmonary circulation; they have the importance of secondary findings.

Normally, the histological demonstration of embolisms of endogenous material does not give rise to any particular problems. The embolic material should be histologically identified as far as possible. In this way, identification of the starting point of the embolism will be promoted.

Aspirations

An aspiration process with the sucking of endogenous or foreign material into the deep respiratory tracts normally presupposes spontaneous breathing movements. The histionic finding of an aspiration is thus to be regarded as an indication of a vital reaction. This evaluation becomes less certain and limited if resuscitation measures with artificial respiration have been undertaken. Here, the artificially inhaled material can be carried to the peripheral sections of the deep respiratory tracts. As a rule, histological evidence of aspiration material in the small bronchi and pulmonary alveoli is important in recognizing an aspiration as a sign of a vital phenomenon. Terminal or agonal aspiration, aspiration in the course of death, usually only brings material into the trachea and larger bronchi. After artificial respiration has been carried out for a long period of time, pulmonary findings must be expected which cannot be distinguished with regard to vital or postmortem origin.

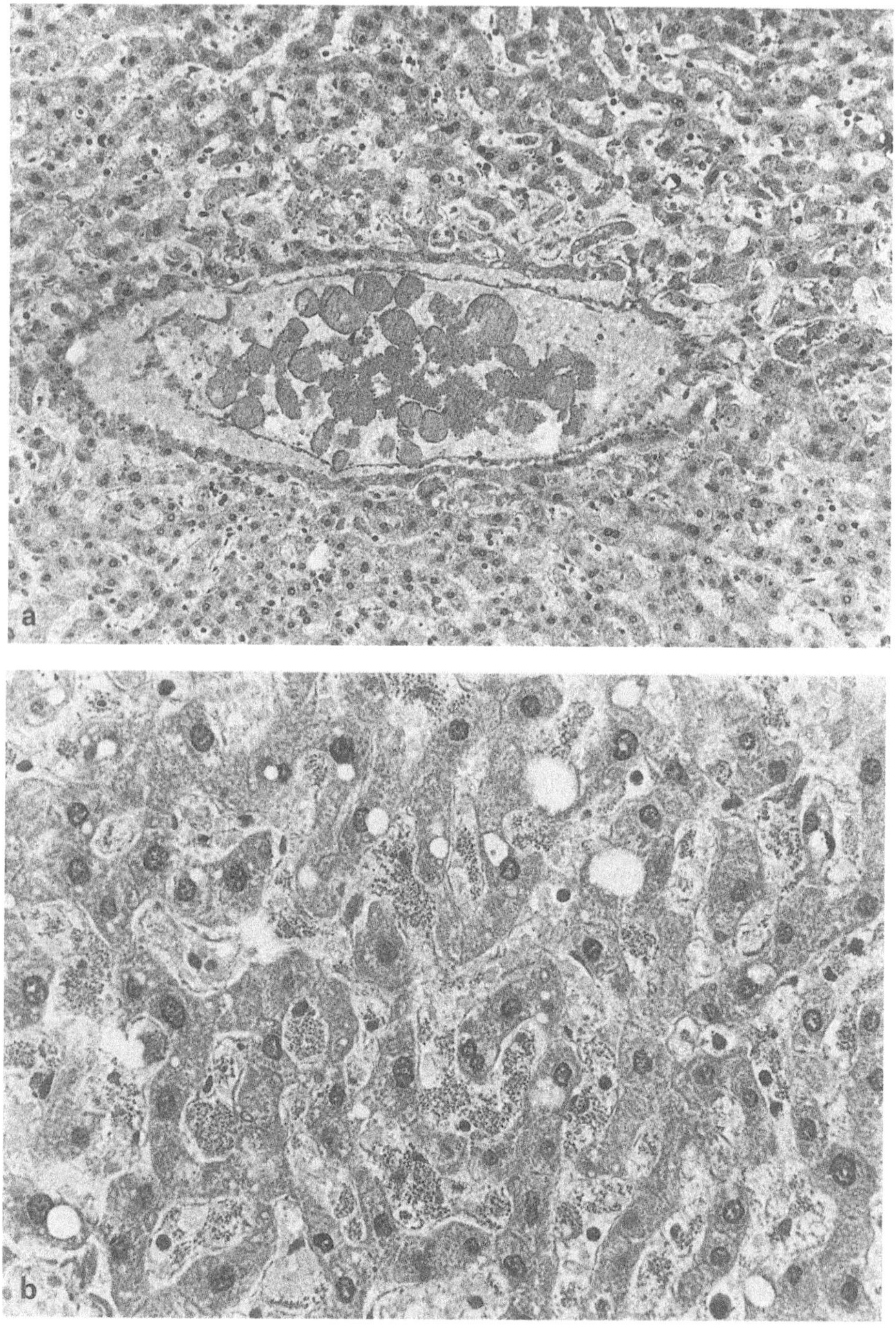

Fig. 73 a, b. Inadvertent introduction of contrast medium into the vagina of a 68-year-old woman during colography: Liver with barium sulfate in the central veins and capillaries. (After Bonte 1980) H and E, 1:250, 1:350

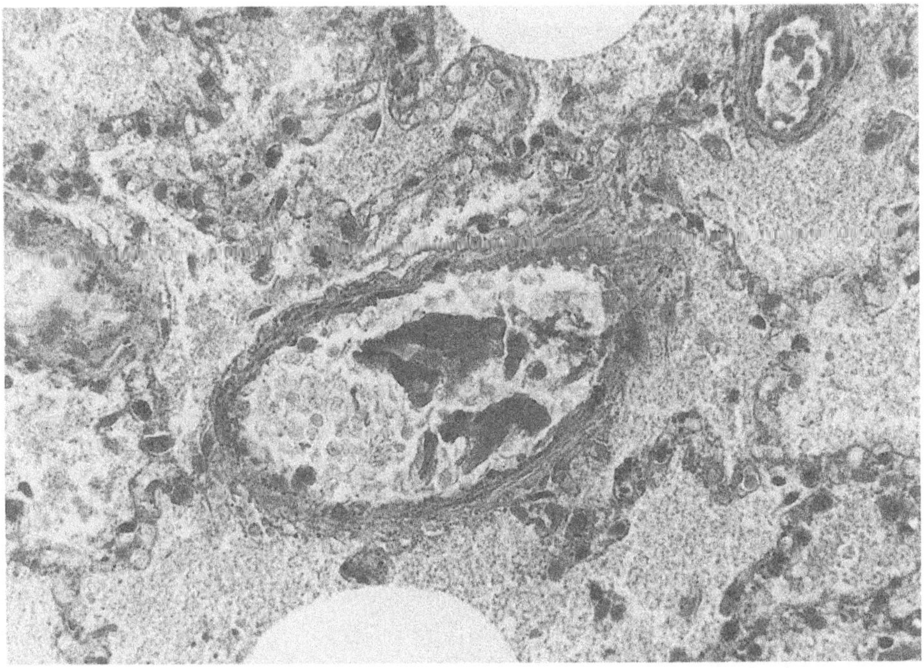

Fig. 74. Pulmonary arteriole with foreign material following an operation on a fractured femur. Subject: 63 years old, ♀. H and E, 1:250

The following come into consideration as aspiration material: Stomach contents following vomiting, blood, mucus, parts of the bronchial mucous membranes, amniotic components, and very diverse foreign material that is capable of being inspired, such as water droplets, fine-grained sand and flour. Soot, aerosols, and particulate admixtures in the inspired air can also be breathed in and histologically detected in pulmonary tissue and, while not actually classed as aspirations, they can be evaluated as vital signs.

Microscopic identification of the aspiration material, which is usually successful, should as far as possible be included in the diagnosis of an aspiration.

Mostly, one finds more or less digested stomach contents, e.g., meat particles, in which occasionally the transverse striation is still identifiable, starchy food components with typical cellulose structures, milk, and bile (Fig. 75). In the histological identification of the material and assessment of the aspiration sequelae, at least H and E, van Gieson, and fat stains should be routinely employed. Difficulties arise in the aspiration diagnosis if there are strong signs of decomposition from stomach juices or postmortem changes. Aspiration foci are also colonized by putrefactive bacteria particularly early after death; with H and E stain, these appear as dark blue, relatively thick plump rods up to 2 µm long and in great numbers. With such findings, which cast doubt on the vital origin, it is best to compare a large number of lung sections from various lobes and pay particular attention to the circumscribed character of the aspirations, which mainly affect several adjacent groups of alveoli or whole lobuli.

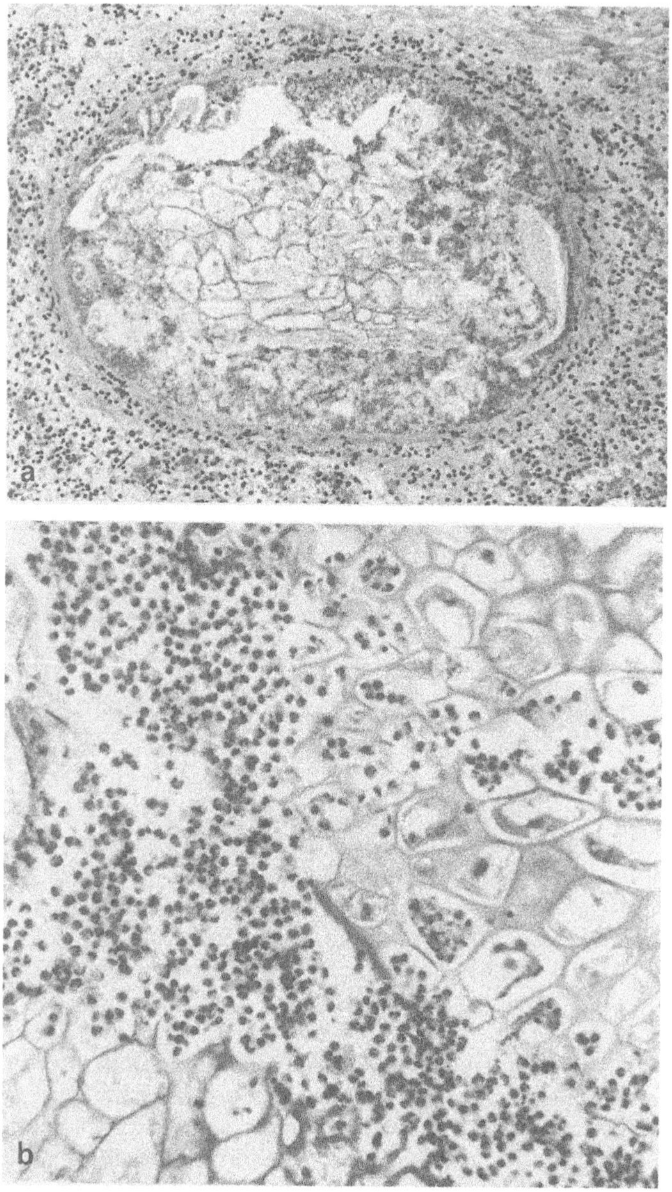

Fig. 75. a Aspiration of stomach contents with cellulose-containing food particles in a bronchus. Onset of aspiration pneumonia. H and E, 1:150. **b** Cellulose-containing aspiration material with leukocytic infiltration. H and E, 1:220.

The same histological criteria for evidence also apply to the aspirations of mucus and parts of organs, e.g., after severe fractures of the base of the skull with the production of a connecting passage between the brain and pharynx. Histological assessment of a blood aspiration, which in massive findings does not usually present any difficulties, is best carried out in combination with macroscopic autopsy

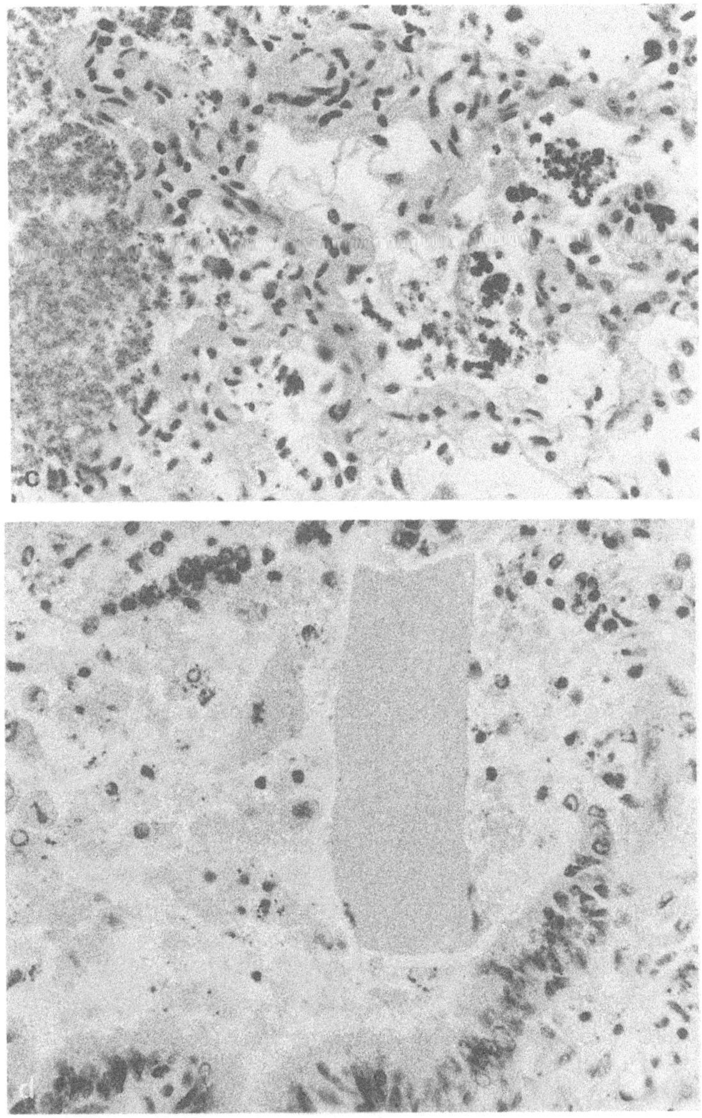

Fig. 75.c Aspiration of stomach contents with dark-green bile particles in the alveoli. H and E, 1:220. **d** Aspiration of stomach contents. Bronchus with fibers of meat (transverse striation still partially recognizable). Accident in the course of anesthesia. H and E, 1:300

evidence. The lung is mainly altered by a strong, acute, vicarious emphysema and contains numerous blood aspiration foci, which on the cut surface are prominent, relatively sharply defined, and dark red; in severe, protracted cases, they can be confluent. Histologically, care should be taken with an indisputable intrabronchial and intra-alveolar localization of aspirated blood. Because of the simultaneous occurrence of acute vascular congestion and engorged capillaries protruding into the

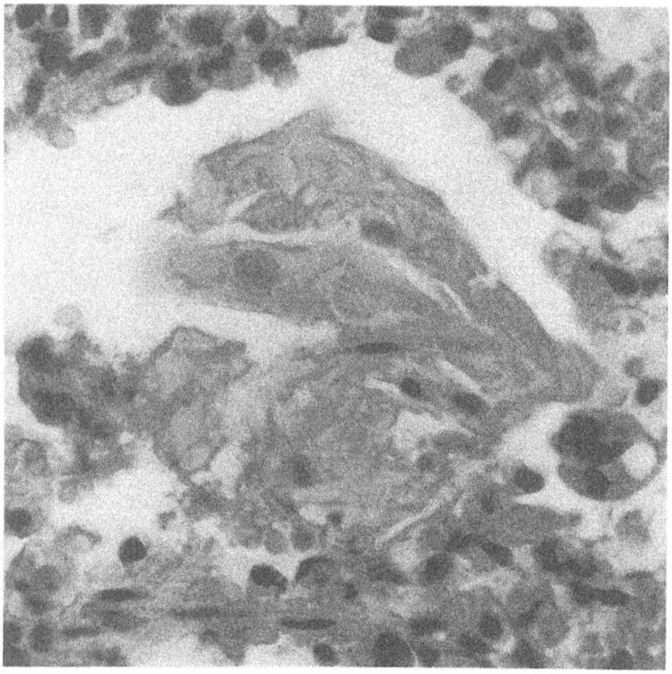

Fig. 76. Amniotic aspiration with particles of epidermis in the alveoli. H and E, 1:350

alveolar lumina, recognition of the alveolar boundaries is particularly important. It is necessary to distinguish in the differential diagnosis between intrapulmonary hemorrhages of various causes, hemorrhagic pulmonary edema, and hemorrhagic pulmonary infarctions and pneumonia, e.g., influenzal pneumonia with hemorrhagic characteristics. With blood aspiration foci that are not completely fresh, making such a distinction can be difficult.

Postmortem filling of the trachea with blood and blood aspirations produced by artificial respiration in human corpses led to blood aspiration foci in the lungs which, without being checked histologically, resembled foci of vital origin (Reinhardt and Zink 1977). With a supine position of the corpse, artificially produced aspiration foci were found virtually exclusively in the dorsal and lateral regions of the lungs. Foci of vital origin, on the other hand, could also be found on the ventral side of the lungs.

In the routine histological examination of stillborn and dead newborn infants, an amniotic aspiration has to be considered. Aspirated components of the amniotic fluid can be detected, e.g., sebum, epidermal epithelia, lanugo hairs, and meconium (Fig. 76). In the sections of the lungs that are affected by the aspiration, regular infiltration of the amniotic fluid into the alveoli can develop. In the absence of visible amniotic components, it is possible for the histological evidence to give the impression of a breathing or partially breathing lung. Among 31 fetuses and 69 neonates, Dell'erba and Vimercati (1966) recorded such a finding twice. In connection with aborticide or infanticide, the evidence of an amniotic aspiration has exceptional, usually vindicatory significance. However, a criminal offence, e.g., deliberately giving birth into a toilet or bucket, cannot be excluded by such evidence.

The *histological changes in aspiration foci* are affected by the survival time, the kind of aspiration material, and the size of the foci. From the behavior of small hemorrhagic pulmonary infarctions, it is known that they can heal completely without a trace (Giese 1960). Experiments on rats by Mueller et al. (1960) revealed a distinct hemolysis 30 min after tracheal introduction of autologous blood. After 4 h, the hemolysis had almost completely developed. The removal of hemolyzed blood ensued either via the bronchi or through phagocytosis. A large increase in the number of macrophages of the bronchi, alveolar septa, and capillaries occurred. The alveolar septa were partly swollen and contained increased numbers of leukocytes. Migration of leukocytes into the alveoli was seldom observed. After a 3-day survival time, the alveoli were clear. After 5–6 days, the alveoli were coated with a thin layer that stained intensely with eosin. Definite traces of hemosiderin were not found until after 4 days, initially in the alveolar epithelia (pneumomonocytes), later in the interstitium; subsequently, there was an obvious migration of hemosiderin-containing macrophages into the alveolar lumina. After about 14 days, a siderous pigment was found only in the peribronchial lymphatic tissue. Comparative experiments have shown that the degradation processes of blood aspiration foci proceed more slowly in humans than in animals. Graev and Fabroni (1962) arrived at similar results.

A basic complication, often fatal, develops through acidic action on pulmonary tissue in the aspiration of stomach contents. The resulting infection of the areas of lung involved is usually rapidly established. The formation of aspiration pneumonia is favored in this manner. These tend to form necroses and abscesses in the central regions and are thus therapeutically not very accessible. Through the aspiration of fat-containing material, e.g., milk, foam cells and findings reminiscent of xanthous pneumonia are seen.

In assessing aspirations as a cause of death, the extent and quality of histological findings can be of decisive importance. Histological evidence of filling-in in several alveolar groups in one visual field argues in favor of a fatal aspiration. These aspirations, which on the whole terminate life acutely, have to be differentiated from those cases in which death does not occur until after days or weeks in association with inflammatory complications. It is here sometimes difficult to demonstrate histologically the aspiration etiology of the pulmonary findings. The following would indicate an aspiration: a heterotopic disproportionate distribution of the foci, early destruction and softening of the pulmonary tissue in the central sections of these foci, and the occurrence of foreign-body giant cells.

A definitive evaluation of aspiration sequelae should always take place in connection with the other investigation findings and established details of the circumstances of death. A critical assessment is particularly important with aspirations involved with anesthesia following resuscitative measures and in all related questions concerning the occurrence of aspirations after traumatic or toxic brain damage.

III. Oxygen Deficiency

1. General, Localized Oxygen Deficiency

A general definition of the injuries caused by oxygen deficiency involves all conditions and sequelae that are caused by impairment or interruption of the oxygen supply or utilization in the tissues. Conversely, the term asphyxiation in forensic medical usage is restricted for practical purposes to such cases in which, e.g., through atmospheric oxygen deficiency, obstruction of the respiratory passages, central interruption of the respiratory function, disturbance of the oxygen supply is induced from outside. In forensic practice, the recognition of death through asphyxiation can present problems if there are no indicative external or internal injuries or obstructions of the respiratory tracts and the conditions of death are not known in detail. In addition, the known macroscopic and histological signs of general damage through oxygen deficiency, e.g., "suffocative hemorrhages," pulmonary emphysema, degenerative cellular changes, fatty degeneration, and increase in lactic acid, are on the whole diverse in character and not conclusive as individual findings (Büchner 1937, 1942, 1944, 1950, 1957; Mueller 1961; Letterer 1959; Kernbach 1963; Ponsold 1961). Similar findings can also arise through injuries leading to impairment of the circulation or ischemia, thereby reducing or interrupting the tissue oxygen supply. The extent of terminal hypoxia is also relevant to the changes detectable postmortem (Jetter 1959).

The distinction has to be made in the histomorphological and histochemical evidence between general changes that appear in the various organs of an individual and localized damage in the form of necrosis. *Hypoxemia,* oxygen deficiency of the blood, can lead to *hypoxia,* oxygen deficiency of the tissue, but together with anemia or ischemia, e.g., in coronary stenosis, hypoxemia can also induce circumscribed tissue damage. *Hypoxidosis* characterizes oxygen deficiency in the tissue and its after effects. Evidence of hypoxidosis is impeded if in rapidly developing suffocation the tissue findings are developed only sparsely, or not at all. In temporary or chronic oxygen deficiency, the injuries can either be reversible or leave behind permanent tissue changes.

The sensitivity of tissues to oxygen deficiency varies; it is particularly dependent on the degree of differentiation, the oxygen requirement, and the functional condition of the cells concerned. The most sensitive tissue is the highly differentiated central nervous system, especially the brain, in which there are again local differences. The shortest survival time is found in the region of the stem ganglia.

It is difficult to differentiate the mainly ischemically induced necroses and necrobioses from reversible functional impairment since the boundaries are on the whole indistinct. The cell does not die suddenly because it possesses protective mechanisms which have to be overcome by the lesion (Holle et al. 1955). Necrosis itself progresses by stages; it is a lengthy and intravital process. It differs from autolysis of structures of the corpse in the different reaction environment, the presence of defense and compensating mechanisms, and in the gradual breaking down of vital reactions. This is connected with the fact that the various biologically active molecular groups within the protoplasm are not inactivated at the same time. Myocardial infarction, the oxygen-deficiency necrosis or necrobiosis of greatest general significance, will be discussed in connection with sudden death (p. 187).

Various metabolic changes accompany oxygen-deficiency damage: fat and lipoid deposition (Büchner 1970; Policard 1955; Schlicht 1955; Bade and Schuhmacher 1964), disorders in proteometabolism, loss of the ability to produce high-energy phosphates (Ponsold 1961), drop in the blood pH (Prokop and Göhler 1975), and increase in the vascular permeability in the form of dysoria (Schürmann and McMahon 1933), with the escape of so-called asphyxial substances (Prokop and Göhler 1975).

The type and cause of oxygen deficiency do not evidently have any bearing on the quality of the tissue damage. It is, therefore, possible to refer to standard reactions of catabiosis (Hölle et al. 1955). Quantitative differences have been observed in animal experiments when strangulation, clamping of the trachea, or ligature of the cervical vessels were performed (Mueller 1961). The environmental temperature is probably significant. In the experimental studies by Tausch and Möller (1973) on the question of cot death by suffocation under bedclothes, there was no case whereby the O_2 or CO_2 concentrations were indicative of external asphyxiation. A hyperthermia effect through accumulation of heat has been discussed in detail as the cause of death. Alterations in oxygen binding and a simultaneous rise in the basal metabolic rate probably bring about a fatal degree of oxygen deficiency in the body.

Schneider (1959) investigated the survival and resuscitation times of the brain, liver, heart, and kidneys and determined the functional impairments of these organs, which can appear a few seconds after interruption of the blood supply. In no case was the energy release under anaerobic conditions sufficient to maintain function, even though these organs are capable of anaerobic glycolysis. The resuscitation time of cranial nerve cells proved to be variable. Complete ischemia of 8–10 min at 37 °C led to final collapse of overall cerebral function, although only a few cells appeared cytomorphologically to be irreversibly damaged at this time. In the liver and kidneys, functional impairment occurs with the same rapidity; the resuscitation time, however, is 3–4 h. After a cardiac arrest of 3–4 min, resuscitation of the whole organism is not possible without auxiliary measures. This is because subsequent to cardiac arrest, the heart muscle is initially so inefficient that it cannot raise the blood pressure above a critical limit. Thus, this exceeds the resuscitation time of the brain even though irreversible damage to the myocardium does not occur at this juncture. A fall in temperature to 15°–17 °C has led to a prolongation of the resuscitation time by a factor of about 6. The focal pattern of the ischemic-hypoxically damaged tissue areas is not explained by vasospasms but by additional thrombocyte aggregates. In support of this is the fact that an increase in filtration pressure is necessary to force blood through a 20 μm-pore filter.

2. Specific Cell and Organ Findings

The histology of the particularly sensitive brain does not yield any findings in which the causation can be determined with certainty. In animal experiments, Lucas and Strangeways (1956) found an enlargement of the pericellular spaces and plasmolysis after 48 h; and after 72-h survival time, there was cellular degeneration, acidophilic behavior, and loss of Nissl substance, to some extent with cellular decay and gliosis. Plasmolysis and fissuration are also present as artefacts. The region of the hippocampus in particular is damaged; the pattern of damage could be correlated with the time-course. The ganglion cell changes corresponded to a chronic and ischemic cellular disorder and to homogenization, in which the nuclei also became acidophilically altered. Recovery of the cells no longer occurred after homogenization. Basically similar findings could, however, also be observed in the cerebellar cortex and Gasser's ganglion of guinea pigs following trichloroethylene poisoning. Kernbach (1963) found shriveled or swollen nuclei, partially with hyperchromatosis or vacuolization of the nucleolus and sometimes also nuclear expulsions, in cortical layers III–V after hanging, drowning, and asphyxia through alimentary bolus. On the whole, the cerebellar cortex, thalamus, and Purkinje cells turned out to be relatively stable to oxygen deficiency in comparison with the hippocampus.

In acute and subacute asphyxiation (e.g., choking, strangulation, thorax compression), the histology of the brain virtually provides only general indications, e.g., high-grade acute congestion, swelling of the capillary endothelia, small localized perivascular extravasation in the cerebral medulla, irregular, largely perivascular edematization, nuclear disaggregation, signs of cytoplasmic vacuoles (Fig. 77), swelling in the external and internal surface cells in the region of the arachnoid, and findings corresponding to sludging. These findings alone do not attain evidence or indicative significance for asphyxiation.

Cerebral tissue damage of more localized ischemic or general hypoxic origin can create problems in histological examinations and evaluations if the subject sur-

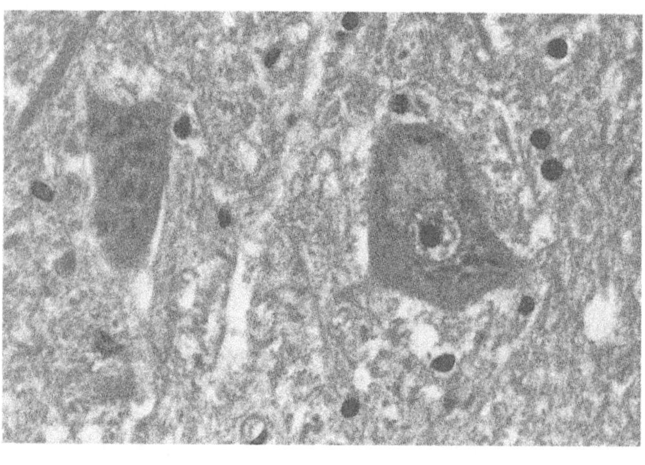

Fig. 77. Ganglion cells with hydropic nuclei and vacuoles in the cytoplasm. Subject: 26 years old, ♀, death as a result of repeated strangulation. H and E, 1:400

vived for a certain length of time and etiological questions require clarification in the light of these findings. In this respect, histomorphological criteria have been compiled, in particular by Colmant (1965). The occurrence of plasmolysis, hyperchromatosis, vesicular nuclei, and glia cell reactions is important (Fig. 78). According to electron-microscopic studies on cat brains by Kalimo et al. (1977), the earliest changes were in the form of clumping of the chromatin; in addition, damage was found to the endoplasmic reticulum, Golgi apparatus, mitochondria, and ribosomes.

Owing to improved resuscitative techniques and intensive care, chemical damage to the brain after survival for a short time is nowadays observed more frequently. The distinction between ischemic and hypoxemic lesion patterns can thus have forensic significance. According to the studies of Eisenmenger et al. (1976), the initial stages of both types of lesions are identical; differences arise in the reactive tissue changes. Lesions due to hypoxemia affect the regions of the brain mainly in the sequence: globus pallidus, striatum, thalamus, hypothalamus. With ischemia, the following lesion order was found: cerebral cortex, Purkinje cells, striatum. The development of laminar and pseudolaminar cerebral cortex necroses is particularly important in ischemias (Fig. 79; cf. Table 7). The medical aspects of brain death and the determination of the time of death in connection with the clinical and morphological cerebral findings were comprehensively discussed by Angstwurm and Kugler (1978).

Vacuoles occur relatively frequently in the epithelia of the liver under the effects of hypoxidosis. These vacuoles are relatively sharply defined, of various sizes, and are located within the cytoplasm, mainly in a perinuclear position (Figs. 80, 81). The liver cells affected do not have any particular localization within the lobules. In severe cases, epithelia in the entire area of a section are almost uniformly affected, in addition to being necrobiotically altered. The vacuoles cannot be stained using the usual cellular and nuclear stains. To be certain of the finding, it is necessary to use a fat stain on a frozen section. Similar vacuoles can also appear in autolysis, but then they occur more as irregularly defined staining defects dispersed over the whole cytoplasm.

According to Ponsold (1961), the vacuoles are caused by an acute effect of hypoxidosis which is still reversible after elimination of the oxygen deficiency. The vacuoles can develop within 3–10 min. In acute hypoxidosis, the cell no longer possesses the energy that is necessary for water elimination. Vacuolar elimination of water within the cytoplasm occurs as a result of inhibition of dehydration. For further details of vacuole formation see Altmann (1944), Policard (1955), Löblich (1962), and Sykes et al. (1976).

We have also seen similar liver cell vacuoles in asthmatics who died of right ventricular failure following an asthmatic attack, and after internal hemorrhages, transfusion and anesthetic accidents, and intoxication of various kinds (carbon tetrachloride, HCN, trichloroethylene, barbiturates). Similar results could also be produced by sucrose injections in rats. These changes should be distinguished from hydropic swelling of the liver epithelia, with diffuse fluid uptake in both the nucleus and cytoplasm, which occasionally can also be observed after asphyxiation (Hambach 1958).

Studies on the submicroscopic structural changes in liver epithelia following

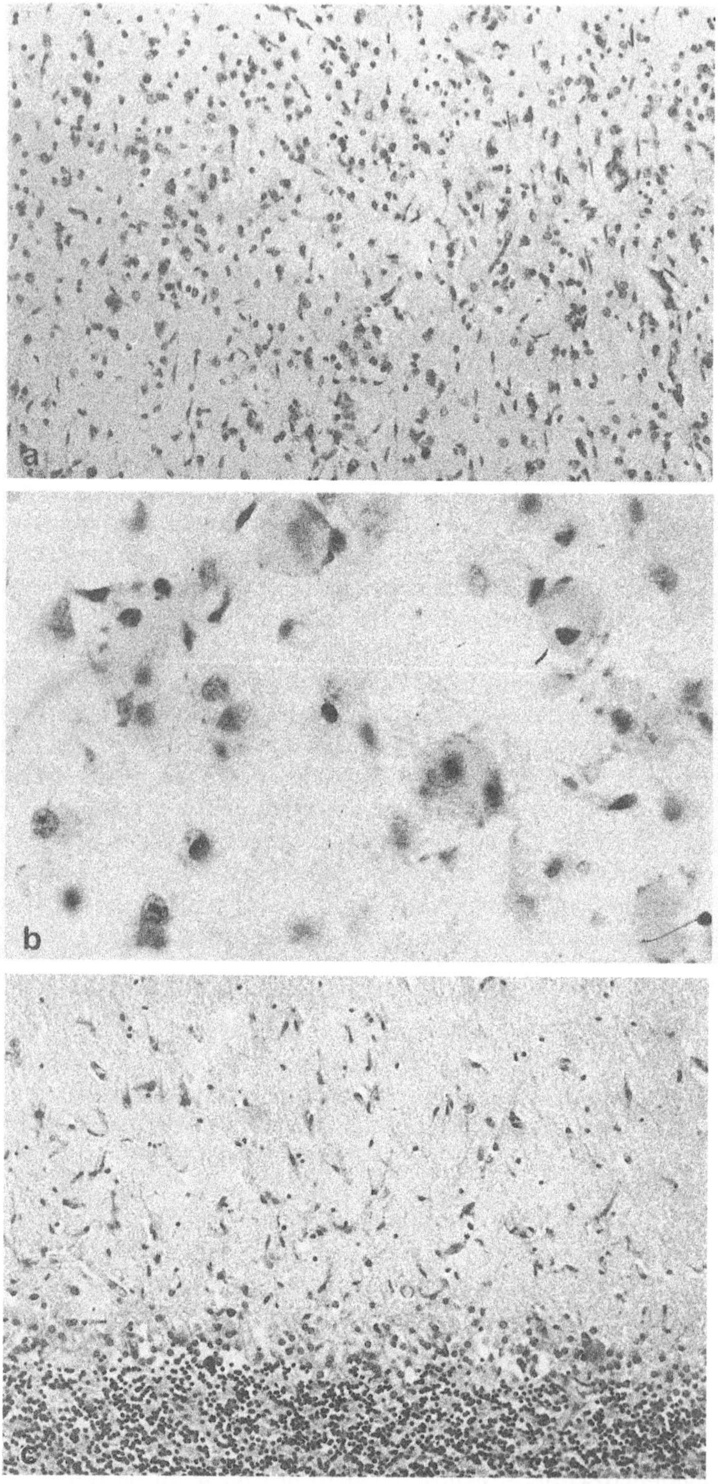

Fig. 78. a–c

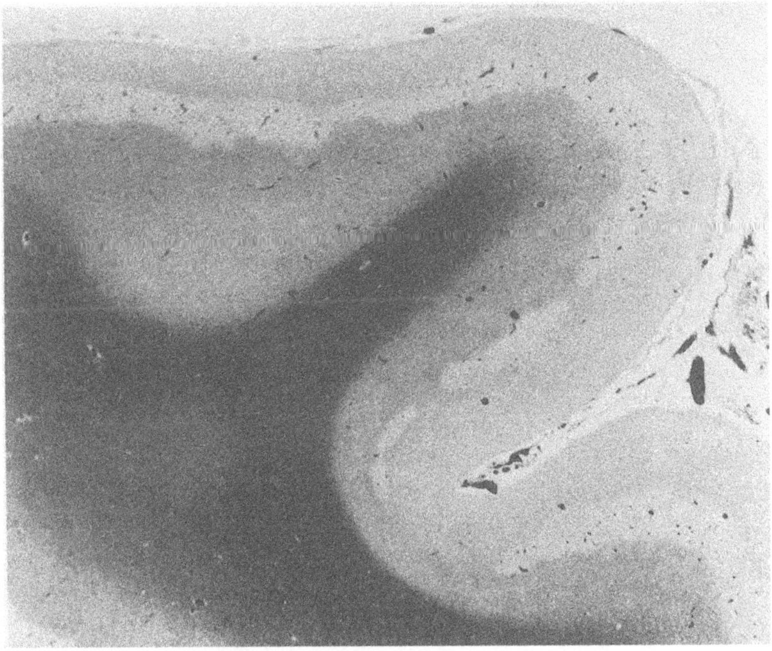

Fig. 79. Laminar cerebral cortex necrosis after post-traumatic loss of consciousness lasting for several weeks. (After Adebahr 1960)

Table 7. Summary of a few important lesion patterns in various forms of cerebral hypoxia and anoxia. (After Kunz 1980)

Form of hypoxia	Cause of hypoxia	Usual localization of hypoxic cerebral injury
Ischemic/oligemic hypoxidosis (short-term interruption or reduction in perfusion)	Cardiac-respiratory standstill, shock, loss of blood, hypotonia	Cerebral cortex, hippocampus, cerebellar cortex, corpus striatum
	Subclavian steal syndrome	Pons, cerebellar cortex, occipital cerebral cortex
Hypoxemic hypoxidosis (perfusion maintained)	Asphyxia, anemia, CO intoxication	Globus pallidus, nucleus dentatus
Nutritive hypoxidosis	Hypoglycemia	Neopallium, corpus striatum
Consumptive hypoxidosis	Epilepsy	Cerebral cortex, hippocampus, cerebellar cortex

◁ **Fig. 78. a** Anoxic damage to the brain. Cortex with early microglial reaction ("rod cells") and depletion of the ganglion cells. Subject survived 4 days. 1:250. **b** Anoxia of the thalamus. Ischemic ganglion cell necroses (so-called homogenizing change) with "microglial envelopment" (neuronophagia). (After Colmant 1965) Nissl's, 1:380. **c** Anoxic damage to the cerebellum. Microglial reaction in the stratum moleculare cerebelli (so-called bush) with destruction of the Purkinje cells. (After Colmant 1965) Nissl's, 1:220

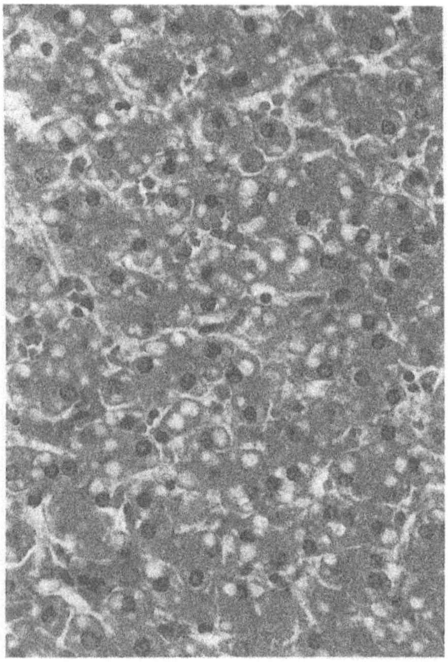

Fig. 80. Liver epithelia with perinuclear fatfree vacuoles. Death after repeated strangulation. Subject: 26 years old, ♀. H and E (control with Sudan stain negative), 1:220

general oxygen deficiency and temporary ischemia by Bade and Schumacher (1964) furnished the following results: 10 min after onset of the circulatory obstruction, changes in the cell membrane and vacuoles appeared. The vacuoles contained very fine well-contrasted elements such as iron and fat particles. It was not until after 30 min that tumefaction and changes in the shape of the mitochondria, swellings in the ergastoplasmic lamellae, clumping and marginal disposition of the chromatin, loss of glycogen, swelling of the endoplasmic reticulum, and ruptures in the cell membranes were seen. In the vacuoles, acid phosphatase could also be detected in the later stages. The vacuoles were more pronounced and the glycogen loss was greater with vascular ligature than with hypoxia from anoxemic blood. At the same time, bile secretion was very much reduced.

An increase in the number of cytolysomes and parenchymal changes occurred 1 h after 70-min hypoxemia, involving round and oval organelles, which contained degenerated cytoplasmic components and acid phosphatase. Later, an increase in the lysosomes, chiefly adjacent to the Golgi area and in the vicinity of the gallbladder capillaries, took place. Transformation of the cytopolysomes into lysosomes is understood to be a physiological phenomenon, which appears particularly clearly as a result of hypoxemic liver cell damage.

With reference to the literature, Bade and Schuhmacher (1964) think it probable that the vacuoles can transform into lysosomes. Following perfusion of the liver in dogs, rabbits, and cats, Schlütz (1954) also found vacuoles in the liver epithelia when the perfusion fluid was copiously admixed with oxygen. Liver cell vacuoles have also been observed in hypothermia and in fatal altitude anoxia. As a general explanation of the findings in humans and animal experiments, Schlütz (1954) sees

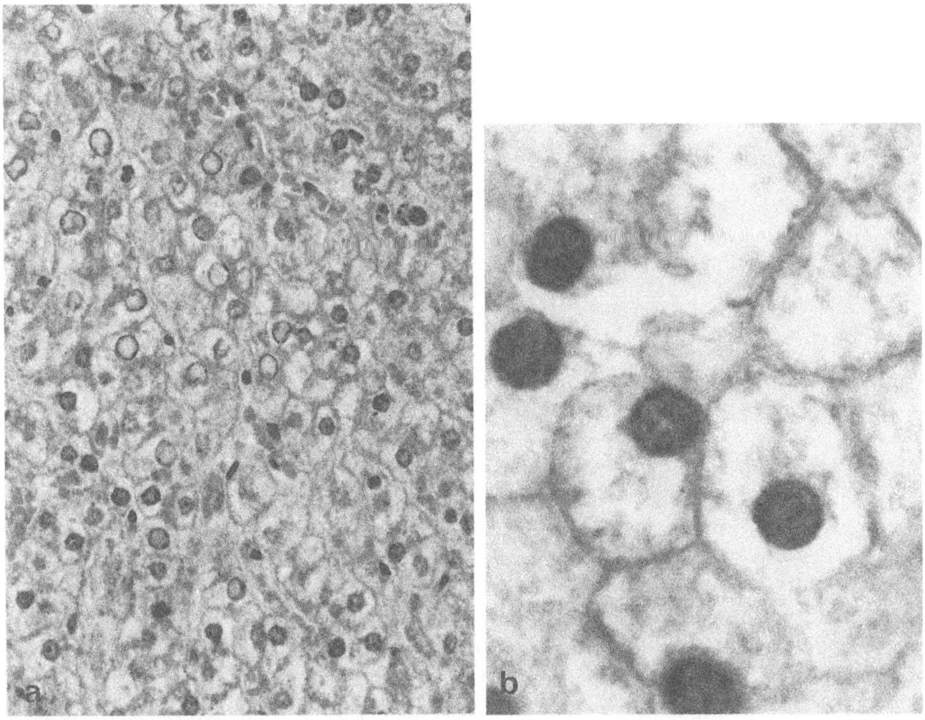

Fig. 81. a Severe protracted anoxic damage to the liver with diffuse epithelial vacuolization and necrobioses. Subject died after 24-h resuscitation, accident during anesthesia, 32 years old, ♂, H and E, 1:320. **b** Same finding as in **a**. 1:800

the cause of vacuolar liver cell degeneration as not being directly the oxygen deficiency, but the increase in carbon dioxide.

Histological-histochemical evidence of neutral fats in the liver epithelia of central lobular areas can be assessed as a general unspecific sign of fatty infiltration through hypoxemia (Sachs 1954). This kind of fatty infiltration has, however, also been found following states of hunger (Schlicht 1955). In oxygen deficiency experiments, peripheral and intermediary neutral fat deposition has also been determined in the liver.

Where death occurred after slow asphyxiation, e.g., burial under sand, we observed sporadic, homogeneous, rounded bodies in the liver epithelia with diameters of 2–4 μm, which displayed distinct primary and secondary fluorescence. These bodies were only weakly PAS-positive, slightly eosinophilic, and phosphatase-, glycogen-, and Sudan-negative. Under the phase-contrast microscope, they had a sharp, almost membranous boundary (Fig. 82) (Janssen 1969). Similar liver findings have been described in alcohol-induced damage (Reppart et al. 1963; Flax and Tisdale 1964; Biavia 1964), as microbodies following anoxia (Oudea 1963), as hyaline-droplet protein accumulation (Schlicht 1963), and as hyaline-droplet deposits, which are probably composed of hemoglobin and an expression of a disorder in the cellular permeability (Beneke and Scomazzoni 1962). The nature of such bodies

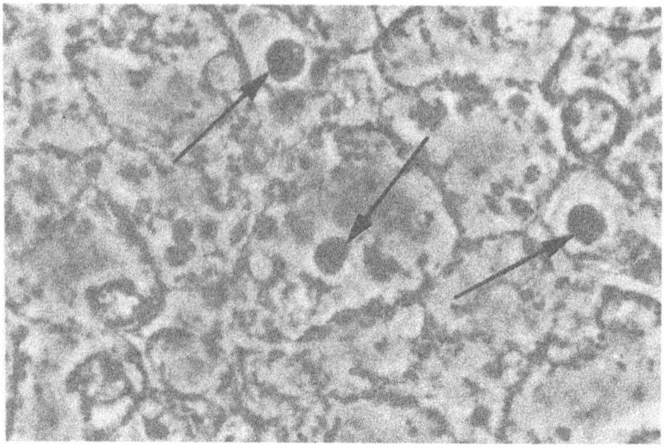

Fig. 82. Liver epithelia with hyaline bodies (↑). Protracted asphyxiation as a result of being buried alive. Subject: 12 years old, ♂. Phase contrast, 1:1000

consequently cannot be entirely explained. Their appearance in an otherwise undamaged liver and their absence in the case of chronic or acute hypoxemia gives these structures a peculiar status. In connection with other pertinent findings, they should be regarded as an indication of subacute oxygen deficiency.

In the cardiac musculature, which is very susceptible to oxygen deficiency, perinuclear unstained vacuoles can also be observed after a relatively short hypoxemia of 10–15 min. In longitudinal section, the cardiac muscle cells affected contain the vacuoles in the perinuclear cuneate space; in transversely cut cells, they are excentrically located in pronounced stages and the cardiac muscle cells may be transformed and take on hollow and cylindrical forms, particularly in central regions. The muscle cell nuclei are variable, sometimes slender, elongated, and pyknotic, sometimes hydropically swollen. The nuclei of the endomysium and intramyocardial perivascular connective tissue are loose and swollen. These changes effect a structural disaggregation of the cardiac muscle, which can progress to hydropic degeneration of the muscle cells.

In contrast, coarsening and condensation of the cardiac muscle cells with reduction in volume can also occur as a result of dehydration. Attenuation of the cardiac muscle fibers develops, which come to resemble so-called collapse cells. In addition, there is strong acidophilia; sometimes, there is also pronounced basophilia of the cardiac muscle cells; both present the picture of basophilic degeneration of cardiac muscle through the storage of basophilic material in the sarcoplasmic halo of the nuclei. The majority of lesions of this kind can be explained as hypoxemic hypoxidosis. The rare cases of substrate-deficiency hypoxidosis of the myocardium, as occur in insulin-hypoglycemia, are in principle similar, though there is a difference in localization. In hypoglycemia, necroses and their precursors are almost always found symmetrically distributed between the left and right ventricles, whereas in acute oxygen deficiency the left ventricle, and especially its inner layer, is clearly more affected than the right (Cain 1962). In experiments on dogs, ischemically damaged cardiac muscle sections could be detected by staining with hematoxylin, basic fuchsin, and picric acid (Cooper 1977). After anoxia for longer than 30 min, the heart muscle was irreversibly damaged.

Electron-microscopic studies on human myocardium showed in the mitochondria after 10–15 min of continuous hypoxia early decreases in the granules, reduction in the matrix density, and minimal alterations in the cristae. In addition, there was chromatin clumping at the nuclear membrane and general cellular edema up to dissociation of the intracellular structures (Burdette and Ashford 1965; Poche 1965). In animal experiments, early disappearance of the well-contrasted glycogen granules and edema of the capillary endothelia, with collapse of the vascular lumen and necroses in the adjacent muscular areas, have often been described (Vogell et al. 1964; Poche 1965; Haster 1964). Premedication with inorganic iodine and persantine led to an increased survival time of heart muscle cells following removal of oxygen and ATP degradation was clearly retarded (Vogell et al. 1964).

The comprehensive studies on oxygen deficiency in rats by Büchner and Onishi (1968) showed electron-microscopically detectable changes in the mitochondria of the heart muscle cells. After 30-min continuous respiration of 9% oxygen, swelling and dissolution of the cristae occurred. Following reduction of the oxygen portion, half of all mitochondria were extensively homogenized after 30 min. These changes are of great importance in the respiratory exchange of the cardiac muscle. The working principle of the cristae mitochondriales is to create in the smallest amount of space a large surface for the respiratory enzymes, respiratory-linked phosphorylation, and deoxidation in the citric acid cycle. These functions would be severely damaged by cristolysis, ligamentous homogenization of the cristae, and of course total homogenization of the mitochondria.

Under the effects of hypoxia, disappearance of the glycogen granules occurred very rapidly in conjunction with high-grade dehiscence of the intercalated discs and filling of the longitudinal fissure by a granular, flocculent, filamentous edema. In contrast to the findings of other authors, we found no visible damage to the capillary walls of heart muscle. According to Büchner and Onishi (1968), all changes in the fine structure of the cardiac muscle are subordinate to the degenerative changes of the mitochondria as a result of anoxic respiration or bleeding. Here, local structurally induced ischemias of the capillaries are of no importance. Histochemically, following acute anoxia in animal experiments, very distinct activation of succinooxidase and succinodehydrogenase could be observed in cardiac muscle, less so in the kidney; cerebral tissue reacted negatively (Wegmann et al. 1959). According to the animal experiments of Bajusz and Jasmin (1964), a histochemically detectable decrease in phosphorylase can be judged as an early indication of an anoxemic myocardial lesion. Spectrophotometric measurements of the enzyme activities of serum, liver, and heart extracts as well as determinations of isoenzymes by means of electrophoresis with diazonium salt revealed significant increases in the activities of S-LDH, S-CPK, and S-ALD. The electrophoretic separation results of GOT isoenzymes likewise showed a significant increase in GOTS and GOTM following asphyxiation. In contrast to oxygen deficiency damage, oxygen intoxication is thought to effect a rise in various enzyme reactions.

The occurrence of neutral fats in cardiac muscle cells is more indicative of chronic anoxic conditions. This finding has to be distinguished from brown atrophy and lipofuscinosis. In severe, atmospherically induced hypoxia, the fatty infiltration

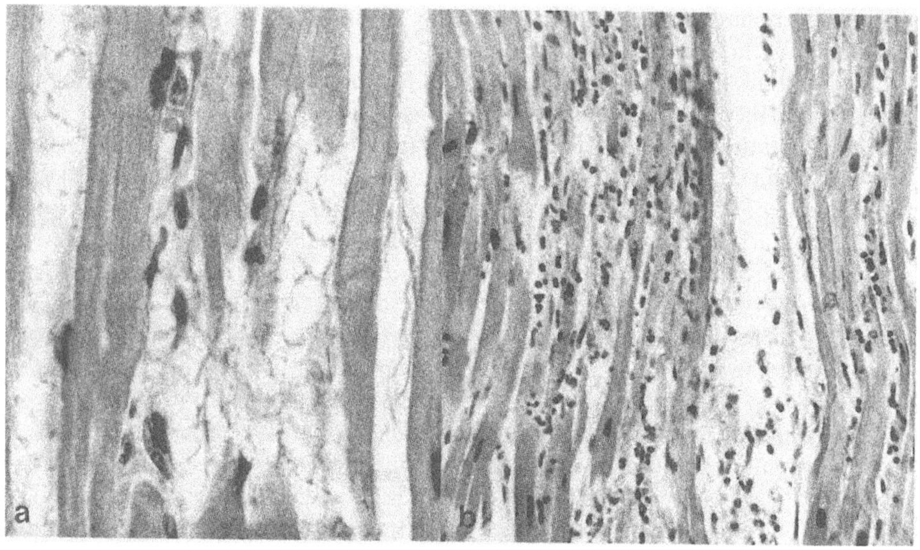

Fig. 83a, b. Circumscribed vacuolar cardiac muscle necroses, partially showing an inflammatory-resorptive reaction. Subject died after 14-h resuscitation, accident in the course of anesthesia, 32 years old, ♂. H and E, 1:300, 1:180

of the myocardium can be similar to that in advanced chronic anemia; connected with this occurrence are disseminated cardiac muscle necroses (Fig. 83), associated with the venous supply area of the cardiac muscle capillaries (Büchner 1970).

In the lungs of acutely or subacutely asphyxiated humans, an acute substantial (vesicular) emphysema is histologically found in most cases. With the appropriate previous damage, this may be in connection with a chronic emphysema. In addition, there is frequently an interstitial emphysema, particularly in young people, with bullous emphysematous expansion in the marginal areas of the lungs. Along with pronounced acute congestion, interstitial and alveolar hemorrhages are also found, which can occupy large sections of pulmonary tissue.

Evidence of an edema as, e.g., produced in animal experiments by Wagner (1966), fits in less well with the primary clinical picture of an asphyxiated lung. In the case of protracted suffocation with gradual failure of the left ventricle, an edema in the region of the pulmonary circulation would be feasible. B. Mueller (1953) and Lange and Latta (1963) previously pointed out such a possibility. In newborn rats, the more frequently occurring pulmonary edema following anoxia was attributed to the physiologically greater permeability of the capillaries in the lungs (Seller and Spector 1964). After repeated oxygen deficiency, Löblich (1962) detected a broadening of the alveolocapillary membrane, including the basal membrane, which attained its greatest extent on day 21 of the experiment. These findings are interpreted as an interstitial edema. The cause of these changes, which on the whole occurred under moderate reduction of oxygen tension, was probably irritation of the terminal vascular system with cytoplasmic edema.

Following slow asphyxiation in four young people who had previously had healthy lungs, we observed abnormal migrations of cells and giant-cell formation in

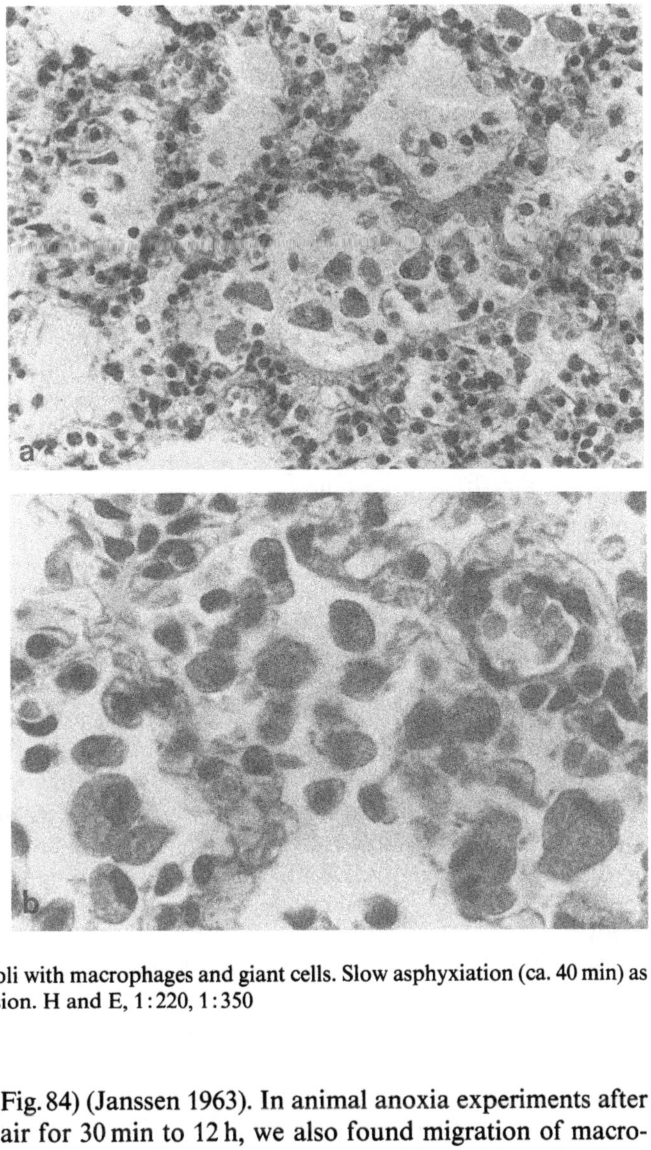

Fig. 84 a, b. Pulmonary alveoli with macrophages and giant cells. Slow asphyxiation (ca. 40 min) as a result of thoracic compression. H and E, 1:220, 1:350

the alveoli of the lungs (Fig. 84) (Janssen 1963). In animal anoxia experiments after graduated exclusion of air for 30 min to 12 h, we also found migration of macrophages with transition to polynuclear giant cells (Janssen and Bärtschi 1964). Histochemically, a weakening of the normally strong phosphatase and lipase reaction could be detected following long asphyxiation leading to death. The distinct form of the cellular changes in the edematic regions of the lungs was particularly remarkable when the animals were not dissected until 12 h after killing by oxygen exclusion. The occurrence of alveolar phagocytes in the edematous pulmonary regions of drowned animals was also observed by Swann (1964). Reh (1969) reported giant cells in the lungs of slowly asphyxiated humans.

The results concerning phagocytic giant cells induced in animal experiments essentially concur with the findings in slowly asphyxiated humans. The cells apparently develop as the last stage of the reaction mechanism caused by oxygen deficiency. Here, it appeared to be important that the oxygen exclusion was continued until death by suffocation and that the macrophage migration with transition to polynuclear giant cells continued after general organ death. This could be recognized when comparing animals dissected immediately after death with those examined later. Induced by the oxygen deficiency, carbon dioxide oversaturation, and the creation of an acidic environment, mobilization of the macrophages continued after the onset of death. Very similar findings were observed by Sedláček and Mráz (1978) in experiments on phagocytosis of India ink in rabbit lungs: 15–30 min postmortem a clear increase in the macrophages of the alveoli occurred by means of mitotic division. Histological evidence in the lungs following oxygen deficiency can thus to a substantial extent also be formed by a supravital reaction.

The cause of the macrophage reactions in the lungs in animal experiments is protracted (subacute) oxygen deficiency with its sequelae and concomitant symptoms. Of course, care should be taken when performing such animal experimental studies to ensure that the changes are not caused by simple reactions to foreign bodies or infections, especially since despite all precautionary measures, infections involving giant cell reactions in the lungs are not so uncommon in smaller laboratory animals.

The development of polynuclear giant cells in pulmonary tissue following oxygen deficiency should not be taken as a degenerative or resorptive reaction but as a process of adaptation. The cell attempts to cope with the more difficult conditions of increasing oxygen deficiency by enlargement of the nuclear surface and amitotic division, which unlike mitosis does not interrupt the cell's performance (Letterer 1959; Wohlgemuth 1962). The relatively short developmental period is explained by the special reactive tendency of this mononuclear phagocyte system (MPS), which should be considered as a unit (Bargmann 1935; Bertalanffy and Leblund 1953; Köberle 1956; Wurm 1956; Bowden 1971). Very similar histological findings develop in the lungs through various finely dispersed foreign bodies and aerosols after considerably longer exposure times (Spector 1974; Evans et al. 1978; Gebbers et al. 1979).

The initial sequelae and damage of subacute oxygen deficiency are at first confined to the cells themselves. It is only later, in our experiments not until after death, that leakage of liquid occurs, which has an increased influence on the cellular changes (cf. Gieseking 1958, 1959; Lange 1909). This sequence supports the interpretation of Büchner (1937, 1942, 1944, 1950, 1957), according to which the primary consequences of hypoxidosis occur in the cell itself, without the influx of blood protein. Conversely, in advanced stages, the findings in the lungs correspond more to the views of Rössle (1944), Policard (1955), Eppinger (1935), and Erich (1956), according to which the damage caused by hypoxidosis can be compared with a serous inflammation. *Following the exclusion of natural possibilities of development, such findings in the lungs of otherwise healthy people represent a practical indication of death by slow asphyxiation.*

The occurrence of intracellular vacuoles is less common in the kidneys after oxygen deficiency than in the liver and cardiac muscle. In addition, difficulties arise in distinguishing them from early autolytic changes in the epithelia of the tubuli. After 14 days hypoxia, a rise in the granulation index could be observed in the juxtaglomerular cells (Oliver and Brody 1965). This process is thought to be connected with an increase in renin formation. Montaldo and Ferrelli (1964) observed in the electron microscope an increased occurrence of vesicles with a diameter of 100 nm in the endothelia of the glomerular capillaries. Otherwise, following oxygen deficiency, the kidneys showed signs of circulatory impairment and transudation with interstitial edema just as all other organs.

Following protracted oxygen deficiency, uncharacteristic changes with increased erythropoiesis and a shift toward the production of immature erythrocytes can be observed in the medullary and extramedullary formation of blood (Saathoff 1950). In consequence of violent respiratory movements in subacute or slow asphyxiation, rupture of muscle fibers and ceraceous degeneration can occur in the musculature of the diaphragm. This is a finding which can also be determined in various forms of poisoning and severe general disorders (Szabò 1940).

It is relatively seldom that conditions of general hypoxia, which lead to necroses of larger groups of cells and tissue regions in a single or several organs, can be survived by an individual. If, however, this does occur, other kinds of injury persist, e.g., defective states arising from carbon monoxide poisoning with cicatricial and cystoid cavity formation, particularly in the brain. Such findings do not have a specific significance for oxygen-deficiency damage.

The histological evidence indicative of oxygen-deficiency damage or death through asphyxiation may be summarized as follows:

1. Fat-free, especially perinuclear, cytoplasmic vacuoles in epithelia of the liver and in cardiac muscle cells, to a lesser extent in epithelia of the renal tubuli.
2. Swelling of endothelial cells in the capillaries of the brain and cardiac muscle.
3. Mobilization and proliferation of alveolar macrophages, occasionally with the formation of polynuclear giant cells (only applicable in healthy lungs).
4. Precipitation of hyaline droplets in epithelia of the liver.
5. Circumscribed hemorrhages in the lungs and brain.
6. Ganglion cell degeneration with shrinking, pyknosis, and disappearance of the Nissl substance, especially in the gyrus hippocampus.
7. Acute alveolar and interstitial pulmonary emphysema, acute vascular congestion of the inner organs – only as a general supplementary finding.
8. As far as possible, electron-microscopic determination of swelling or dissolution of the cristae mitochondriales, chiefly in liver and cardiac muscle cells, and depletion of glycogen.

IV. Shock

1. Fundamentals and General Histomorphology

Clinical and pathoanatomical research of shock has, especially in the last 20 years, yielded new findings which have been important in elucidating causes of death. From the forensic point of view, histologically detectable evidence that testifies to previous shock has particular bearing if the case history and detailed circumstances of the death are not known.

States of shock are caused by very diverse injuries, e.g., traumatization, burns, blood loss, intoxication, infection, heart failure. The pathological mechanisms involved are predominantly impairment in the microcirculation of the terminal vascular system, alteration of the blood coagulability, and disturbance of the tissue oxygen supply. These factors substantially influence the tissue effects of shock. Findings associated with shock are not modern phenomena, but their frequency has clearly increased due to the consequences of advances in intensive care and the greater chance of survival.

A uniform mode of action thus underlies shock-induced tissue damage. The manifestation of the individual components is basically determined by quantitative and chronological factors. Shock becomes clinically irreversible if the oxygen debt of the organism exceeds 120 ml/kg body weight (Guyton and Cromwell 1961). Certain tissue damage can be correlated with this "point of no return." Factors influencing the outcome of the histological examination are the time of examination in the course of shock, the organ examined, the animal species in experimental studies, and, to a certain extent, the kind of shock. The findings are pronounced in varying degrees in the individual organs, such that it is possible to refer to "shock organs", which tend to be affected most by the damage from the shock. In humans, chiefly the lungs, kidneys, and intestines are regarded as shock organs. The primary damage to an individual organ, which consequently becomes the starting point of universal shock, has to be conceptually distinguished from these shock organs. An example of this is acute pancreatitis, which generally induces severe shock. The very comprehensive literature, which also has to be considered in evaluating histological evidence, can here only be reflected in examples and summaries: Hardaway et al. (1961, 1965, 1966, 1967), Sandritter (1966, 1967), M. Schneider (1963, 1964, 1967), Robb (1965), Lederer and Mittermayer (1967), Lasch et al. (1966, 1967, 1971), Beneke (1970), Seifert (1970), Remmele et al. (1971, 1973), Lutz (1972), Rolffs et al. (1972), Umbach (1971), and Heene and Lasch (1977).

A general basic finding is impairment of the blood flow in the organs affected. The arterioles, capillaries, and venules are distended and generally engorged with blood. In the lumina of the terminal vascular system, aggregation of erythrocytes occurs, which is frequently linked with thrombocytic accumulation, i.e., sludging. Such changes in the vascular contents, which are still reversible, lead to homogeneous packed columns of blood (rouleaux) in the sinusoids of the liver (Gelin and Shoemaker 1961) and in the capillaries of the intestines, kidneys, and brain. Care should be taken in distinguishing them from postmortem intravascular homogenization of blood, e.g., in the region of hypostases. Differentiation with azan or Lepehne's stain is recommended in such cases.

The endothelial cells of blood vessels react quickly to the effects of shock. In animal experiments, there were numerous endothelial cells in the circulating blood 15 min after onset of endotoxin shock and an increase in DNA synthesis of the endothelial cells could be observed as a sign of active regeneration. In the hours that followed, severe defects to the endothelial cells occurred with cytoplasmic protrusions, crater formation, degenerative changes to the organelles, lacerations of the plasma membrane, and thrombocyte aggregates at the intima, probably to cover the damage (Freudenberg 1977, 1978). The highest proliferative quotients were found in the vascular endothelia of the pulmonary veins, capillaries of the lung and kidney, and sinusoids of the liver (Witte 1978). Thrombogenesis of the detached endothelia, which were charged with blackish granules, was observed by Fazekas (1965).

Following states of shock, the observed damage to the tunica media of coronary arteries is probably connected with states of collapse and sustained hypertonia. Histologically, this involves necroses with encroachment on to the intima, occasionally even with disruption of the vascular wall or formation of parietal thrombi. In animal experiments, this process was interpreted as anoxic trophopathy of the muscle cells in the media and intimal cushions of muscular arteries (Faria 1962, 1963). In organs with loose periadventitial tissue, pronounced perivascular edema almost always occurs.

A very important finding for the histological diagnosis of shock is the occurrence of hyaline globules and thrombi in the terminal vascular system (Figs. 85, 86). The structures termed shock bodies ("globular clots") are rounded, sometimes oval, red, and up to 200 µm in size; they are generally surrounded by a protein coat, which often shows a halolike, fibrillar, radial pattern. They stain in an identical manner to hemoglobin and are probably composed of aggregated fibrin degradation products (Harms 1971 a). In our experience, they have a distinct primary fluorescence. Shock bodies probably develop intravascularly by the increased release of serotonine.

The development of microthrombi, which are also designated as hyaline thrombi, is connected with an increase in activity of the coagulation system. Hardaway (1961) termed this system a disseminated intravascular coagulation syndrome. The equilibrium between thrombogenesis and thrombus dissolution, described as latent coagulation by Lasch, is thereby disturbed. The circulatory disorder in the terminal vascular system makes a substantial causal contribution to hypercoagulability. Disseminated intravascular coagulation does not involve the simultaneous appearance of fibrinous thrombi in all vessels of the human organism; many organs are often unaffected. Harms and Lehmann (1969) found such microthrombi in 47% of cases after clinically established shock. They were most frequent, up to 88% of cases, in endotoxin shock (Remmele and Harms 1968). Multiple intracapillary fibrin throm-

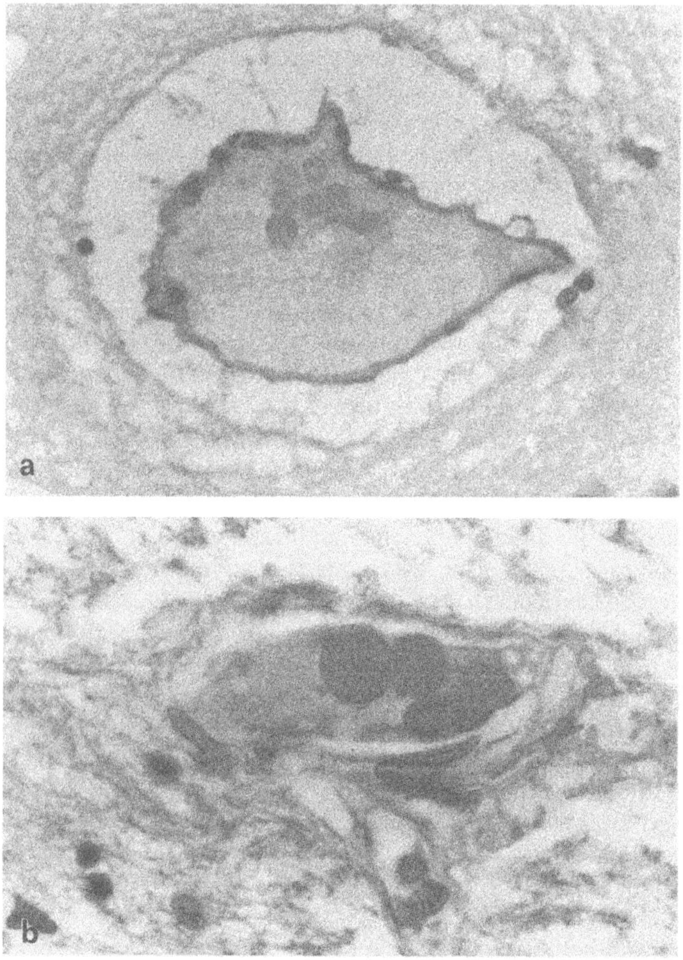

Fig. 85. a Severely dilated cerebral capillary with multiple shock bodies, sludging, and perivascular edema. H and E, 1:280. **b** Cerebral capillary with large shock bodies and swelling of the endothelial cells. H and E, 1:320

bi were also detected following 13 fatal cases of hypobaryopathy (Nayak et al. 1964).

Hyaline thrombi are seen electron microscopically and histochemically to be composed of thrombocytes and fibrin (Bohler and Bibighaus 1967; Prose et al. 1965; Lapp 1971). In about 35% of all fatal cases of shock with microthrombi, they are evident in the liver, predominantly in the sinusoids, central veins, and branches of the hepatic veins (Beneke 1970 – references). More recent studies (e.g., Remmele and Goebel 1973) have revealed that the tendency is greater in the lungs, with 27.1% of all cases; less affected by microthrombosis were the kidneys with 15.2% and the liver with 17.1%. The differences in the data concerning the frequency of microthrombi in shock are probably explained by varying duration of survival and different postmortem times of examination. After longer periods of survival, part of the

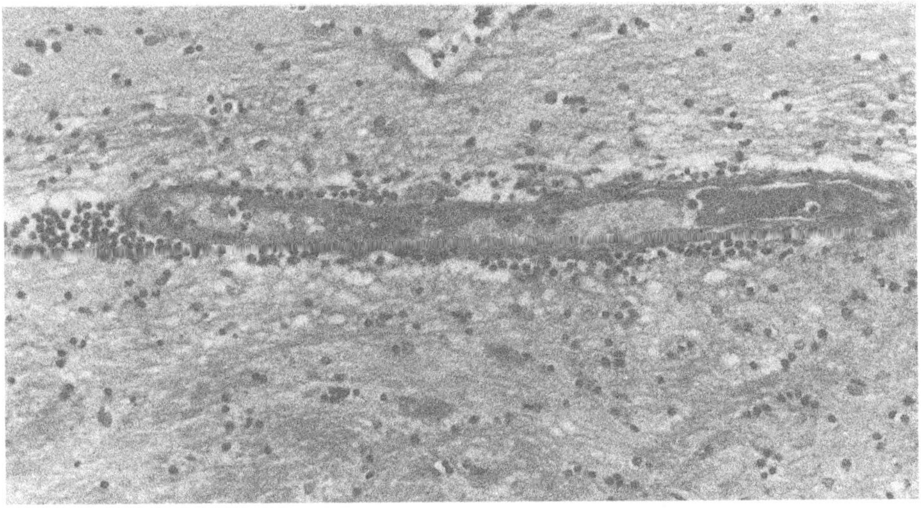

Fig. 86. Cerebral arteriole with fibrin thrombus, sludging, and perivascular round cell infiltration. Subject survived 6 days, 77 years old, ♂, automobile accident. H and E, 1:220

intravascular coagulum can be eliminated by fibrinolysis. The same also occurs with longer postmortem periods through postmortem fibrinolysis (Harms 1971 a). This diagnostically important finding can thus be lost by delayed autopsy, a circumstance which clearly underlines the necessity of an early postmortem examination.

The microthrombi are best stained by the PAS reaction, the trichrome stain according to Goldner, PTAH, and, in particular, the staining method according to Ladewig, a modification of the Mallory-Heidenhain method. It is possible with Ladewig's stain for the fibrin to appear bright red and be clearly differentiated from the orange-colored erythrocytes. The granular portion of the microthrombi originating from the blood platelets is stained blue. The shock bodies also take on an intense blue color (Harms 1971). Care should be taken in differentiating microthrombi of intravital origin from coagula developed postmortem (Boyd 1967; Remmele and Harms 1968). In this regard, the recognition of postmortem hemolysis with hyalinization of the vascular contents is important, as is the absence of fibrin precipitation. Microthrombi of intravital origin consist of long fibers parallel to the vascular wall and bloodstream. They are compact and sometimes straddle small vascular bifurcations. In the case of survival, the thrombi become organized in a fibrous manner (Fig. 87); they can later be detected as so-called Siegmund's nodules.

Reticulohistiocytary cells have particular importance in the course of shock. Their effect is dependent on whether the microcirculatory impairment is irreversible or whether it can be surmounted. Reticulohistiocytary cells eliminate from the blood by phagocytosis the coagulative substances activated in shock. In model experiments, Spaet (1962) was able to demonstrate this faculty of the RHS on Kupffer's cells: following injections of thrombokinase into the portal vein, defibrination of the blood failed to occur, whereas the same quantity injected into the aorta did give rise to defibrination. It was possible to demonstrate with radioactively labeled thrombokinase that Kupffer's cells effect the elimination of activated clotting sub-

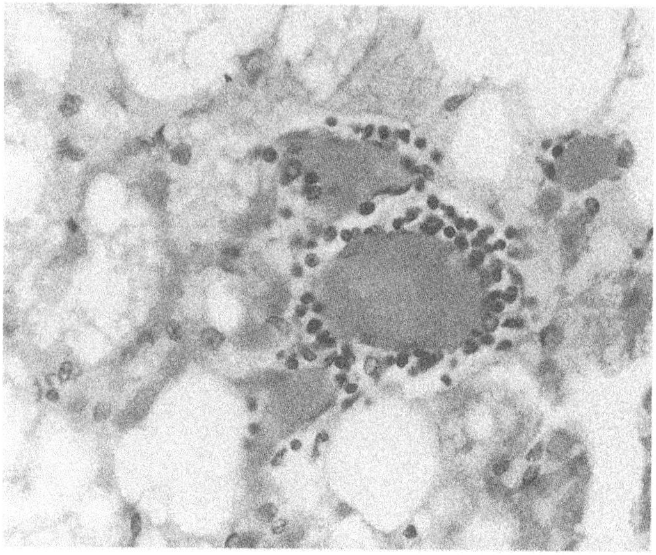

Fig. 87. Cellular disintegration of microthrombi in the capillaries of the mesentery. Burn shock. Subject survived 4 days. H and E, 1:280

stances from the blood in the manner of clearance. Kief and Vitak (1971) were able to show in experimentally induced coagulative shock on rat livers that liver cells also perform a similar function in peripheral sections of the lobules. This is indicated by intracellular evidence of fibrinogen, fibrin monomers, and fibrin. Similar results have been found following hemorrhagic shock and after bilateral high ligature of the lower extremities.

Specific measurements of RHS functions have demonstrated that the phagocytic capacity of these cells is clearly curtailed in various forms of shock. This restriction in function is caused by a whole chain of reactions, set in motion by the slowing of the circulation and insufficient blood supply. Kupffer's cells are already swollen shortly after the onset of shock. They detach themselves from their tissue structure and become necrotic, such that the number available for phagocytosis is reduced. In addition, the stellate cells have to deal with phagocytosis of lipids, the level of which is increased during shock. Experimentally, following endotoxin injections, an increase of the lipids in the serum and, simultaneously, a breakdown of the depot fat could be observed (Kovats et al. 1961). This process was seen histologically to lead to fatty infiltration of the stellate cells. The reduction in phagocytic capacity indirectly promotes the increased intravascular tendency to coagulate in the peripheral circulation. Thus the circulatory disorder, at first only functional, becomes a fixed anatomical feature. In states of shock induced by infections, bacterial elimination is negatively influenced by damage to the RHS cells. In this manner, bacillemia can be transformed into sepsis through the effects of shock (Adebahr 1971).

In many states of shock, the intensified activation of the coagulation system in the peripheral circulation leads, via a rapid consumption of thrombocytes and clotting factors, to an acute tendency to hemorrhage. These hemorrhages arising from consumption coagulopathy (Lasch 1959; Lasch et al. 1961, 1963, 1966, 1967, 1971) can appear at very diverse sites in the human organism, sometimes specifically in the vicinity of microthrombi. Histologically, we observed these shock-induced hemorrhages predominantly in the lungs, brain, and adrenal glands. The differentiation and presentation of a "microembolism syndrome" (Saldeen 1972) is not necessary in the light of present understanding of shock; the reasons for this are evident in the shock pathogenesis.

The effects of shock on the parenchymal cells of affected organs are largely caused by the reduction in blood flow. Histologically, these effects are largely identical to hypoxic lesions; thus far, the early morphological changes can essentially only be detected in animal experiments by electron-microscopic observation. They affect all parts of the cell and, like oxygen-deficiency damage, are reversible in their initial stages. Following hemorrhagic shock, the mitochondria in rat livers were swollen and rounded. However, disorders in the enzyme systems of energy production, e.g., oxidative phosphorylation, could not be determined (De Palma et al. 1970). The mitochondria of the liver proved to be resistant to shock hypoxia in the early stages.

A longer state of shock, lasting continuously for about 10 h, can lead to clinically and histologically detectable cell and tissue damage (Bywaters 1948; Ellenberg and Osserman 1951; Wilson et al. 1938). It is possible that autoantibodies against DNA appearing in the blood serum during shock contribute to the formation of parenchymal necroses (Nick and Dodd 1967; Nick 1968). Specific histological necrotic findings which morphologically indicate shock as the causative factor have so far not been in evidence.

2. Specific Organ Findings in Shock

Lungs. The frequency and expression of findings concerning pulmonary damage due to shock have been particularly influenced by the development of modern intensive care. The shock lung syndrome is an acute disorder of the lung parenchyma, which in healing leads to pulmonary fibrosis. It is determined by impairment of the following functions – microcirculation of the lungs, change in the permeability at the alveolar wall, and change in the surfactant system of the alveoli (Wichert and Riesner 1977). Other lung parenchymal disorders with a similar course and comparable histomorphology are paraquat poisoning, bromium carbamite intoxication, and the bleomycin lung (Mittermayer et al. 1972). Similar findings in the lungs also arise following sustained perfusion or resuscitation (Baer and Osborn 1960; Veith et al. 1968; Webster and Blum 1972).

Histological examination of the shock lung provides characteristic findings, which, however, do not in themselves prove a shock etiology (Hardaway et al. 1967). In the initial phase of shock, a pronounced interstitial and intra-alveolar edema occurs, with dilation of the perivascular lymph vessels and widening of the interalveolar connective tissue; in addition, there is high-grade vascular congestion, circumscribed escape of erythrocytes, and atelectasis. In states of shock that were survived for long periods of time, the interstitial edema was superimposed by increasing activation of the local connective tissue cells and the occurrence of monocytic cells. In-

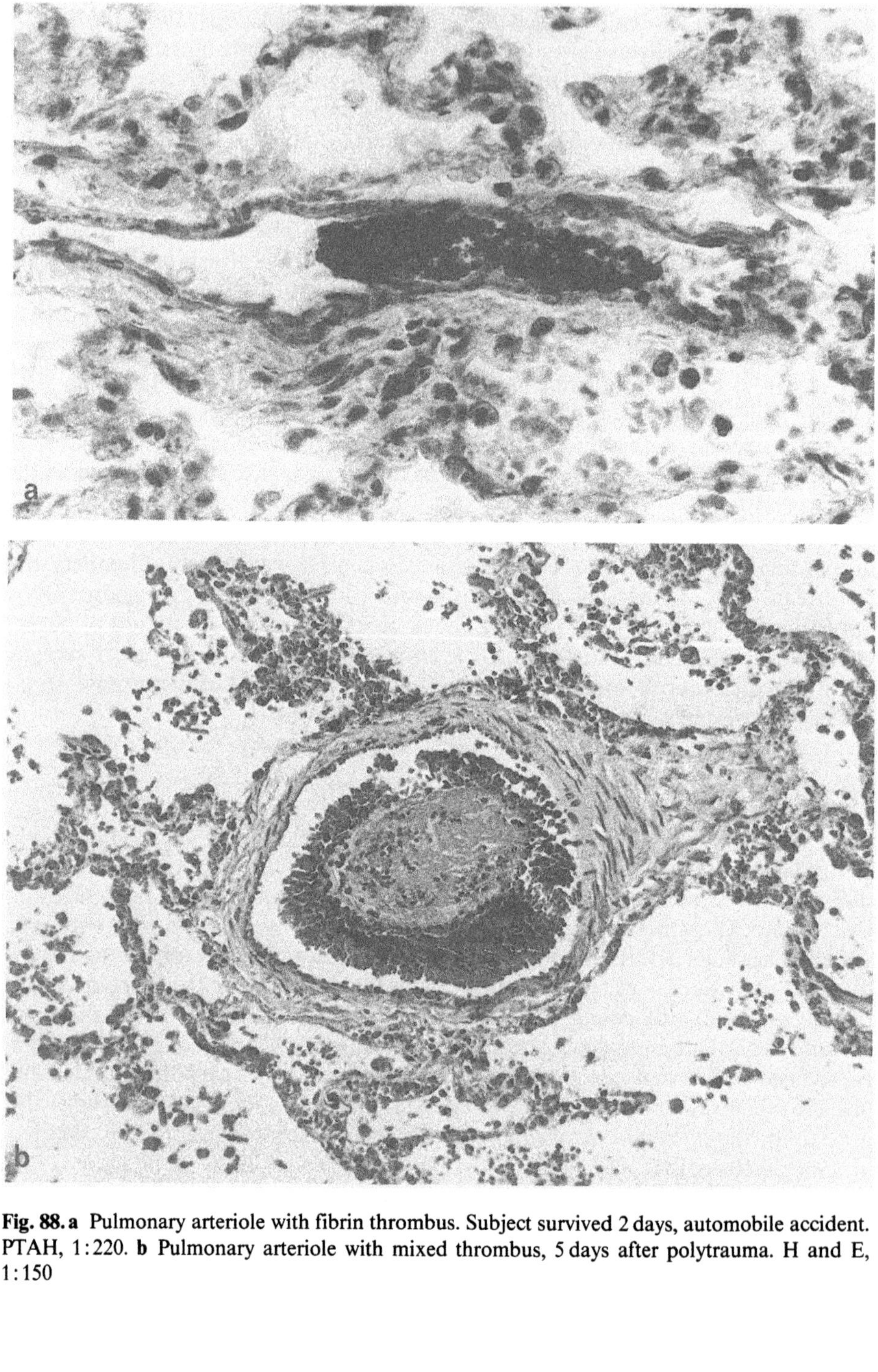

Fig. 88. a Pulmonary arteriole with fibrin thrombus. Subject survived 2 days, automobile accident. PTAH, 1:220. **b** Pulmonary arteriole with mixed thrombus, 5 days after polytrauma. H and E, 1:150

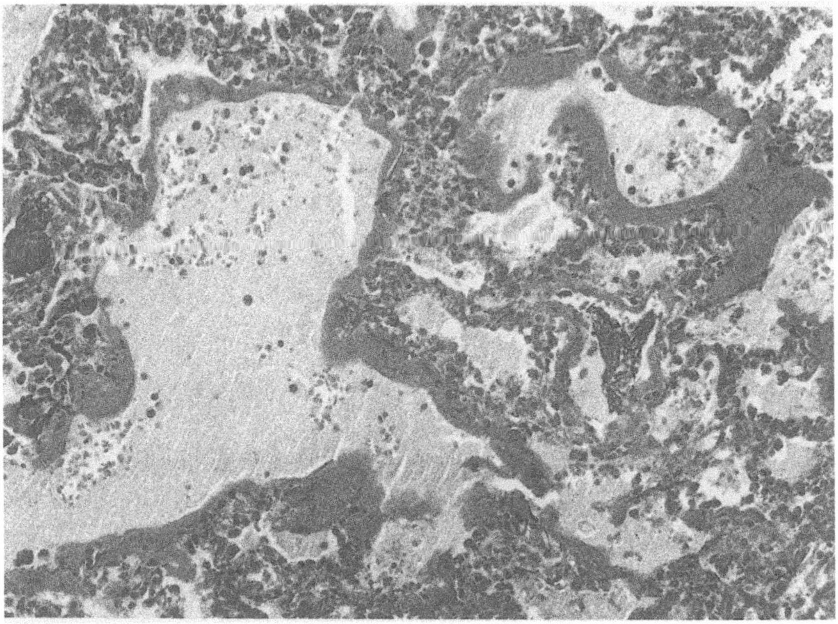

Fig. 89. Typical hyaline membranes of the lung after protracted shock; subject received intensive artificial respiration. Subject survived 12 days, 15 years old, ♀. PTAH, 1:220

travascular precipitation of the characteristic fibrinous coagulum occurs approximately at the same time as the beginning of the regionally confined atelectasis (Fig. 88); it is the result of a shock-induced generalized hypercoagulability of the plasma with disseminated intravascular clotting. According to Remmele and Goebel (1973 – references), over 27% of all fatal cases of shock are affected by this.

The formation of pulmonary hyaline membranes and their connection with shock were extensively clarified in studies by the group around Bleyl (1969, 1970, 1971 a). According to them, the membrane syndrome of neonates develops from asphyxial circulation shock (Dawes 1961, 1966), elicited in utero and continuing perinatally, with hypercoagulability of the plasma, using up of coagulation factors, and subsequent microthrombus formation. Intrauterine asphyxiation with "inadequate capillary perfusion" (Hardaway 1966) can thus not only lead to intravascular polymerization of fibrin monomers and coagula, but, under additional conditions of pulmonary hyperperfusion, also to extravasation of plasmatic fibrin monomers and extravascular polymerization to pulmonary hyaline membranes (Fig. 89). Hitherto, the hyaline membrane syndrome in neonates has been basically attributed to a congenital deficiency of antiatelectase factor (surfactant) in the lungs (Campiche 1963; Grünwald 1963; Reynolds and Strang 1966). This is a lipoprotein with dipalmitoyllecithin and sphingomyelin, which as a substance active on the interface of the intra-alveolar interior surface prevents collapse of the pulmonary alveoli in expiration. The causes of antiatelectase factor deficiency in neonates have largely been attributed to pulmonary immaturity (Reynolds and Strang 1966; Benzer et al. 1969). Typical hyaline membranes have also been detected in the lungs of adults following

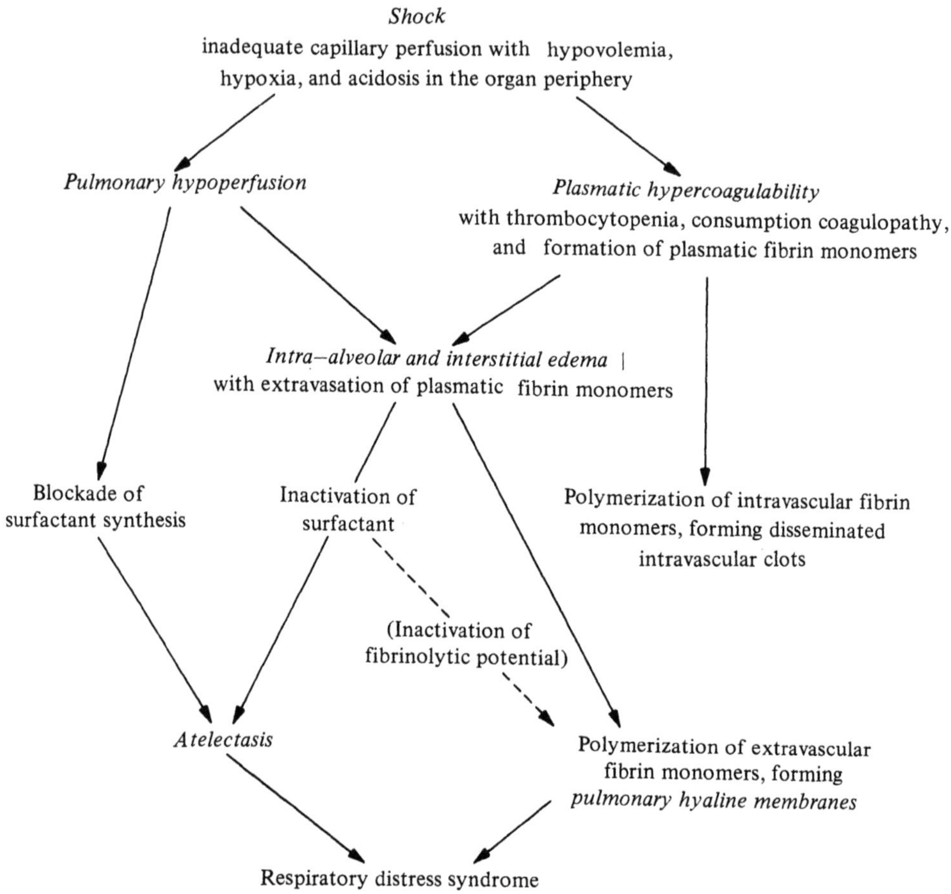

Fig. 90. Pathogenesis of respiratory distress syndrome as a result of shock with the formation of pulmonary hyaline membranes. (After Bleyl 1970)

variously induced states of shock (e.g., Bleyl 1970); the majority tended to be found in the bronchioli terminales, just as in neonates. The membranes occurred in combination with intra-alveolar and interstitial edema. Chiefly affected were the subpleural regions of the lungs. The blockade of surfactant synthesis can also be explained in view of identical histological findings and evidence of similar pathogenic mechanisms in the formation of hyaline membranes as a result of shock in adults and neonates (Bleyl 1970). The lungs in respiratory distress syndrome with hyaline membranes in neonates can thus be considered shock lungs as a parallel to the "respiratory distress syndrome" in adults (Fig. 90). The connections between changes in the lungs following artificial respiration with pure oxygen and mechanical positive pressure respiration have been pointed out by Northway et al. (1967) and Nolte (1968).

The development of post-traumatic shock lung syndrome has also recently been registered in continuous biopsy studies (Schlag et al. 1980). According to them, posttraumatic progressive lung failure without direct pulmonary trauma can be di-

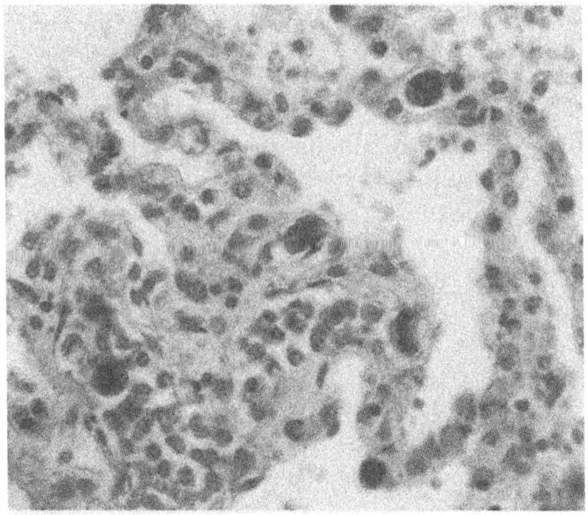

Fig. 91. Multiple megakaryocytes in the pulmonary capillaries in post-traumatic shock survived for 4 days. H and E, 1:250

vided into two main phases: (1) Early changes – massive leukostasis of polymorphonuclear granulocytes in the pulmonary circulation, swellings of the endothelial cells, fat globuli, and the onset of interstitial edema. (2) After 24–72 h, the actual shock lung or fat embolism syndrome occurs with pronounced interstitial edema and subsequent fibrosis, considerable changes in the alveolar epithelium, and increased occurrence of phagocytozing macrophages in the alveoli. The much-feared fibrosis of the lungs, which usually leads to death, can sometimes be reversible. The absence of previous lung conditions and intact alveolar basal membranes are among the preconditions for ascertainment by biopsy (Hassenstein et al. 1980).

In differentiating postmortem shock lungs from normal lungs, the weight of the lungs has been particularly considered as a diagnostic criterion and has been supplemented by histological, morphometric, and biochemical investigations (Joachim et al. 1978). Normal lungs had an average weight of 234 g; after the effects of shock for 1 week, the lungs had an average weight of 774 g. The maximum weight was 1124 g. The correlating histological findings were chiefly determined by the interstitial edema.

Evidence of megakaryocytes with a naked nucleus in the capillaries of the alveolar septa is a finding in the lungs following death from shock which occurs in roughly one case in three (Fig. 91) (Remmele and Goebel 1972). This probably involves a bone marrow reaction elicited by shock-induced hypoxidosis.

In cases where a pulmonary edema is already present, the occurrence of shock is thought to have a favorable effect. Such observations in humans could be confirmed in animal experiments by the beneficial influence of formalin shock on artificially produced pulmonary edema (Szám 1967).

Liver. In the liver parenchyma, shock damage is chiefly manifest in two forms of cellular necroses, which can also appear as stages in the course of a disease: disseminated individual and group necroses, or centrolubular necroses. The former are distributed diffusely in the hepatic lobules without any recognizable systematic pattern. The latter are induced by "light zonal degeneration;" this involves edema of the liver epithelia, loss of cytoplasmic basophilia, and reduced stainability with eosin. Occasionally, the degeneration begins by dissociation of the hepatic cells in the center of the liver lobules, whereby the individual epithelia are released from the tissue structure. From point of view of the differential diagnosis of autopsy material, early autolysis should always be taken into account as it can lead to central acinar dissociation of the epithelial cytoplasm and nuclei even in good preparations. With further development, coagulation necrosis forms in the center of the light zonal degeneration; it extends toward the lobule periphery and is sharply defined against the surviving parenchyma. No notable inflammatory reactions can be determined. Confluence of the necroses can occur, causing interlobular bridges to develop (Fig. 92).

In the livers from 1000 random autopsies, Müller et al. (1970) found initial uncharacteristic changes in terms of shock damage of the first stage in 43 individuals who had died 3–24 h after a circulatory collapse: considerable dilation of the central acinar sinusoids, fat-free vacuoles in the hepatic cells, single necroses demarcated by leukocytes, and reticular necroses (Korb et al. 1969). In addition, numerous fibrin thrombi in the sinusoids, sporadic hyaline swellings in the walls of the arteria hepatica, and basal vacuoles in the epithelia of the bile duct were found. In 63 cases in which 12 h to several days had elapsed between circulatory crisis and death, typical zonally confluent necroses corresponding to the second stage of shock necrosis were evident. Using different material involving variously induced forms of shock, Ellenberg and Osserman (1951) found fully formed necroses of the central hepatic lobules in 34.4% of cases.

The decomposing liver epithelia are removed about 48 h after the onset of shock-induced necrosis. The reticular fiber network usually remains undamaged. If the lesion is survived, a phase of repair can follow whereby the parenchymal defects are replaced by regenerated liver cells, which advance along the preserved reticular network to the central vein (Killip and Payne 1960). The shock-induced necroses also lead to clinically evident disorders in liver function and high transaminase levels. These provide the indication for bioptic investigation and lead to the detection of the reparative healing processes.

Duration and severity of the shock, irrespective of its etiology, have an influence on the extent of damage to the liver. Determination of etiology and forensic evaluation of the histological findings in the liver are rendered more complicated in that central liver cell necroses must also be taken into account in every long-term premortal circulatory failure (Sandritter and Lasch 1967; Scheuer 1968; Sherlock 1965; Thaler 1969). In postmortem examinations the second stage of confluent necroses is predominantly found; the reparative stage, conversely, is found only in liver biopsies (Müller et al. 1970). It is probable that autopsy tends to be performed largely on those cases involving a severe circulatory collapse which could not be therapeutically treated. From animal experimental studies, it can be concluded that survival of the shock within 10–14 days leads to repair of the hepatic cell defects. If death occurs after this time, the parenchymal necroses can no longer be detected.

The differential diagnosis of shock liver and chronic stasis liver can be difficult. In the histological diagnosis of shock, particular care should be taken with the fol-

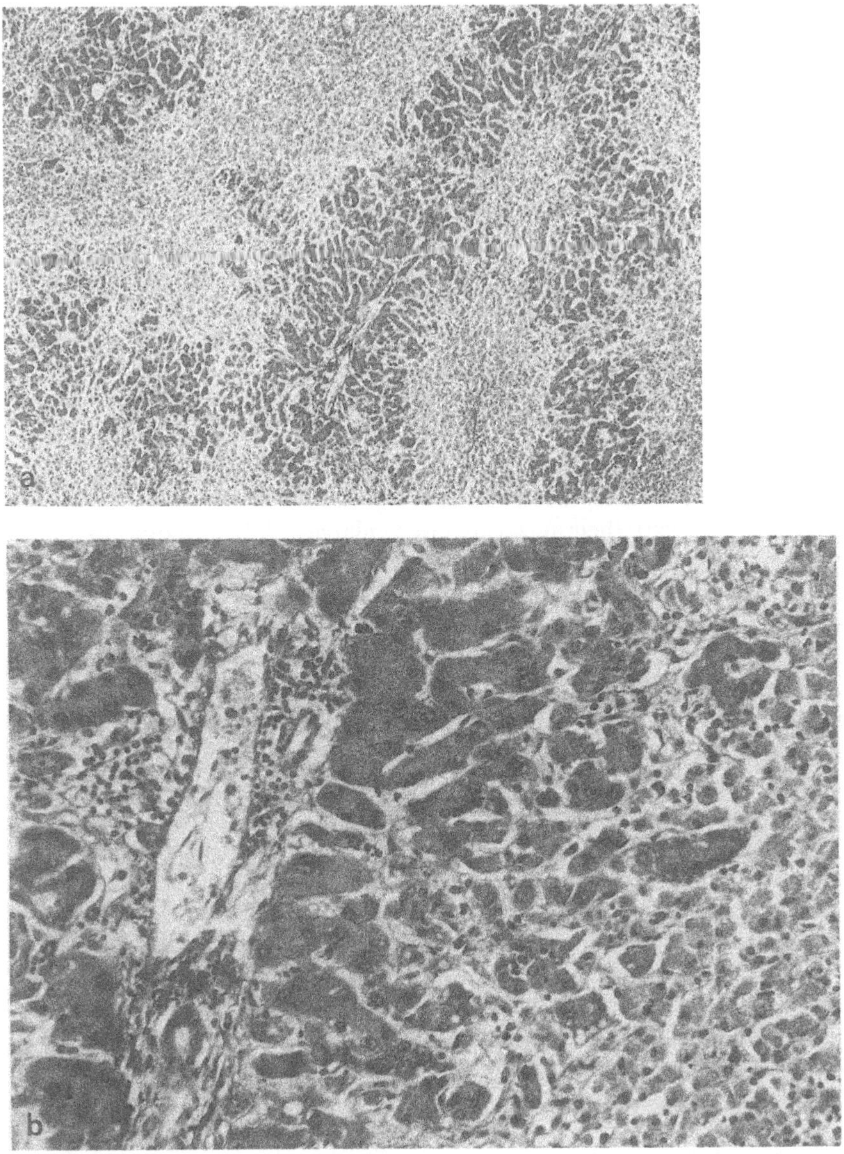

Fig. 92. a, b Confluent centrolobular shock necroses of the liver (nuclei and Kupffer's cells still partially preserved). Subject survived 10 days. H and E, 1:80, 1:220

lowing – extensive necroses of the acinar centers of the lobules, neglible or completely absent hyperemia, microthrombi chiefly in the peripheral sinusoids of the lobules and in the intrahepatic branches of the vena portae. In many cases, however, a secondary shock event cannot be histologically differentiated from pre-existing congestion of the liver (Remmele and Loeper 1973). Misinterpretations can arise in hepatic eclampsia (eclampsia sine eclampsia) with the histological findings of a consumption coagulopathy; the same applies to the Shwartzmann phenomenon and amniotic embolisms (Ryvarden 1972).

Kidneys. The pathogenesis of the shock kidney (van Slyke 1948) is based on a reduction in blood flow and the associated lack of nourishment. Hemodynamic shock damage to the kidneys seldom leads to death; usually it only does so in combination with other, in particular toxic, lesions. The findings in connection with shock kidney can be reversible. Observations of histological renal changes corresponding to a shock kidney but which did not give rise to any clinical shock symptoms during life should be pointed out (Wollheim 1952; Balslov and Jorgensen 1963). The pathophysiology of the "kidney in shock" was extensively reported by Leber and Schütterle (1971).

Histologically, collapse, swellings of endothelial and surface cells broadening of the basal membrane, and impairment of the loops are found in the glomeruli (Staemmler 1957; Suda 1962; Rollhäuser and Vogell 1960). In the region of the proximal convoluted tubules, the epithelia are at first distinctly swollen and later flattened (Zollinger 1966); their nuclei are often enlarged. Polynucleosis also occurs as a sign of epithelial regeneration; this finding can be observed in approximately every eighth case of premortal shock (Remmele 1975). The renal interstitium presents an edema which sometimes has an inflammatory character (Spühler and Zollinger 1941; Rotter 1959; Randerath and Bohle 1959). Marked expansion of the tubuli with flattening of the epithelia deserves particular attention (Fig. 93). This finding in the kidney is regarded as a typical indication of shock by many authors. Expansion of the tubulus can, however, be absent in very severe shock and be present without shock having occurred (Zollinger 1966). Intravascular fibrin precipitation occurs in the kidney in about 7% of cases (Loew et al. 1971). The vasa recta usually exhibit severe stasis of the blood. The juxtaglomerular cells (myoepithelia) are unchanged after hemodynamic shock. Interstitial edema in the region of the renal capillaries leads in parts to compression of the tubuli and blood vessels, which, however, can also be locally dilated as a result of compression of distal sections.

The hemodynamic effects on the kidney are probably also determined by general vasoconstriction of nervous origin (Zollinger 1966 – references): The associated ischemia of the renal cortex is absent following denervation of the kidney (Franklin et al. 1949). The histological findings in the kidneys in a state of shock are also influenced by traumatic and hypoxia-induced histolysis as well as by damage due to blood, muscle, or icteric pigments (Zollinger 1952; Koslowski 1960). The studies of Knisely (1961) and Fajers and Gelin (1959) were specifically concerned with the direct effects of sludging on renal tissue.

One particular complication in shock concerns necrosis of the renal cortex. This is an acute necrotizing process accompanied by hemorrhages which almost only affects the cortical tissue; the medulla, renal pelvis, capsule, and a narrow subcapsular portion of the cortex are unaffected. The loops of the glomeruli and contiguous arterioles generally contain fibrinous thrombi. Calcified centers can be recognized within the necrotic masses. In the early stage of cortical necrosis, the glomeruli are extremely dilated. In later phases, the glomerular changes may resemble glomerulonephritis. Similar findings are also oberserved in microangiopathies with glomerular involvement and secondary cortical necrosis: The tubuli are necrotic and rup-

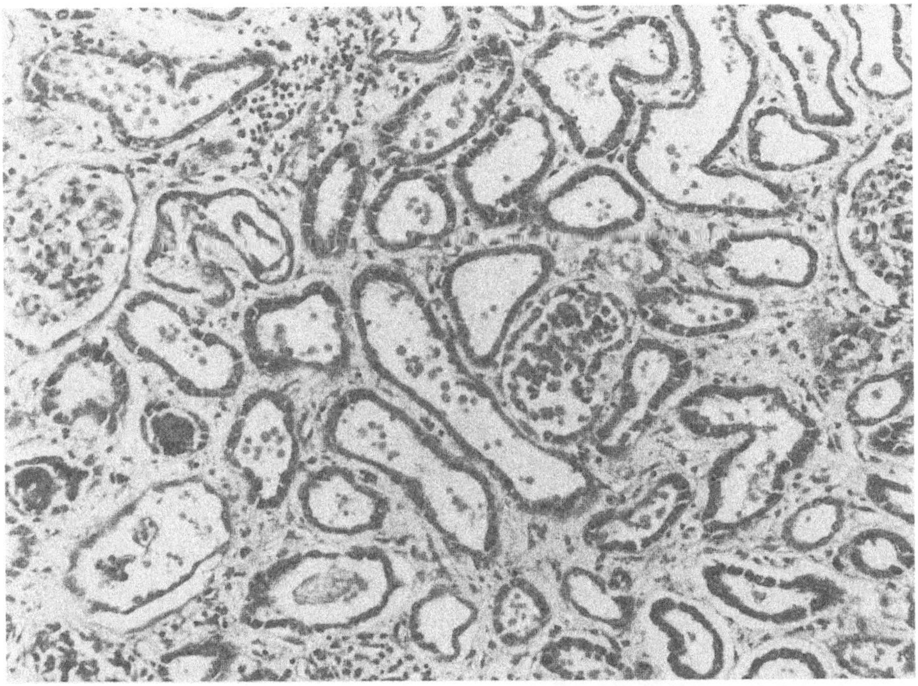

Fig. 93. Shock kidney with dilation of the convoluted tubules, flattening of the tubular epithelia, interstitial edema, and collapse of the glomerular loops. Isolated fine granular casts. Subject survived 7 days, severe burns. H and E, 1:280

tures of the basal membrane are evident. The interstitium is impregnated by hemorrhages and infiltrated by leukocytes in the marginal areas of the necroses. The prognosis for necroses of the renal cortex, which commonly occur bilaterally, is distinctly poor: Those affected die after 8 h to 15 days. Occasionally, however, the necrosis can be survived if it does not reach the full stage but can still lead to death after months or years, appearing clinically as severe cirrhosis of the kidney with extensive cortical calcification.

The factors inducing necrosis of the renal cortex are diverse (Zollinger 1966). Of prime importance is pregnancy, especially with retroplacental hematoma, secondly, children with shock or infections. Other causes are endotoxin shock, coagulopathies of various origin, microangiopathies, and, more rarely, arteriography and renal vein thromboses in neonates.

Concentrations of nucleated cells in the venous limb of the vaṣa recta of the renal cortex are important in the diagnosis; they were evident in over 70% of all fatal cases of shock (Remmele et al. 1964; Lowe et al. 1971). Involved here are lymphocytes, monocytes, plasma cells, plasmacyte precursor cells, and myelopoietic cells, particularly promyelocytes, myelocytes, normoblasts, and megakaryocytes. The cells originate from the bone marrow or extramedullary hematopoietic centers in shock and are transported via the blood system into the renal vessels. Circulatory collapse probably plays a pathogenic role in this. Leukosis and leukemic reactions should be considered in differential diagnosis.

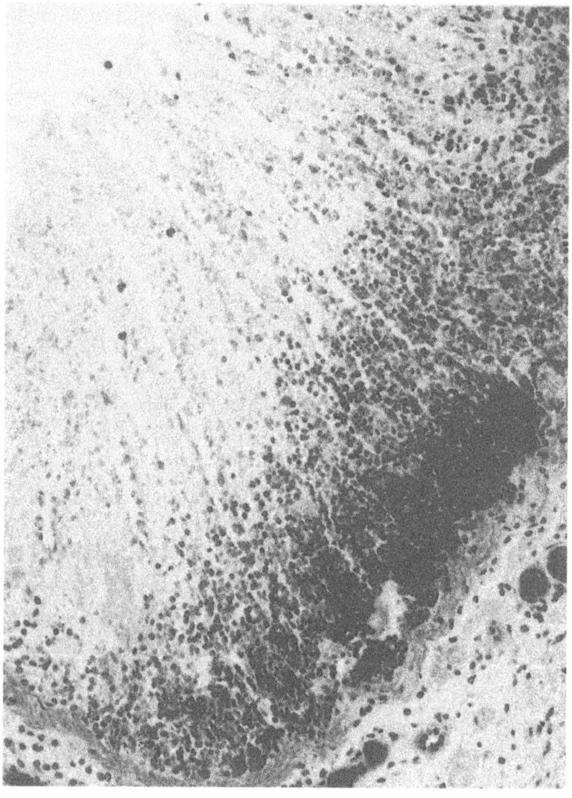

Fig. 94. Small intestine with fibrin thrombi in the vessels of the submucosa and hemorrhage and necrosis of the mucosa. Subject survived 7 days, severe burns. Goldner's, 1:150

Following allogenic kidney transplantation, disseminated intravascular clots can sporadically occur which resemble the findings in shock. It has been demonstrated in clinical studies that products of fibrinogen splitting in the serum may be detected significantly earlier than the usual clinical criteria of a rejection reaction, such that this finding can be taken as an early sign of an impending kidney rejection (Zühlke et al. 1972).

Gastrointestinal Tract. Following severe states of shock of about 4–5-h duration, edema of the villi with desquamated epithelia is found, especially in the small intestine. It should be taken into account that the mucosal epithelia can be detached very early postmortem by autolysis in the villous apical region. Fibrin thrombi and shock bodies are frequently found in the vessels of the submucosa following shock (Fig. 94).

The acute occurrence of erosions and ulcers have a particular significance in shock (Fig. 95) (Rotter 1971; Klein et al. 1971; Rösch 1974); the frequency is between 3% and 14% of all fatal cases (Remmele 1975). Forensic investigations carried out on 18583 autopsies over a period of 26 years revealed 3.9% (719 cases) to have acute esophagogastroduodenal ulceration, which was the cause of death in 85 cases (Kringsholm et al. 1979). Two-thirds of the stress lesions are in the stomach,

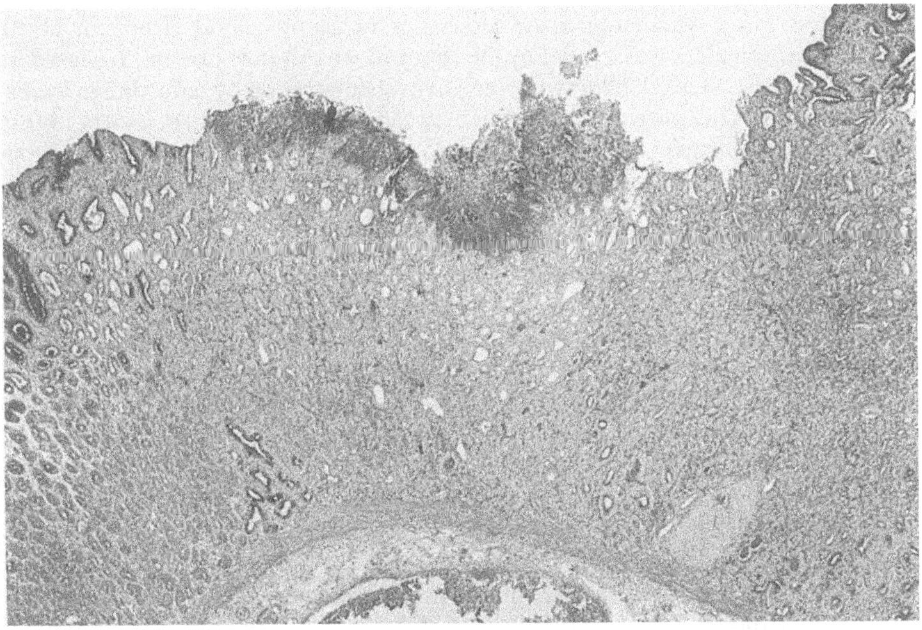

Fig. 95. Shock erosion of the stomach mucosa with hemorrhages and fibrin precipitation. Subject survived 7 days, severe burns. PAS, 1:80

chiefly in the form of multiple hemorrhagic erosions, and one-third are localized in the duodenum, almost exclusively as acute ulceration with a high proportion of erosive hemorrhages (Berndt et al. 1978). Surface erosion of the mucosa is only conspicuous in obduction material if it was a source of hemorrhage and, accordingly, covered with hematinized blood. A histological classification by Oehlert et al. (1978) distinguishes between completely superficial erosions of the mucosal folds, incomplete erosions with a diameter of 0.1–0.5 cm, and complete erosions which extend down as far as the muscularis mucosae without breaking through it. These are circumscribed coagulation necroses, sharply demarcated from their surroundings, and restricted to the mucosa; they heal quickly and without scar formation. Acute ulcers ("stress ulcers") rapidly permeate the mucosa and submucosa as far as the muscularis propria and lead relatively frequently to hemorrhages and perforations. The clinical prognosis is regarded as poor; mortality is between 40% and 60% (Berndt et al. 1978). The shock-induced microcirculatory changes in the gastroduodenal vascular system, with apical necroses of the mucosal cells, increases in the acidity of the stomach juices, and changes in the mucosal barrier through gastroduodenal reflux, are pathogenetically significant. The increase in gastroduodenal stress lesions observed in recent years is attributed to longer survival times in connection with intensive care (Schulz and Albert 1976).

The forensic histological investigation and appraisement of such mucosal defects orients itself particularly to determining their age in the tissue. In several sections from the peripheral region and base of these defects, a check has to be made with the appropriate stains for visualizing cicatricial tissue, fibrin, and signs of inflammation to see whether an acute process or a chronic callous ulcer is involved, i.e., whether the ulcer was caused by the shock or was already present. It should be noted that corticosteroid therapy can lead to acute ulceration by reduction in the tissue resistance. A histological distinction between shock and "cortisone ulcus" is not possible. If corticosteroid therapy was employed to control shock then a causal connection should be evident in the assessment between the cause of shock and the ulcus with its sequelae.

Heart. The histologically detectable effects of shock to the heart have largely been investigated in animal experiments. Following hemorrhagic shock in dog hearts, subendocardial hemorrhages, necroses, and "zonal lesions" were found, which are defined as decreased or absent succinodehydrogenase and cytochrome oxidase activity close to the intercalated discs (Martin et al. 1963, 1964, 1966). In the surroundings of these enzyme deficits, increased enzyme staining was found. Electron-microscopic studies have revealed that the zonal lesions are to a large extent reversible. Pathogenetically, contraction of the myofibrils in paraintercalary parenchymal cell regions is regarded as a primary alteration, which leads to displacement of the mitochondria into adjacent unaltered areas of cytoplasm. In this way, an energetically unfavorable situation arises simultaneously by withdrawal of the ATP source, with subsequent structural disorganization up to fully developed lesion. This kind of lesion is thought to appear only in oligemic hypotension and to differ from other known lesion symptoms. Disseminated fine fibrotic foci were detected in the musculature of rabbit hearts after shock (Pokk 1963). In humans following severe states of shock, the findings were confined to circumscribed myocardial necroses, which are probably connected with the tissue hypoxia and histologically do not present any specific characteristics (Fig. 96). The clinically observed behavior of serum transaminases is probably influenced by this parenchymal damage (Sandritter and Lasch 1967; Müller et al. 1970).

Pancreas. It is only seldom that the histionic effects of shock to the pancreas become evident as a particular clinical picture. After 1 h, hypoxemia and ischemia can lead to acinar necroses as a result of shock to the excretory part of the gland (Seifert 1970). Similar findings can, however, also develop in terminal pancreatitis due to agonal circulatory impairment. Hypoxemic shock factors then become particularly effective if the pancreas had been previously damaged. The role of the pancreas is better known when it is the primary cause of shock through acute inflammation with histolysis and general intoxication.

Pituitary. In connection with states of shock, necroses have frequently been described in the anterior pituitary in the form of microinfarctions with and without thrombi. In 72 of 825 pituitaries, Saeger and Hanke (1978) found necroses in the anterior lobe with the characteristic structure of an anemic infarction. Fresh or somewhat older necroses were found in 28 of 134 proven cases of shock, but there were no scars. Microinfarctions probably develop in the anterior lobe in shock-induced hypercoagulability of the blood as a result of microthrombi in the adenohypophyseal sinusoids. The findings concerning actually proven microthrombi are variable.

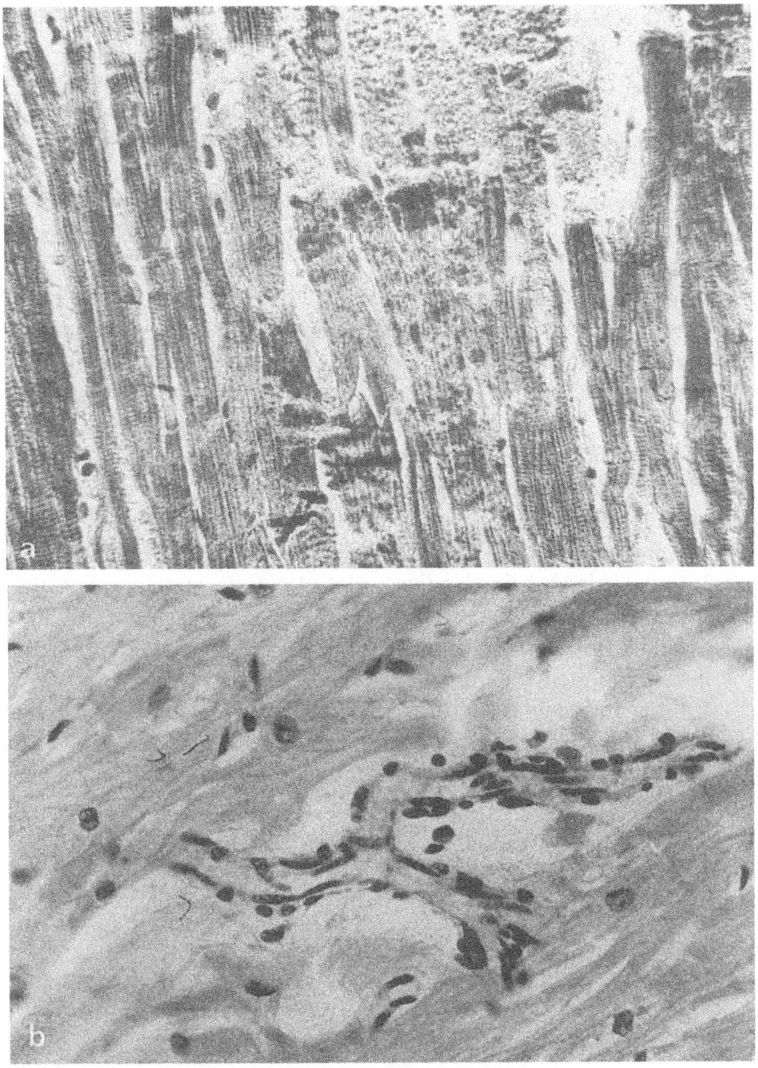

Fig. 96. a. Onset of fibrillar necrosis of the myocardium. Subject survived 3 days, automobile accident. PTAH, 1:320. **b** Same subject as in **a.** Capillaries with swelling and pyknosis of endothelial cell nuclei

Histologically evident effects of shock have also been observed in other organs and tissues. In the skeletal musculature, the capillary endothelia react in the form of swelling and rarefaction of their cell structures, with constriction of the vascular lumen. Subsequently, edematization of the perivascular tissue and escape of plasmatic components, erythrocytes, and granulocytes into the muscular interstitium occur. These changes can probably be attributed to hypoxia. Muscle biopsies are recommended in the clinical assessment of the course of shock.

Shock can also be elicited by blunt muscular trauma. Myotoxin, containing ADP and ATP, is released as a result. Both ADP and ATP induce thrombocyte aggregates and, in connection with traumatically released tissue thrombokinase, the development of thromboembolic shock (Marx et al. 1966).

Fifty-one cases involving intubations were histologically examined to see whether a shock trachea is also possible. It was shown that the upper respiratory tracts are also a point of attack for shock-induced circulatory and microvascular disorders (Heymer and Fischer 1980).

Neurogenous shock is of particular interest since the pathogenic agent attacks the central organ itself, which both regulates and is itself regulated (references in Schmidt and Potthoff 1976).

A synoptic evaluation of all findings that have thus far been determined in tissues and organs reveals that the histological examination can contribute to the verification of shock and shock death. It is important that the individual findings are brought into relation with one another and correlatively assessed.

Diagnosis of Shock. The following histological findings can be indicative of shock.

1) Sludging (aggregations of erythrocytes and thrombocytes) in the dilated arterioles, capillaries, and venules, particularly of the lung, gastrointestinal tract, kidney, liver, and brain.
2) Intravascular hyaline bodies – globular clots, shock bodies and microthrombi, predominantly in the terminal vascular system (particularly in the lung).
3) Swelling and necroses of capillary endothelia and reticulohistiocytary cells, especially in the liver sinusoids.
4) Intimal and medial necroses, particularly in the coronary arteries.
5) Isolated and group necroses of parenchymal cells in the liver and kidneys; centroacinar necroses of the liver lobules, which also become confluent.
6) Bilateral necroses of the renal cortex.
7) Villous edema with epithelial loss in the small intestine.
8) Generalized and local hemorrhages as an expression of consumption coagulopathy in consequence of disseminated intravascular clotting.
9) Acute erosion and ulceration of the mucous membrane in the esophagus, stomach, and small intestine.
10) Widening of the renal tubuli.
11) Multiple megakaryocytes in the pulmonary capillaries.

3. Allergies

General. A presentation of the histomorphology of injuries and fatalities due to an allergic event has to take into account the close connections with shock. However, in allergies, histionic changes are found which do not have a direct relation to the effects of shock and impairment of the microcirculation in the terminal vascular system. There are also allergic changes without shock.

The morphological effects of an antigen-antibody reaction are basically influenced by two preconditions:

1) Function and structure of the tissue or environment in which the reaction takes place; 2) a complex body of factors, which include the chemical character and degree of purity of the antigen, its route of entry and chronological and quantitative

circumstances of entry, the individual, and the human constitution (Letterer 1962). The strength of the stimulus is particularly important since it affects the cellular findings connected with the reaction. The form of the reaction is primarily explained by the complex structural quality of the reacting substances. The cell can participate actively or passively in an antigen-antibody process. Strong stimuli have cytotoxic effects, under some circumstances they may be negligibly anabolic and activating. The first reaction of a cell is a surface membrane reaction and not until the second reaction is the cytoplasm involved. The surface reaction is in the form of agglutination; the cytoplasmic reaction takes the form of swelling, necrosis, and cytolysis. In tissue reactions, the behavior of the arterioles and capillaries is decisive, whereby the contractility of the muscle cells has a significant influence. The vascular-free intima reaction adopts the form of endarteritis with insudative inflammation; the media and adventitia show periarteritis, exsudation, and proliferation. According to Letterer (1962) three types of tissue reaction pattern can be distinguished: (1) Arthus' phenomenon, as the so-called early reaction; (2) the tuberculin type, as the so-called late reaction; (3) primarily granulating reaction. The morphological pattern of the early reaction is determined by the capillary, that of the late reaction by the cell. For the organism as a whole, there are two forms of the reaction – anaphylactic shock and serum sickness.

Histological Findings. The histological manifestations of cellular sensitization can be seen in the tuberculin skin reaction in animal experiment. In the 1st h after intracutaneous injection, neutrophilic leukocytes are diffusely scattered in the subcutaneous tissue. After this, there is a gradual increase in the numbers of monocytes, histiocytes, and lymphocytes in the vicinity of subcutaneous veins, which show strong leukostasis. Mononuclear cells almost completely dominate the findings. After 24 h, there are signs of nuclear destruction in the polynuclear cells. Occasionally, lipophagic foci and fat and muscle necroses can be detected in the subcutaneous tissue 1–2 h after antigen injection (Kolin et al. 1965). The pathogenesis and morphogenesis of such cellular sensitivity reactions occur in two phases (two-step reaction): (1) Specific phase – conjunction of sensitized cell and antigen with the release of biologically active substances, mediators, which attack and destroy the surrounding cells; (2) nonspecific inflammatory reactions as a result of the substances released, which produce permeability in the vessels and migration of leukocytes.

In animal experiments, the early histological consequences of antigenic stimulation affect reactions in the white splenic pulp, which appear within a few hours. They begin with a depletion in the lymphocytes in the marginal regions of the Malpighian corpuscles. An increase in macrophage activity in the germinal centers then follows (Congdon 1964). Continuance of the stimulation leads to dissolution of the germinal centers and proliferation of new cells with basophilic cytoplasm and vesicular nuclei. This process can encroach onto the red pulp; at the same time there is a strong increase in the number of plasma cells. The kind of antigen involved also affects the extent and character of the reaction. Further experimental studies on the histological detection of immunological processes concern investigations on the lymph nodes, the lungs of guinea pigs (Morgenroth 1970), the pancreas (Freytag et al. 1970), and immunologically treated acute leukosis in infancy (Lange and Kornhuber 1970).

The role of eosinophilic leukocytes has not yet been entirely explained. Their increased appearance is generally known in the interstices of various organs, especially the spleen, lymph nodes, lungs, and cardiac muscle, in people suffering from allergies, asthma, vermination, etc. In the splenic blood of corpses, between 41 000 and 46000 eosinophils/mm^3 are normal (Voigt 1966). Following stress or anaphylactic or allergic shock, wide dispersions of 7200–167000/mm^3 have been found. An "allergic constitution" is present if more than 100000 eosinophilic leukocytes/mm^3 can be determined in the splenic blood of the corpse. Eosinophilia can also be found during the life time of such individuals. Allergic fatalities where the counts are lower than the norm are perhaps explained by an "immune reaction." In animal experiments following reinjections of antigens giving rise to complete antibodies, edemas with local eosinophilia occurred; these failed to appear when incomplete antibodies were formed (Archer 1965). The edematous formation can be hindered by eosinophilic extract, known to have a bradykinin antagonism. Eosinophils are probably not involved in antibody formation, especially since in their maturation RNA- and PAS-positive cells disappear from the cytoplasm – in contrast to the behavior of lymphocytes and plasma cells. Eosinophilic leukocytes are probably more involved in a reduction in the effects of local antigen-antibody reactions.

Allergy Death. Histological determination of an allergic etiology for shock fatalities is difficult. Where there is no known sensitization, the causative or contributory significance of an allergy can usually only be supposed. The detection of tissue mast cells has indicative value. In 12 of 13 cases in which death occurred directly after intramuscular injection of drugs in allergic shock, Ambrosi et al. (1968) found numerous mast cells in diverse organs – liver, kidneys, cardiac muscle, lungs, sporadically also in the perivascular tissue of the skin, spleen, pancreas, thymus, adrenal glands, tonsils, and pituitary body. The mast cell reactions are unusually transient. The presence of plasma cells and pyroninophilic monocytic elements suggests increased immune reactivity. Otherwise, decreases in the fat content and degenerative changes in the adrenal cortex were found, frequently also previous chronic, usually degenerative damage, to the heart and liver (Okumura 1969).

The histologically detectable effects of shock in penicillin allergy and anaphylaxia through bacteremia commonly yield similar findings in the brain and lungs (Bankl and Jellinger 1968; Waisbren and Arena 1965). As a result, shock and allergy findings cannot be differentiated with certainty. Common to all these cases is the frequent occurrence of hyaline thrombi in the terminal vascular system and the tendency to hemorrhage. In the further diagnosis of a fatal penicillin accident, antigen-antibody complexes and antibodies following depot penicillin therapy can also be detected. The evidence is obtained by immunohistological investigations on the basal membranes of the proximal renal tubuli and the eluate of kidney tissue (Dirnhofer et al. 1978). Inflammatory reactions to the immunological process could not be histologically detected. This form of reaction is pathogenetically interpreted as a form of serum sickness. Even after longer postmortem times, the application of immunohistological investigatory methods is believed to permit the detection of previous sensitization to penicillin. The tissue and serum to be examined should, however, be deep-frozen directly after the autopsy. Kent and Ekker (1965) demonstrated that anaphylactic shock in guinea pigs is due to a reaction with intracellular antibodies and not due to the formation of complexes with antibodies circulating in the blood.

Death from Insect Stings. The presentation of the histological effects of insect stings within the context of allergies has to differentiate between acute fatal cases following one or several stings and those cases that occurred after a great many stings, e.g., attack by insect swarms (Janssen 1966 – references). After numerous insect stings, the following can be found in the autopsy – pulmonary and cerebral edema, hyperemia of the inner organs, petechial hemorrhages in the skin and serous coats, softening foci in the brain, and toxic parenchymal lesions. Histologically, in isolated cases, cuneate skin necroses have been found as far as the subcutis in the region of stings, in addition to necroses of the spleen follicle, fatty degenerations of the liver, kidneys, and myocardium, and necrobiotic softening foci in the cerebral cortex and striatum, with diffuse oligodendroglial and macroglial proliferation. Extensive hemorrhagic infarctions of the cerebral cortex, splenic arterial thromboses, and splenic infarctions have also been observed as direct toxic effects of insect poison (Day 1962).

Of particular interest are fatalities due to a single or a small number of insect stings; where the previous history is unknown, their clarification can be forensically significant. According to the reports published in the literature, fatal insect stings appear to be increasing in frequency. In the USA, the number of annual fatalities from direct anaphylactic reactions following insect stings is estimated at 200. Of the deaths through insect stings thus far investigated, 88% occurred within the 1st h after the sting. The examination of puncture sites by Wegelin (1933, 1948), Halperin (1936), and Jensen (1962) on the corpses of humans who died following a single sting revealed a puncture channel extending into the corium. In some cases, small hemorrhages and focal necroses were found here which sporadically stretched as far as the fatty tissue of the subcutis, presenting an edematous disaggregation and leukocytic permeation of the connective tissue in the vicinity of the puncture. The capillaries were markedly dilated. In some cases, circumscribed necroses of the adjacent sweat glands occurred. Frequently, no tissue reactions were evident in the region of the puncture sites. The macroscopic and histological findings are uncharacteristic in the inner organs: acute vascular congestion and cyanosis; hyperemia and cyanosis of the mucous membranes in the pharynx and larynx; cerebral edema; pulmonary emphysema; subepicardial, subendocardial, and subpleural petechial hemorrhages; hemorrhages in the pia mater, cerebral tissue, and mucous membranes of the pharynx, trachea, and esophagus; isolated hemorrhages in the mucous membrane of the renal pelvis; perivascular hemorrhages in the liver; fresh small hemorrhagic infarctions in the lungs; hemorrhages and necroses in the medulla oblongata and adrenal cortex.

The processes of immunity and allergy have a particular significance in explaining sudden death from single insect stings. A distinction has to be made here between a local reaction and a general effect. The striking similarity in the local reaction following bee, wasp, and hornet stings, which is that of an immediate allergic reaction, is due to the fact that in the sting of these insects, to a certain extent, the same active principles are injected as are released in an antigen-antibody reaction in the tissue (e.g., histamine, serotonine, kinin, phospholipase A and B). An urtica with a white center and sometimes a small central hemorrhage forms within a short period of time in the punctured cells. The adjacent tissue is, according to the site on the body, more or less strongly inflamed, reddened, and swollen; in well-vascularized regions, extensive edema is formed. In sensitized individuals, the local reaction can be more pronounced following repeated stinging. In these cases, in addition to the toxic components, the allergic components, protein components, of the insect poison become effective. According to Rajka (1959), 2% of the population are sensitized to insect poisons. The processes and types of reaction that play a role in this have been the object of numerous studies (references in Janssen 1966).

Evidence of a fatal insect sting is particularly difficult if the local reaction is only very weak or not recognizable at all. In this regard, it has also been discussed whether in an insect sting the poison may be directly injected intravascularly. The occurrence of the anaphylactic general reaction would then be considerably accelerated. Rapid conductance of the poison through the vascular system would explain the absence of the local reaction. The presence of free antibodies against insect antigens can be detected by application of the Prausnitz-Küstner reaction. In this, the serum of an individual allergic to insect poison is injected intracutaneously into, e.g., a guinea pig. After about 24 h, an insect antigen is injected into the same site on the skin, after which in a positive case a distinct allergic weal response develops.

Occasionally, deaths from single insect stings can be important in the context of legal accident insurance (Störmer 1961).

V. Histological Contribution Toward Identification

General. Occasionally, the application of histological methods of investigation can contribute to the identification of corpses of unknown persons or to the clarification of the kind and origin of parts of the corpse and pieces of tissue that otherwise can not be differentiated. This involves procedures that are also employed in trace chemistry. There is no need for histological identification to be considered an independent subject area; it is more a question of applying histological methods and knowledge in examining material for the presence of specific features, permitting further inferences as to identity. These investigations can be regarded as screening using histological methods.

The possibilities and methods of sex determination by means of nuclear morphological features in body tissues and traces of secretory products have been comprehensively presented by Helmer (1970) with regard to forensic considerations. Hienz (1959, 1971) discussed this theme from the pathoanatomical and clinical points of view. Nuclear sex determination through the evidence of Barr bodies in the female chromosome complement and by staining of the Y-bodies with quinacrine derivatives and visualization under the fluorescent microscope (Degenhardt et al. 1972) has been developed to such an extent in recent years that its employment with histological and cytological material has become routinely possible. Kovács et al. (1972) were able to demonstrate Y-bodies in the organs of corpses in over 15% of all male organs investigated. Following fluorescent staining of loosened hair root cell nuclei of females, Sperling and Schwinger (1973) were able to render the Barr body very conspicuous. Restaining with diamond fuchsin led to minor variations in localization; after fluorescent staining, the Barr body appeared larger and less sharply defined than after staining with diamond fuchsin. A full discussion of nuclear morphological sex determination in this context will be dispensed with, and the reader is referred to the book by Helmer (1970).

1. Determination of Type and Organ

The possibility in forensic practice of clarifying the type and origin of parts of a corpse and pieces of tissue by histological investigation is slight. However, use should be made of this procedure in every case. If parts of a corpse are found in a highly putrified or decomposed state, then sometimes only histological examination can allow diagnosis of the organ to be made. Use of stains specifically for visualization of the siver-stainable fibrous framework (among others Gomory's, Bielschowski's) is recommended. Occasionally, a simple hemalum stain is sufficient for reproducing the outlines of the cell and fiber contours. Even with extensively altered organs that are already liquefying, it is still possible to identify the basic structures and the tissues to which they belong. Thus, it was still possible for us to identify liver, lungs, and kidneys 4–5 months PM. Even cerebral tissue can be recognized in section or teased-out preparation, particularly in its vascular structure, despite complete macroscopic destruction.

With regard to sex determination, there is thought to be a detectable difference in the skin. In men, the papillae are wide and short; in women, they are narrow and long (Mueller 1953). We have not been able to obtain practically utilizable results using this distinction.

In one case, it was possible to recognize chorionic villi in a catheter taken as evidence 3 years after having been used for abortions (Zanaldi 1966). The blood-encrusted tissue was found in the lumen of the catheter tip and it had been shaped to a certain extent by the bore of the catheter. It had possibly been fixed by a disinfectant that happened to be in the instrument.

The histomorphological means of distinguishing human from animal bones in sections or transverse microsections involves measuring the Haversian canals (B. Mueller 1953; Rämsch and Zerndt 1963). Recent examinations have shown positive differential findings in the region of the upper femoral diaphysis. The canal width is measured after maceration and decalcification of 10- to 15- µm-thick sections, which are stained with thionin and examined in a projection microscope. One hundred visual fields are counted. A diameter of 40 µm is rarely exceeded in human bone; the average is about 50 µm. The diameter of the canals in domestic animals is 10–20 µm. The number of canals per visual field is lower in humans than in animals. In humans, the central sections of bone contain on average larger and wider canals, whereas narrower canals predominate in the periphery. In animals, wide and narrow canals are irregularly distributed over central and peripheral areas of the bone. The bone most similar to that of humans is found in horses, although it has a different lamellar pattern (see B. Mueller 1953). A study of the paper by Knese (1970) on the structure and ultrastructure of osseous tissue is recommended to the investigator who is concerned with these problems. Knese's comprehensive presentation of the variable lamellar system with respect to its behavior in polarized light and the various courses of collagenous fibers in the individual skeletal elements provides excellent basic information concerning species and age-specific characteristics of problematic skeletal remains. There may be further possibilities of evaluating the origin of osseous tissue by means of fluorescent tetracycline labeling according to the method of Frost and determining the biological half-life of the osteons. For determinations of the postmortem time of skeletal remains see Berg and Specht (1958).

2. Individual Characteristics

Age determination by means of histological sections can normally only be an estimate (Leutert and Rother 1978). A comparison of tissues from individuals of different ages, with large intervals between the age-groups, however, does provide a basis for a rough age classification for the practised histologist. In an infantile brain, for example, the cerebral cortex is incompletely differentiated and a clear distinction of the various nerve cell layers is not possible. The occurrence of lipofuscin deposition in the ganglia and drusen in medullary and cortical tissue has been particularly investigated with regard to the recognition of cerebral tissue of old people; both findings indicate older age. It should, however, be remembered that lipofuscin can also occur in a very finely dispersed form in the ganglion cells of children. In older individuals, the intracellular form of distribution involves accumulation at several sites. A precise age-related distinction from the occurrence of drusen in younger people has thus far not been possible (Mueller 1953). Systematic studies of senile brains by Schwartz (1964) revealed copious amyloid deposits in plaques and vascular walls to be the basis of senile changes. These were seen as a Congo-red-positive, doubly refractive material that was bright green and glistened following staining with thioflavine S. Nerve cells with Alzheimer's basket cell changes often showed fluorescence. Very fluorescent material was situated intramurally in the meningeal and cortical arteries, whereby the latter were frequently surrounded by a loose, striated bright halo. By means of fluorescence microscopy, the early senile changes in the brain can be detected particularly well.

In the myocardium of neonates and small children, the cardiac muscles are very tightly packed. The cell nuclei are more slender and elongated, and the interstitium is on the whole sparse and delicately formed. In adults, on the other hand, the cardiac muscle cells are substantially richer in cytoplasm, the average lateral distance between nucleus and cell membrane is greater than in children, and the nuclei are more oval and the ends tend to be somewhat blunt. The myocardial interstitium of older individuals is, on average, wider than in adolescents and it contains more collagenous fibers even in the absence of pathogenic changes.

The presence of arteriosclerosis is no certain criterion of advanced age in the individual concerned. This arterial disorder also occurs in adolescents and even children (Janssen 1957, 1968). High-grade stenoses of the coronary arteries can even be observed in neonates as a result of arteriopathia calcificans infantum (Janssen 1963).

In the infantile kidney, the glomeruli appear relatively small and rich in cells. The tubuli contorti are tightly packed and the nuclei of the tubular epithelia are closer together than in the kidneys of adults. Similarly, the collecting tubules are so tightly packed that an interstitium is barely recognizable.

In contrast to the brain, cardiac muscle, and kidneys, no histological age-dependent differences emerge so distinctly in the liver during the period of growth. The lobes and liver cell strands are well differentiated comparatively early. The average size of liver cell nuclei remains relatively constant in the first 60 years of life, but then increases in people over 60 years old. Moreover, the average liver cell size increases with advancing age to a greater extent than the increase in nuclear size. There is a statistically significant correlation between the cellular enlargement and the decrease in the total weight of the liver (Watanabe et al. 1978). In premature infants, hematopoietic foci in the liver, just as in the spleen, indicate early age of the individual. However, it should also be borne in mind in this respect that pathogenic conditions with extramedullary hematopoiesis can also induce similar findings in the liver and spleen.

The lungs of neonates and small children can be differentiated from those of adults with particular clarity in their general histological aspect. Here too, the width and fiber content of the interstitium can be correlated with age, particularly near the larger bronchi and vessels. Planimetric studies on serial sections from the lungs of 36 males and females aged 3 weeks to 75 years by Fuest et al. (1965) revealed an increase in alveolar size during the course of life. In the first 10 years, the alveoli are smaller in the superior lobe than in the inferior. Between the ages of 20 and 30 years, the alveoli have practically the same size in all lobes; after the 30th year, the alveoli in the superior lobes are larger than those in the inferior. The width of the alveolar capillary network corresponds to the size of the alveoli. With advanced age, a reduction in the capillary network is frequently found in the superior lobes, which at the same time accompanies dilation of the capillaries. After the age of 45–50 years, an increase in collagen can be observed in the form of increased thickening of the fibers and also in terms of numbers, particularly in the superior lobes; the capillary membranes are then normally thickened.

The level of coal dust deposition in pulmonary tissue has been repeatedly observed. Systematic observations on 1000 autopsies by Shibata et al. (1963) revealed an increase with advancing age in the amount of deposition, which could be arranged into six different grades. No clear distinction could be made between the sexes. According to our own studies, the results of which were obtained by more empirical means, anthracosis in big-city dwellers of the same age and living in roughly the same environment has an extraordinarily large range. In addition, there are the histological differences that are particularly distinct between urban and rural populations, with the result that where it is not known what kind of an environment an individual came from, the evaluation of anthracosis only has a rough orientational value in age estimation.

In the spleen, micrometric measurement of the thinnest part of the capsule by Shibata and Hirota (1962) showed statistically significant differences for each 10-year age-group. In individuals under 5 years old, the capsule was on average 22 μm thick; in people over 50 years old, the thickness was 100 μm. Putrefaction at room temperature for up to 6 days had no affect on the values.

Serial tests on the evaluation of prenatal age from the histological structural pattern of the spine by Camba (1958, 1960) revealed a number of criteria which allow age determination to within approximately 1 month. The development of the mesenchyme, prechondral tissue and cartilage, with the onset of central cellular hypertrophy, centers of ossification, occurrence of the first bony tissue, and character of the notochord were assessed.

By means of amniotic cytology, Rauchfuss and Widmaier (1971) discovered a highly significant difference for the time before and after the 37th week of pregnancy. This time had been exceeded in every case where there was a content of more than 10% orange-colored cells following staining with Nile blue sulfate. The application of this method should be very simple as it does not presuppose any special knowledge of histology.

The use of histological methods in forensic odontology also offers certain possibilities in age determination. The longitudinal section technique based on the method developed by Gustafson (1950) has been practised by many authors. Wear, character of the dentine, attachment in the tooth socket, cement accumulation, changes to the root of the tooth, arrangement and width of the dental canaliculi, and the nature of the lines in the enamel and dentine are examined. With this method, which we are unable to judge from our own experience but which has encountered criticism (Saunders 1965), the age of people with teeth can be assessed relatively accurately to within about 5 years (Dechaume et al. 1960; Schröder 1971).

One method of age determination of bone from a border area of histology, microradiography (Breitenecker 1959 – references; Dobryak and Kirichinsk 1964), involves the degree of mineralization of older and younger osteons in cross sections of the compact substance. In this way, criteria toward the estimation of age can be established (cf. Göring 1970). A method of age determination of human bones based on the diameter of the Haversian canals was developed by Balthazard and Lebron.

Histology makes an important contribution in identification by detecting individual characteristics which cannot always be reliably diagnosed macroscopically. These include previous illnesses, florid diseases, such as tuberculosis, malaria, and syphilis, with their various forms and organic manifestations, and foreign-body granulomas after old injuries involving the inclusion of inflammatory foreign substances. Occasionally, the histological examination can clarify the nature and origin of the material. Thus, a foreign body was found close to a fistula in the femoral musculature of a man 15 years after the accident that gave rise to it. Botanical consultation identified it as a rare kind of wood found in Siberia; the man had in fact been there as a prisoner and had been injured by splinters of wood in an accident.

Foreign-body granulomas in the skin are also found after the introduction of dyes or punctures in order to produce tattoos. After the removal of tattoos in living subjects so as to impede identification, scars and particles of dye can be histologically identified in the upper layers of the corium. Where the corpse has become very putrefactive, particularly if it has been in water for a long period of time, the identification of scars and tattoos is much more difficult. Scars reaching the corium and subcutis can sometimes be histologically identified particularly well by means of van Gieson's and van Gieson's elastica stains. On the other hand, in one particular case of an unidentified highly putrefactive corpse found in water, following histological investigation circumscribed blue patternlike markings in the manner of tattoos on the forearms proved to be colonizations of blue chromogenic bacteria and fungi, which had partly penetrated the sebaceous and sweat glands.

Mention should also be made of the histological identification of skin pigmentation in colored people when the corpse has undergone considerable postmortem changes. Despite detachment of the epidermis, the melanin can still be detected quite well in the upper layers of the stratum papillare. Exogenous pigments, e.g., in argyria, can also be registered in various places of deposition, especially in the skin.

Reference should also be made to the possibility of determining the type of ABO blood group in pieces of organ and histological sections which have been formalin-fixed for a long time (Slavik and Meluzin 1972; Tröger and Jungwirth 1975). By means of the absorption-elution method, it was possible to make a clear determination of the blood group, e.g., in preparations of heart, lung, liver, kidney, spleen, and brain that had been preserved for up to 10 years.

C. Special Section

I. Sudden Death from Natural Causes

1. Preliminary Note

From a forensic point of view, a question that needs to be clarified is whether death in sudden and unexpected fatalities was due to an internal or external cause. Death that is solely dependent on an internal cause and not affected or induced by an extrinsic agent is defined as natural death. Sudden death cannot be precisely delimited with regard to time. In practice, the course of dying is frequently not observed, and the description given by other people cannot always be totally relied upon. Thus, reference is made to unexpected death, which signifies that these cases require further explanation.

An understanding of the natural causes that suddenly lead to death and the ability to diagnose them are the basic prerequisites for the identification and assessment of unnatural death. In investigating unnatural death, it is necessary to establish whether an internal cause that could explain the occurrence of death at the time in question can be excluded with the required reliability. It should be borne in mind that despite autopsy and careful histological and toxicological investigations, some cases of death remain unclear. Their number is given as between 0.8% and 10% (Du Chesne 1978). These are either natural causes of death that cannot as yet be morphologically identified, or the causes are evident to such a slight extent that they are disregarded or underestimated.

Statistical analyses of a large number of autopsy records reveals a distinct predominance of certain groups of diseases, in particular of the cardiac and vascular system, respiratory organs, brain, and digestive system, as causes of sudden natural death (Janssen and Naeve 1975 – references). These natural disorders account for over 90% of all cases of sudden and unexpected death. An acquaintance with their histology is assumed and it will not be specially discussed here. For the purposes of forensic histology, however, it would be appropriate to draw attention to a few main points, since these involve diagnostic problems and are frequently encountered in forensic practice.

2. Diagnostic Problems

Early Recognition of Myocardial Infarction. Histomorphological evidence, gained as early as possible, of myocardial infarction is of central importance in proving cardiac death. According to definition, infarction involves a large coagulation necrosis or the resulting condition in the myocardium, induced by a long-term circulatory deficiency (ischemia) of a circumscribed section of cardiac muscle (Hort 1969). The difficulty of proving a myocardial infarction is due to the fact that the formation of coagulation necroses in cardiac musculature requires a certain survival time of the individual concerned. One task of research is to increase the sensitivity and reliability of the histomorphological methods of identification such that, as far as possible, myocardial infarctions that lead immediately to death may also be recognized. With the present limits of establishing evidence, it is to be expected that there are cases of death from cardiac infarction that can be neither proven nor disproven. Particular difficulties emerge in chronologically arranging the morphological signs of infarction. This is due to the fact that in the majority of cases in humans, the definite onset of infarction and the beginning of cardiac muscle necrosis cannot be precisely detected and are often inferred only from the statements made by the individual concerned. On the other hand, there are also infarctions that are survived for a longer period of time and then suddenly lead to death without any particular symptoms or signs. Finally, early diagnosis is often made more difficult by autolytic effects, especially in forensic medical practice where the autopsy is, unfortunately, carried out very late. The above circumstances explain why it is that the basic established knowledge concerning the morphologically detectable early stages of myocardial infarction has been obtained from animal experimental studies under definable conditions.

In the histomorphological examination of the heart, the times of death and autopsy should be taken into account in addition to the macroscopic findings from the myocardium. The changes should be detected at as many circumscribed sites of cardiac muscle as possible by the comparative examination of various cardiac muscle sections (Doerr 1981). A standardized pattern of removal is recommended, with at least eight sectional sites from the walls of both ventricles and auricles.

In the following section, there is a summary of the important hitherto established early changes. Electron microscopically, translucence of the ground substance of the cytoplasm, decrease in the small granules, and widening of the tubuli in the endoplasmic reticulum have been observed in cardiac muscle cells 10 min after cardiac arrest (Meessen and Poche 1963). Thirty minutes after onset of hypoxia, there were distinct changes in the mitochondria with swelling and dissolution of the cristae (Büchner and Onishi 1968). After 30–60 min, the glycogen content of the necrotic cardiac muscle can be seen histochemically to be perceptibly reduced (Neoral et al. 1959; Shnitka and Nachlas 1963). The enzymes dissolved in the cytoplasm of heart muscle cells (SGOT, LDH) pass into the blood serum about 2 h after the onset of infarction. Mitochondrial enzymes, e.g., succinodehydrogenase, on average do not leave the cell until after 2–4 h. Enzyme-histochemical investigations into the early recognition and determination of the time of myocardial infarctions have so far led to varied results. Utilizable findings have in the main only been achieved with early autopsy a few hours after death. A systematic examination of the enzymes histochemically detectable in 1964 and investigation of the quantitative and qualitative activity changes in experimental cardiac infarction by Hecht did not produce any forensically utilizable results. Later studies of phosphorylase activity yielded variable results: Jääskeläinen (1968 – references) found a distinct reduction 2–5 min after ligature of the coronary arteries, and after 10 min enzymatic activity could no longer be detected. Sakurai (1977) did not find a focal loss in the phosphorylase activity until after 90 min, phosphorylase was eliminated by autolysis 2–3 h PM in undamaged cardiac muscle. This method indicating sensitive and early changes only appears to be appropriate for experiments. Utilizable results on human autopsy material have been provided by studies of cytochrome oxidase and succinodehydrogenase; after myocardial infarctions that had been survived for 1–2 h, decreases in enzymatic activity and formazan formation were detectable. According to our own investigations, which did not permit any reliable chronological ordering of the findings, we would accept that the checking of these two enzymes is the most suitable method for an attempt at an early diagnosis of myocardial infarction, as long as strong autolysis is not present.

The hematoxylin – basic fuchsin – picric acid (HBFP) method developed by Lie for the selective staining of ischemically damaged cardiac muscle fibers has been investigated and modified many times. Its practical applicability has been both positively and negatively rated in the literature (Tausch 1974; Rajs and Jakobsson 1976b; Sakurai 1977; Reempts et al. 1976; Knight 1979; Gregersen 1979; Saukko 1981). In experiments with HBFP, a dark red staining of the damaged myocardial fibers occurred within the 1st h after the onset of ischemia, sometimes even after 5 min. This method is forensically unsuitable owing to the occurrence of false-positive and false-negative results.

The tartaric acid–Kresylecht violet–inclusion stain was recommended by Holczabek (1970, 1973) for detecting fine necroses beginning in the region of a myocardial infarction. In contrast to the undamaged musculature, which is stained blue-violet to red-violet, the damaged muscle areas appear extremely pale or sky to light blue. Experimentally, the damaged areas of muscle could be clearly distinguished after 1 h with this technique. Occasionally, it is possible with normal H and E stain to visualize the eosinophilia in the marginal areas of fresh infarctions before the first interstitial reactions. The hyaline transverse striation of the muscle cells shows a similar stainability following hypoxic damage (Adebahr 1966; Hirvonen 1976). A comparable effect is also possible with PTAH stain. After acridine orange fluorochromatization on unfixed sections, damaged cardiac muscle cells can be distinguished by a clear green fluorescence; in animal experiments this occurred as early as 2–3 h after the onset of anoxia (Korb and Knorr 1962; Korb 1964; Korb and Totowic 1967).

A simple and reliable histological method was introduced by Hort (1964, 1965). This involves measuring the intervals of transverse striation in cardiac muscle fibers in unstained sections using an eyepiece micrometer on a phase-contrast microscope. The straining of the cardiac muscle fibers in the region of a fresh cardiac infarction can be determined 15 min after the interruption of blood supply by the comparative investigation of several sections of cardiac muscle. The average distance between the muscle bands is normally 1.3 μm; in the region of an infarction, it increases to 2.25 μm. We found the same results in human infarction hearts with a survival time of 1–2 h. Noteworthy here were also the pronounced edema, which could be discerned particularly well with phase-contrast microscopy, and the occurrence of circumscribed fibrous contractions. The measurements on the heart have to be carried out with rigor mortis already having set in (Böhm 1981).

In all, the possibilities for early recognition of a myocardial infarction have improved in recent decades. However, it must be borne in mind that in the case of a short survival time, an infarction cannot be excluded with certainty by negative findings in the examination.

After a survival time of 6–7 h, whereby macroscopically a pallor becomes distinct on the myocardial cut surface, histologically general eosinophilia of the muscle fibers and depletion of the cardiac muscle nuclei can be seen. The transverse striation of the heart muscle cells is preserved for a relatively long time. Subsequently, after about 8 h – the accounts are variable – leukocytic migration into the peripheral zone of the infarction occurs, which reaches a peak after approximately 5–6 days. Abscesslike liquefaction with myocytolysis, myomalacia, and rupture of the whole ventricular wall can also occur. In the event of survival, the infarction necrosis is removed by granular tissue and replaced by an increasingly fibrous scar tissue.

Coronary thrombosis. Since the introduction of regular histological investigations on the coronary arterial system, the diagnosis of coronary thromboses has perceptibly increased in frequency (Krauland 1966, 1972). Histological examination has often been held to be superfluous in cases where macroscopically the coronary arteries appeared unobstructed or a coronary thrombosis found during the autopsy seemed to be unequivocal. The histological finding is, however, indispensable as a check and when offering evidence, particularly in disputed cases. An autochthonous coronary thrombosis has to be distinguished from postmortem clots, embolisms, and ruptures of the walls without thrombosis. It has to be expected that a coronary thrombosis in its initial phases may go unnoticed by the naked eye.

In the preparation for histological examination, the coronary arteries should not be cut open but laminated by sections transverse to the vascular axis. The sites of the sections must be recorded; for this a schematic diagram is frequently used. In systematic histological investigations of the entire coronary arterial system, combination with coronary angiography is recommended for the detection of vascular occlusions and stenoses. The adventitia and adjacent vascular area should also be incorporated as far as possible in the examination at the sites where the individual sections were made.

The morphology of coronary occlusions is so diverse that pathoanatomical and histopathological findings only have a limited value in statistical evaluation and clinical treatment (Krauland 1966). The histological examination of coronary thromboses concentrates on age determination of the clots, which mainly arise through striation (cf. p. 103). It is important to investigate the nature of the arterial wall, from which the causes of the coronary thrombosis can usually be deduced. Arteriosclerosis is clearly of prime importance with its extremely variable forms, changes, and signs of organization. An acquaintance with the histomorphology here is assumed (Krauland 1966; Janssen 1968; Liebegott 1969); this includes knowledge of other inflammatory and degenerative lesions of the coronary arterial system (Doerr 1979).

Occasionally, it is difficult to recognize fibrin-rich flat thromboses beginning above arteriosclerotic ruptures of covering plates and parietal hemorrhages. H and E, elastica van Gieson, PTAH, and iron stains are recommended for routine use.

Myocarditis. Histological diagnosis of myocarditis is based on the morphological evidence of an inflammatory exudate or cellular proliferation (Doerr 1981). The inflammation occurs in the vascular connective tissue of the myocardium, i.e., in the cardiac muscle interstitium. Inflammations that primarily emanate from a lesion of the cardiac muscle parenchyma, and afterwards include the interstitium, have to be pathogenetically differentiated from those forms that initially attack the vascular connective tissue. Further, the differentiation has to be made between inflammatory myocardial disorders, which as independent events exclusively or predominantly affect the heart, and inflammatory reactions in the region of the myocardium, which appear in the context of a general disorder or damage to other organs.

The causes of fatal myocardial insufficiency in myocarditis are attributed to a reduction in the contractility of cardiac muscle and disturbances in the excitation process in the heart (Zebe and Mall 1979). The commonest and clinically most significant inflammatory cardiac muscle disorders are rheumatic, bacterial, and viral myocarditis. The differential diagnosis of myocarditis should particularly consider the histionic consequences of coronary heart diseases and primary cardiomyopathies.

The center of interest here does not lie in cases of fully expressed myocarditis and the various causes and forms (Janssen and Naeve 1975) but in problematic discrete conditions and initial phases. The forensic significance of myocarditis as a cause of sudden natural death lies in the fact that, in particular, young, seemingly healthy individuals can unexpectedly die without any special preliminary signs emerging in their daily lives, and that it can coincide with forensically irrelevant circumstances. In cases of cot death, myocarditis must practically always be considered (Noren et al. 1977; Thurner 1977). Myocarditis can easily be overlooked in autopsies where no detailed histological examination is performed. Histological investigations are occasionally dispensed with when the events causing death, e.g., in road and industrial accidents, appear sufficiently certain from the injury findings.

Macroscopic cardiac muscle findings can be deceptive with regard to two features. First, there are cases of moycarditis in which the cardiac muscle appears firm and has a normal color; second, in autopsies performed early that the cardiac musculature has been found to display a loose and patchy character. The macroscopic nature of the myocardium is probably influenced by the terminal metabolism and circulation. Finally, in the examination it should be borne in mind that myocarditis frequently appears focally and its diagnosis without histological control leaves a good deal to chance. Assessment and evaluation of the myocardial interstitium can sometimes be difficult in inflammatory general disorders and other extracardial lesions.

For the identification or exclusion of myocarditis, a standardized procedure is recommended with the routine examination of particular section sites; at least eight sites should be examined in the region of both ventricles, including the conductive system. This method also permits topographic visualization of any localized inflammatory findings that may be present. Otherwise, no particular technique is required. As a rule, thin paraffin sections suffice, with H and E, Goldner's, and van Gieson's stains. The Ladewig staining method has proven useful in the identification of early changes in the myocardium (Althoff 1980). For continuous cell differentiation, the Giemsa stain is recommended.

With stronger reactions of the vascular connective tissue, swelling and increase in the number of cardiac histiocytic elements, endothelia, and mast cells, various interpretations arise as to whether this is autonomic myocarditis or a "co-reaction" of extracardial disorders. These changes are frequently accompanied by interstitial edema with enlargement of the perfusion section between the capillary wall and cardiac muscle cell. In addition to a qualitative differentiation of the cells located in the interstitium, a quantitative verification is required. A method of counting and evaluating the nuclei of the interstitium compared with the number of muscle cell nuclei was developed by Klages and Gerken (1972). Use of this technique can facilitate the identification or exclusion of myocarditis.

Commotio Cordis. There are no unequivocal anatomical and histomorphological findings in commotio cordis. In a case where this condition is suspected, a histological status examination of the entire heart is recommended with several section sites, particularly in the regions located toward the anterior chest wall.

Unequal blood distribution within the cardiac muscle can be an indication of previous commotio cordis. Disproportionate distention of the cardiac muscle fibers, detectable under the phase-contrast microscope, also has indicative significance, although this can be a sign of a fresh myocardial infarction in the case of stenoses of the coronary arteries. The investigation should include a histological examination of the conduction system. All signs of a long-standing reduced cardiac performance should be noted as these can lead to "hypersensitivity of the heart to trauma" (Krauland 1954; Bratzke 1980). The diagnosis of commotio cordis can only be forensically advocated if the heart is on the whole healthy and an appropriately strong trauma damaging the pericardial sections of the chest wall preceded death by a short time.

The change to commotio cordis is occasionally smooth. Histological evidence for it can be adduced by discontinuous tissue in the region of the heart. Fiber contusions can be recognized by consolidation of the fibrillar structure and increased stainability. Hemorrhages with dissociation of the cardiac muscle cells have indicative value. Maculate changes in the cardiac muscle in the form of myocarditis can also occur as a result of direct traumatic violence to the thorax (Plueckharn and Cameron 1968). The late sequelae following contusio cordis are very diverse and histologically uncharacteristic (Behrenhoff 1966; Staak 1968; Walther 1972; Rajs and Jakobsson 1976a).

Conduction System. Cardiac death which cannot be explained by other examination findings may sometimes be attributable to relatively discrete changes in the conduction system. The evaluation and assessment of the functional significance of such mainly circumscribed findings is not easy. Changes and lesions in the conduction system can be divided into three groups – age-dependent changes, ischemic changes as a result of arteriosclerosis, and lesions as part of more or less generalized pathological processes (Voigt 1976; Voigt and Steinmetz 1977). The age-dependent changes are wholly unspecific; they comprise diffuse fibroses, increase in the elastic fibers, pigment deposition, and nerve cell degeneration. The chronic ischemic lesions lead to more localized fibroses. In this connection, the character of the blood vessels belonging to this region, in particular the sinoatrial node artery, have to be considered; fibrous swellings of the intima, hyperplasia of the muscularis, and constriction of the vascular lumen can be found. The diseases that can damage the conduction system include all general disorders that have an effect on other parts of the heart, especially infections, inflammations, granulomas, and tumors.

Particular attention should be paid to the conduction system in the case of sudden death of unknown origin, even in infancy (Ferris 1972, 1974; Lie et al. 1971). In sick sinus syndrome, other cardiac rhythm disorders, and hypertrophic and congestive cardiomyopathy, disturbances in the normal tissue texture have been detected in the region of the sinoatrial node in addition to fibroses with the loss of specific muscle fibers (Knieriem et al. 1980).

Aneurysms. Here, the histological examination concentrates on distinguishing between traumatically and naturally incurred aneurysms and clarifying the question of a traumatic or spontaneous aneurysmal rupture. Aneurysms of the arteries of the base of the brain are of major importance; of less interest here are aneurysms of other vascular regions. Natural aneurysm formation is explained by congenital weaknesses in the vascular wall, lacunal development in the normal structure of the elastica and media, and numerous vascular diseases, e.g., arteriosclerosis, medionecrosis, calcinosis, and inflammations. Identification and assessment of the etiology and pathogenesis of an aneurysm becomes difficult when the formation dates back a long time and subsequent reparative and degenerative processes, e.g., secondary arteriosclerosis, cicatrization, trophopathy, thromboses, inflammations, and organizational processes, are superimposed upon the original finding.

Traumatically induced aneurysm, which is only survived by several weeks or at most a few months, can be identified by the following histological findings: circumscribed, nondegeneratively incurred interruption of parts of the vascular wall, mainly of the elastica interna, with widening of the unaffected, continuous vascular wall layers. The wall of such a false aneurysm thus does not contain an elastica interna in an ideal histological case, but only intima and parts of the muscularis and adventitia.

Histological identification of a traumatically incurred aneurysmal rupture is carried out by careful serial sections from the aneurysmal wall in the marginal areas of the rupture site. It is presupposed that a trauma occurred which was capable in terms of type, localization, serverity, and time of inducing the aneurysm in question. If an aneurysmal wall can then be identified in the rupture fissure as being sufficiently nourished, multilayered, and histologically appears resistant, such a finding constitutes a forensically utilizable basis for a traumatic aneurysmal rupture. If, on the other hand, significant degenerative changes and fresh malacia, e.g., puriform softened parietal thromboses, are found in the region of the rupture site, then such changes are highly indicative of a spontaneous nontraumatic aneurysmal rupture (Klages 1970; Weiler 1980).

Careful pretreatment of the preparation is important in the histological examination. This includes spraying the tissue in question with a 4% formalin solution or carefully plugging the aneurysmal sac with formalin-soaked cotton wool, which is removed again prior to embedding. The preparation is best carried out on sections parallel to the longitudinal axis of the vessel. For staining, H and E, van Gieson, elastica van Gieson, and PTAH are recommended. The possibility of aneurysmal ruptures occuring gradually at different times with inflammatory reactions of varying age should be considered. Further, it is important to assess and determine the age of parietal thromboses which are usually present.

Hepatosis – Acute Atrophy. Histological identification and assessment of acute damage to the liver parenchyma generally does not give rise to any diagnostic difficulties in autopsies performed early with organs that are not excessively autolytic. Certain diagnosis, however, becomes problematic if strong autolysis is already present and the hepatosis is still in its initial phase. This can lead to difficulties in the differential diagnosis with regard to vascular and biliary congestion, eclampsia, shock changes, and exogenous and endogenous intoxications, e.g., as a result of poisoning or burns. Examination of the liver, taking in several central and peripheral sites, is recommended by means of paraffin sections and different stains – H and E, Goldner's, elastica van Gieson, and visualizing the fibers by silver-staining.

In advanced autolysis with extensive disappearance of the lobe borders and reduction in the stainability of the nucleus and cytoplasm, the presence of an acute hepatosis can sometimes neither be confirmed nor excluded. Inflammatory changes to the interstitium and biliary congestion remain for a comparatively long time.

The histological diagnosis of hepatosis is forensically significant in that such an acute liver disorder can explain the sudden natural death of a person even without other morbid organ damage.

II. Pregnancy – Abortion – Aborticide
(Forensic Gynecology)

1. Pregnancy – Death of the Mother

From the forensic point of view, the question sometimes needs to be clarified as to whether pregnancy is or was present. In the case of living subjects, a histological examination cannot be undertaken solely for forensic reasons. For medical reasons, however, tissue material may be obtained from the uterus by curettage and histologically examined; an expert opinion on the histological finding may later be called for. Parts of the endometrium and uterine contents come under consideration as findings.

Only parts of the fetus and chorionic villi are proof of a pregnancy having taken place (Fig. 97). Prior to the increase in the number of abortions through nonmedical indications, it was relatively seldom that curettage material from an intact pregnancy could be examined; the material predominantly originated from curettages which were performed in a status post abortum or abortus incipiens, particularly the latter if the fetus had been fatally injured for some time or had already died.

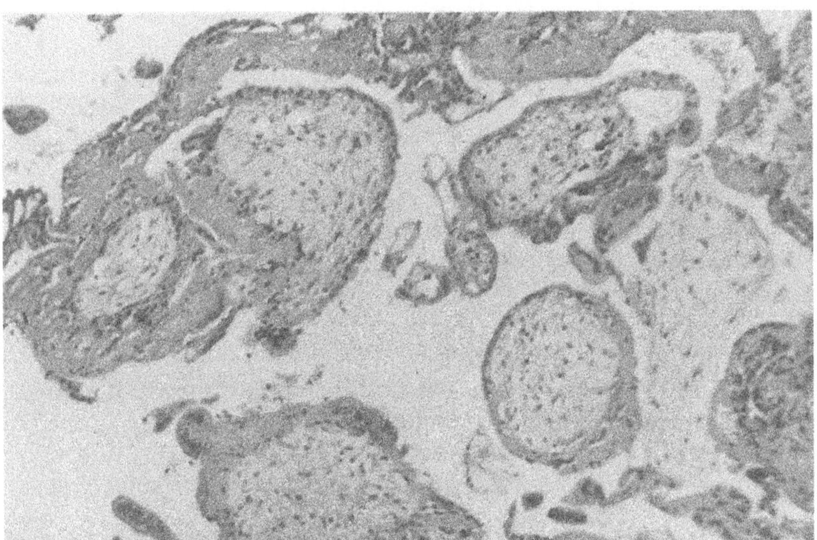

Fig. 97. Status post abortum with relatively well preserved chorionic villi (curettage material). H and E, 1:150

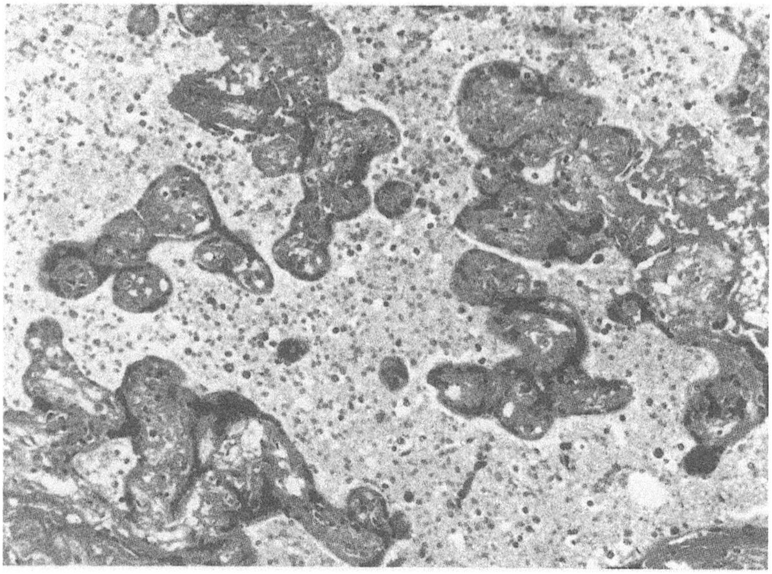

Fig. 98. Placental remains with regressively altered chorionic villi (autopsy material). PTAH, 1:150

Where pregnancy has taken place, a large number of curettages contain only inflammatory or regressively changed tissue components; here, identifying evidence of pregnancy requires a certain amount of practice and experience. The diagnosis of well-preserved and normally structured chorionic villi should not create any difficulties. Conversely, chorionic villi that are hyalinized, extensively broken down, or evident only as shadows (Fig. 98) and which can be found only by serial sections of the curettage material, can provide problems. Here, the histologist with experience of gynopathology directs his attention to the remaining components of the curettage material that may indicate a foregone pregnancy. This includes, e.g., decidual stromal transformation of the endometrium if it contains large cells, has a broad structure, and is in the form of decidua compacta.

The presence of a decidua alone is no proof of pregnancy; it is an expression of the hormonal activity of the corpus luteum. A decidua can also form without pregnancy in persistence or hyperactivity of the corpus luteum and in various hormonally active ovarian tumours. The development of a decidua without pregnancy has been recognized for some time and does not merit particular consideration from a clinical point of view (Spechter 1953).

The significance of the Arias-Stella reaction is disputed. It involves atypical glandular changes in the mucosa of the corpus uteri. It has to be inferred from many studies that an Arias-Stella reaction does not in itself represent evidence of pregnancy (Bellinvia and Aragona 1963; Schönfeldt et al. 1964; Dallenbach 1966).

If, in an unclarified case of death, it is suspected that a pregnancy may have occurred or if macroscopic findings suggest such a possibility even without the presence of a fetus, then the following histological examinations are advised: checking the interior surface of the uterus, especially in the region of the fundus and angles of the Fallopian tubes, for placental remains. A basic requirement is an extensive col-

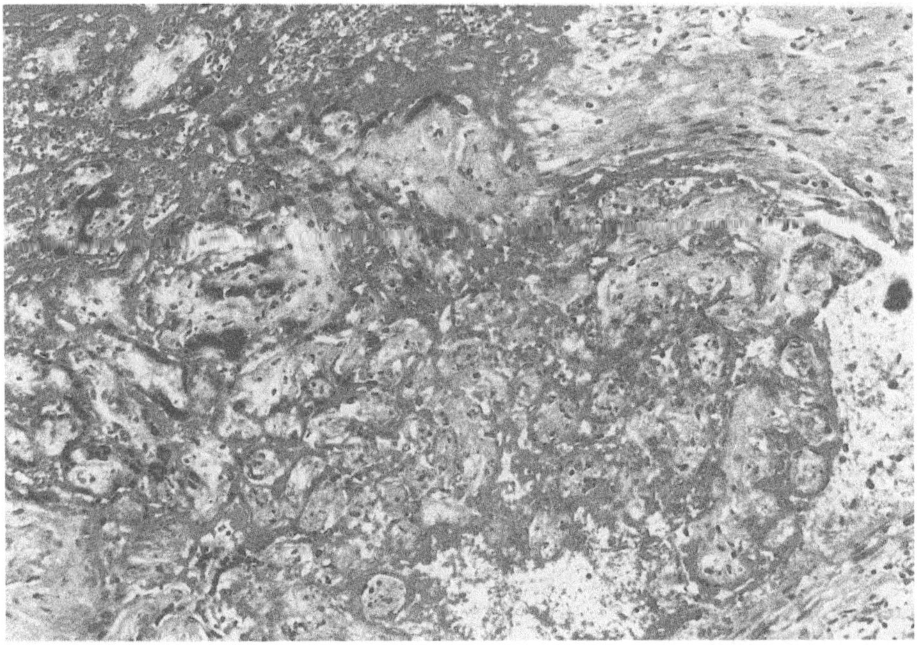

Fig. 99. Uterine wall with regressively altered placental remains. Puerperal sepsis, exitus 14 days post partum. PTAH, 1:150

lection of samples from the whole uterus, including the vagina, parametria, and adnexa. Suspicious material adhering to the placental remains should first be precisely described with regard to its locality and size. It should be borne in mind that with histologically proven placental remains and unequivocal chorionic villi, such structures are often significantly enlarged through blood coagula, fibrin, and inflammatory deposits. The relationship between placental remains and secondary deposits must be clearly presented in the macroscopic and histological report. These details constitute important morphological evidence and may later be called upon with regard to questions of correlation in legal proceedings requiring the opinion of a medical examiner.

Sections for visualizing placental remains should be made serially, perpendicular to the interior surface of the uterus. The myometrium must be sectioned as far as its medial areas, otherwise chorionic villi located deep in the uterine wall in cases of placenta increta will not be detected. It should be borne in mind with older placental remains that parts of the placenta can be subject to considerable regressive changes and show signs of degradation corresponding to the time elapsed since fetal death (Fig. 99). A rough estimate of this interval is possible with the appropriate experience. Remains of chorionic villi can still be identified 2–3 months after a pregnancy with Giemsa stain. There are not as yet any systematic studies concerning chronological determination by histological means.

After a pregnancy, choreal migratory cells may frequently be detected in the uterine musculature and sometimes also in the lymphatic vessels of the parametri-

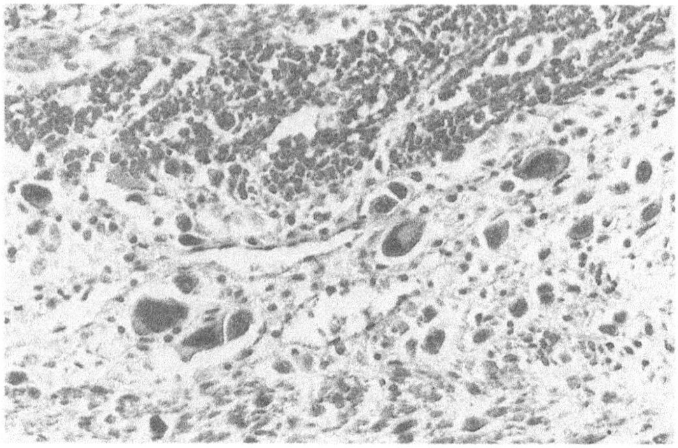

Fig. 100. Choreal migratory cells in the uterine wall; 1 day post partum. H and E, 1:220

um (Fig. 100). These are large, mainly mononuclear cells which originate in the syncytial surface layer of the villi. They can also appear in the uterine wall in a normal pregnancy. Using Giemsa stain, they can be distinguished from the myometrium comparatively well.

Histological investigations of the corpus luteum graviditatis are usually not very productive from a forensic point of view. Histological identification of a corpus luteum in the secretory and desquamative phase or a persistent corpus luteum cannot be made with certainty in the initial stages of pregnancy. In advanced pregnancy, beyond the 3rd – 4th month, the corpus luteum graviditatis can be determined with certainty in most cases by its typical structure in the outer zone. The possibilities for histological identification are considerably restricted even a few days after pregnancy by the regressive changes that commence directly after parturition or fetal death.

A further possibility is offered by histological examination of the anterior lobe of the pituitary for pregnancy cells. These appear at the end of pregnancy and during lactation. The fine granules in the cytoplasm, which are typical for these cells, can be visualized by the use of appropriate stains, e. g., with performic acid – alcian blue and periodic acid – Schiff (PAS) orange (Fig. 101). By counting these cells and comparing this number with the normal cellular proportion in the anterior pituitary, a particularly reliable diagnosis of pregnancy may be achieved. Here again, the signs of retrogression, which set in comparatively rapidly after parturition, fetal death, or end of lactation, must be considered (Glatthaar 1962).

Without other specific findings, histological investigations of the mammary glands for signs of lactation only have indicative value for a pregnancy even when lactation is fully in progress. Milk secretion can be set into operation in a woman by various hormonal influences, for example, hormone-active tumors, hormone therapy, even without gravidity.

Histology of Causes of Death Through Natural Pregnancy Complications. Particular attention has to be paid to the histological changes of the liver in eclampsia. According to the generally accepted interpretation, this involves acute damage to the

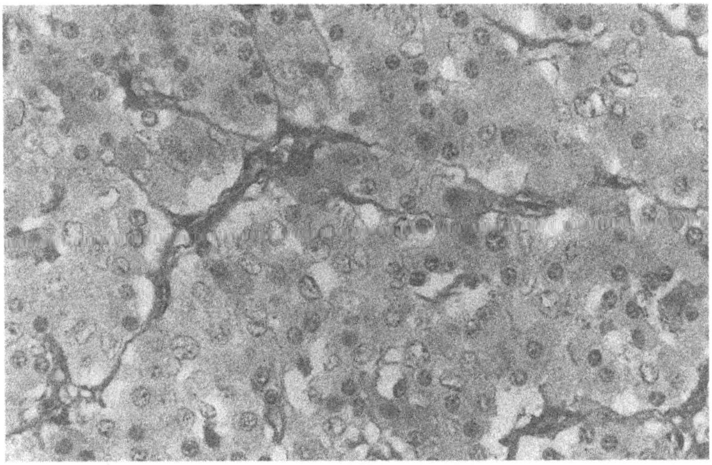

Fig. 101. Anterior lobe of the pituitary in gravidity (very fine granulation of the epithelia difficult to recognize). Performic acid-alcian blue and PAS-orange G, 1:350

liver parenchyma caused by a pregnancy intoxication. Rapid destruction of liver cells occurs, originating from the lobule centers. The partly necrobiotic liver epithelia are on the whole very fatty. The rapid parenchymal collapse also leads to dilation of the liver sinusoids and the necrotic zones filling with blood. Histologically, the symptoms resemble acute hepatosis. Inflammatory changes do not appear until after an appropriate survival time. With regard to differential diagnosis, exogenous intoxication, e.g., carbon tetrachloride or phosphorus poisoning, must be considered. Bioptic, histological, and electron-microscopic studies performed in parallel on kidneys in gestational toxicosis showed diffuse unspecific changes to the glomeruli with protein-like precipitates and sedimentation of fibrinous material (Yamazaki 1965).

The spreading of necroses in the region of the anterior pituitary in complications of pregnancy and complicated deliveries has been known for some time (Simonds 1914; Sheehan 1937). Spontaneous necroses with extensive destruction of large areas of this important endocrine organ can occur particularly in the terminal phase of pregnancy. Intravascular fibrinous thrombi or metabolic disturbances in diabetes (Dorfman et al. 1979) have been cited as causes of such tissue destruction. Similar pituitary findings are also observed in connection with Sheehan's syndrome.

Malignant tumors that arise from the often previously malignant degenerated placenta (hydatiform mole) can be the cause of natural death during or after pregnancy. Important here is the very malignant choriocarcinoma, which emanates from the epithelium of the chorionic villi and can lead to metastases in various organs within a short time. The diagnosis can be confirmed by the typical histological evidence.

In the case of death through exsanguination in an ectopic pregnancy, e.g., in the region of the adnexa or in the free abdominal cavity, the macroscopic findings are usually very distinct. Nonetheless, even here, histological documentation of the cause of death is recommended by taking sections from the peripheral areas of the site of implantation along with evidence of fetal components, in particular parts of the placenta.

2. Miscarriage – Abortion

Histological examination findings can have a decisive significance for proof of an abortion when other evidence, e.g., parts of the embryo or fetus or macroscopically detectable parts of the placenta, is not at hand. The investigation is performed on abortion or curettage material. Histological evidence for abortion is identical with that for a pregnancy having taken place, as described above. To identify with certainty an abortion in progress or a status post abortum, it is necessary for there at least to be evidence of chorionic villi. Usually, these are well mixed with blood clots and decidual components altered by necrosis and inflammation. Leukocytic inflammation of decidually transformed endometrium, which is almost always present, has indicative value but in itself is not proof.

Other than through chance findings, the cause of abortion cannot be determined by the histological examination of abortion and curettage material alone. The presence of specific inflammations, e.g., tuberculosis, could adequately explain the cause of an abortion. Otherwise, embryo- and fetopathy as causes of abortion should be dealt with and assessed by an appropriately experienced pathologist. Further natural causes of spontaneous abortions, for instance those that are genetically or hormonally dependent, cannot be entered into here.

The reliable identification of an artificial termination of pregnancy and differentiating this from a spontaneous abortion is usually not possible by the histological examination of abortion and curettage material alone. It is conceivable that foreign bodies could be detected as signs of an induced abortion in rare cases. The presence of pronounced endometritis post abortum can indicate an abortive operation complicated by infection; in itself, however, it is not proof of an artificial termination of pregnancy.

The evidence of well-preserved components of pregnancy without concomitant inflammatory symptoms may be taken to indicate curettage of an intact fetus. Otherwise, the question of whether an abortion was brought about by artificial means can only be clarified in connection with the case history, course of disease, clinical investigatory findings, and the results of inquiries.

The following histological examinations on the corpse should be considered in ascertaining whether death was incurred by spontaneous or artificial abortion: evidence of the route of propagation of infection, if present, through systematic sections of the endometrium, myometrium, parametrium, adnexa, ovarian veins, lungs, liver, spleen, and regional lymph nodes; investigation for histomorphological indications of shock (cf. p. 156), especially disseminated intravascular fibrin thrombi; histochemical evidence of material that could have been applied to elicit an abortion; in addition, sections from the uterus, kidneys, lungs, and brain and staining with Sudan black, Sudan III, and Nile blue sulfate.

Evidence of intravascular fat-positive substances can contribute to the detection of soap-abortion (Weinig and Schwerd 1951; Schwerd 1959). A negative result with the fat stains does not argue against such a soap-abortion, since the fat substances can be eliminated in the case of longer survival times (Dreese 1968).

Connected with the search for morphological criteria, the anamnestic, clinical, bacteriological, and histomorphological indications for the presence of a general Shwartzman's phenomenon should be considered. It appears that this syndrome and renal complications have increased in recent decades as causes of death following abortion; in contrast, infections due to pyogenic organisms were more frequent in earlier years. This change in the fatal complications that occur after abortion is possibly connected with the increased use of antibiotics (Krecke 1964; Adebahr 1964). The endotoxins liberated during intensive antibiotic therapy which flow into the bloodstream can have the effect of "preparatory injections." The morphological findings in general Shwartzman's phenomenon after abortion and infection with gram-negative pathogens are not fundamentally different from other generalized infections with the morphological character of endotoxin shock. The important findings are damage to the kidneys and adrenals, with the development of bilateral cortical necroses, changes in blood coagulation and blood lipids, and the incidence of fatal cases with evidence of a Waterhouse-Friedrichsen syndrome. In young women, such findings should always be reason to look for signs of a previous pregnancy and abortive operations (Tabbara et al. 1962; Huth et al. 1964; Josey et al. 1966; Adebahr 1964).

In one particular case, Adelson (1963) found histological evidence of abundant amniotic components in the terminal bronchi and alveoli of both lungs in a young woman after criminal abortion with perforation of the uterus and rupture of the jejunum. It was assumed that amniotic fluid had entered the jejunum via the uterine perforation and from there made its way into the lungs by antiperistalsis, vomiting, and aspiration.

3. Aborticide and Perinatal Death

In clarifying aborticide and cases of perinatal death, the histological investigations of the medical examiner are particularly concerned with the question of whether the child lived. Frequently, also, the question of the cause of the child's death cannot be satisfactorily answered without histological examination.

The Problem of Live or Still Birth

In tackling this problem histological, histochemical, and biochemical investigations of the lungs, umbilical ring, and umbilical vessels can make a contribution.

In the case of a newly born infant either stillborn or found dead, the state of the lungs is of particular forensic interest. For centuries, the result of the classic pulmonary docimasia has had decisive significance. Nowadays, forensic medicine endeavors to secure and extend the diagnostic possibilities. Critical objections have to be settled which arise, e.g., from artificial respiration of a newborn child, putrefaction-induced changes in the lungs, and liquid infiltration of the pulmonary tissue.

Even in unborn children taken dead from the uterus of the dead mother, partial infiltration of air into the lungs could be detected (Meixner 1926). The cause of this partial aeration was explained by postmortem entry of air into the lungs as a result of manipulations to the corpse of the child during autopsy. Nowadays, in a time of widespread enlightenment and instruction in resuscitative measures, it has to be expected that actual or alleged postmortem aerations of the lungs will be increasingly encountered. Forensic practice does show, however, that a clear-cut positive pulmonary docimasia, in which the entire breathing apparatus, including the heart and cervical organs, is supported by the lungs, is still valid as a strong sign that the child lived. Care must be taken in the autopsy prior to the removal of the lungs and cervical organs that the trachea is first ligatured and that the lungs do not show any pronounced signs of putrefaction. The assessment becomes difficult if partly aerated lungs or signs of putrefaction and gas formation are present in the pulmonary tissue. All lobes of the lungs must then be histologically examined for further clarification. Of particular significance here is the comparative histomorphological evaluation of elastic fibers in aerated and nonaerated lungs (Prokop 1971 – references). According to Plank (1965), histological examination of nonaerated lungs in stillborn babies is best performed with prior in situ fixation.

The view is predominantly held that artificial respiration cannot cause the alveoli of the lungs of stillborn neonates to be perfectly and uniformly aerated. Artificial respiration usually leads to the formation of irregularly sized alveoli, in parts expanded; such findings resemble putrefaction. The ventilated lungs of neonates that lived at least 17 min could be well differentiated from these findings (Hirvonen et al. 1969). According to the present level of knowledge and possibilities for examination, ventilation of the lungs alone cannot be taken as a certain indication of a live birth. Under various circumstances, lungs originally aerated can become devoid of air: conversely, the lungs of stillborn neonates can appear aerated. It is not possible to be certain in all cases. A critical and correlative assessment of the histological and macroscopic findings is required with regard to the histology of pulmonary development (Buris et al. 1979).

The pulmonary tissue of immature stillborn infants with a body weight of less than 800 g is characterized by a glandlike quality of the alveoli. It is not until further development that the beginnings of irregular alveolarization become evident. In stillborn infants over 2500 g and in fully developed fetuses taken from the uterus of dead mothers, the alveolar formation is largely uniform. The alveolar walls are seen with convoluted surfaces, which bear highly capillarized pulvinate or club-like ramifications; they have been termed "crumpled alveoli" (Essbach 1961). In this condition, the elastic fibers are not strained and the argyrophilic fibers run in a slightly undulatory manner. The elastic fibers behave like rubber bands, i.e., in both the tense (aerated) and relaxed (atelactic, nonaerated) condition they appear straight and nonundulatory. The form of the elastic fibers is thus impracticable as a morphological criterion for a "vital test" (Prokop 1971). The connections between the development of elastic fibers, aeration, and maturity of the fetus have already been studied by Goldbach (1956) and Ogawa et al. (1962).

Similarly diffcult to assess is a liquid infiltration of the lungs, which can occur by intrauterine inhalation of amniotic fluid and, therefore, is to be regarded as physiological (Plank 1965). However, as a source of amniotic fluid, the lung itself also comes into consideration; this is indicated by fluid-infiltrated lungs in cases of congenital occlusion of the larynx and trachea. Thus, the term fetal atelectasis cannot be applied to the fluid-infiltrated lungs of stillborn infants; the designations "apneumatosis pulmonum" or "status fetalis pulmonum" are suggested. The misgivings against the use of pulmonary docimasia by Raubitschek (1955), who based his objections on animal experiments with the introduction of amniotic fluid into pulmonary tissue, have generally not been accepted.

Histological identification of a fluid infiltration in pulmonary tissue can be problematic if the liquid does not contain any recognizable admixtures of bodies, e.g., amniotic components, as then the alveolar lumina appear unstained. An infiltration of fluid developing during childbirth does, however, normally give rise to alternating atelectic and infiltrated areas of the lungs. Physiological intrauterine infiltration of fluid also affects more circumscribed areas of lung and does not lead to the uniform total infiltration of whole pulmonary lobes.

The influence of autolysis and putrefaction can lead to the disappearance of air or regeneration of gas within the pulmonary tissue. A good contrast staining of the lung structures present, with visualization of the argyrophilic fibers, e.g., with Gomori's or Bielschowsky's stain, is required for the histological identification of such postmortem changes. If no severe tissue destruction has set in, it is possible in this manner to determine whether the putrefactive bubbles are partially located in the pulmonary interstitium or have led to a disproportionate expansion of the alveoli with bacterial colonization.

Comparative histological studies on fresh and artificially mummified lungs revealed relatively well-preserved alveolar structures in the subpleural sections. An infiltration of the alveoli could also be detected in the mummified tissue. Histological examination of the sections of the lungs close to the surface is, therefore, recommended for mummified neonate corpses (Tomaszewska and Sawa 1973).

The filling of the bronchioli respiratorii and alveolar ducts is thought only to occur in live-born infants. Similarly, hyaline membranes have only been observed in the lungs of children who lived (Kuoda et al. 1965a, b).

Thickenings of the intima protruding into the vascular lumen have only been detected in the small and intermediate pulmonary arteries of stillborn children. They were particularly localized in the vascular ramifications and were composed of light, round cells, partly with pyknotic nuclei (Mityayeva 1970).

Small hematoxylin particles are occasionally found in the lungs of live-born immature neonates. These are chiefly located in the terminal ramifications of the bronchioles, sometimes also in the alveoli. They are round homogeneous bodies which are intensely stained by basic dyes and are also Feulgen-positive, pyroninophilic, and weakly PAS-positive. These particles may also be enclosed together with other nuclear material in hyaline membranes. It is assumed that these hematoxylin particles are composed of mucopolysaccharides, lipoproteins, and nuclear substances. The particles are probably formed from the nuclei of necrotic epithelia of the terminal respiratory tracts or from hyaline membranes (Bayer et al. 1962; Link 1964). The hematoxylin particles have not been observed in stillborn or mature neonates.

The evidence of starch particles in the fluid pressed out of the lungs can as a kind of a preliminary test, indicate a vital aspiration. At the same time, the lungs should be histologically investigated for starch particles in the respiratory tracts and the stomach contents examined for comparison (Petersohn 1964).

Histochemical studies of the alkaline and acidic phosphomonoesterases in the skin, lungs, liver, and kidneys show an increase in enzymatic activity with the beginning of respiration. This finding is possibly stimulated by the process of childbirth (Lo Menzo and Chiara 1966). Alkaline phosphatase could not be detected in stillborn infants. Contrary to other assertions made in the literature, evidence of enzymes was not found until after 8-h breathing (Ruthig 1973). Free and total histamine was evident in distinctly higher concentrations in the lungs of live-born children than in those stillborn (Fazekas et al. 1973). Histamine determination is thought to be suitable for application in forensic practice.

Umbilical Cord and Ring. Evidence of inflammatory changes in the region of the umbilical ring at the boundary between the skin of the umbilical cord and the epidermis of the abdominal skin shows that the child had lived. A critical assessment of all studies published thus far, however, reveals that in a given case such a demarcating inflammation has to be evaluated in conjunction with the maturity of the child and, as far as is known, the duration of birth.

For the histological examination, the whole navel should be removed together with a 1- to 2-cm-long piece of the umbilical cord and, if possible, a piece just as long of the umbilical vessels running intra-abdominally and within the abdominal walls. The investigation should be carried out by serial sections made parallel to the longitudinal axis of the umbilical cord at the level of the border with the navel skin. Any good nuclear stain would be suitable for visualizing the tissues.

At least two to three polymorphonuclear leukocytes per visual field under intermediate magnification, are held to be the first sign of an inflammation and are, on the whole, located closely beneath the epidermis at the boundary of the umbilical cord skin. If there is doubt as to the type and inflammatory nature of the cellular elements then a peroxidase reaction is recommended, which can also be carried out easily on paraffin sections. Extravascular fibrin deposits and infiltrative hemorrhages are rare. The further stages of demarcation develop in the form generally familiar in inflammations, first of all with reduction in the polymorphonuclear leukocytes, then appearance of mononuclear cells, budding of capillaries from the region of the subepidermal navel skin, and finally the development of typical granular tissue.

In stillborn premature infants, no signs have thus far been detected of inflammation at the umbilical ring (Fritz 1935; Fazekas et al. 1969 – references). Even with stillborn mature infants, no cases have hitherto been known of the beginnings of demarcating inflammation. In post-term stillborn infants, e.g., infants suffocated during birth, sporadic leukocytes were detected at the amnion–navel skin boundary in a number of the cases investigated. An observation by Fritz (1935) on a mature neonated should be noted. The infant was delivered after a 72-h birth and showed cardiac activity only for 15 min without respiring. A large leukocytic infiltration was found histologically at the border between the navel skin and the umbilical cord; the infiltration had already developed wedgelike into the deeper areas and had also reached the vascular walls in this region. In this case of a practically stillborn child, the very distinct demarcatory inflammation has to be taken in connection with the protracted birth. Comparable findings have, however, thus far only been observed in mature or post-term neonates. With such rare findings, the presence of a periumbilical demarcatory inflammation cannot in itself be taken as certain evidence of a child having lived without knowledge of the duration of birth.

The studies published so far show that in living premature infants, the inflammatory demarcation border develops more slowly than in mature neonates and cannot be detected until after a survival time of 7 h. In mature neonates, the first signs of a demarcatory inflammation were seen after the child had lived for 3 h. In all, therefore, a histologically substantiated periumbilical demarcatory inflammation can only be judged as an indication, the evidence value of which becomes increasingly important with the shortening of the duration of labor and reduction in the maturity of the child.

The histological nature of the umbilical vessels should be taken into account particularly in the initial section of their intra-abdominal course. The presence of a definite thrombotic vascular occlusion with signs of incipient organization establishes, independent of all other examination findings, a survival time of at least several days. Only positive evidence of a thrombosis can be accepted, since from personal experience even after longer periods of survival thromboses do not necessarily occur in this vascular region.

Histochemical determinations of alkaline and acid phosphatase and fluorescent-microscopic studies of the umbilical ring have revealed an increase in the positive reactions dependent on survival time of the neonate (Lo Menzo 1969; Lo Menzo and Chiara 1968 a, b). Utilizable reactions could not be observed until after a survival time of 12 h; this method thus cannot be applied in the determination of the time of death below this limit.

Further investigations, which do not directly contribute to clarifying whether a child had lived but which make a study of disorders and injuries to the umbilical cord, concern the occurrence of degeneration and calcification (Perrin and Kahn-Vander Bel 1965) and the pathomechanisms and findings in the case of traumatic omphalotomy and in the formation of the umbilical ring (Riemann 1963; Toshimitsu 1972; Fazekas and Kosa 1970).

The Problem of the Cause of Death

A careful examination of diseases and birth injuries that could have caused or contributed to death has naturally to be included in medico legal investigations of perinatal death where there is the suspicion of infanticide.

A frequent cause of death associated with birth is the aspiration of amniotic fluid. Histologically, this can be recognized as lethal if the alveoli of the larger connected sections of the lung are filled with fluid and amniotic components. There are, however, no criteria applicable to all cases for establishing the extent of infiltration in pulmonary sections that would be fatal. It may be assumed that individual circumscribed aspiration foci cannot explain the death of an otherwise healthy infant during or shortly after birth. If infected amniotic fluid was inhaled, smaller aspiration foci can also become the starting point of fatal aspiration pneumonia.

The diagnosis of an amniotic aspiration is based on the histological evidence of amniotic components in the alveoli (Fig. 102). This involves sections from the central and peripheral areas of all pulmonary lobes. Evidence of neutral fats along with

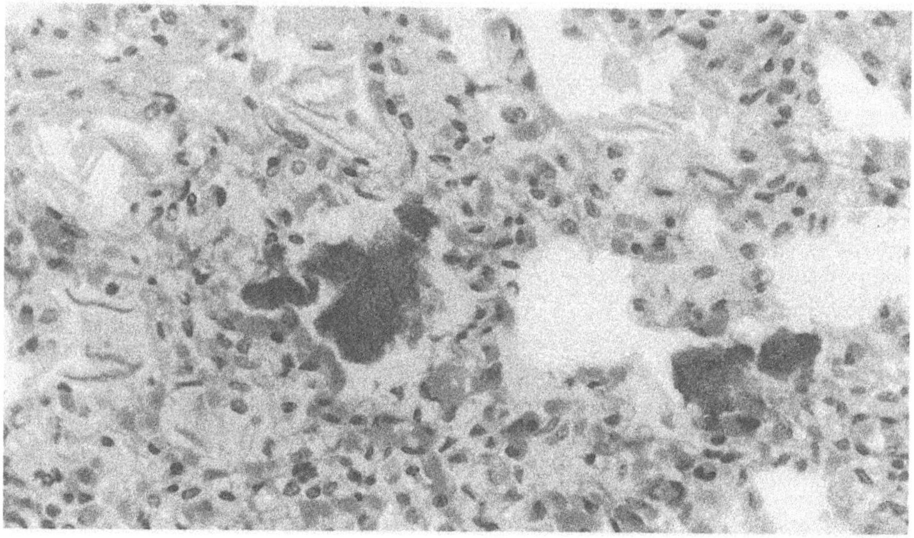

Fig. 102. Aspiration of amniotic fluid with intra-alveolar epidermal components and bacterial clumps. H and E, 1:220

visualization of the nucleus should be taken into account when staining the sections. Sudan III, Sudan black, and Nile blue sulfate can be used. In the affected alveoli, there are fatty parts of the vernix caseosa, desquamated epidermal sections, lanugo hairs, and a largely fine-granular meconium, which can also be recognized by its dark green quality without special staining. The finding of amniotic components can also be facilitated by simple fluorescent microscopy (Mascia 1970). A synopsis of the diagnosis and medicolegal evaluation of amniotic aspiration is provided by Caroff and Celestin (1973).

Without amniotic components, the assessment of a fluid infiltration of the alveoli can pose forensic-medical problems in neonates if there is no detailed knowledge of the circumstances of birth. It is possible for a partial infiltration of the pulmonary tissue to take place in utero; conversely, a similar finding is produced if a child is asphyxiated immediately after delivery by the respiratory orifices being submerged in water. From the histological consideration alone, the manner of death cannot be proven. In such cases, a critical and reserved assessment of the investigation findings in conjunction with a careful ascertainment of the case history is advisable.

In the following section, a few further examples will be given of the extremely numerous diseases and possibilities of injury in perinatal death without outside intervention that can be uncovered or substantiated by histological examination. Otherwise, reference is made to the relevant papers and studies by Essbach (1961), Potter (1953), Töndury (1962), and Skogrand and Harnaes (1960).

Disorders and abnormalities of the placenta: these involve amniotic syndrome, chorioamnionitis with massive infiltration of leukocytes, the appearance of massive fibrin deposits, placental dysfunction syndrome, and qualitative and quantitative alterations in the chorionic villi with the formation of necroses and fibrous changes

(Benirschke 1962; Pisarski et al. 1963; Hoppe and Mildner 1971; Widder 1978; Höpker and Ohlendorf 1979).

Findings in the lungs: these comprise perinatal pulmonary hemorrhages of unclear etiology. They may be observed in connection with an infection, cardiac defects, intracranial hemorrhages, and in kernicterus (Mahnke 1973; Esterly and Oppenheimer 1966; Skogrand and Harnaes 1960). Histologically, these are seen as intra-alveolar and interstitial hemorrhages; sometimes, it is difficult to distinguish them from blood aspirations during birth. Occasionally, thrombotic occlusions occur in the small peripheral pulmonary vessels without a simultaneous cardiac defect. The pathogenesis of these thromboses is unclear; a shock etiology is thought to be responsible. The thromboses, which are sometimes partially organized in stillborn babies, are restricted to the lungs. In the vascular areas affected, the walls contain peculiar homogeneous eosinophilic inclusions. There is a certain similarity to the pulmonary vessel findings observed in Shwartzman's phenomenon of rats (Groniowski 1963).

After mechanical positive pressure respiration of asphyxiated neonates, interstitial and mediastinal emphysema, subpleural vesicles, vesicle ruptures, pneumothorax, and retropneumoperitoneum were observed (Jobba 1970). Histologically, periarterial transport of the gas could be seen.

There is extensive literature on pulmonary hyaline membranes, which tend to appear in neonates and premature babies. The membranes can be observed a short time after birth. They appear as membranous linings of the alveolar inner surfaces (Fig. 103). The occurrence of the membranes requires respiration prior to death. The hyaline membranes can, therefore, according to Grosser (1962) also be regarded as evidence that a child had lived. According to the studies of Bleyl et al. (1969, 1970, 1971), the membrane syndrome of neonates is explained as a shock process induced by asphyxiation beginning within the uterus and continuing post partum; it leads to the expulsion of plasmatic fibrin monomers with intra-alveolar polymerization of the pulmonary hyaline membranes (cf. G. Müller 1963). A further pulmonary disorder that appears very early and comes into question as a cause of perinatal death is infantile interstitial plasma pneumonia (pneumocystis pneumonia). The causative agent of this disease has been recognized as *Pneumocystis carinii*. Clinical studies and the pathology of this disorder were comprehensively presented by Pliess et al. (1970). Congenital pneumocystis pneumonia has also been sporadically observed; this was probably caused by a transplacental infection (Pawlica 1962).

Various lesions, hemorrhages, and necroses in the region of the central nervous system are important as causes of death. They frequently develop in premature births as a result of various complications during the pregnancy and delivery or directly after birth. They occur mainly as traumatic and anoxic lesions of the infant (Ross and Dimmette 1965). The difference between the macroscopic and histological findings is sometimes striking. The frequency, localization, and etiology of hemorrhages in the spinal canal, cerebrum, and subependymal layer of the cerebral ventricle have been extensively investigated (Volbert and Schweitzer 1954; Grönert 1954; Dominok 1964; Ross and Dimmette 1965). In the case of the frequent subependymal hemorrhages, histological findings indicate that they originate in the outer half of the subependymal matrix of the transverse sinus. They also spread over the whole of the head and tail of the nucleus caudatus and appear in the anterior

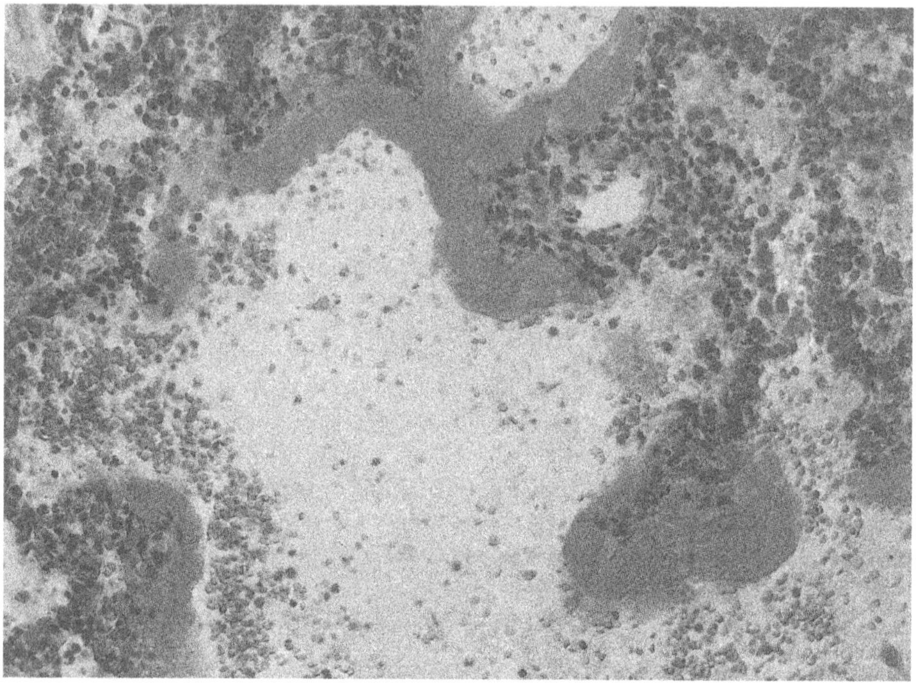

Fig. 103. Premature birth, lung with hyaline membranes and hemorrhages. Subject survived 5 days. PTAH, 1:250

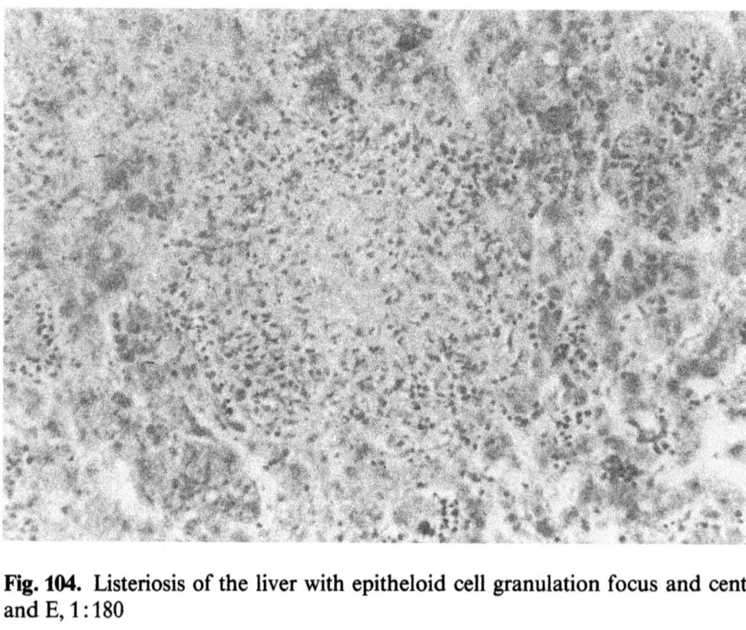

Fig. 104. Listeriosis of the liver with epitheloid cell granulation focus and central necrobiosis. H and E, 1:180

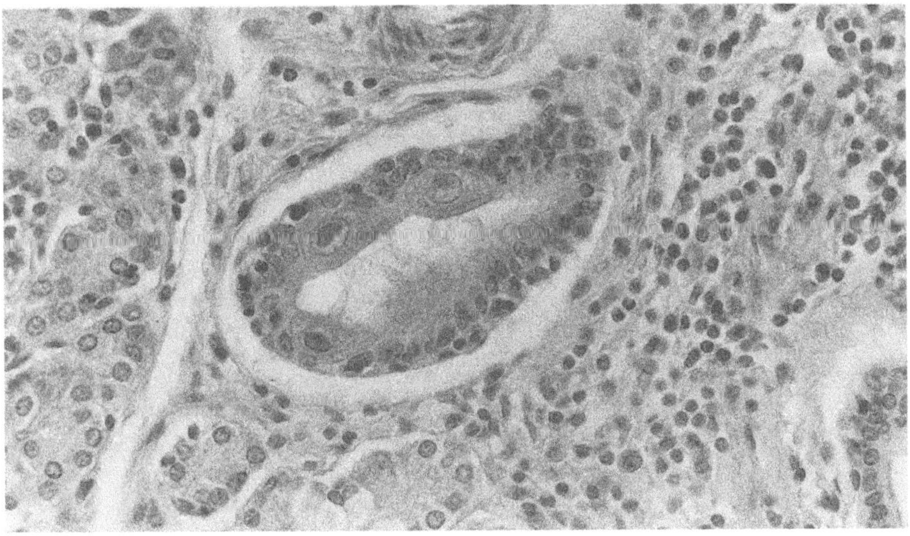

Fig. 105. Cytomegaly with typical giant cells and nuclear inclusions in the epithelia of a salivary gland. H and E, 1:280

portion of the stria terminalis. They are less common in the posterior or inferior horn of the lateral ventricle. Cellular reactions have also occasionally been observed in connection with these hemorrhages.

Fatty infiltration has been regularly detected in cardiac muscle fibers, predominantly in the right ventricular septum, of neonates who died as a result of asphyxiation or hindrance of gaseous interchange in the lung and who presented signs of cardiac failure during the autopsy (Scott 1961). Hypoxia and simultaneous strain on the right heart were considered to be the cause. The conduction system, with visualization of degenerative cellular changes, necroses, macrophages, and the replacement of specific conduction cells by collagenous fibers has also been histologically investigated (Valdes-Dapena et al. 1973).

The occurrence of adrenal hemorrhages, mainly traumatically or hypoxically induced can, particularly when bilateral, lead to the death of the fetus or neonate through acute adrenal insufficiency in the perinatal period. Adrenal hemorrhages that are predominantly localized in the medulla have to be histologically checked, since, from the macroscopic finding alone, it is not infrequent for them to be mistaken for regression hemorrhages at the medulla-cortex boundary or postmortem softening of the medulla with subsequent postmortem infiltrative bleeding via the central vein, so-called red softening (Janssen 1962).

Infectious general disorders also come into consideration as natural causes of death in the perinatal period – cytomegaly (Robertson and Sundelin 1962; Seiffert and Oehme 1957) and listeriosis (Reiss and Knolle 1963; Janssen and Naeve 1975). Listeriosis (Fig. 104), here caused by anthropozoonosis, occurs mainly as a result of infection after the first half of pregnancy in the form of fetopathy. An increase in this disease has been observed in middle Europe since 1950. Cytomegaly, on the other hand, involves a viral disorder, which leads to typical cell inclusions and giant-cell formation particularly in the acini and efferent ducts of the exocrine glands (Fig. 105). The histology of both disorders is characterized by specific findings. In the case of dead infants, the diagnosis can only be confirmed by an extensive histological status investigation of all inner organs.

Proving or excluding natural perinatal death of an infant makes high demands on the knowledge and ability of the investigator. Here, there is a special area of problems which exhibit a gradual transition to sudden infant death syndrome (SIDS). Problems and findings of SIDS will not be entered into here. A comprehensive presentation is found in Althoff (1980). The histology of unnatural injuries in connection with infanticide is to be found in the appropriate sections of this book (e.g., asphyxiation, p. 144; strangulation, p. 214; mechanically induced tissue damage, p. 67).

III. Injuries Caused by Atmospheric Effects

These involve the effects of positive and negative atmospheric pressure and the consequences of too-rapid a reduction in pressure (decompression sickness). In principle, they are lesions that show similarities to the sequelae of air and gas embolisms. Of major interest are the injuries incurred by ventilatory disorders in the respiratory system, circulatory lesions due to gas bubbles in the bloodstream, and histomorphological evidence of shock.

An acquaintance with the pathophysiology and macroscopic autopsy findings in the case of death from rapidly increasing or decreasing positive pressure must here be assumed (references in Mueller 1975). Extent and form of the organic sequelae are related to the duration of exposure to positive pressure and the speed of reduction of this pressure (Fati and Pennarola 1972).

Histological examination of the lungs practically always shows a high-grade acute vascular congestion with septal hemorrhages and extravasation into the alveoli. There is, in addition, a predominantly diffuse acute alveolar emphysema with elongation and lacerations of the septa, negligible swellings and signs of detachment in the pneumonocytes, focal chiefly subpleural atelectases, which alternate with subpleural bullous emphysemal regions, and sometimes also a circumscribed protein-deficient intra-alveolar edema. In the case of positive barotrauma with collapse obstruction of the small and peripheral respiratory passages, these passages show isolated parietal ruptures and hemorrhages. The consequences are penetration of air into the pulmonary interstitium and under the pleura, pleural ruptures, pneumothorax, extensive subcutaneous emphysema, and air embolisms in the systemic circulation (Unterdorfer 1979). Occasionally, following fat staining of the blood vessels with Sudan III or Nile blue sulfate, there are findings in the form of lipemia that resemble decompensated diabetes. The origin of such Sudan-positive substances, which can also be detected in other capillary regions of the heart and brain, has not yet been clarified; mobilization of neutral fats from the bone marrow and fatty tissue by the effect of suction through pressure reduction is assumed to be responsible.

Difficulties are encountered with direct evidence of the liberated nitrogen gas bubbles, which appear largely in the venous system, and the histological diagnosis of air embolisms (cf. p. 123). The results of one experiment, carried out on people who died acutely and could be dissected shortly after death, appear promising (Adebahr 1972). In the case of five patients with fatal decompression sickness as a result of positive-pressure treatment who died 2–38 h after the decompression, Richter and Löblich (1978) found very small "gas nuclei" and larger intra- and extracellular gas vesicles in all organs examined. Vacuoles and interruptions in the rouleaux in the capillaries are, however, to be evaluated with care since postmortem changes in the intravascular blood content and early gas bubble formation, even without evidence of putrefactive bacteria, can only be excluded with difficulty. The occurrence of vacuoles in the intravascular blood and right ventricle, together with a peripheral aggregation of thrombocytes, leukocytes, and erythrocytes, was regarded by Adebahr (1972) as proof that the gas bubbles had an intravital origin (further references in Pioch 1961).

The circulatory and histionic effects of arterial gas embolisms in the organs of the systemic circulation have to be given particular consideration. Predominantly affected are the brain and cardiac muscle. The findings include circumscribed hemorrhages, sometimes in the form of ring or spherical hemorrhages, in the gray and white matter and fine, maculate hemorrhages and necrobioses of the myocardium (Möttönen and Karkola 1971). It is uncommon for radiologically detectable skeletal changes to develop (Wünsche and Scheele 1976). Experiments on rats with different levels of positive-pressure decompression revealed histologically detectable scar and cyst formation in the skeletal system. In animal experiments, Leithoff et al. (1972) demonstrated that in the case of explosive decompression, gas bubbles appeared predominantly in pericardial veins and in the atria. The morphological effects could be reduced by immediate recompression.

Changes in the blood and hematogenic tissue in the case of a rapid rise and fall in pressure are manifest as thrombopenia, an increase in the number of megakaryocytes, and an increase in the nuclear volume (Barres et al. 1978). Scanning electron-microscopic studies revealed compaction of the fibrin network and changes in the shape of the thrombocytes (Schneider and Fien 1978).

Severe impairment of the peripheral circulation and shock occur in lesions caused by acute decompression, negative pressure, and arterial gas embolisms produced by explosion. In the terminal vascular system, intravascular aggregations of thrombocytes and erythrocytes and small fibrinous thrombi form (cf. p. 156). Similar findings were also observed by Adebahr (1972) in the case of air embolism, diving accidents, and decompression sickness as an expression of the associated normovolemic shock.

It was possible to demonstrate in animal experiments that sufficient oxygen supply during decompression restricts the damage to the lungs, central nervous system, and myocardium to a degree that is nonfatal (Nikolaeva 1959). As a result of protracted oxygen respiration, the findings that normally appear in the lungs of guinea pigs following decompression sickness, acute meteorism, septal lacerations, thinning of the septa, hemorrhages, atelectases, and intravascular gas formation, could be prevented (Haberer et al. 1972). A protective effect can thus be assigned to oxygen. Protracted hyperbaric oxygen administration can, on the other hand, lead to incipient oxygen intoxication.

Negative atmospheric pressure and lowering of the partial pressure of oxygen can produce histologically detectable damage that is basically comparable with the tissue effects of oxygen deficiency. Here also, the duration of the change from normal to negative pressure and the exposure time under negative pressure phase are of importance. A rapid sinking to blood oxygen saturation levels of less than 80% would be expected to cause histologically detectable lesions, corresponding to a height of more than 5000 m (Mueller 1975). In fatal cases, acute ganglion changes, necrobioses and necroses in the cerebral cortex, nucleus caudatus, medulla oblongata, and cerebellum should be histologically examined (Peters 1970). Pulmonary edema and acute vacuolar degeneration of cardiac-muscle and liver cells have also been described (Pioch 1961).

Explosions with fatal shock waves tend to produce uncharacteristic lacerations of the alveolar septa and pulmonary hemorrhages. Gas embolisms have also been observed in this context in animal experiments.

IV. Strangulation: Hanging – Choking – Throttling

1. General

In the case of corpses with indications of strangulation, particularly suicidal hanging, an autopsy and extensive histological and biochemical investigations are frequently dispensed with if the circumstances of death and external examination of the body do not present any inconsistancies. For a forensic and scientific clarification of these cases, however, such a procedure is unsatisfactory. Homicide with subsequent hanging to create the impression of suicide would remain undiscovered or could not be refuted. Therefore, with regard to medicolegal considerations, a thorough examination of these cases is necessary.

The histological contribution to the diagnosis of death by strangulation is particularly concerned with the question of whether the compression of the soft parts of the neck occurred before or after the death of the victim.

2. Findings in the Neck

The histological nature of rope marks, signs of throttling, and strangulation marks demand particular care. An acquaintance with the cutaneous and subcutaneous changes in the region of the neck caused by pressure and abrasion as a result of applying various implements for strangulation, as well as knowledge of the lesions created by strangling, must here be assumed. Basically, the injuries are cutaneous and subcutaneous lesions as a result of blunt trauma. The character with regard to the form and color of the strangulation marks and signs of throttling has been explained as being largely due to a desiccation effect following epidermal damage. Observations involving impervious strangulation implements remaining on the skin for a long period of time have suggested that drying out through loss of liquid to the outside is improbable, or only possible to a minor extent. In addition, histological studies have provided evidence that in the region of strangulation marks, the tissue fluid is forced inward as a result of compression (Simon and Müller 1976a, b). This is supported by evidence of electrolyte displacements with a variable sodium concentration in the area of strangulation marks.

A great many studies over the past 80 years have been concerned with the detection of vital reactions in the region of cervical injuries. Here, principally the same difficulties exist as with all injuries that are only survived for a short time: On the whole, this time is insufficient for reactions to develop that can be reliably distinguished from lesions of postmortem origin. It has been known, at the latest, since the basic studies by Robert Schulz (1896) that practically all findings observed in vital strangulation can also occur in cervical injuries produced postmortem. Even today, a positive distinction is not possible in every case; a synoptic evaluation of all investigation findings is therefore necessary. For a thorough histological examination of cervical injuries, the following requirements have to be met:

a) Precise registration should be made of the external and internal findings recognizable with the naked eye, as far as possible with a sketch and indication of the sites of removal. Particular consideration should be given to hypostasis and postmortem effects that hinder or prevent the recognition of hemorrhages (cf. p. 26).
b) In the fixation, pieces of skin and hypodermis removed should be mounted in such a way as to match the natural state.
c) Histological examination should be made of: parts of the skin and hypodermis, both heavily and lightly damaged by the process of strangulation; hemorrhages and tissue severance in the region of the larynx, hyoid bone, and retrolingual region; the cervical lymph nodes above, in, and below the region of the strangulation marks. Undamaged skin should also be taken from the neck for the purposes of comparative histochemical examination.

In all cases of death by strangulation in which it is asserted that injury was incurred without the intention of murder on the part of the accused, it is recommended that bilateral preparations and serial sections be made of the carotid ganglion, including the surrounding soft parts (Schollmeyer 1961; Niedorf 1970). Particular attention should be paid to the carotid ganglion following attacks made on the neck where there are no macroscopically recognizable traces and after injuries to one side of the neck only, e.g., after karate blows.

The following factors need to be visualized by histological staining: nature of the cells and nuclei in damaged areas of tissue (H and E, hemalum), the components of hemorrhages (azan, Lepehne's, Weigert's fibrin stain, PTAH), fibrous elements (elastica van Gieson, Gomori's), crushed but not destroyed musculature (eryochromocyanin, Janssen et al. 1968), changes in the fatty tissue (Sudan III, Sudan black).

The early enzymatic changes are histochemically significant; less so are the changes to the tissue elements. According to Pioch (1969), the test for unspecific esterases (alpha-naphthyl-esterase reaction) in the strangulation mark is suitable for distinguishing a positive reaction as evidence of intravital strangling.

The following histomorphological findings can be identified in the region of the neck following strangulation:

Plethora of the vessels in the marginal zones above and below the strangulation mark.

Hemorrhages in the cutaneous and subcutaneous tissue and in the deep soft parts near the strangulation mark and area of throttling as a direct consequence of the traumatic violence.

Tissue ruptures with hemorrhages, e.g., in the cervical and hyoglossal musculature (Koops et al. 1982a).

Incipient inflammatory reactions around lesions after protracted agony.

Hemorrhages in oblique ridges and on the ridges of skin between two strangulation marks.

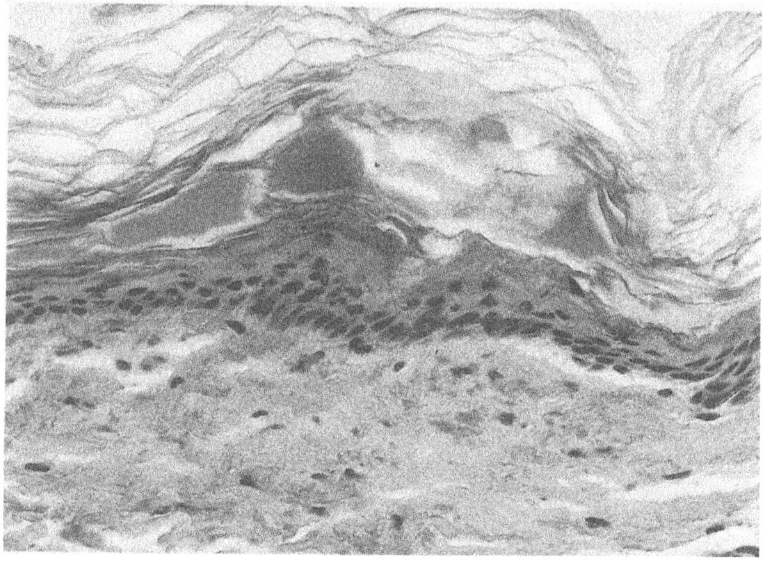

Fig. 106. Periphery of a strangulation mark with escape of fluid (homogeneous, stained dark) in the basal layers of the stratum corneum, flattening of the basal epidermal layers. PTAH, 1:300

Formation of intraepidermal liquid-filled vesicles (Fig. 106).

Metachromasia of the cutaneous and subcutaneous connective tissue (Mallory stain, Orsós 1935).

Contusion of fatty tissue cells and emulsification of their cell contents (Blum 1937). Care should be taken not to confuse this with brown adipose tissue!

Increased stain uptake of contused musculature without destruction or ruptures (eryochromocyanin stain, Janssen et al. 1968).

Swelling of the nerve axis cylinders and nerve endings.

"Intercolloidal crystals" in the thyreoid gland (Nanetti 1972).

Hemorrhages in the cervical lymph nodes (Jankovich and Incze 1933; Schulz 1936).

"Waxlike degeneration" in the musculature in the form of Zenker's necrosis (Orsós 1935; Bonnet and Pedace 1972).

Hemorrhages and ruptures in the carotid ganglion and surrounding fatty connective tissue (Schollmeyer 1961). Such findings have to be evaluated critically in the case of a general heavy vascular congestion. Isolated acute lesions of the carotid ganglion as a cause of death (carotid sinus reflex) in otherwise healthy people should be assessed with extreme caution (Mueller 1975).

Displacement of epidermal fragments and foreign bodies into the subcutis in the region of strangulation marks (Klein 1956).

The following findings indicate intravital strangulation:

Distinct hyperemia of the skin, confined to the peripheral zones of a strangulation mark.

Hemorrhages with the beginnings of inflammatory reactions around strangulation injuries.

Positive alpha-naphthyl-esterase reaction of the skin and integumentary appendages in the region of the strangulation mark.

3. Consequences to the Inner Organs

Evidence of death by strangulation, compression of the soft parts of the neck, is largely based on the detection of the sequelae of obstructive asphyxiation brought about by this mode of killing; these involve disorders in the blood circulation and respiration. According to recent research results, acute and agonal reactions of the circulatory and respiratory system have particular bearing. The secondary effects on the spinal column and skeletal musculature should also be taken into account. Assessment of the histopathological examination findings should always be made in conjunction with a consideration of the macroscopic findings.

The mechanically caused disorder in the blood circulation is largely manifest in the appearance of hemorrhages due to passive hyperemia in the soft parts above the strangulation site. It is debatable whether oxygen deficiency of the capillary walls plays a role in the local development of these hemorrhages. The diapedesis probably occurs as a result of overdistention of the capillaries. Regular ruptures of the capillary walls, however, can not be demonstrated in histological serial sections (Henn et al. 1973). A critical consideration should be made of influences through previous cardio circulatory disturbances, postmortem hypostasis, and displacement of traumatically incurred hemorrhages (Prokop and Wabnitz 1970; Reh and Haarhof 1975; Janssen 1967). Histological evidence of highly dilated venules with simultaneously constricted arterioles above the strangulation mark is thought to be indicative of vital hanging (Bedrin et al. 1973).

Severe obstruction also leads to hemorrhages from the nose and ears, which can be histologically traced to preformed gaps in the basal membrane of the nasal mucosa and burst subepidermal hematomas (Stichnoth 1954; Bschor 1964).

The histopathologically detectable effects of oxygen deficiency in the tissues are dependent on the effectiveness of the strangulation process, the duration of agony, and the sensitivity of the tissue concerned. Characteristic findings, which do not, however, in themselves have the significance of proof, are predominantly detected in the liver, cardiac muscle, brain, and lungs (see p. 144). In cases of delayed death from strangulation, which can also be incurred by thromboses of the large cervical vessels (Kaeser 1955), ischemic changes in the nerve cells of the brain are a prominent feature. Two forms can be recognized: in the first, death occurs after sustained unconsciousness; in other rare cases, the individuals affected first of all regain consciousness until renewed cerebral functional loss leads to death, days or months after strangulation (interval form). Histologically, severe ischemic nerve cell lesions in the cerebral cortex and frontal sections of the brain stem are found in both forms (Wünscher and Möbius 1960). The caudal brain stem is largely unaffected. Secondary processes induced by oxygen deficiency, such as edema and swellings, do not normally in themselves have causal significance in delayed death from strangulation. It is probable that in the interval following elimination of the partial depriva-

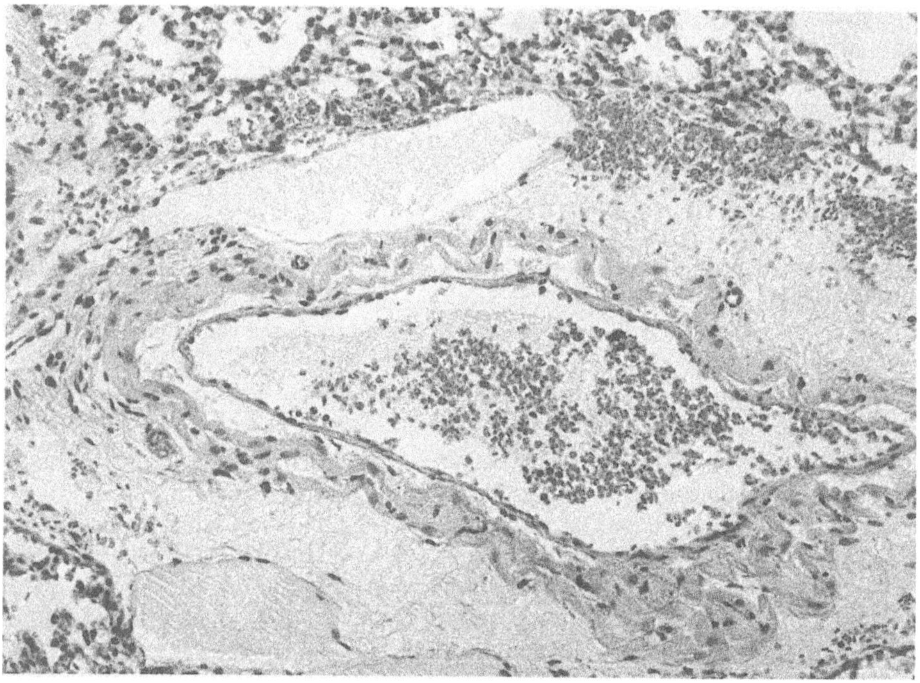

Fig. 107. Rat lung, strangulation. Massive partly hemorrhagic perivascular edema with dehiscence of the vascular coats. Pronounced dilation of the lymph tract. H and E, 1:100

tion of blood supply to the damaged nerve cells, there is initially recovery, clinically manifest as an intermission, until the impaired cells fail under renewed functional loss. In such cases, changes in the retina, nervus opticus, and cervical region of the nervus vagus have been detected (Permyakow 1968).

The indirect and secondary effects of the strangulation process have also to be macroscopically noted and histologically checked. Mention should be made here of hemorrhages, which probably develop during "asphyxial convulsions," on the periosteum of the claviculae at the lower points of attachment of the sternocleidomastoid muscles (Laiho et al. 1968), the musculature of the axilla and upper region of the back, and the musculus pectoralis major (Aguiar and Nunes 1962, 1963). "Simon's hemorrhages" (ventral intervertebral hemorrhages) following death by hanging also deserve consideration; they tend to appear in the region of the lumbar spine and are more frequent in younger people (Simon 1968). Similar hemorrhages can, however, also develop postmortem through putrefaction and vitally through traumatic effects, with stretching and hyperextension of the vertebral column (Geserick et al. 1976a, b).

The macroscopic and histological evidence of an air embolism in death by strangulation has hitherto been variously assessed as proof of a vital reaction. Andrä (1981) demonstrated by systematic studies on a great number of corpses that air embolisms following strangulation cannot be reliably detected and do not signify proof of an intravital hanging.

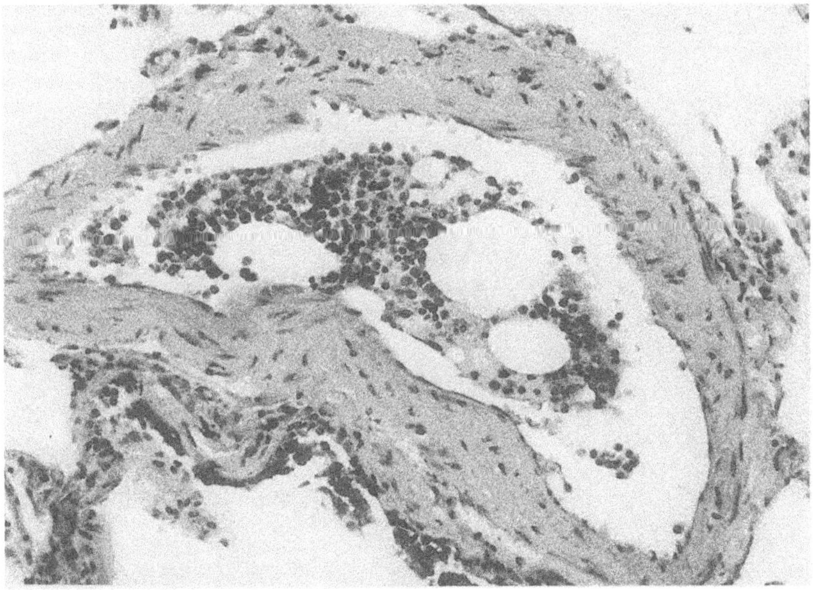

Fig. 108. Hanging. Pulmonary arteriole with an embolus composed of the hematogenic bone marrow with the typical structure. H and E, 1:380

The vital reactions in the circulation and respiratory system have attained particular significance in recent years. Thus, the Hamburg working group around Brinkmann has systematically studied the pathophysiological processes that occur in the pulmonary vascular system and pulmonary tissue during strangulation. The object of these animal experiments and comparative pathological studies in humans was the compilation of findings utilizing histopathological staining methods and forensic-medical assessments. The histological investigation of the lungs (semithin section technique, toluidine blue and Giemsa stain) of 30 cases of suicidal hanging and two cases of choking in humans revealed remarkable changes in the vascular contents. In the arterial pulmonary vessels, fragments of fatty and bone-marrow tissue were found which in parts had the character of tissue embolisms. In addition, disseminated accumulations of cells were evident in the capillaries and venules (Figs. 107–109). These findings are related to vital reactions in the pulmonary vascular system, which can be explained by an interaction of several factors: suffocative convulsions with mechanical alteration of the bone marrow, damage due to hypoxidosis in the vascular epithelia of the sinusoids of the bone marrow, and early effects of shock on the bone marrow. The pulmonary vascular system thus proves itself to be a "target organ of strangulation agony" (Brinkmann 1978a; Brinkmann and Püschel 1981).

In animal experiments, a variable character was observed in the blood pressure of the pulmonary vascular system and in the mechanics of breathing with different endotracheal pressure conditions in the case of killing by strangulation or isolated occlusion of the trachea (Brinkmann et al. 1981b). These disturbed regulations of respiration and circulation had a particular reaction pattern, which enabled them to

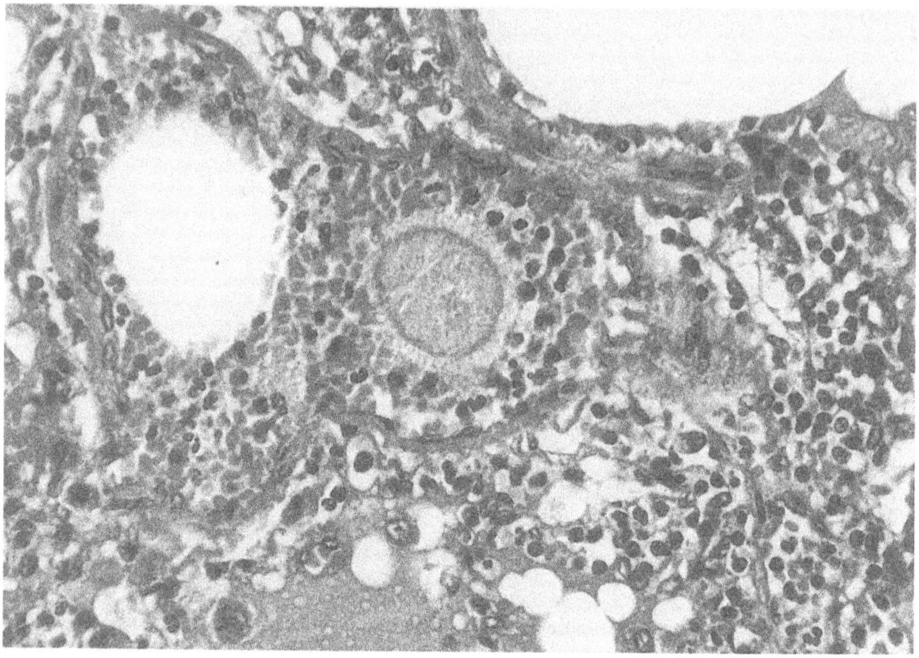

Fig. 109. Mixed microthrombi composed of fibrin, thrombocytes, and myelocytes. There is also disseminated intravascular myelocytosis. Swelling of the nuclei of the vascular endothelia. Suicide by hanging. H and E, 1:380

be distinguished from other forms of death. Accordingly, specific morphological changes can also be expected in the parenchyma of the lungs. Studies on rats and rabbits, with appropriate controls, showed a pronounced hemorrhagic syndrome, which extended to all compartments of the lungs, to be a qualitatively and quantitatively prominent finding in strangulation. By means of semithin sections and electron microscopy, a distinct alveolar septal edema could be demonstrated which did not occur in other forms of killing with short agony (Figs. 110–113) (Brinkmann and Püschel 1981).

Further investigations concerning these problems involve the frequency of pulmonary edema in death by hanging (Pollak 1975), the question of acute emphysema in strangulation (Nasemann and Brinkmann 1982), the pathology of hanging with particular consideration of vital reactions (Kleiber et al. 1982), the findings in suicidal strangulation (Koops and Brinkmann 1982), the pathophysiology and pathomorphology of death by thoracic compression and traumatic asphyxia (Brinkmann 1978, Hambeck and Püschel 1981), and arterial obstruction in cervical compression (Brinkmann et al. 1981 a).

Forensic-medical research into strangulation ultimately concentrates on the question of whether compression of the soft parts of the neck occurred when the victim was alive or dead. To that end, it should be borne in mind that according to earlier studies in some fatal cases of strangulation no vital reactions were detectable (Roer and Koopmann 1938). In prospective studies on 222 cases of suicidal

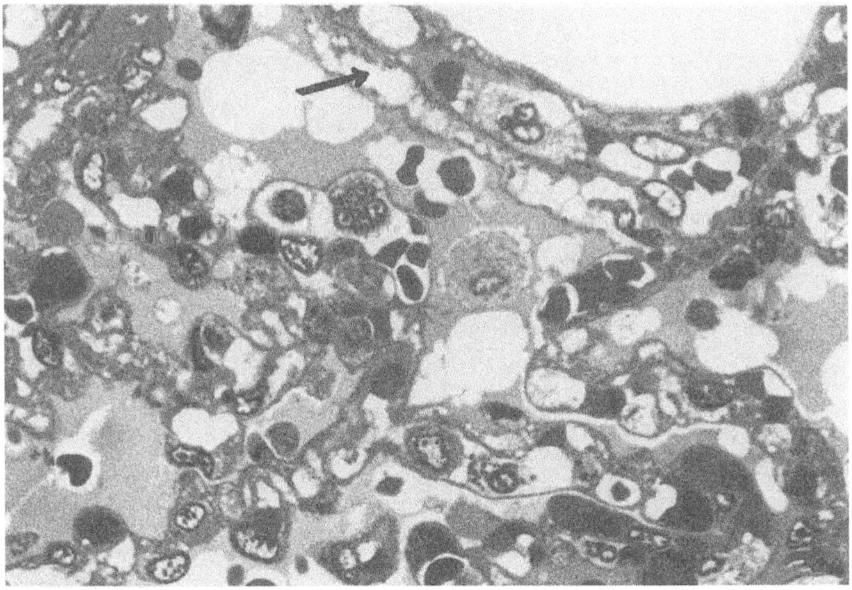

Fig. 110. Hanging. Intra-alveolar hemorrhagic edema and, in particular, alveolar-septal edema (↑). Semi-thin section, toluidine blue, × 730

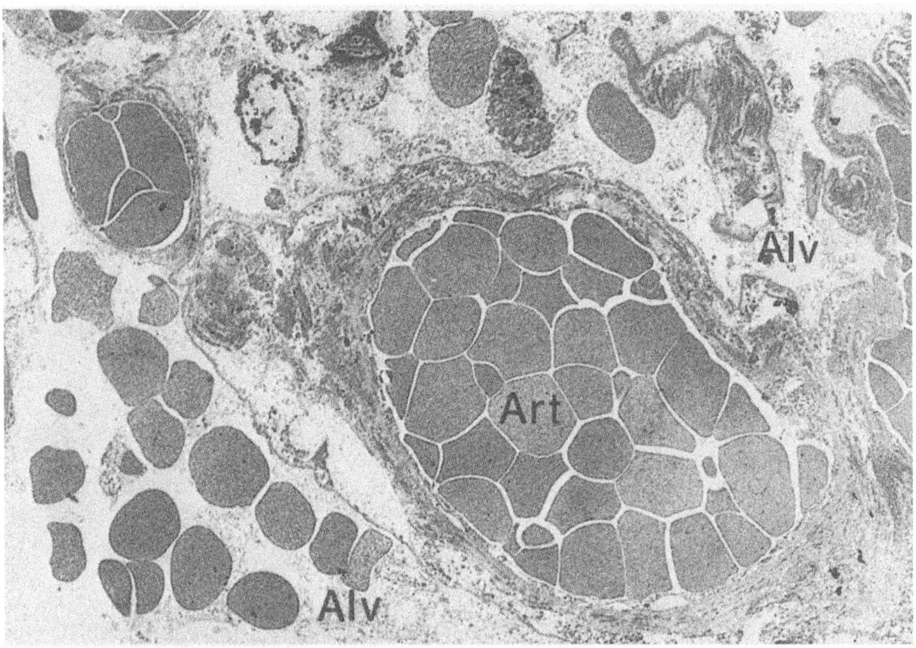

Fig. 111. Strangulation. Arterioles and capillaries engorged with erythrocytes. Intra-alveolar hemorrhagic edema. Edema of the endothelium and distinct periarteriolar edema. Electron microscope (EM), × 1100

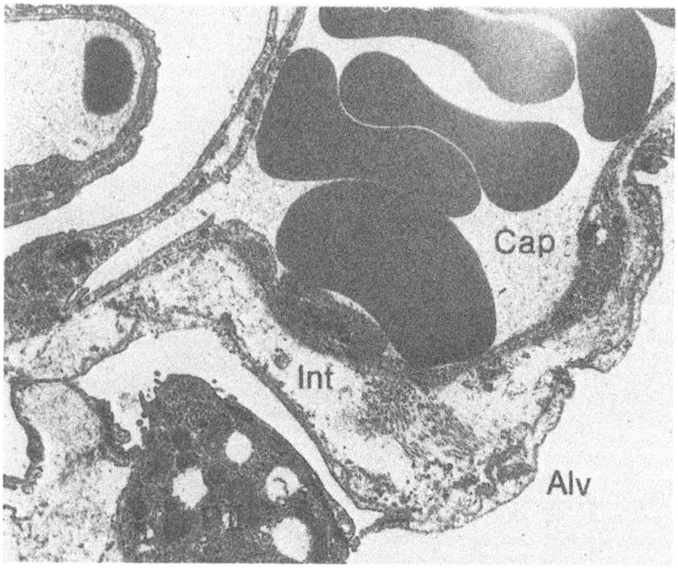

Fig. 112. Rat, strangulation. Pronounced alveolar-septal edema. EM, ×4400

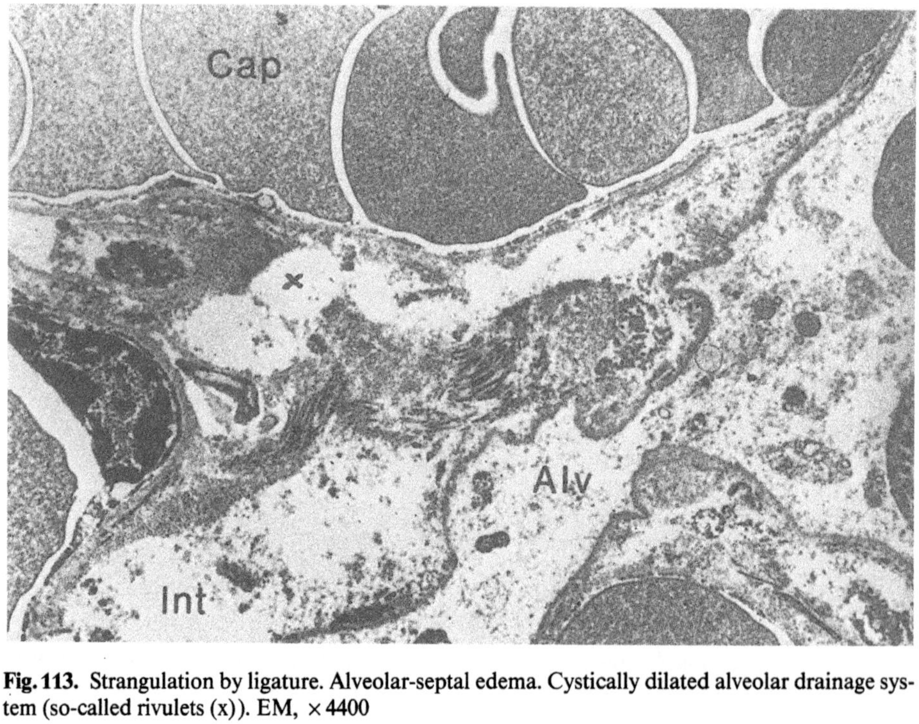

Fig. 113. Strangulation by ligature. Alveolar-septal edema. Cystically dilated alveolar drainage system (so-called rivulets (x)). EM, ×4400

hanging, no vital reactions whatsoever could be recognized in 2% (Kleiber et al. 1982).

The histological proof or disproof of vital reactions is an important part of the final assessment of a case of strangulation. *An intravital strangulation may be regarded as proven if in the pulmonary vascular system there are vital reactions in the form of bone-marrow embolisms and if in the parenchyma of the lungs a hemorrhagic syndrome connected with an alveolar septal edema is evident.*

Strong doubts as to an intravital strangulation are appropriate if the above histological changes in the lungs are absent, no positive histological or histochemical evidence of strangulation marks is at hand present, and the blood-biochemical investigations (catecholamine – Berg 1966; Berg and Bonte 1973) argue against death by strangulation.

V. Drowning – Changes to Corpses Found in Water

1. Changes in Water

The histologically detectable natural changes to human corpses found in water occupy a special area of histothanatology. An acquaintance with these changes is an important requirement in assessing the time the body spent in water (water time) and in the diagnosis of death through drowning. In this regard, it should be borne in mind that the same or similar changes to the skin of corpses can also develop out of water through the effects of damp.

The wrinkling and whitish discoloration of *water-soaked skin* affects the skin free of sebaceous glands on the palms of the hands, the soles of the feet, around the finger tips and toes, and in the region of the nipples. Histologically, this change is due to water uptake and swelling of the epidermal epithelia. The water intake brings about a loosening of the stratum corneum with fibrillation of the corneal lamellae and the appearance of vacuoles in the epithelia of the basal epidermal layers. Loss of the cell and nuclear boundaries and keratohyalin plaques occurs. With further wrinkling, the epidermis detaches itself from the corium. Histologically, the remains of the stratum germinativum (basal) can sometimes be recognized in the detached skin. The stratum granulosum remains discernible for a comparatively long time.

Systematic histological investigations on the wrinkling associated with water-soaked skin, taking into consideration water temperature, kind of water, water movement, age of individual, and thickness of the epidermis, did not reveal a regular connection between the length of time spent in water and the time of appearance of morphological changes in the structure of the epidermis (Schleyer 1951). There have been cases in which the stratum corneum was already clearly loosened before an externally recognizable wrinkling washed appearance of the skin was present. Conversely, it is possible that formation of the typical wrinkling may occur without histological changes in the stratum corneum.

The wrinkling of the epidermis is explained by a contraction in the elastic fiber network in the upper layers of the corium. The fact that this wrinkling only forms on skin surfaces with thick horny layers indicates that the strength of the stratum corneum plays a part in its development (Schleyer 1951).

The *corium* is changed by swelling and loosening, roughly parallel with the development of wrinkling. The reaction of the thick-bundled elastic fibers in the corium to the effects of water has also been investigated for criteria in determining the time spent in water. The elastic fiber system is thought to be particularly stable toward putrefactive influences, acids, and temperature changes. Experiments by Ökrös (1968) revealed a dwindling of the elastic fibers in the abdominal and dorsal skin after 3–10 weeks in water. Good stainability of the elastic fibers in the stratum papillare of the soles of the feet indicated that a corpse was in water for no longer than 1 week (Dierkes 1938). Moderate stainability of the fibers and distinct creasing of the skin without epidermal detachment indicated a period in water of 2–3 weeks; poor or no stainability of the elastic papillary network indicated a duration in water of more than 4 weeks.

In tissue material fixed in formol and stained according to the method of Weigert, it was possible to detect a dependence of the fibrous character on the age of the individual concerned (Goldbach and Hinüber 1956). The question also arose of the influence of the means of fixation on the stainability or stability of the elastic fibers. In infancy, the fibers are probably more adversely affected than in adulthood. The elastic fibers can be visualized better in an unfixed state in about 90% of the material in children.

The *elastic fibers of the pulmonary tissue* do not show a distinct reduction in stainability and structure until the corpse has been in water for over 2 months. Beyond this time, the very diverse findings cannot be systematically presented (Kunz 1960). A histologically well-preserved pulmonary elastica does, however, indicate a period in the water of less than 2 months.

A histological investigation of the structure and stainability of elastic fibers can, on the whole, only have a supportive role in the determination of the time a corpse spent in water.

It is relatively seldom that corpses found in water develop so-called lime soap nodules (Nippe 1913) on the intima of veins, in particular the hepatic veins, and on the endocardium. Similarly disposed nodule formations, composed of calcium phosphate, calcium carbonate, neutral fat, and proteinaceous substances, have been described in the skin of corpses found in water by Klauer and Walcher (1937). These studies carried out with gelatin-frozen sections revealed characteristic crystalline drusen with coarse needles and spearlike projections to the surface of the cutis, which in these regions was denuded of epidermis. The formation of these nodules is explained by a conjunction of phosphate ions, which derive from the putrefactive process, and calcium ions from the water.

The occurrence of struvite crystals in the skin is thought to be an indication that a corpse spent a long time in sea-water (Cherkavsky and Stukochenko 1965). Evidence of particularly large crystals connected to one another is thought to indicate that the corpse was in the water for over 9 months.

The formation of *adipocere,* occasionally observed in the region of the cutis-subcutis boundary, can also appear outside water if the corpse is in a damp and cool environment with extensive exclusion of air. In the diagnosis of adipocere formation, the initial phases in particular have to be histologically checked (cf. p. 45). Adipocere formation is not suitable for the determination of the postmortem time especially since earlier conceptions with regard to the time necessary for it to develop have had to be considerably reduced in recent years. However, a minimum time of 3–4 weeks prior to the first histologically detectable development of adipocere may be assumed.

Occasionally, chromogenic bacteria *(Bacillus prodigiosus and B. violaceum)* occur in the cutis of corpses found in water after a period of at least 1–2 weeks (Berg 1975). The bacteria can proliferate in the integumentary appendages and be arranged in patterns such that they can give the impression of tattoos (Janssen 1969).

Generally, it can be said of the histological investigation of corpses found in water that recognition of morbid or unnatural changes that occurred prior to the effects of water is sometimes not as hopeless as might be feared from the macroscopic findings of considerably altered corpses. The structures of the inner organs, especially liver, kidneys, cardiac muscle, and musculature, can still be very well preserved even after a corpse has been in water for several months. On the other hand, the internal structure of the spleen is usually completely destroyed after 1–2 weeks.

After a longer period of time in water, it is also worthwhile to distinguish between vital and postmortem lesions in corpses. Inflammatory reactions with incipient structural change are preserved just as long in water as the structures in the tissues concerned (Bargagna and Selvaggio 1963).

The absence of histologically detectable reactions in the peripheral regions of injuries in corpses found in water does not exclude the possibility that lesions of vital origin are involved. The identification of injuries to corpses produced postmortem, through drifting in water, ships' propellers, etc., is determined by the macroscopic evidence. However, in cases where there is doubt as to a postmortem origin of these injuries in water, a histological check should be undertaken.

The changes in the lungs of corpses found in water will be presented and discussed in connection with the differential diagnosis of drowning.

2. Histological Contribution to the Diagnosis of Death by Drowning

Evidence of death by drowning is dependent on the macroscopic findings in the respiratory system and histologically detectable damage symptomatic of general acute oxygen deficiency, i.e., asphyxiation, in consequence of the inhalation of water or other liquids and obstruction of the deep respiratory tracts. Here, the histological contribution concentrates on changes brought about by the process of drowning and the medium in which it takes place. As far as they are ascertainable, the following should be taken into account in the histological diagnosis: Depth of water in which the corpse was lying, water temperature, fresh or salt water, impurities in water, resuscitative measures, general state of preservation of corpse, previous illnesses, and other earlier injuries that could have caused death or contributed to its occurrence.

The *drowned lung* is the focus of attention of the histological diagnostic efforts. At least one central and one peripheral section should be investigated from every lobe of the lung. It is important for the material to be carefully removed with a sharp knife, not with scissors, without causing contusion. Through incompetent handling of the lungs, even a classic emphysema aquosum can to some extent be "squeezed from" the pulmonary tissue. The routine histological examination involves paraffin sections with H and E and Gomori's stains as well as frozen sections with Sudan III.

An important histological finding in the lungs is the acute dilation of the alveoli with extension, elongation, and thinning of the septa and compression of the alveolar capillaries (Fig. 114). The intensity of the alveolar expansion can be considerably affected by the manner and duration of the drowning process, age-dependent com-

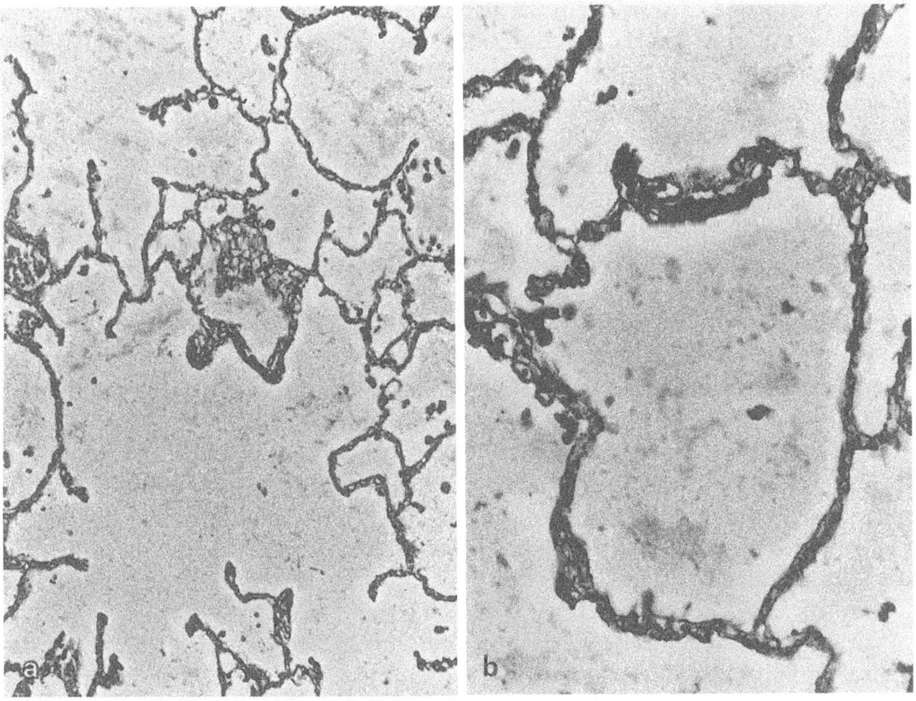

Fig. 114. a, b Drowned lung with dilation of the alveoli, elongation and disruption of the septa. Gomori's, 1:180, 1:300

pliance, and previous pulmonary disorders (pleural adhesion, chronic emphysema, chronic vascular congestion). Findings in the lungs very similar to the clinical picture of drowning can develop through hydrostatic effects in corpses lying in more than 4 m of water. The efforts of Reh (1970) to detect specific histological characteristics of a drowned lung should especially be pointed out. His systematic serial tests and animal experiments were concerned with the nature of the reticular fiber structure (cf. Böhm 1973). The criteria and characteristics for classification presented by Reh, the distinction of typical and atypical drowning, and his division into phases I–IV has not been universally accepted by other investigators. In 18 of 57 cases, Heinen and Dotzauer (1973) were able to demonstrate the reticular fiber regarded by Reh as specific for a drowned lung although the corpses examined had not been in water. Alveolar expansion with the corresponding change in the reticular fiber structure has, thus, become very doubtful as a diagnostic criterion of a drowned lung. According to our experience, which includes corpses found in both rivers and seawater and subjected to various processes of drowning and postmortem conditions, it is only possible histologically to speak of a "so-called drowned lung." Where drowning occurred over a relatively long period and the victims came to the surface several times and inhaled air, the histologically detectable expansion of the alveoli was most pronounced. Very similar findings were also observed, however, if the victims were immediately pushed under water by building materials in harbor accidents. We considered that as long as the blood circulation persists, CO_2 is released and leads to expansion of the alveolar lumina. We have been led to conclude that there are only quantitative differences between acute ventilatory emphysema formation and alveolar expansion incurred by inhalation of liquid. Provided that no liquid is evident in the alveolar lumina there are no specific differential criteria.

Further studies on drowned lungs (references in Reh 1970; Mueller 1975) have revealed the following basically unspecific findings: Swelling and intracytoplasmic vesicular formation; detachment of pneumonocytes, swelling, and vesicular formation of the capillary endothelia in the alveolar septa; intralobular hemorrhages; perivascular and peribronchial edema; and general hemolysis (De Bernardi et al. 1965; Caroff et al. 1968).

Studies into the differentiation of rapid and slow drowning have largely shown only quantitative differences. In the case of rapid drowning, emphysematous expansion, partial ruptures in the alveolar septa, empty alveolar spaces, and dilation of the capillaries were found. In the case of slow drowning, there were basically similar findings, though quantitatively less pronounced, and the additional evidence of acidophilic substances in some alveoli and reduction of the PAS reaction in the stroma. In animal experiments, the glycogen content in both forms of drowning appeared to be distinctly reduced. It was possible to demonstrate in studies using dyes that the liquid in drowning always advances as far as the alveoli (Recine and Falchi 1963; Recine and Filauro 1963; Fazzari 1963).

In the differentiation between drowning in freshwater and saltwater by histological and histochemical examination, the various osmotic effects of the drowning medium are of significance. Reidbord and Spitz (1966) were able to detect light microscopically a broadening of the alveolar septa and collapsed capillaries without erythrocytes after drowning in freshwater. Electron-microscopic studies revealed discontinuities in the plasma membranes of numerous cells, such that cell organelles were found in the vascular lumina and alveolar septa. The mitochondria and endoplasmic reticulum were swollen. Conversely, the structure in the lungs was well preserved after drowning in seawater. Experimental studies on rats involving active aspiration of watery liquids of various osmolarities revealed histologically and electron-microscopically detectable differences of diagnostic significance (Brinkmann and Butenuth 1982): The pneumonocytes of the alveoli and endothelia of the lung parenchymal capillaries showed variably pronounced vesicular transformations after freshwater drowning, in addition there was a general hyperhydration of the organism with hydrops and interstitial edema (Figs. 115–117). After the effects of salt water, there was a highly altered rheological state and damage to the epithelia; this form of lesion is termed villous transformation (Fig. 118). Only negligible changes were evident in the case of drowning in an isotonic environment. These findings after drowning in liquids of different osmolarity can be explained by hemodynamically disordered regulation and agonal chemical changes during the drowning process (Püschel et al. 1982; Madert et al. 1982; Hughes 1977). Studies of the primary fluorescence of pulmonary tissue have shown different findings according to the effects of fresh- or saltwater (Santini 1966). The peroxidase of the pulmonary tissue was perceptibly increased in saltwater drowning as against freshwater influences (Spitz et al. 1969); the peroxidase was evident for up to 5 h postmortem.

With fresh corpses found in water, it is sometimes possible histologically to detect aspirated water particles in the deep respiratory tracts and alveoli. If the corpse

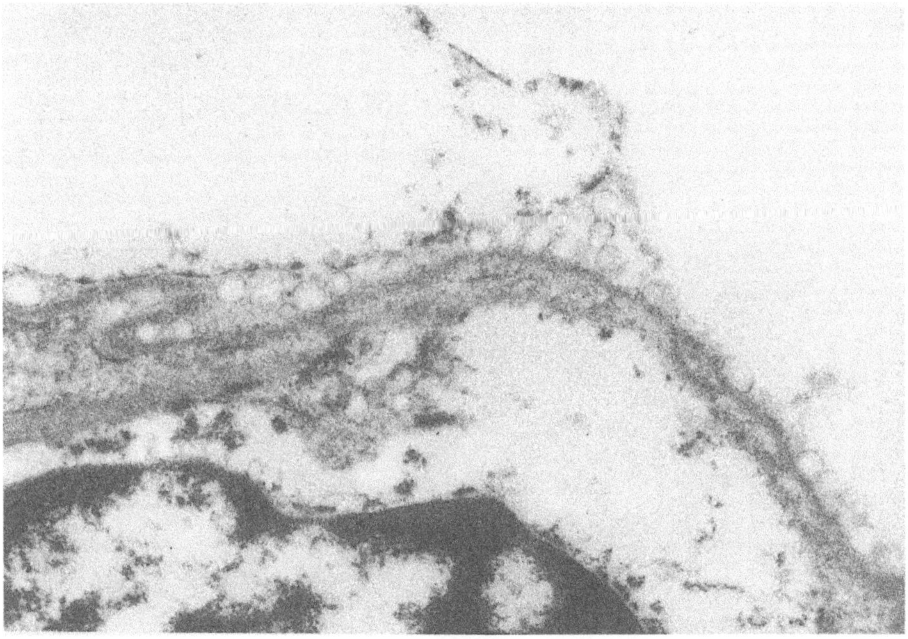

Fig. 115. Drowning in fresh water: Vesicularization of the alveolar epithelium. EM, ×12000

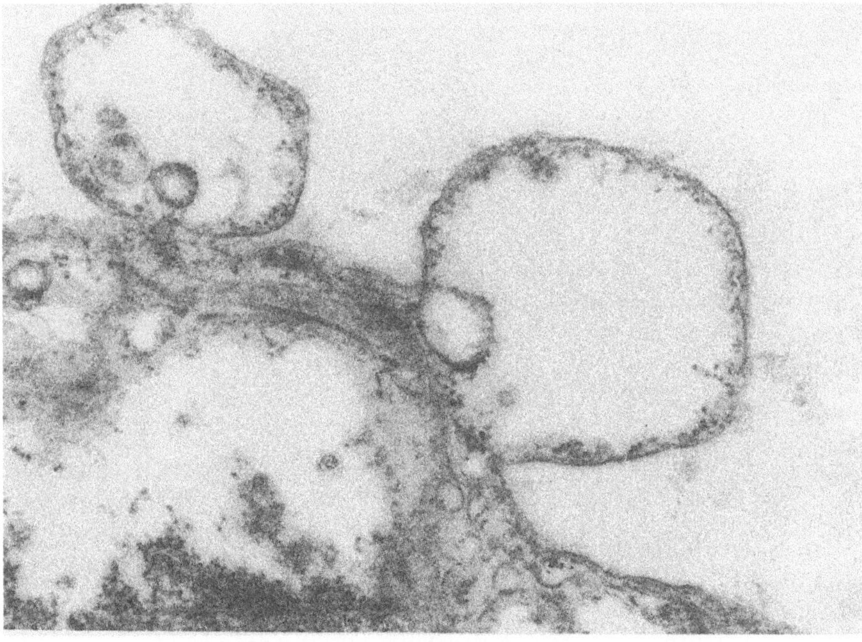

Fig. 116. Drowning in fresh water: Pronounced large vacuolar swelling of the alveolar epithelium. EM, ×20000

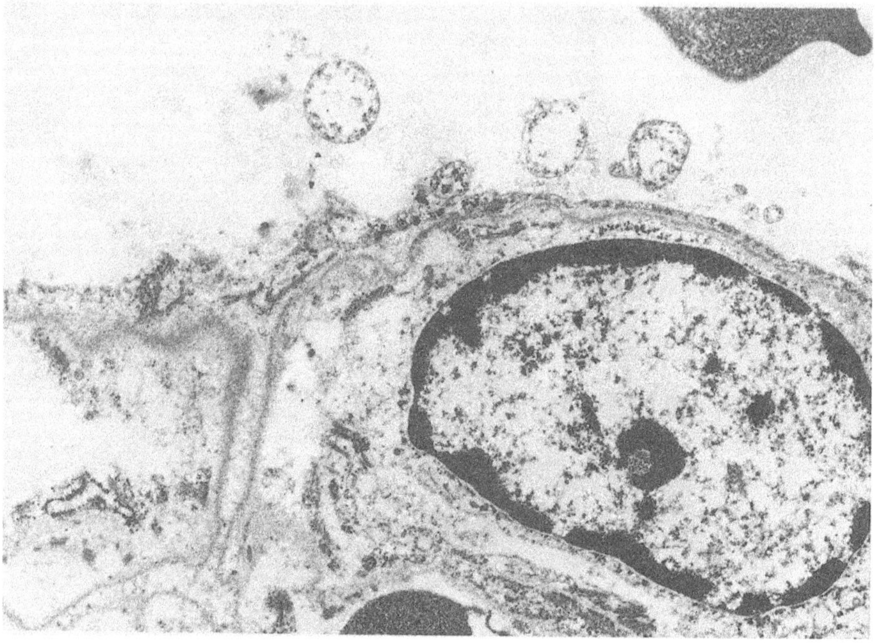

Fig. 117. Drowning in fresh water: Detachment of rounded, swollen and vacuolized cell sections of the alveolar epithelium. EM, × 7 000

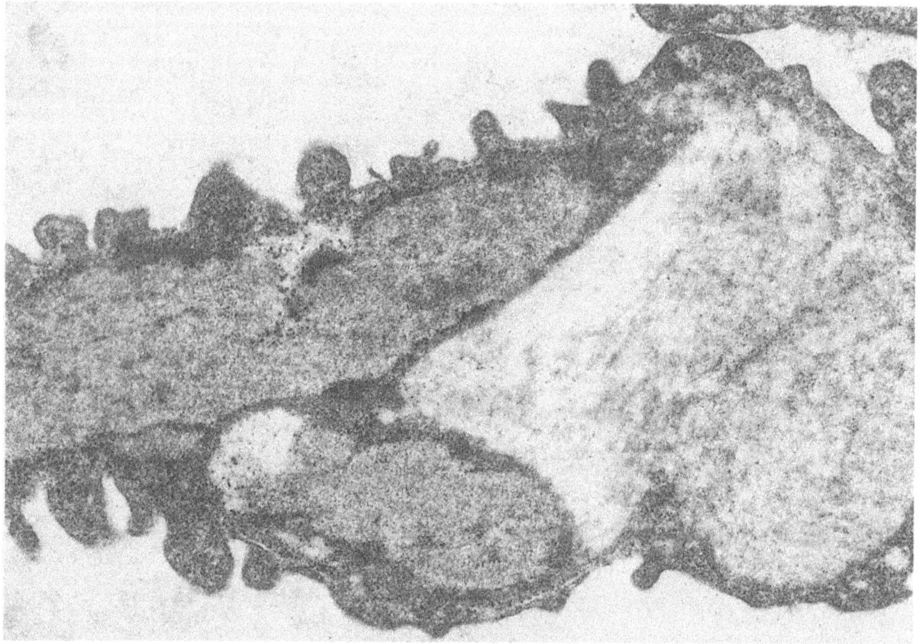

Fig. 118. Drowning in salt water: General compaction of the matrix. Villous transformation of the alveolar epithelium. Circumscribed rupture of the basal membrane. EM, × 12 000

was in shallow water of up to 3 m for only a short time, less than a day, it is possible for a vital intrusion of liquid into the alveoli, i.e., drowning, to be detected according to the investigations of Reh (1970). This intrusion normally involves components of plants and algae, which are conspicuous because of their natural green or brown color. Aspiration of the stomach contents and bile should be considered from the point of view of differential diagnosis.

In the case of putrefied corpses found in water where there is extensive destruction of pulmonary tissue, histological examination of the lungs can make a valuable diagnostic contribution in visualizing the alveolar reticular fiber structure. If the fibers are not completely destroyed, the degree of expansion of the alveoli can be detected. Acute expansion of the alveoli distributed over large sections of the lungs indicates that a death by drowning is possible. However, a check should be made as to whether such a finding in the lungs could have arisen through other means of partial or total obstruction of the respiratory tracts, e.g., aspirations, severe bronchitis, exogenous respiratory embarassment, prior to the influx of water.

Histological investigation of corpses found in water should not, as often happens, be confined to the lungs. In routine practice, the liver, cardiac muscle, and kidneys have to be examined for signs of acute oxygen deficiency and asphyxiation. Histoenzymatic studies of cardiac muscle have revealed an early disappearance of phosphorylase activity after experimental drowning (Vimercati et al. 1976). In the case of rapid death of drowning, distinct enlargement of the liver sinusoids and vesicular discharge (visible electron microscopically) in the vascular epithelia of the kidneys were observed (Montaldo 1963, 1964). Histological studies toward substantiating splenic anemia by counting the erythrocytes in the case of death by asphyxiation and drowning were carried out by Gatti (1963).

Histological examination of hemorrhages in the musculature of the neck and chest wall is also recommended. In the case of uneven putrefaction with, in parts, a good state of preservation, reddish patches can develop through hemoglobin imbibition which can be confused with the muscular hemorrhages that appear in connection with drowning (Wachholz 1907; Mueller 1975). The same applies to Paltauf's spots (subpleural hemorrhages), which cannot be macroscopically identified with certainty. In the peripheral areas of hypostasis in the lungs, postmortem intra- and subpleural hemoglobin patches can also develop. Only extravascular evidence of erythrocytes in these areas is proof of the existence of a hemorrhage.

The differentiation between death by drowning and other causes of death in the water, particularly if the macroscopic signs of drowning are only slightly developed or absent, requires a complete histological status examination. Special consideration should be made of previous disorders of the cardiac muscle, liver, adrenal glands, kidneys, and thyroid. In our experience, the presence of higher grade adiposis hepatica in unsatisfactorily explained cases of death, e.g., after trivial trauma or in water, is relatively common. Although the connections between adiposis hepatica and death following a relatively negligible exogenous stress have thus far not been proven, this empirical observation should be taken into account and a histological check made. In some cases of "muscular weakness in water," a histomorphologically detectable hypoplasia and deficient vascular supply to the adrenal glands are thought to have had causative significance (Patti 1954).

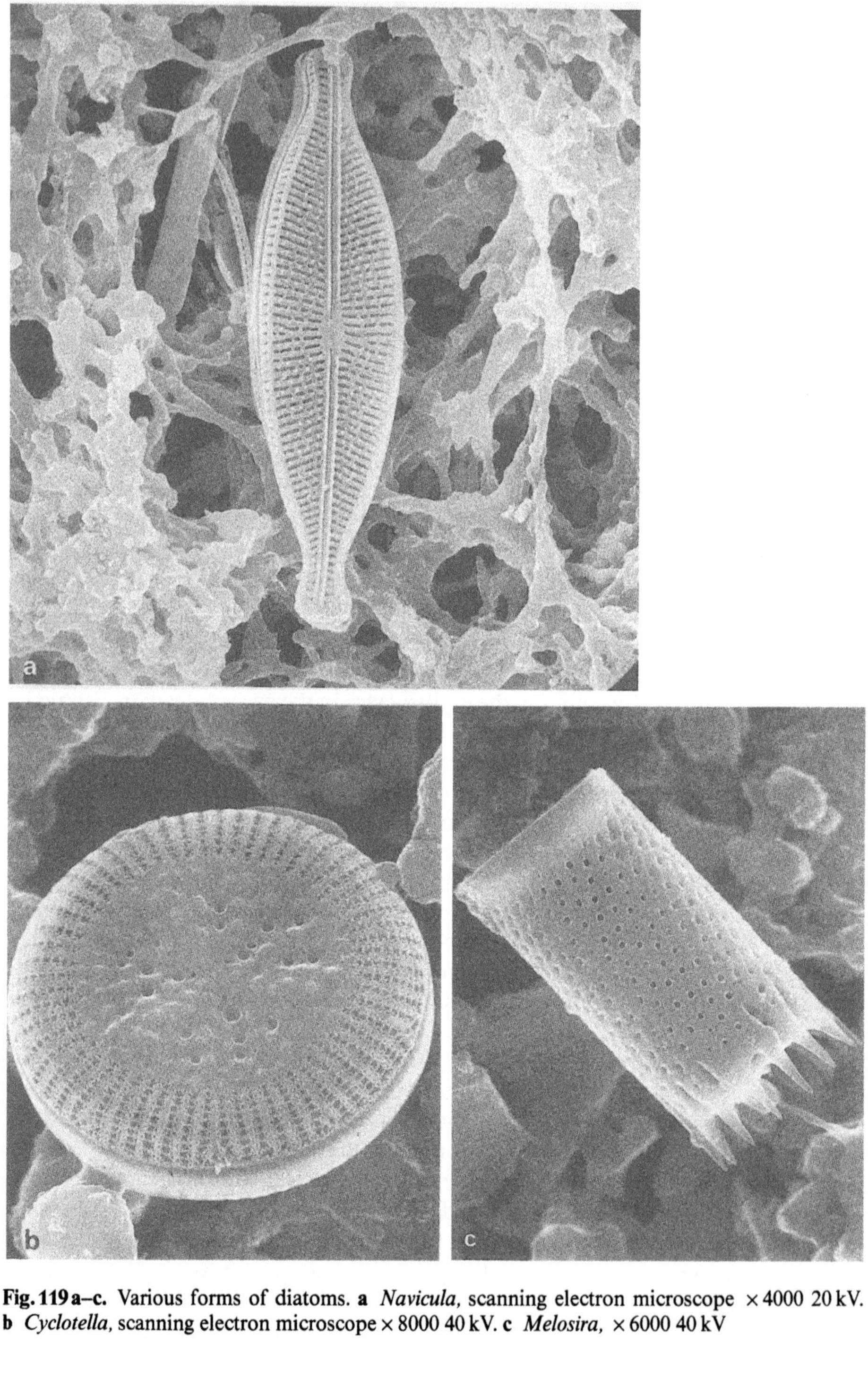

Fig. 119 a–c. Various forms of diatoms. **a** *Navicula*, scanning electron microscope × 4000 20 kV. **b** *Cyclotella*, scanning electron microscope × 8000 40 kV. **c** *Melosira*, × 6000 40 kV

The importance of evidence of diatoms in the organs and tissues of the systemic circulation has been disputed for some time. Histologically, the detection of diatoms is extremely difficult and usually only an accidental finding. With improvement in the methods of processing organs for the extraction and microscopic assessment of diatoms, the diagnostic value of this method has evidently improved despite differences in investigation findings (Fig. 119) (Schellmann and Sperl 1979; Terazawa and Takatori 1980; Udermann and Schuhmann 1975; Fukui et al. 1980; Timperman and Thomas 1980).

A *summary* of all investigation results thus far published shows that the individual findings that occur in connection with death through drowning can also be caused by other exogenous or morbid effects or by the water in which the corpse lies. Examination of a corpse found in water without detailed knowledge of circumstances and preceding events can only attain a higher degree of probability by evaluation of the individual findings; it cannot achieve certainty in the forensic sense. The histological contribution to the diagnosis of death by drowning concentrates on the state of alveolar expansion, identification or exclusion of previous disorders, evaluation of resuscitative measures, detection of signs indicating asphyxiation, and impairment of the findings through autolysis and putrefaction.

VI. Injuries Caused by Heat and Cold

1. Local and General Heat Injuries – Burned Corpses

The presentation of histomorphologically and histochemically detectable heat injuries will follow the usual divisions and approaches, whereby forensically utilizable criteria will be particularly emphasized. Of especial importance are the tissue lesions that are directly incurred by the effects of heat, with their general organic sequelae, and the question of vital or postmortem origin.

Cutaneous and Subcutaneous Lesions

The manner of heat transmission by radiation, the action of flames, or contact with solid and fluid substances are significant to the form of heat injury, although they are similar to one another in their effects. The well-known staging into four or six grades of heat injuries follows qualitative and quantitative criteria.

First Stage: Erythema. This, the mildest form of heat injury, which appears intravitally on the areas of skin affected as a reddening and swelling, has thus far only been histologically investigated in a few cases. A characteristic feature is distension and hyperemia of the blood vessels, particularly the capillaries in the region of the stratum papillare of the cutis, lasting on average 2–4 days. The surrounding connective tissue disaggregates and is frequently interspersed with a proteinaceous edema; expulsion of leukocytes occurs only sporadically. The upper subepidermal connective tissue is predominantly affected, and the findings correspond to the symptoms of a mild serous inflammation. Swellings in the connective tissue fibers of the underlying cutis are rarely observed. In the region of the epidermis, intracellular intake of fluid with disaggregation of the nuclear chromatin can temporarily occur in the stratum germinativum and stratum granulosum (Fig. 120).

The histological findings of erythema can be visualized by simple general stains, e.g., H and E. The findings recede within a few days, 8 days at the most, in an individual who survives and heal without leaving a trace. Erythema can be similarly produced postmortem in a weaker form by the effects of heat on the skin of the corpse. In the region of livor mortis, the histological identification of heat erythema can become difficult; when severe hypostasis is superimposed it may be impossible. In our own experiments, we were able to produce distension of the subepidermal blood vessels, sometimes also with increased congestion, in the skin of a 1- to 4-h-old corpse by contact warming of 50–60 °C outside areas of livor mortis. Such skin

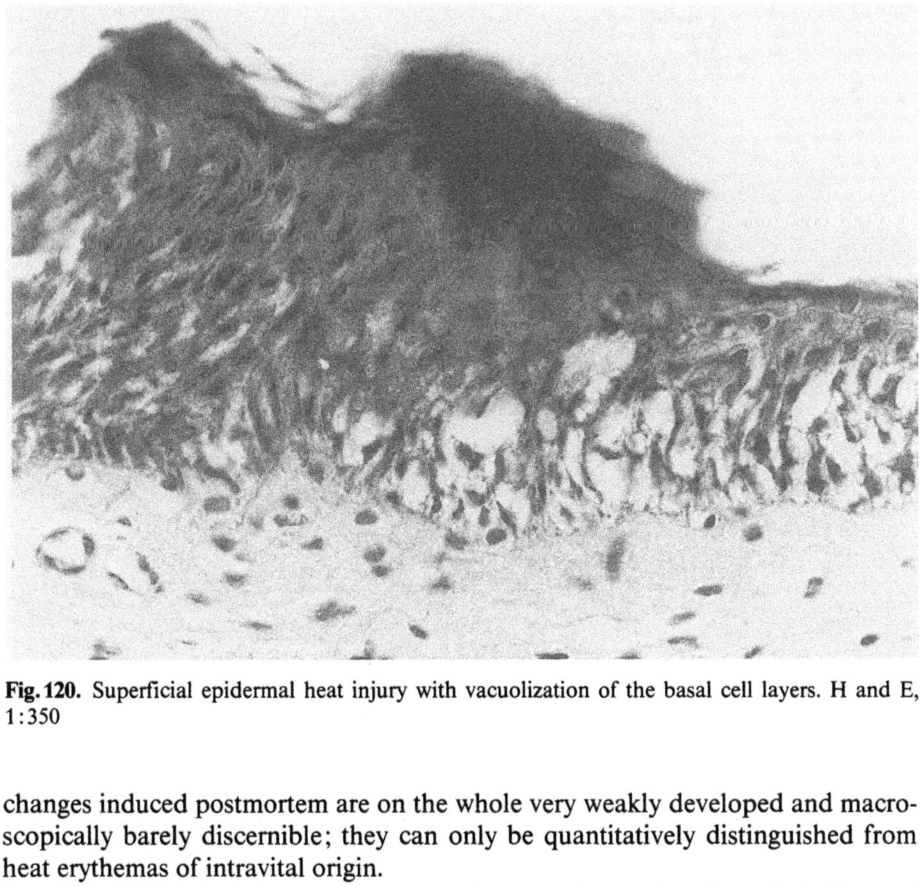

Fig. 120. Superficial epidermal heat injury with vacuolization of the basal cell layers. H and E, 1:350

changes induced postmortem are on the whole very weakly developed and macroscopically barely discernible; they can only be quantitatively distinguished from heat erythemas of intravital origin.

The finding of erythema is thus not reliable evidence of the intravital effects of heat.

Second Stage: Vesiculation. Numerous investigations and animal experimental studies have been carried out to study the histological visualization and forensic assessment of burn blisters, and the literature on this subject is very extensive. Histologically, these blisters are mainly unicameral serum-filled vesicles, which as a sign of inflammatory reaction mostly contain only a few lymphocytes, monocytes, and polymorphonuclear neutrophilic and eosinophilic leukocytes. In the case of fresh burn blisters, the cellular and nuclear outlines can be easily recognized using general stains on the raised areas of epidermis (Fig. 121). Soon after development, desiccation gives rise to the corresponding changes. The detachment of the upper epidermal areas mainly extends through the basal-cell layer (Fig. 122a); thus, remains of the stratum basale and fibrin deposits are found in the vesical fundus. Occasionally, the vesicles contain copious fibrin and diathermally coagulated material (Fig. 122b). The deeper parts of the stratum papillare and underlying upper layers of the corium undergo acute inflammatory change. Of particular importance here are hyperemia and edema, and to a lesser extent inflammatory cell infiltrates. In the peripheral areas of the vesicle, the epithelia of the undetached epidermis are swollen

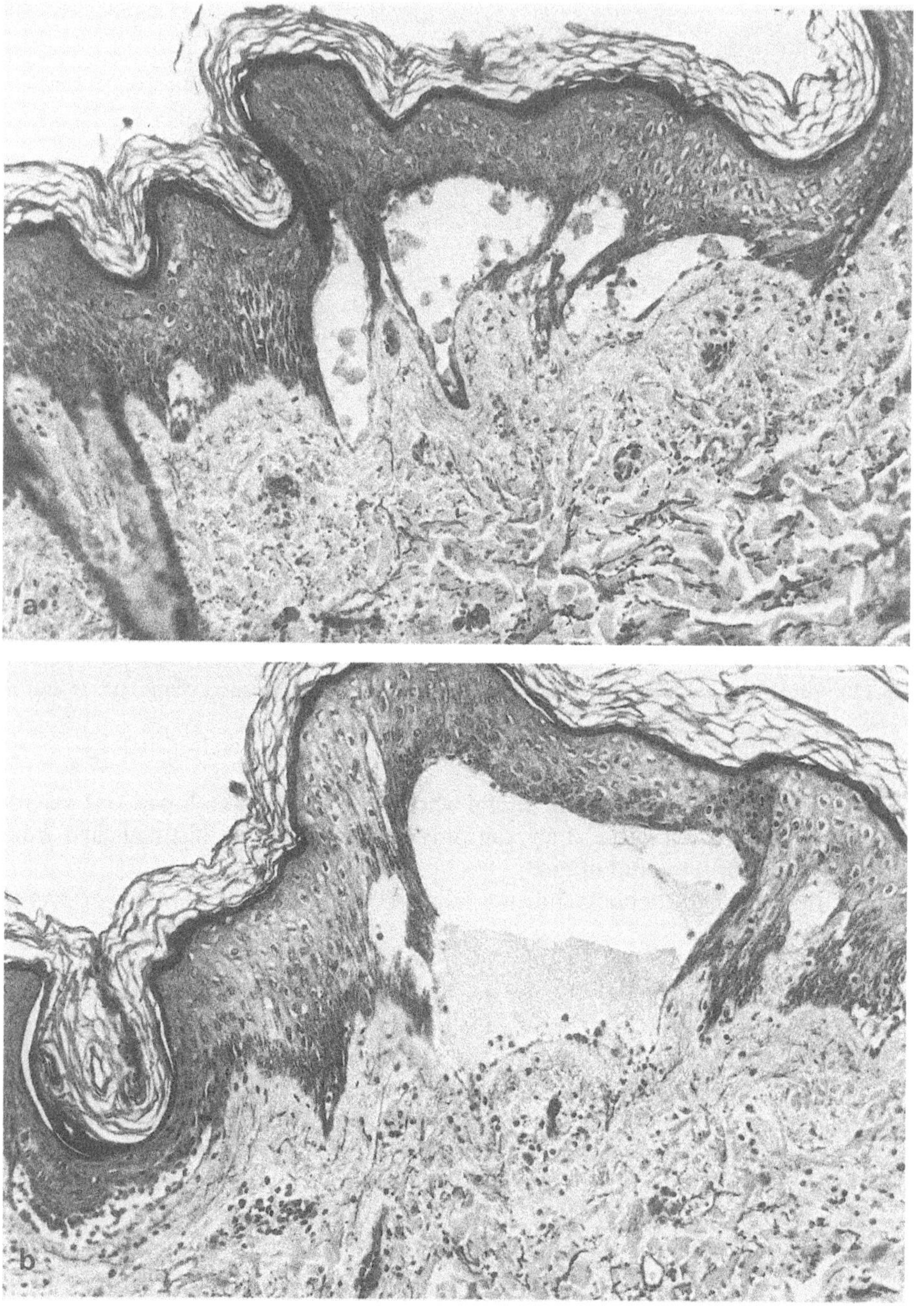

Fig. 121. a, b Epidermal burn (stage 1 to 2) with microvesicles. H and E, 1:250

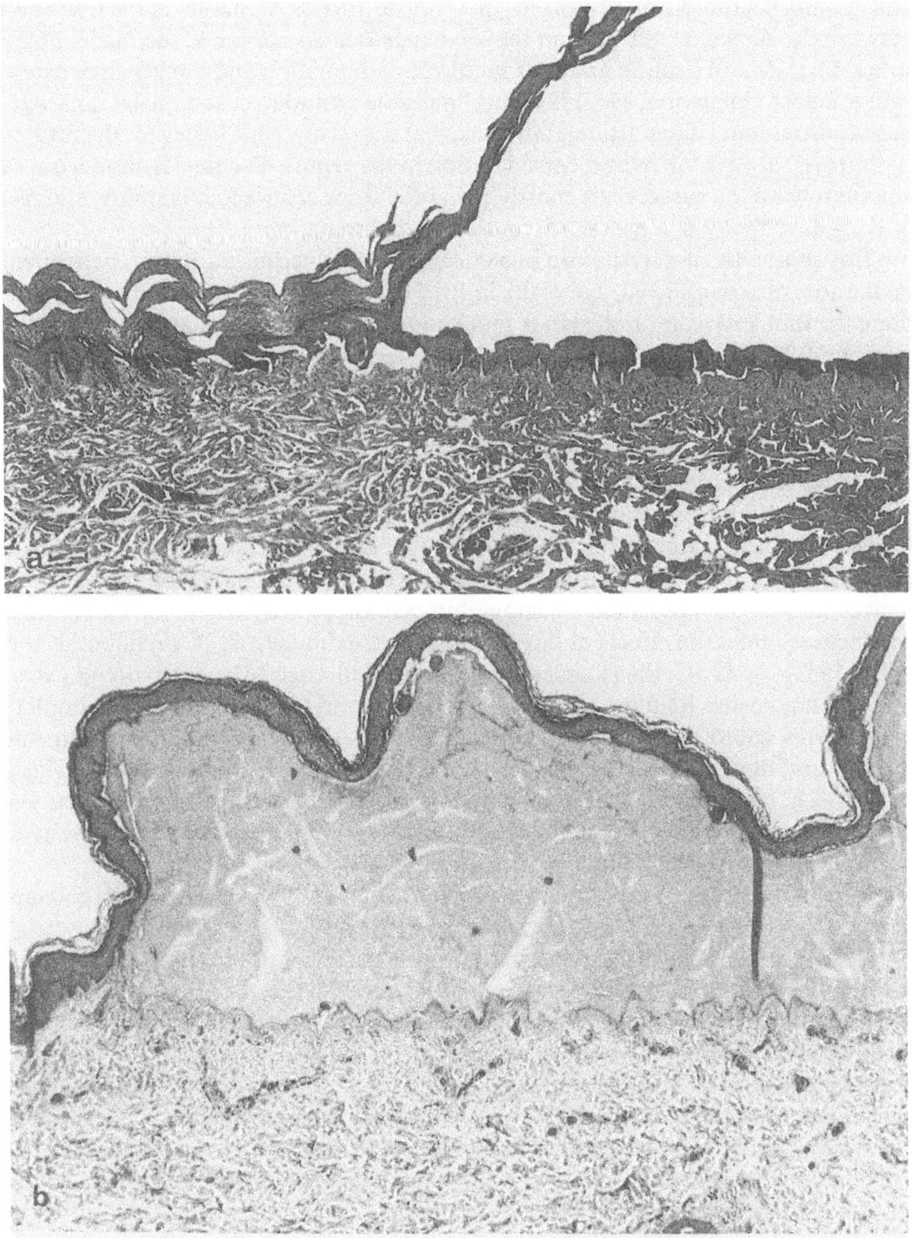

Fig. 122. a Intraepidermal heat blister, evacuated. H and E, 1:80. **b** Heat blister with detachment of the epidermis. Questionable postmortem origin in the case of a fire in an enclosed room and death through CO intoxication. Subject 72 years old, ♂. H and E, 1:80

and in parts necrobiotically changed; their nuclei are less stainable. In the transition between the damaged margin and the unchanged cutaneous area, the nuclei of the stratum basale and stratum granulosum display attenuation and longitudinal extension (nuclear elongation, Fig. 123). This "palisade attitude" of the nuclei no longer has the differential diagnostic significance that was at one time believed; the finding is, however, always taken into consideration in the report. The nuclei, drawn out to a point toward the surface, are mostly pyknotic, show reduced stainability, and frequently have finely disaggregated, restructured chromatin.

This prototype of a fresh burn blister can, undergo certain variations dependent on the area of skin affected, age of the individual, and kind of heat involved. In children, the thin and water-rich skin is much more reactive to thermal injury than the skin of adults. Clinically, the deep-reaching effects beneath burn blisters are sometimes underestimated (Koslowski 1965). In the case of more intense thermal effects, the vesicular detachment can involve the whole epidermis including the stratum germinativum (Pearson 1965). Histologically, in these cases, the base of the blister is seen to be composed of the partially destroyed stratum papillare of the cutis. The vessels, which are initially contracted and later dilated and extremely congested, contain clumped erythrocytes. Thermal damage to the red corpuscles has already been extensively studied. Thermal fragmentation with decomposition of the erythrocytes into larger and smaller hemoglobin-containing particles is well known: It commences under the effects of direct heat at approximately 48 °C (Schubothe and Gross 1953). At 52 °C, the fragmentation had ended after 24 h; hemoglobin extrusion did not ensue. Reunion of the fragments to form larger particles or complete erythrocytes could not be observed. A distinction should be made between this reaction and thermal hemolysis, which begins later than the fragmentation and lasts about 1–2 h. It is assumed that fragmentation and hemolysis are different processes, differing in the way they attack the blood cell. Both phenomena can also, however, be induced by postmortem thermal effects on fresh corpses.

Sometimes, pronounced disaggregation and increased basophilia of the collagenous fibers can be found under burn blisters in the upper layers of the cutis.

A *differential diagnostic comparison* of burn blisters and blisters subsequent to barbiturate poisoning reveals a great similarity between the two. Both types of blisters are characterized by signs of an acute, largely serous inflammation. In the case of barbiturate blisters, the nuclear elongation in the peripheral areas is less pronounced developed (Schollmeyer 1961). Just as in all forms of blister development, the nuclear changes in the marginal areas are explained by stretching and pulling of the tissue. Clumping and fragmentation of the erythrocytes and increased tissue basophilia are absent in the vicinity of barbiturate blisters. Consequently, despite the great similarity, a histological distinction between these two etiologically different types of blisters is possible. Blisters produced artificially by cold could not be histologically distinguished from burn blisters. In humans, they developed between the basal cells and basal membrane (Pearson 1965). Histologically, identifying putrefactive blisters does not present any problems. The whole epidermis is always detached, and the cutis exposed; there are no signs of hyperemia and inflammation; the vesicular content is practically devoid of protein and does not contain any cells. In the marginal areas, indications of cellular and nuclear elongation can occur through raising and stretching of the epidermis commencing in the lower layers.

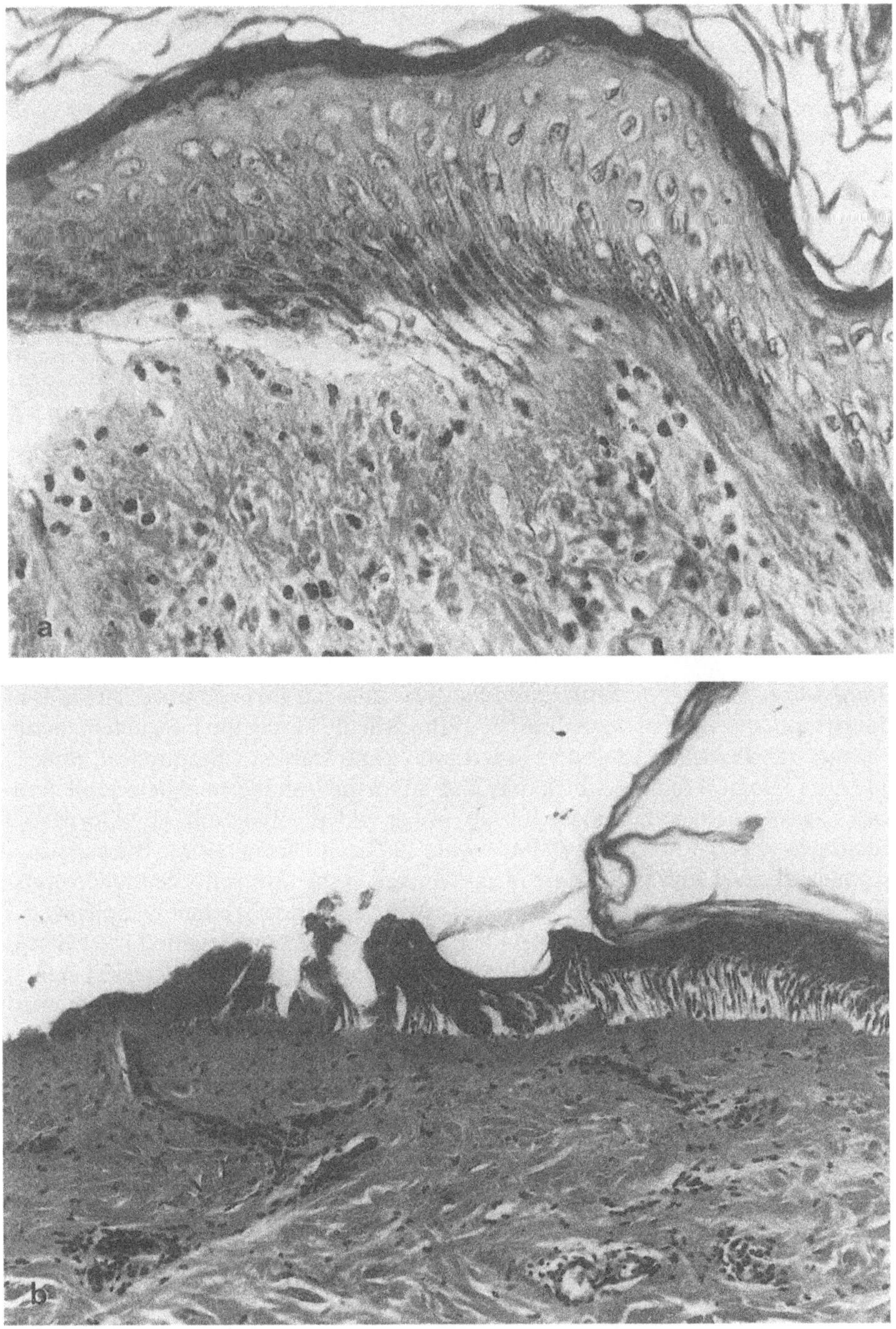

Fig. 123. a, b Elongation of the basal epidermal cells in the proximity of second and third degree burns. H and E, 1:250, 1:150

Skin diseases with vesiculation should also be taken into account with regard to differential diagnosis; anamnesis and clinical and histological findings are important in the differentiation. In Lyell's syndrome, the laminar detachment of the whole epidermis from the corium in the region of the cleft does not show any cellular reaction. In the stratum granulosum, circumscribed eosinophilic necroses are found, which encroach onto the upper layers and lead to total necrosis of the epidermis. The eosinophilic necroses also affect the corium and integumentary appendages (Metter and Schulz 1978).

Burn blisters with fibrin and leukocytes and vascular reactions in the adjacent tissue are now generally regarded as evidence of a vital reaction (Pioch 1966b). Vesicular raising of the epidermis may be brought about by the effects of heat a short time after death, though this does not give unequivocal inflammatory reactions. As far as can be assessed from the literature, there is only one case report, concerning a victim of an air crash by Janezig-Jelacic (1954), of postmortem formation of fibrin- and leukocyte-containing burn blisters. The value of burn blisters with inflammatory signs as evidence of a vital reaction has not diminished despite this report.

The healing of burn blisters is usually effected within 10–12 days if no particular infectious complications arise. The vesicular content is resorbed, and the detached epidermis dries up and is shed. Proceeding from the marginal areas, new epithelization follows, often under the burn blisters, after a few days and covers the epidermal defect.

Third Stage: Necroses of the Skin and Subcutis. This category comprises all kinds of destruction and signs of devitalization of the skin, including the integumentary appendages and subcutis, caused by heat (burning and scalding). Biophysical, clinical, and chronological factors, which may also affect the histologically detectable findings, cannot be entered into here. Details are provided in the studies by Moritz and Henriques (1947), Moritz (1954), Price et al. (1953), and Klein (1975). The most conspicuous finding with third-degree heat damage to the skin is the central coagulation necrosis of the cutis (Fig. 124). The overlying epidermis is either completely destroyed and no longer present or evident as a homogeneous liquefied layer that is fully detached from the cutis. These epidermal remains show an increased stainability with general dyes. At the periphery of the areas affected by heat, the liquefied epidermis passes into epidermal sections that are also largely unstructured, though more extensive and often faveolate. Externally adjacent to these, in the lower, undifferentiated epidermal layers there are the familiar longitudinally elongated cells and nuclei. Beyond these cells, in the neighboring epidermal zone, there are the graded forms of slight thermal damage passing into undamaged tissue: swelling of the cells and nuclei, loss of basophilic cytoplasmic granulation, intracytoplasmic vacuoles partly with basophilic contents, pyknosis of the nuclei, destruction of the nuclear chromatin, and karyorrhexis. Altogether, these cell changes in the outer transitional zone are to be judged as the beginnings of devitalization, i.e., necrobiosis.

The cutis located in the center of the thermal damage under the destroyed or liquefied epidermis is necrotic. Histological detection of such necrosis immediately or a short time after it was caused can be difficult, especially in the case of scalding or long-term, medium-grade contact heat. The stainability of the nuclei in the inte-

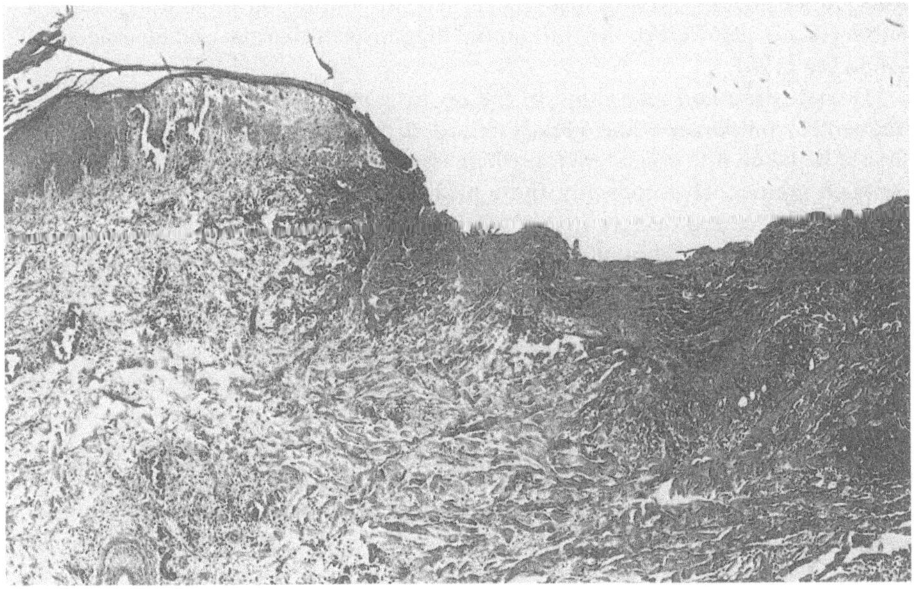

Fig. 124. Deep intradermal burn with areas of inflammation. Subject survived 10 days. H and E, 1:80

gumentary appendages is not diminished until after 12–24 h if there is no coarse structural damage. The collagenous and elastic fibers of the cutis may sometimes be distinct for days. The most conspicuous finding is early edema, which appears after minutes; it is most pronounced in the peripheral zones of the devitalized cutical area. The superficial blood vessels are frequently contracted, the deeper vessels dilated. Clumped erythrocytes, thermal fragmentation, signs of hemolysis, and regular occlusions through thermal coagulation are found in the vessels. Particular difficulties are encountered in demarcating the necrosis of the cutis and subcutis with regard to depth and lateral extent, which is of great significance in the clinical assessment. The nuclei of the vascular musculature and endothelia are also stainable for some time. Apart from uncharacteristic swelling and edema, initially there are no signs of irreversible tissue damage. In deep-reaching thermal lesions, the characteristic delayed appearance of inflammatory reactions should be noted. A borderline leukocytic infiltration does not occur until 6–24 h after the heat injury was first incurred. Fibrin deposits and hemorrhages are rarely found.

The damaged fatty tissue in the subcutis contains circumscribed liquefaction with cell collapse and extracellular fine- and coarse-grained de-emulsified neutral fat. Heat-damaged skeletal musculature appears faded with general stains. The cell membranes and sarcoplasmic borders are blurred. The endomysium is swollen and the transverse striation of the muscle cells is no longer recognizable directly after the injury (Masshoff 1957).

In the case of skin burns through contact with metallic objects, "thermal metallization" can occur similar to that seen with electric skin injuries. These metallic traces, which tend to be located on the surface of the affected dermal area, can be detected particularly well in histological section with the silver-staining method of Timm (Pioch 1966b). For the differential diagnosis of thermal and electric metallization see p. 261.

Demarcation and resorption of the necrosis and subsequent tissue repairs are frequently complicated and greatly retarded by wound infections, a factor that should be taken into consideration when assessing healing and other states following such injuries. Histologically, these healing processes, which are terminated by considerable scarred defects, do not offer any characteristic features.

One problem of central importance concerns the histological and histochemical differentiation between burns of vital and postmortem origin. The differential diagnostic difficulties become particularly apparent in fresh third-degree burns. All the essential histological criteria of this stage can also appear after death or be experimentally induced. An evaluation by Pioch (1966b) of his own histological studies and of the pertinent literature disclosed that identification of the vital nature of thermal cutaneous and subcutaneous lesions using conventional histological staining techniques is largely dependent on the occurrence of inflammatory changes. These are, however, not normally evident in a histological preparation until a matter of hours after the injury.

The same conclusions were obtained in experimental studies carried out with modern histochemical methods on volunteers and corpses (Nedwich et al. 1964; Graev 1964; Cutotiu et al. 1965).

The significance of histochemical examination in forensic practice was systematically studied by Pioch (1966b) with burns of intravital and postmortem origin in mice and guinea pigs. Since these studies, no essentially new findings toward the identification of intravital thermal skin lesions have been reported, and there has been no broader application and scrutiny of animal experimental results in forensic practice. The results of the studies by Pioch (1966b, 1971) toward the identification of intravital heat injuries in synoptic form are as follows:

Reduction of glycogen in the integumentary appendages, onset 5–15 min after localized burn trauma (PAS stain). Loss of glycogen through decomposition beginning soon after death and through the fixation process should be critically taken into account.

Transformation and degradation of proteins in the marginal zones of the damaged region. Evidence of tryptophan by the Ninhydrin(alloxan)-Schiff test and rosindol reaction. As early as 15–30 min after the heat injury was caused, a positive zone regularly formed, demarcating the tissue affected. Subsequent reaction zones offered additional markers for age determination of the burn.

Karyolysis can be detected in the indistinct damaged epidermal periphery 30–45 min after trauma by means of a nucleic acid test (Feulgen's test), with the appearance of Feulgen-positive particles in the epidermis, cutis, and cells of the integumentary appendages.

Reduction or loss of various desmoenzymes. Evidence of a negative vital reaction, just as in mechanical injuries. The evidence of unspecific esterases has proven to be especially suitable; using this method an increased enzyme reaction was apparent 15 min after vital burning, demarcating the necrotic periphery.

The results from animal experimental studies are a good guide to among the histologically and histochemically detectable reactions following intravital heat inju-

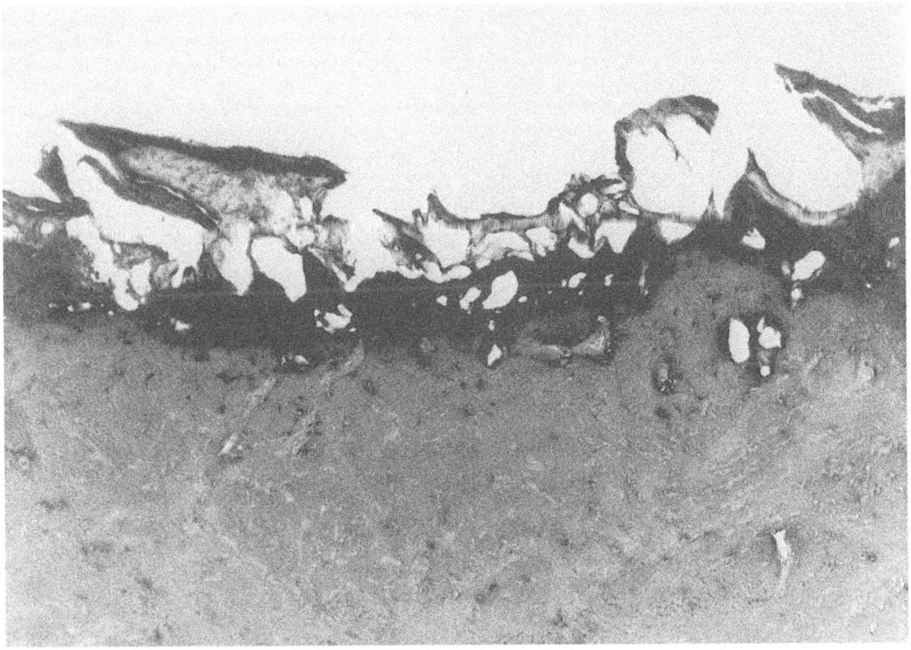

Fig. 125. Postmortem burn: Cavity formation and charring of the epidermis, homogenization of the corium. Azan, 1:80

ries. They do not, however, allow any direct inferences to be made with regard to the time-course of reactions in humans.

The histological identification of heat injuries of postmortem origin involves problems similar to those in the diagnosis of intravital burns produced shortly before death. Experimental studies on the skin of human corpses with heat from a contact or flame source between 100 °C and 300 °C on the skin with periods of application of 5–20 s revealed some histological indications for the presence of postmortem thermal lesions (Naeve 1981). The presence of a postmortem heat injury was indicated by the occurrence of: (1) blisters and empty cavities in the epidermis (Fig. 125); (2) bandlike parallel structures in the subcutaneous fatty tissue (Fig. 126) (following higher grade effects of heat); (3) marginal vesicles in the vessels.

The determination of a postmortem heat injury was substantiated when the following histological criteria were absent or only negligibly developed: (1) Hyperemia (outside areas of postmortem lividity); (2) dilation of blood vessels; (3) vascular wall edema; (4) negligible extent of thermal coagulation in the blood vessels of the corium; (5) erythrocytic fragmentation; (6) metachromasia.

Biochemical animal experimental studies by Fazekas et al. (1973) were concerned with detecting histamine in the skin after vital and postmortem burns. A high level of free histamine (70.9% ± 10.3%) is thought to be proof of a vital origin.

Fourth Stage: Deep Burns and Charring. The fourth and severest grade of burns comprises the deep effects that extend as far as the bones, usually accompanied by

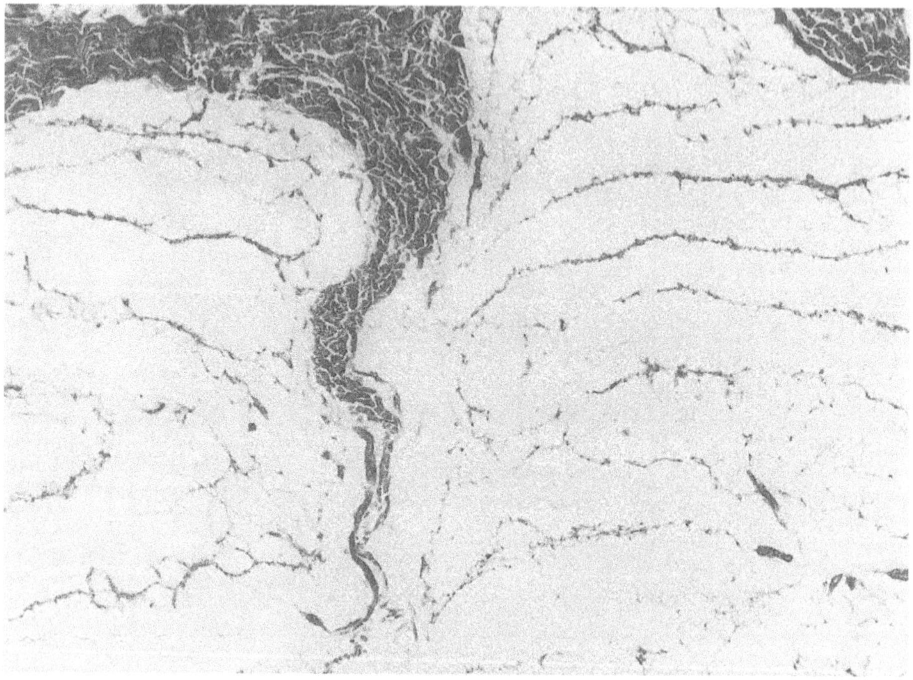

Fig. 126. Deep postmortem skin burn. Transformation of the subcutaneous fatty tissue through rupture of the fibrous septa that run vertically to the surface. Azan, 1:60

carbonization, and leading to the large-scale destruction of whole extremities and sections of the body. Only high temperatures, usually brought about by the effects of direct flame, are capable of producing such severe burns. Scalding does not, therefore, come into consideration. From a medico legal point of view, this group of heat injuries does not present any special problems and considerations. Further particular points will be discussed with reference to the examination of burned corpses, which will be dealt with later.

General Heat Injuries

The general effects of heat injuries to the skin and subcutaneous soft parts concern the appearance of the inner organs, the histomorphology of burn shock, and the problems of acute death through burning (Könn and Brandt 1974; Schickedanz et al. 1975). The present level of knowledge permits many sequelae to be distinguished in the inner organs as an expression of acute or protracted shock. The prominent lesions in individual organs and functional systems as a result of external heat injury, require the presentation of a specific organ histology, even where many of these findings are understood to be components of universal shock.

The common feature of the effects to the inner organs is a histologically detectable, morbid permeability of the capillary walls to blood plasma and corpuscles

(Zinck 1940). Proteinaceous edema develops together with a widening of the interstitial spaces. This finding corresponds to a serous inflammation and is pathogenetically explained by dysoria of the vascular walls. The interposition of protein-rich fluid between the capillary wall and parenchyma leads to an increase in the oxygen diffusion and parenchymal hypoxia. Many authorities regard this histomorphologically distinctive process as being responsible for the nature of parenchymal lesions and the onset of morphological changes attributable to burns.

The damage to the inner organs probably results from protein degradation substances, which enter the circulation from the burn. They either directly affect the vascular walls and parenchymal cells or do so via a lesion of the vasomotorium. Particular efforts have been concerned with evidence of a burn toxin and isoantibodies (Truss 1968; Rittenbury 1970; Haferkamp 1962; Haferkamp et al. 1963; Schoenenberger et al. 1976; Kremer et al. 1979). A toxin develops in the skin as a result of burns, which has been isolated and electron-microscopically visualized; it is a polymer that accumulates in the inner organs and effects the destruction of parenchymal cells. Under standardized conditions, thermal energy induces a lipid-protein complex in the skin which has toxic effects. In animal experiments, these effects are due to inhibition of oxidative phosphorylation and massive suppression of all ATP-dependent steps of glycogen synthesis.

The extent of the damage to the inner organs described in the following section is not always dependent on the size of the cutaneous and subcutaneous lesions (Delarue et al. 1962; Klein 1975). Numerous complications are also of substantial influence (Sevitt 1979).

Liver. Following extensive burns, distinct pericapillary edema and a lymphocytic-monocytic infiltration of Glisson's triangles occur in the lobules of the liver after a few hours. In the peripheral lobule sections, the liver epithelia are opague and swollen; there is a fine-droplet separation of the cytoplasm and distension of the nuclei (Zinck 1940; Reh 1960). Pyknotic giant nuclei and polymorphonuclear liver epithelia are also found. In less severe burns, the swollen liver parenchyma is diffusely opague, the epithelia are sometimes dissociated, and the capillary walls appear distended through the accumulation of proteinaceous fluid in Disse's spaces (Fig. 127). In this stage, this finding can resemble acute Basedow's disease or the initial phases of acute yellow atrophy. With extensive burns and severe systemic damage, centroacinar and intermediary coagulation necroses of liver cells also occur, which can become confluent and lead to collapse of the intervening parenchymal sections. The necrobiotic liver cells generally contain fine to medium-sized droplets of fat. After a child was severely scalded, Lindlar and Berger (1962) found a diffuse infiltration of large droplets of fat in the liver and characteristic polynuclear giant cells with pigment accumulation and phagocytic plaquelike products; chemically, these were mainly composed of amino acids. Following scalding, animal experimental and enzyme-histochemical studies revealed an early alteration in various enzymes in the liver epithelia of the lobule periphery at a stage when histologically only negligible fatty infiltration was evident. NAD cytochrome-c oxidase, isocitric acid dehydrogenase, and ATPase were particularly impaired; alkaline phosphatase and a few esterases were, on the other hand, increased (Hermann et al. 1965). These findings indicate damage to the energy metabolism of the cells.

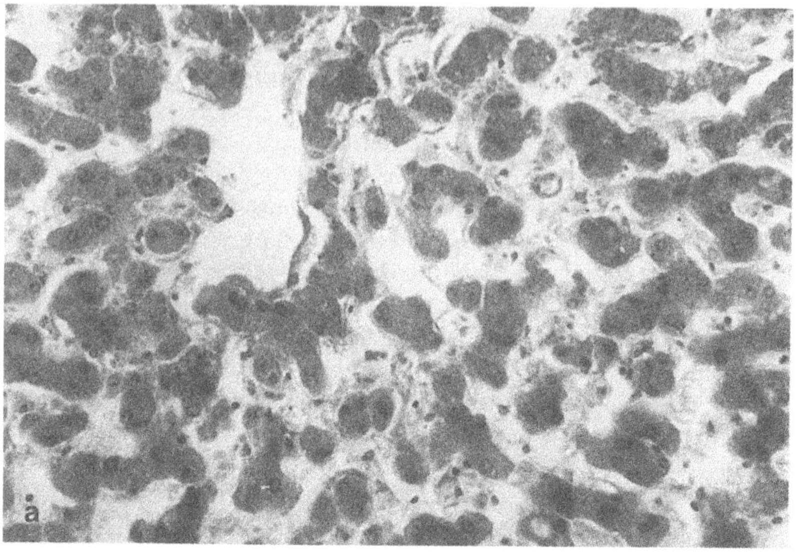

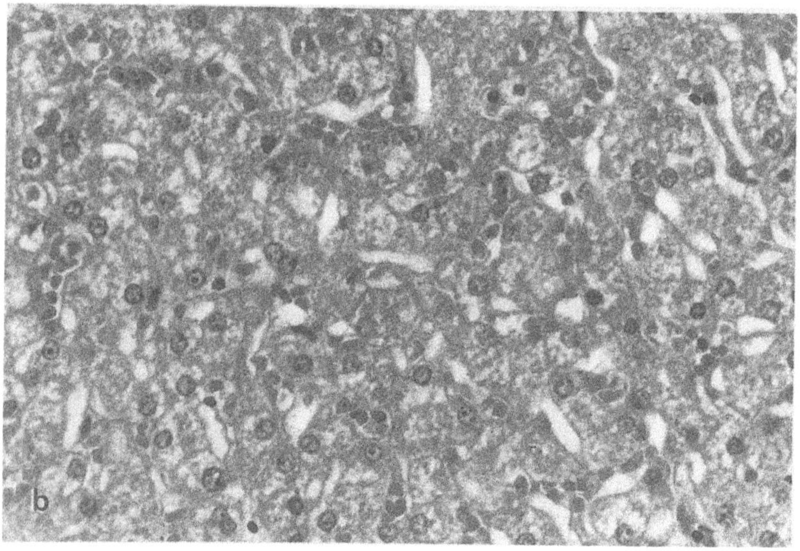

Fig. 127. a Dissociation of the hepatic cell strands, widening of the intertrabecular spaces as a result of edema, reaction of Kupffer's cells after burning (beginning of so-called serous hepatitis). H and E, 1:220. **b** Opaque swelling and vacuolar transformation of the liver epithelia, pronounced widening of Disse's spaces following burning. H and E, 1:350

Kidneys. Systematic histological investigations of the kidneys after fatal burns mainly showed the following unspecific findings (Zinck 1940; Reh 1960; Pinchuk 1964; McCaninch et al. 1964): pronounced general hyperemia and congestion of the vessels, opaque swelling and hyaline-droplet degeneration in the epithelia of the tubules, hemoglobin casts, broadening of Bowman's capsule, detachment of the tubular epithelia from the basal membrane, regressive changes in the tubular epithelia

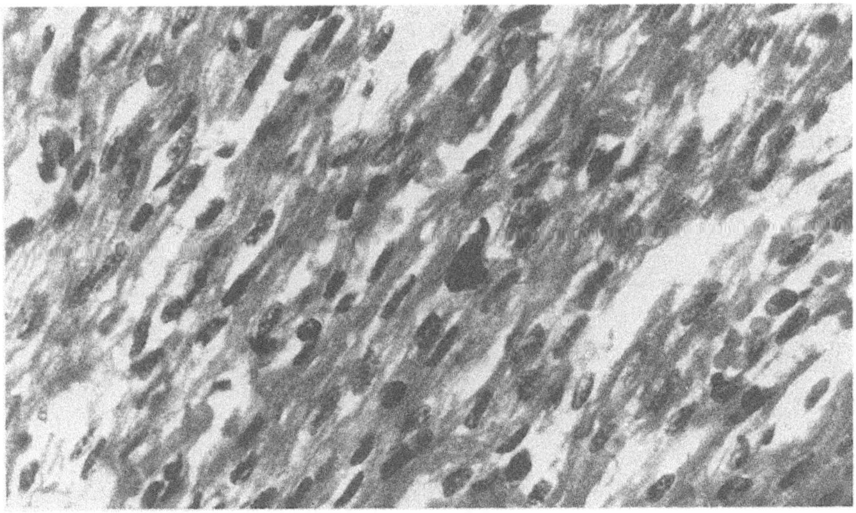

Fig. 128. Myocardium (right ventricle) with interstitial edema, narrowing of the muscle fibers, dehiscence of the muscle cell nuclei. Intracapillary megakaryocyte. Subject survived burn 4 days. H and E, 1:280

up to the extent of necrotizing nephrosis, an abundance of cells in the glomeruli, collapse of the glomerular loops, glomerulohistolysis and serous capsular space exudates, disappearance of glomeruli, protein casts, and septic focal infiltrates and liquefaction. In cases of delayed death, the kidneys, unlike the liver, were always affected by the burns. Occasionally, epithelial and interstitial calcium deposits are found after 1–2 days, chiefly in the region of the papillae. In cases of previous injury with fixed hypertension or nephrosclerosis, even negligible burns led to extensive necroses of the tubular epithelia (Pinchuk 1964).

Heart. Changes in the form of serous myocarditis occur early together with fibrous edema and swelling of the transverse striation and intercalated discs (Fig. 128). In addition, pale focal areas and homogenization are seen, particularly in the musculature of the right ventricular septum. In later stages, disseminated, perivascular, cardiac muscle fiber necroses occur with circumscribed resorptive cell reactions. As in diphtheria, extensive deparenchymization can take place in the inner and intermediate muscular areas and in the region of the papillary muscle. In many cases, especially in young children, well-developed perivascular accumulations of histiocytes and fat-free vacuoles are found in the cardiac muscle cells, probably as an expression of hypoxic damage.

Lungs. There is the early development of general interstitial edema (Fig. 129), focal intra-alveolar edema, intra-alveolar hemorrhages, and swelling and disaggregation of the vascular walls, particularly near arterioles, which is connected with pronounced swelling of the endothelial cells (Hagedorn et al. 1975). Sochor and Mallory (1963) investigating severe burns, chiefly in the head region found pseudomembranous tracheobronchitis, bronchiolitis, interstitial and alveolar hemorrhages,

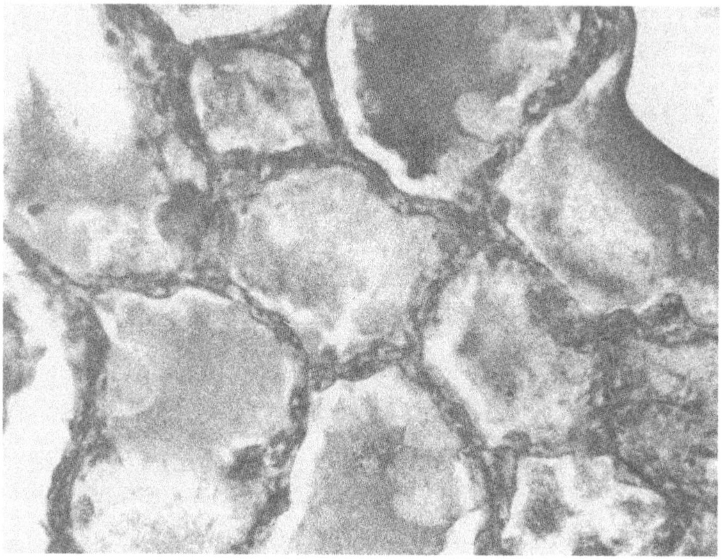

Fig. 129. Protein-rich intra-alveolar pulmonary edema; 3 days after burning. H and E, 1:280

fibrin thrombi in the small arteries and arterioles, focal atelectases, bronchopneumonia, and acute emphysema. Bronchopneumonia was accompanied by severe necrotizing bronchiolitis.

Brain. An important finding here is often the very pronounced edema. Extensive fibrillolysis and cell shadow formation, acute swellings and homogenization of ganglion cells are also found. Vacuolar degeneration and dissipation of cell processes occur. Particularly affected are the nucleus dentatus, the olive, Purkinje cells, the pons, and large areas of the cerebral cortex (Zinck 1940). In the case of neonates who died within 2 days as a result of burns, histologically regressive changes were found in the motor pyramidal cells of the third and fifth cell layers of motor regions of the motor cerebral cortex; there were also homogenized cell changes in the Purkinje cells, olive, and nucleus dentatus. Investigation of the thermoregulatory center in rostral and caudal areas of the hypothalamus revealed relatively sparse ganglion cell changes with intercellular edema and acute cellular swelling (Schmitt and Schröter 1962).

Adrenal Glands. Histological findings suggest a distinct dependence on the survival time after burn trauma as well as on the general reactive state of the organism. Hyperplasia of the outer adrenal cortex and increased production of aldosterone and adrenalin were found when death occurred in the first few hours after burning (Fain 1964). The hyperplasia also affected the inner cortical layer when death occurred later. Lipid and cholesterol levels were reduced. After 2–4 days, a reversal of these findings and dystrophic changes were evident. Olbrycht and Ramult (1924) found extensive hemorrhages and necroses in the cortex and defects in the chromaffin medullary substance following scalding. In animal experiments, Kuwabara (1954) detected a positive effect of artifical hibernation with reduced damage and exhaustion of the adrenal cortex.

Pancreas. This organ has not been histologically examined to any great extent specifically with regard to burns, but it has been investigated in connection with conditions of shock. Fibrinous thrombi in the capillaries and arterioles, circumscribed hemorrhages, necrobioses of individual parenchymal cells, and sometimes also grouped necroses are found after burns.

Stomach and Intestine. With ulcers of the stomach and duodenum that have fatal complications, it is recommended, just as with shock ulcers, to undertake a scrupulous histological examination. With regard to later forensic considerations, it is particularly necessary to obtain the data for an age determination of the ulcer and superficial erosions. It is important to decide whether the hemorrhage or perforation arose from a previous ulcer or from a stress ulcer that developed in connection with shock as a result of the burn and subsequent therapy. After proper removal and mounting of the stomach or intestinal wall with the complete ulcer, the floor and marginal areas of the defect are examined by vertical sections using general and connective tissue stains. Fresh ulcers developing acutely after burning penetrate the mucosa (often as if punched through), including the muscularis mucosae as far as deep into the submucosa. The peripheral areas are largely unreactive and do not show any scar formation whatsoever in these ulcers which develop within a few hours. When a finding is substantiated in this manner, a causal connection with a directly preceding heat injury may be inferred. The same applies to the likewise acutely developed erosions, which are usually multiple and superficial, extending as far as the muscularis mucosae.

It is difficult to assess the causality of hemorrhages and perforations from older, callous, penetrating ulcers. It would, then, be perfectly possible for the ulcer to have existed prior to the burn. A hemorrhage from such a chronic ulcer can be induced by a systemic injury after the burn. A spontaneous ulcerous hemorrhage cannot be excluded in most cases with the required forensic degree of certainty.

The frequency of gastrointestinal ulceration is estimated to be about 25% following a burn (Curling's ulcer) (Drüner and Grözinger 1972).

The histopathology of burn shock essentially embraces all the findings presented in Chap. C IV; they are frequently superimposed by the sequelae of impairment to the inner organs caused by the burn. Postmortem identification of burn shock is basically founded on a synoptic evaluation of the individual findings. A "morphological shock syndrome" (Remmele 1975; Sellés 1965) is present when there are the following changes: Intravascular microthrombi in lung, liver, kidney, and gastrointestinal tract; epithelial necroses in the liver and kidney; distension of the renal tubuli; intravascular accumulations of myelopoietic cells in the kidneys; mucosal erosion of the gastrointestinal tract.

Death following exposure to superheated steam and inhalatory scalding gives rise to findings with a distinctive character. Studies by Brinkmann et al. (1979) and Püschel et al. (1980) on 27 victims of a boiler explosion who died at different intervals after the accident gave the following findings: ruptures with hemorrhages and escape of fibrin in pulmonary tissue, heat swellings and vesicular detachment of the

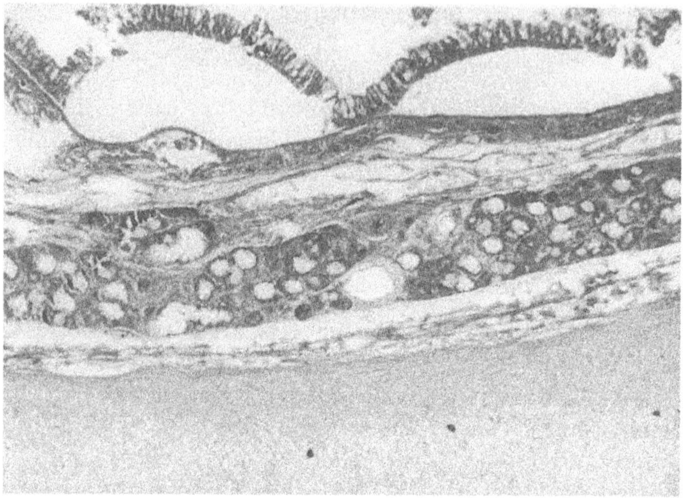

Fig. 130. Heat swelling and vesicular detachment of the tracheal epithelium following inhalation of superheated steam. Goldner's, 1:80

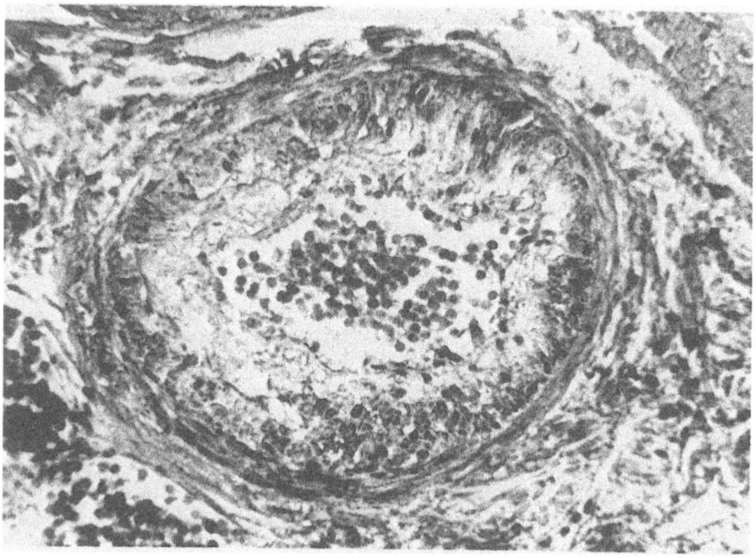

Fig. 131. Small pulmonary vein with intimal swelling and constriction of the lumen after subject had survived effects of superheated steam for 2 days. H and E, 1:200

epithelium in the trachea and bronchi (Fig. 130), pronounced intra-alveolar and perivascular edema in the lungs, intimal and septal swellings and aggregations in the small vessels of the lungs (Figs. 131, 132), high-grade parietal swellings of the small arteries and arterioles in the cortex of the kidneys, signs of hypoxia in the alveolar epithelium and parenchymatous organs, sporadically also complete de-

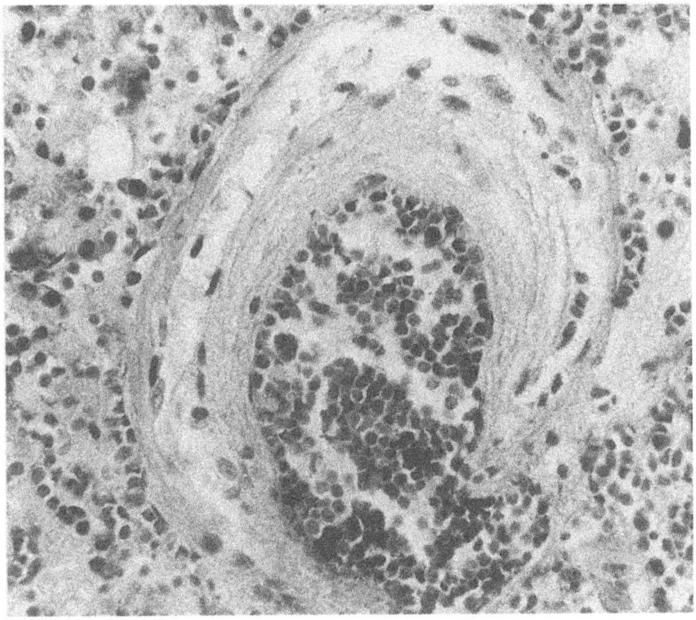

Fig. 132. Small pulmonary arterial branch with splitting of the vascular wall and infiltrative bleeding. Subject had survived effects of superheated steam for 2 days. H and E, 1:200

struction of the tracheobronchial mucosa with inflammatory reaction and parietal edema (Fig. 133). The histological findings in all victims, even those who died immediately, were explained as vital reactions and the result of a general oxygen deficiency and fulminant shock following massive exposure to heat and inhalation of superheated steam. There were no indications a reflex death.

Burned Corpses

These are human corpses that either intravitally or postmorten were subject to the effects of heat. Of forensic-histological significance are: evidence of injury by heat prior to death, the clarification of the cause of death, taking into account previous diseases, and the detection of some largely specific findings incurred by the effects of heat.

The investigation of vital and postmortem injuries due to heat is impeded by the fact that the thermal effects frequently continue beyond the time of death and thus destroy valuable tissue findings. This particularly applies to the determination of the cause of death. However, histological examinations even in extensively carbonized remains of corpses are more useful than is generally accepted.

One group of histological examinations is concerned with traces in the respiratory system that develop by the active inhalation of hot air, steam, or particles of soot. Generally, it can be assumed that no hot air, flames, or soot particles penetrate into the deep respiratory tracts after death and lead to alterations in the mucosa, as

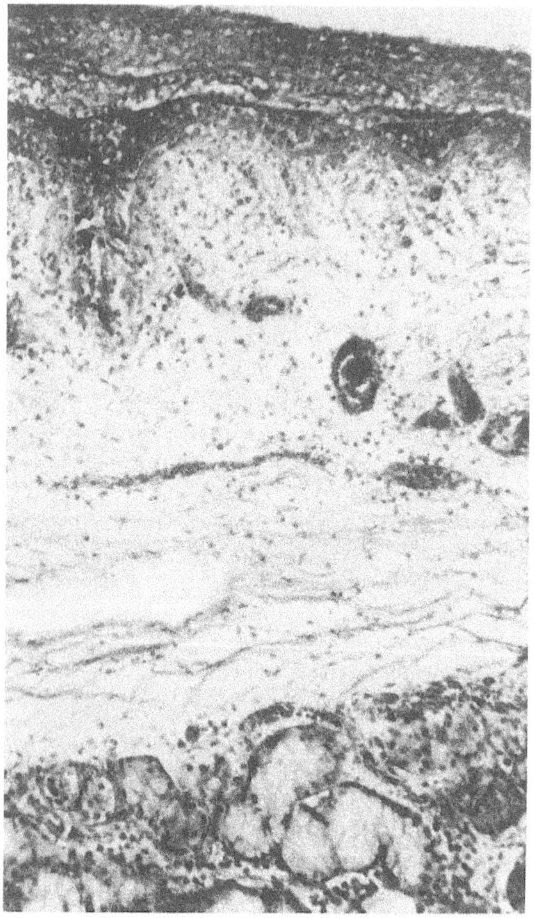

Fig. 133. Trachea with fibrinous necrosis of the upper mucosal layers, parietal edema, and inflammatory reaction. Subject survived effects of super-heated steam for 3 days PTAH, 1:120

long as these tracts are not themselves damaged by the effects of the heat. Histological sections from all levels of the tracheobronchial tree and all lobes of the lungs should be included for evidence of vital inhalation of heat. A normal general stain is sufficient. Particular consideration should be made of changes in the deep sections of the lungs, i.e., in bronchi of the second and third order and in the lung tissue itself. These changes include: swellings and superficial coagulation necroses of the multilayered cylindrical epithelium, elongation of the epithelial nuclei and a palisade arrangement (Fig. 134), evaginations of the superficial glandulae mucosa, fragmentations and clumpings of the erythrocytes in the mucosal vessels, edema of the submucosa, and general mucosal hyperemia. These findings together signify strong evidence of vital inhalation of heat.

In the parenchyma of the lungs maculate hemorrhagic edema can be found after the inhalation of hot air. Within the edema, there are mobilized and swollen pneumonocytes and macrophages with brown, granular, and plaquelike pigments, probably derived from hemoglobin. After guinea pigs were exposed to hot air, inflam-

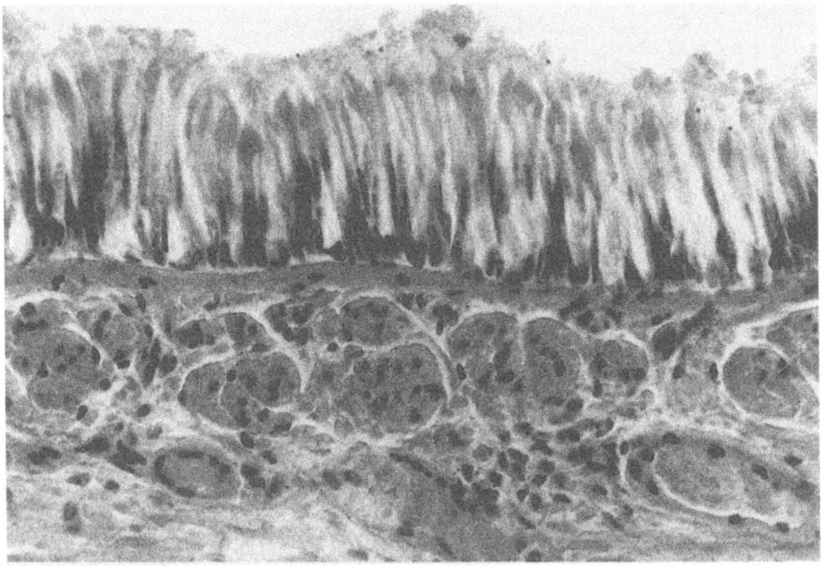

Fig. 134. Nuclear elongation and palisade arrangement of the bronchial epithelia following death through scalding and respiration of hot steam. H and E, 1:400

matory changes in the lung parenchyma and marked signs of destruction of the elastic fibers were found (Goldbach 1956). When the animals were exposed to hot air postmortem, comparable changes could only be detected in a very much reduced form in the areas of lung near the hilus. Circulation of superheated steam in the tracheobronchial system in anesthetized dogs following tracheotomy showed a frothy-hemorrhagic pulmonary edema and a gelatinous fluid impregnation of the mediastinum.

The significance of soot particles in the mucosa of the deep respiratory tracts and in the alveoli is generally known. In the case of acute death as a result of fire and the effects of smoke, these particles are not incorporated into the tissue; evidence of vital exposure and the inhalation of these products is when they are lying loosely on the mucous membrane or embedded in the mucus (Fig. 135). The same applies to the histological evidence of soot in the alveoli. Here, care should be taken that no confusion with anthracotic particles arises, perhaps through an unsuitable type of incision. A particularly critical approach is requisite in the histological localization of the products of fire within the respiratory system in the case of direct effect of fire on the organs of the thorax (Petersohn 1959).

Through the effects of fire on the lungs of neonates, evidence as to whether a child may have lived may be thwarted by destruction of the air-containing pulmonary sections (Olbrycht 1927).

It is only rarely that evidence of vital reactions can be obtained from the soft parts of burned corpses; the attempt should, however, be made. Even with severely burned corpses, there are still sections of soft parts in covered and less exposed sites that can successfully be examined using histological and histochemical methods.

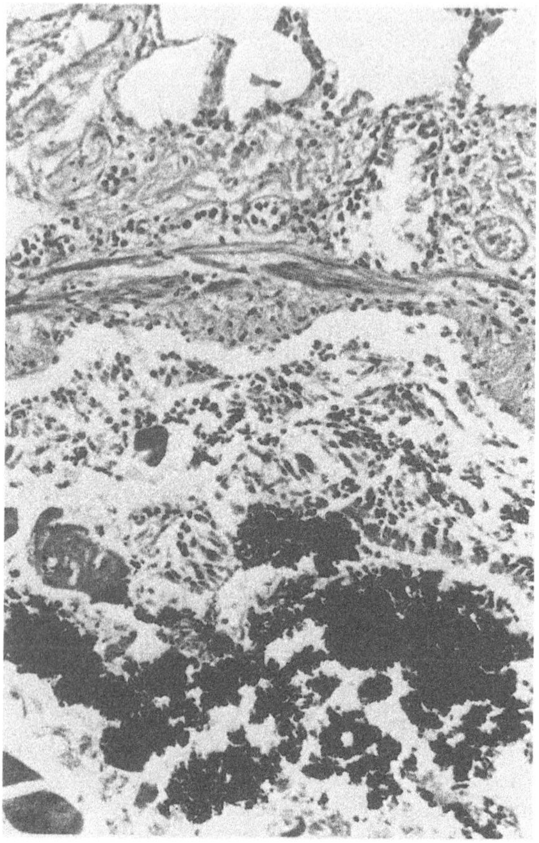

Fig. 135. Inspired rust particles in the lumen of a large bronchus in a case of death through burning. H and E, 1:180

Occasionally, a 6- to 8-mm-wide red zone is found in the marginal areas of burns of postmortem origin. Between this zone and the periphery of the burned area of skin, there is a pale dermal strip several millimeters wide. Histologically, this red band consists of distended blood-filled vessels in the upper layers of the cutis and subcutis. Such findings can also be produced experimentally in human corpses.

A fat embolism should be assessed with care as a sign of a vital reaction in burned corpses. An aggregation of neutral fats in the pulmonary vessels could also be produced experimentally postmortem through the effects of heat on whole corpses or on exposed livers (Schollmeyer 1962). When the pulmonary vessels were ligatured prior to the application of heat, the occurrence of fine droplets of neutral fats appeared only in the tissue of the burned zone. From our own investigations of burned lungs, this fat was exclusively located extravascularly in the connective tissue of the pleura and in the adjacent interlobular septa (Fig. 136). There is general agreement that a traumatic fat embolism of the lungs with the infiltration of neutral fats (in the form of large droplets or sausage- or antler-shaped, pressed into the pulmonary vessels) can be differentiated without any difficulty from a postmortem fat embolism caused by burning. A coarse-particulate fat embolism is always evidence

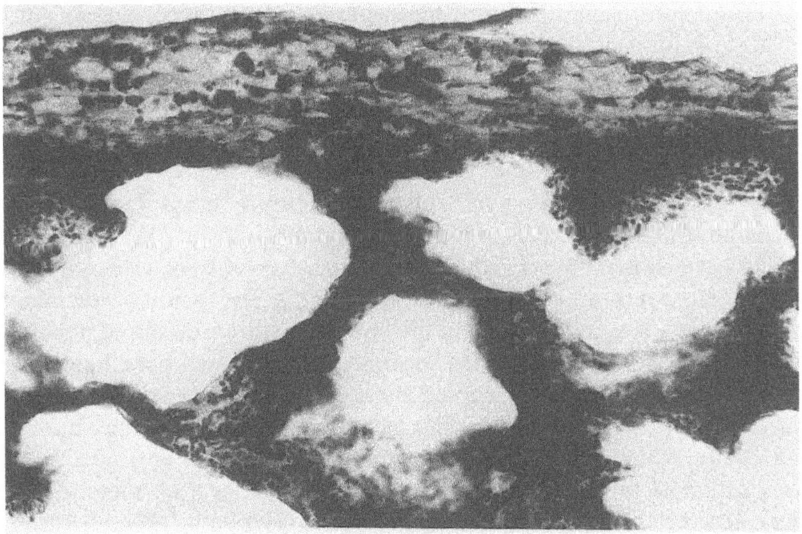

Fig. 136. Deep burn with exposure of the lung surface. Sudan-positive material located extravascularly in pleural connective tissue (dark particles). 1:220

of a vital, traumatically caused embolism even in a severely damaged burned corpse (Eidlin 1965).

In the examination of burned corpses, all natural morbid causes of sudden death have to be taken into consideration. Despite advanced destruction of a corpse by fire, the possiblity of histologically detecting morbid organ changes is quite good in our experience. No special procedures need to be considered for the examination; success is chiefly determined by the state of preservation of the organs concerned and by the heat resistance of the pathological finding. Old cardiac muscle scars, arteriosclerotic vascular changes, hemosiderin deposits, and foreign-body granulomas can sometimes still be distinguished quite well.

It is not uncommon for the brain also to be in a state permitting histological examination despite external carbonization and partial destruction in the central areas. Through fluid loss and shrinking, compaction occurs with preservation of the original structures (Dotzauer and Jacob 1952). Changes in the cerebral vascular apparatus and perivascular brain tissue should be noted. Intravascular coagulation processes with the formation of fibrin globules, perivascular areas of demyelinization bound by glial cells, and homogenization of the vascular walls have been observed (Jacob 1956).

An epidural *burn hematoma,* developed postmortem after strong local effects of heat on the skull, can on the whole be macroscopically distinguished from similar intravital hematomas. With an increased blood content and negligible fat components, there is, however, the possibility of making a false judgement; histological examination is necessary here to check the findings. Histologically, the burn hematoma appears as a structure that is predominantly composed of liquefied fat and gelatinous masses and only contains a few components of blood.

Histological examination of *burned human bones* according to our experience involves certain problems. It is difficult to prepare histological sections from the hard, thermally altered bones. Experimental studies have shown that with increasing exposure to heat, the mechanical stability of bone becomes distinctly reduced. The minimum stability is attained at about 400 °C. With a further increase in temperature up to 800 °C, there is an increase in the bone strength until it becomes twice that of the original value. The increase in strength is due to a stabilization of the bone structure (sintering). With temperatures of over 700 °C, fusion of the crystals of bone mineral occurs; the lamellar structure of bone gives way to a more homogeneous composition (Hermann 1973, 1975). The fusion of the mineral crystals necessitates a loss in volume and the characteristic shrinking of bone of 10%–25% occurs. In undecalcified grinded sections, the calcinated bone has a homogeneous surface, which is only interrupted by the Haversian canals and osteocyte clefts. Wada (1909) established a staining technique for distinguishing human from animal bones, which has frequently been unable to provide any utilizable results. The application of microradiography is better; it permits a histological assessment of the osteons to be made even in burned bones (Hermann 1973). Scanning electron-microscopic studies showed typical changes in the periosteal surface at temperatures up to 700 °C, and with even higher temperatures also on the fracture surfaces of the compact tissue (Harsányi 1977).

2. General Heat Damage – Heat Death

The identification of death through heat without definite signs of burning or scalding can be exceptionally difficult if details of the circumstances and events leading up to death are unknown. With small children in particular, forensically utilizable evidence then becomes virtually impossible.

The examination of "heat death" requires a carefully investigated histological general status. The findings registered cannot in themselves prove death by heat injury.

The classification of general heat injuries according to etiological, clinical, and pathophysiological aspects cannot be sufficiently differentiated in the histomorphologically detectable effects on the organs. A subdivision into sunstroke, heat stroke, and heat exhaustion is thus not necessary here. Moreover, a comparison of general heat injuries with the effects of thermal lesions on the inner organs ("burning sickness", general hyperpyrexia) shows that there are no qualitative differences. After burns, therefore, the same findings can be determined as after death through general heat injuries.

The following histologically detectable consequences of a heat injury of hyperpyrexia tend to appear in individual organs:

Brain. High-grade general hyperemia, sporadic fine-maculate hemorrhages in the cerebral medulla, extravasation in the pia mater and arachnoidea, marked cerebral edema, circumscribed necroses in the paraventricular cerebral sections; in the cerebral vessels the same findings as in shock.

Lungs. High-grade vascular congestion, focal hemorrhagic and proteinaceous edema, interstitial edema with widening of the alveolar septa, hemorrhages in the subpleural connective tissue and signs of shock.

Liver. Serous inflammation, opaque swelling of the liver cells, enlargement and mobilization of Kupffer's cells, signs indicative of shock.

Kidneys. Strong hyperemia, interstitial edema, opaque swelling of the epithelia in the renal tubules, signs indicative of shock.

Cardiac Muscle. Serous inflammation with widening of the interstitium, swelling and enlargement of the nuclei in the connective tissue, individual and grouped necroses of cardiac muscle cells. The cardiac muscle necroses are the consequence of oxygen deficiency (Fischer 1965).

Adrenal Glands. Interstitial edema, necroses of the epithelial cells of the cortex, reduction in the lipoids of the cortical outer zone, occurrence of phospholipids in the inner zone, signs of increased activity in the medulla (Bellieni 1959).

In cases of death through hyperthermia in early infancy, histological studies have also revealed perifollicular hemorrhages in the spleen and in individual lymph node groups of the abdominal cavity (Klein and Mueller 1964). In the main, however, only unspecific petechial hemorrhages under the pleura, pericardium, and endocardium and in the thymus are found (Goodyear 1979).

Toward a clarification of the cell damage through the effects of heat, experimental studies have also been carried out with different conditions of temperature and oxygen. They led to the hypothesis that cells under hypoxia are more heat-sensitive than under anoxic conditions (Bass et al. 1978 – comprehensive references). After 3-h continuous heat of 43 °C under hypoxia, ruptures of the plasma membrane, nuclear evaginations, and granular transformation of the membrane vesicle and cellular contents were evident. With the scanning electron microscope, rounding of the cells and a reduction in the microvilli could be observed.

In the hepatic cells of rats kept for 80 min in a water bath at 41 °C under urethan anesthesia, vesicular transformation of the endoplasmic reticulum and detachment of the ribosomes, a very low-grade swelling of the mitochondria, and an increase in the number of autophagosomes were found electron microscopically. These findings proved to be reversible.

In humans, however, fatal cases are also encountered which from a precise knowledge of the circumstances are caused by hyperthermia, but which do not present any diagnostically utilizable findings. In such cases, the cause of death cannot be clarified with certainty; only the morphological signs of cardiovascular failure, general cyanosis, vascular congestion, and sometimes agonal vomiting with terminal aspiration of the stomach contents are evident (Maulhardt 1975).

A rare, probably genetically conditioned disease is malignant hyperthermia, which mainly manifests itself in connection with narcosis and in earlier times, before the introduction of modern methods of treatment, was fatal in a relatively high percentage of cases. Histomorphological studies of this disease have been largely

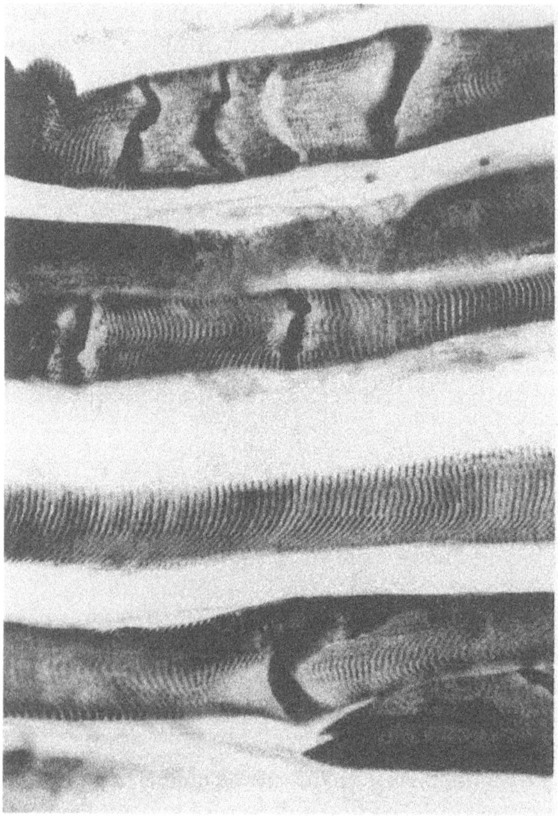

Fig. 137. Malignant hyperthermia. Skeletal musculature with hypercontraction necroses. Subject 24 years old, ♂. PTAH, 1:380

devoted to a careful examination of the skeletal musculature. Here were found various changes to the muscle fibers and sarcolemma. Hypercontraction necroses and plaquelike signs of decomposition are characteristic (Fig. 137) (Brinkmann and Püschel 1977 – extensive references).

A synopsis of all findings and indications makes it clear that the determination of death through heat without burning or scalding can only be attained by a coordinated evaluation of all available findings and a subtle examination. In the presentation of the evidence, the forensic expert opinion will seldom exceed a high degree of probability. The assessment is impeded by previous diseases, and it is not rare for these to come under consideration as the cause of natural death.

3. Death from Hypothermia

In the histological examination of frost bite, it should be taken into account that postmortem effects of cold can also lead to the formation of ice in the tissues of parenchymatous organs and in the skeletal musculature in human corpses. Such postmortem frost effects cause cavity development and considerable tissue destruction with detremental effects on the histological collation of data. Occasionally, the damage is attributable to inexpert storage of corpses or parts of corpses at too low a temperature (under 0 °C). There have been cases of medical novices zealously exaggerating the low temperature necessary for an optimal conserving effect.

Local Frostbite. This develops predominantly at circumscribed sites of the skin in contact with cold-emitting conductors and in acral regions exposed to the cold, such as the auricles, nose, point of the chin, and extremities. Locally confined frostbite, e.g., through liquid nitrogen on the skin of volunteers (Pearson 1965), gave rise to the eruption of blisters, which histologically could not be distinguished from heat blisters. For an understanding of local frostbite, experimental studies on the associated vessels and organ sections are of importance (Thorban 1963). The vascular changes in rabbits that appeared after freezing were induced by the associated nervous apparatus. The damage to peripheral nerves by cold causes a disturbance in the vascular wall innervation. An influx of liquid into the deeper layers with trophopathy of the vascular wall occurs by means of an increase in the intimal permeability. The peripheral nervous system is the most sensitive to low-temperature stimuli. Thus, the condition of the skin alone cannot be evaluated as an indicator of the actual cold injury.

The studies of Fischer and Müller (1971) and Shafer and Thomsen (1955) indicate the clinically significant delayed effects following peripheral freezing.

Histological and histochemical studies by Laiho and Hirvonen (1971) on intravital and postmortem frostbite in the skin and fatty tissue of guinea pigs revealed many individual findings that could not be reliably distinguished from heat injuries to the epidermis, cutis, subcutis, vascular system of the skin, and vascular contents. In contrast to mechanical injuries, the first histochemically detectable reactions to frostbite in the skin developed later (1 h after causation) than in fatty tissue (30 min after causation).

An unusual fatal complication of peripheral cold injury concerned a severe fat embolism of the lungs when both lower extremities were frozen (Hardmeier 1963). After excluding bone fractures and contusion of fatty tissue, the embolism must be explained as a release of fat through necrosis in the region of freezing.

General Frostbite (Fatal Hypothermia). The findings in fatal hypothermia are on the whole slight and uncharacteristic (Hirvonen 1976). Occasionally, pronounced shock findings also occur. In such cases, the inner sequelae are comparable with those after external heat injuries. It has to be accepted that from the autopsy findings alone, e.g., in infanticide through hypothermia (Hering and Dietz 1960), the cause of death cannot be definitely determined without details of the circumstances (Trube-Becker 1967).

The assessment of large serial studies of cases of hypothermic death showed the following results: cutaneous and subcutaneous edema on the face and extremities, erythema and blisters at the sites in contact with the cold source (heels), coarse-maculate hemorrhages of the mucosa of the stomach and small intestine, fat necroses in the pancreas, hemorrhagic pancreatitis, microinfarcts in almost all inner organs, induced by erythrocytic agglutination in the small blood vessels, and bronchopneumonia as a frequent terminal complication. Intrapulmonary hemorrhages were detected in the majority of cases in children (Mant 1964, 1969; H. Müller 1971). In addition, depletion of glycogen in the liver, fatty degeneration of the epithelia of the proximal renal tubules, escape of protein in Bowman's capsule, and hemorrhages under the endocardium and pleura were evident.

A relatively specific vital sign of death through hypothermia, muscular hemorrhages in the body core, especially in the musculus iliopsoas, was described by Dirnhofer and Sigrist (1979) and confirmed by Schneider and Klug (1980). Histologically, this involves diapedetic hemorrhages as a result of a disturbance in permeability of the terminal vascular system in the region of the musculature. Further, signs of a hypoxic vascular wall lesion in the form of vacuolar degeneration were found in the cells of the medial layer.

According to experimental studies on white mice, cold-induced pneumonia can be prevented by operative removal of the cervical sympathicus and by hypophysectomy. The same effect could also be attained by prior histamine application (Senger 1955). In humans and animals following general frostbite in cardiac muscle, degenerative changes in cardiac muscle fibers could be observed, with eosinophilia, edematic swelling, vacuolar formation, nuclear pyknosis, and focal necroses (Müller 1975; Shuda 1964, Sarajas 1964). In the adrenal glands, lipoid depletion of the cortex and vacuoles in the medulla occurred. In animal experiments, distribution and quantity of lipoids in the cortex were pathologically changed after hypothermia (Löfgren 1963). Colloid resorption, capillary hyperemia, and epithelial desquamation were found in the thyroid after hypothermic death as an expression of a negative feedback via the pituitary (Simon and Müller 1961). Experimental hypothermia on the uterus and ovaries of rats showed necroses and an increased occurrence of follicular cysts in the endometrial epithelium and stroma. With very low temperatures, circumscribed cold lesions in the brains of rabbits and rats led to deep necroses, and with increasing survival time to a granular tissue wall (Feldmann et al. 1976; Breining et al. 1977). From numerous animal experimental studies, it has been shown that the brown adipose tissue takes on a particular thermogenetic role in acclimatization to cold. In exposure to cold, the lipids of the brown fat cells become mobilized, whereas white fatty tissue does not react to cold stress (Hirvonen and Elfving 1973; Cameron and Smith 1964).

A summary and critical evaluation of all macroscopic and histomorphological findings in hypothermic death shows that the organ changes, which are sometimes present but not always very distinct, basically concur with the findings after states of shock, just as in death through burning and heat. According to Mueller (1975), these findings are not in themselves sufficient for forensic evidence of hypothermic death. The definite exclusion of a violent or natural death and the determination of the events leading up to death are important.

VII. Injuries Caused by Electricity

1. General

An understanding of histologically detectable injuries caused by electricity is facilitated by a knowledge of the electrophysical conditions, which are well summarized by Sellier (1975).

Research into tissue damage caused by electricity was for a long time dominated by the notion of a specific electrogenesis. Jellinek (1932, 1955, 1961, 1964) in particular took the view that electric current in tissues leads to specific changes. He criticized the belief that the microscopically detectable changes following the effects of electricity should only be considered the result of Joule heat, as then all electric lesions would have to be interpreted simply as burns caused by electricity (Jellinek 1964). A specific effective principle involving transport of metal ions into the deeper tissue layers under the contact site has similarly been supposed to account for the development of metallization following contact with metallic conductors (Schrader 1920).

In the recent literature, many authors have concerned themselves with the question of specific tissue lesions through the effects of electric current. The studies have concentrated on forensically utilizable histomorphological evidence of the electric origin of tissue damage. The cardinal problem involves a reliable differential diagnostic distinction between electric lesions and burns caused by heat.

2. Electric Lesions – Burns Caused by Heat

The development of an electric lesion is dependent on many electrophysical factors, in particular the current density under the point of contact and the part of the body affected. The diverse histomorphological nature of the epidermis and cutis, with differences in the thickness of the horny layer and fibrous ramification of the corium in the soles of the feet and palms of the hand compared with other areas of the body, affects the macroscopic and microscopic evidence. Qualitative and quantitative differences are seen particularly in the region of the wall-like margin of an electric lesion; these differences do not form or form only slightly in areas of skin with a thin stratum corneum.

Depending on the current strength and duration of the effect, lesions in the skin and subcutis display principally the same histomorphogenesis as a local heat injury. With short-term effects of electricity involving negligible heat development, only swelling and homogenization occur, with increased stain-binding in the upper

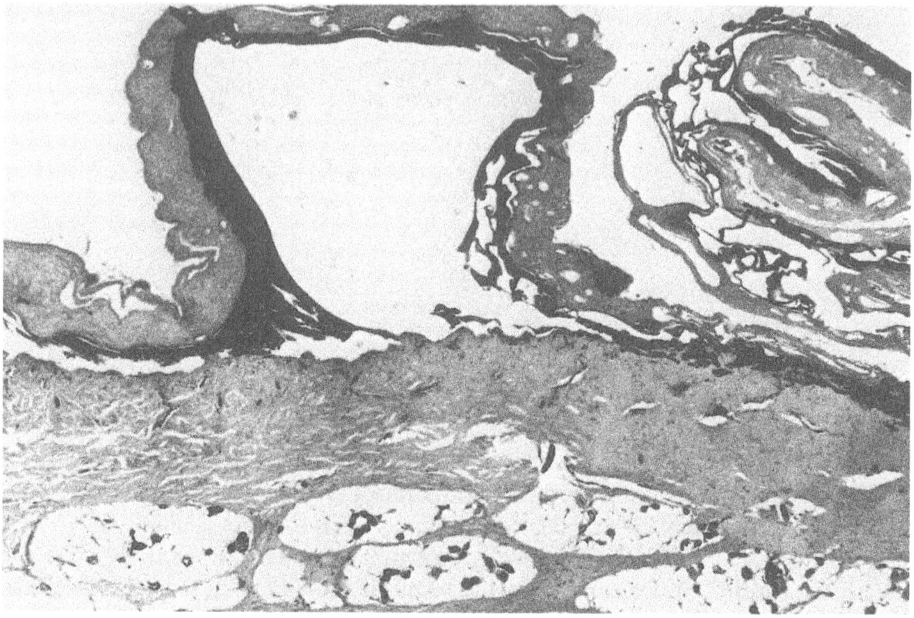

Fig. 138. Electric lesion with vesicular and festoon-like detachment of the epidermis. H and E, 1:80

horny layers. In the middle epidermal layers, the cytoplasm of the cells is homogenized, the nuclei appear vesicular and swollen, and the keratin is clumped and discolored yellow. Electron microscopically, the nuclei appear particularly changed; they are deformed, contain clumped chromatin, homogeneous areas, and fine-granular regions (Thomsen et al. 1981a, b). In the central areas of the affected epidermis, there are also slight depressions, attenuation, and channel-like discontinuities with black-charred margins. These findings correspond to the electric lesions visible on the skin with the naked eye or with a magnifying glass (Böhm 1967; Sellier 1975). Burn blisters can also develop, containing proteinaceous fluid and leukocytes, without lesions forming on the epidermis in the case of survival after injuries incurred by electricity (Fig. 138).

With strong thermal effects through electricity, the epidermis is extensively destroyed in the center of the site affected by the current and detached from the papillary body (Fig. 139). In the peripheral areas, the epidermis is thickened, festoon-like, homogenized, and interspersed with vesicular cavities. These findings are particularly prominent when the contact sites are on the palms of the hands and soles of the feet. In the wall-like marginal regions, the lower epidermal layers of the center appear compacted toward the exterior, thickened, and with elongation of the basal epithelial cones. In this marginal zone, the basal epithelial layers frequently contain the familiar longitudinal nuclear elongation. The elongated nuclei are pyknotic, mostly tightly packed, and have fasicular radiations in the direction of the underlying papillary body (Fig. 140a). The same nuclear changes are also found in the integumentary appendages, especially in the hair follicles (Fig. 140b). The arrangement

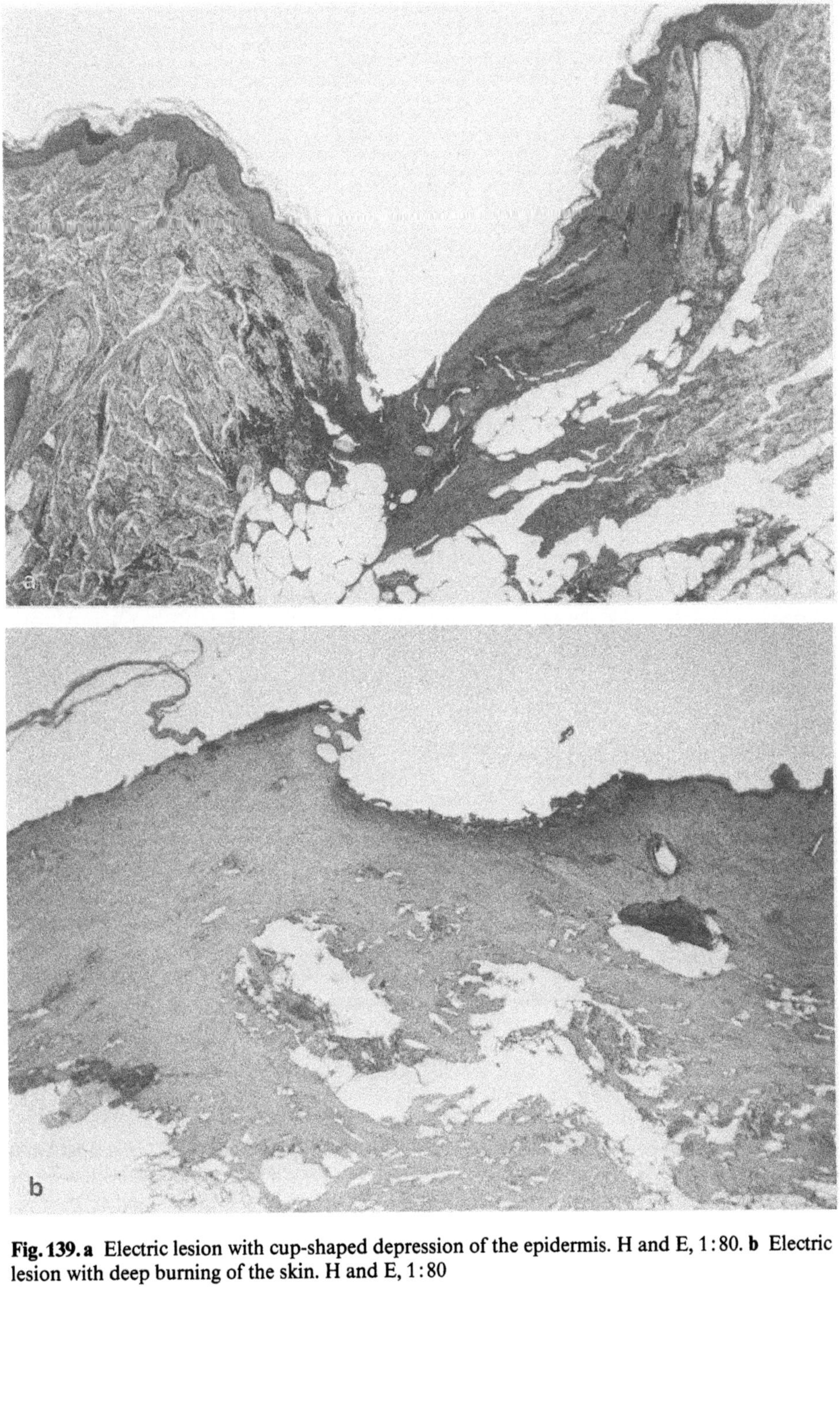

Fig. 139. a Electric lesion with cup-shaped depression of the epidermis. H and E, 1:80. **b** Electric lesion with deep burning of the skin. H and E, 1:80

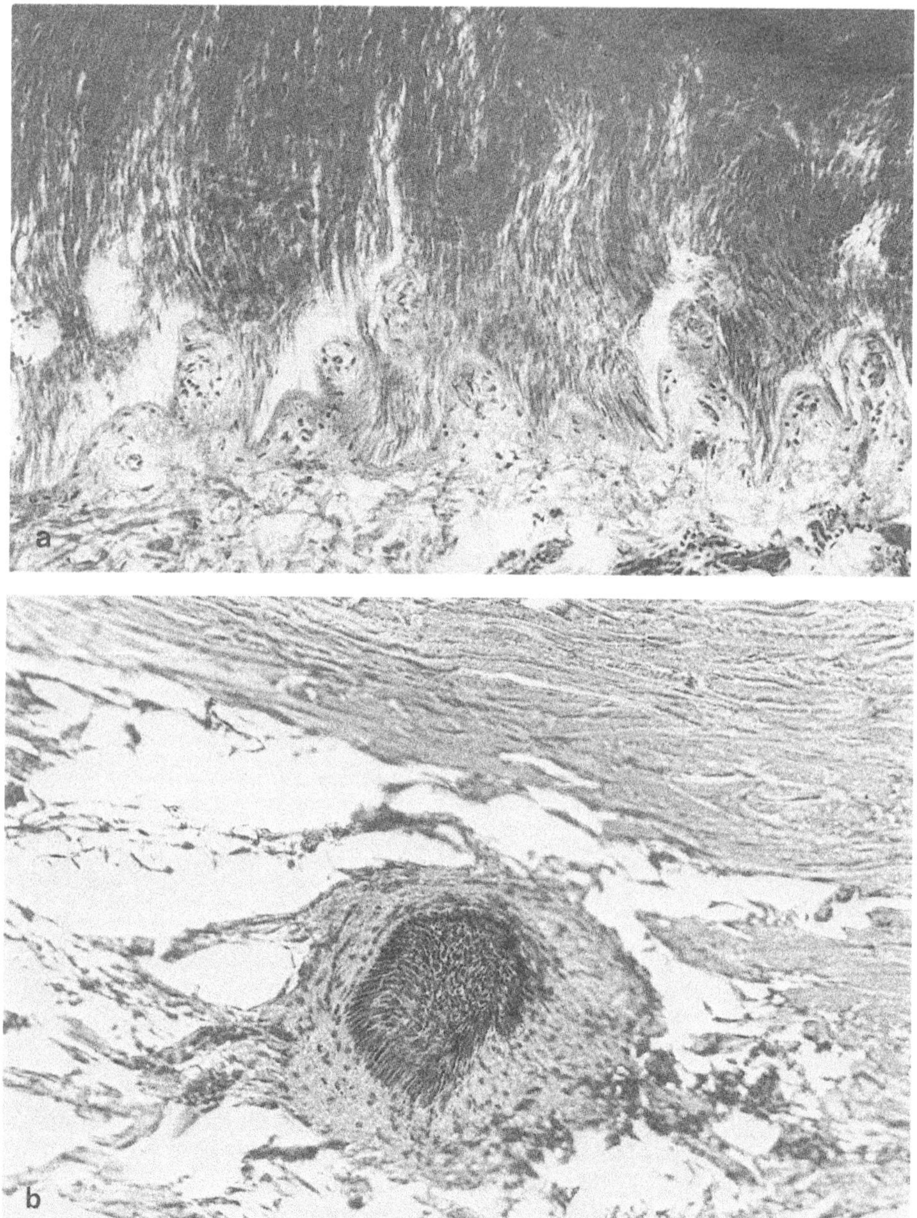

Fig. 140. a Periphery of an electric lesion with elongation of the cell nuclei (palisade arrangement) in the stratum basale. H and E, 1:200. **b** Elongation of the epithelial nuclei of a hair root under an electric lesion. H and E, 1:180

of the elongated nuclei can present many variations – whorls, spirals, loops, palisades, and streaked elongations.

The patterns of the nuclei in the peripheral areas of electric lesions have been investigated by many authors for a specific electrogenesis (Schäffner 1965; Marziano and Lo Menzo 1965; Somogyi et al. 1965, 1966 a, b; Canale et al. 1966; Rozsa et al. 1971). Jellinek (1964) and his school took the view that the nuclear elongations of the epidermal cells are attributable to an electric polarization effect. This concept was also confirmed by Heinlein (1962) in a model experiment. Conversely, numerous experiments in recent times have conclusively demonstrated that unspecific changes are responsible. Similar nuclear elongations are also found in the marginal regions of burns caused by heat, blunt dermal injuries, cauterization, desiccation, and blisters following barbiturate poisoning and freezing. The only differences are quantitative and these do not have forensic evidence value. Nuclear changes can thus no longer be adduced as evidence of an electric injury.

The lesions affecting deeper regions following severe electric injury are comparable with those after local third-degree burns (cf. p. 240). Electric injuries also give rise to pronounced necroses, coagulations of the corium, and superficial carbonization, or swellings of the collagenous fibers and changes in the blood in adjacent vessels. Histochemically, reduced activity in various enzymes could be detected in the epidermis and cutis. Particularly affected are NAD-diaphorase and acid and alkaline phosphatase (Pioch 1966; Lo Menzo 1965). Just as with deep heat injuries, in lesions incurred by electricity the connective tissue structures are only slightly impaired and are difficult to differentiate from undamaged tissue.

Somogyi et al. (1965) by means of fluorescence microscopy divided electric burns into three grades of severity: 1) Circumscribed minimal epithelial damage and swelling of the connective tissue fibers; 2) destruction of the epidermis, swelling, homogenization, and reduced stain-binding ability of the connective tissue – though increased stainability with basic stains; 3) coagulation and homogenization of all kinds of tissue with strong cavity formation and loss of nuclear staining.

Particular consideration should be given to the non-uniform distribution of swellings, necroses, and hemorrhages in the corium under the area of electric contact. These changes are more evident near the integumentary appendages. This variable intensity of tissue damage permits the inference that the electric current follows the path of least resistance in the subepidermal vascular connective tissue, leaving behind traces of its passage. These are relatively discrete indicators of a lesion caused by electricity and in forensic practice can only be distinguished from marks caused by heat when they are particularly distinct.

In this connection, care should always be taken in the histological examination that the extent of the electric tissue damage under the contact surface is completely embraced in its depth and lateral extent by serial sections perpendicular to the skin surface.

In the differential diagnosis of lesions caused by electricity and heat, the form of the damaged zone in the deeper parts of the affected tissue should be given particular attention (Schrader 1920; Kawamura 1921; G. Schmidt 1964; Böhm 1968). Electric injuries produced experimentally in corpses and isolated pieces of skin, stained with Congo red and alcian blue on formalin-fixed material, led to different kinds of lesions with cuneate and rounded shapes. The necrosis produced by an electric cur-

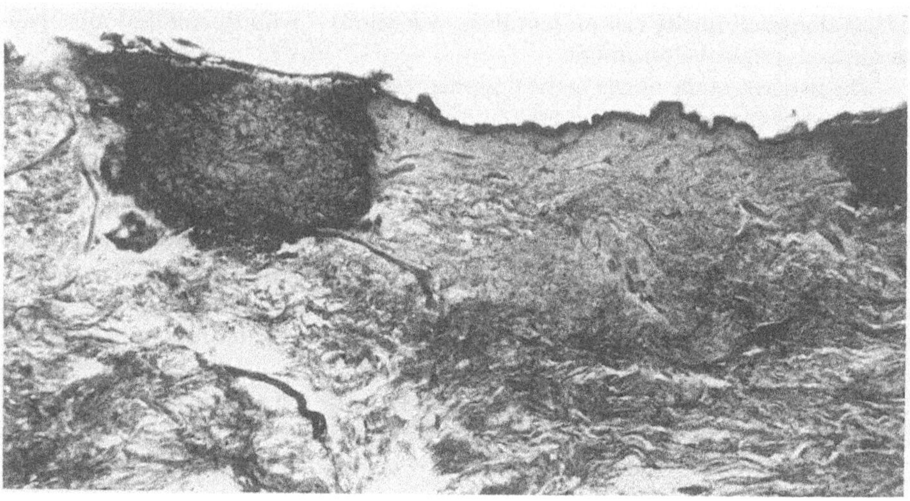

Fig. 141. Spherical and cuneate necroses experimentally produced by electric current. Congo red-alcian blue, 1:80

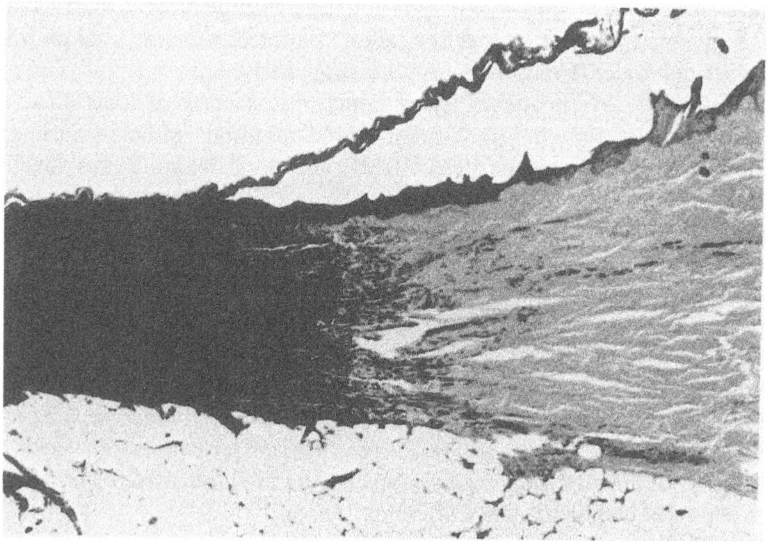

Fig. 142. Necrosis of the corium produced by electric current with diffuse lateral demarcation. Goldner's, 1:100

rent was stained by Congo red but not by alcian blue (Fig. 141). The limits of the necroses against the undamaged tissue were indistinct (Fig. 142). In serial sections, ramifications of the necroses were found toward the sides and base, with lattice-like formations (Böhm 1968). In contrast, thermal necroses are sharply delimited; when produced experimentally by contact heat they are plate-like or patelliform.

With electric lesions caused by broad electrodes, numerous parietal micronecroses developed, which were interpreted as burns caused by an electric arc. In histological section they have a spherical form (Böhm 1968).

Histochemical investigations of NAD-diaphorase, which is especially sensitive to the effects of heat, led to evidence of necrotic foci in the form of an inverted cone (Pioch 1966). Thus, the form of a burn does not allow a certain differential diagnosis to be made between thermally or electrically caused injuries.

The *metallization* of an electric lesion deserves particular consideration as a differential diagnostic criterion in a micromorphological investigation. Similar findings can develop in thermal skin burns by contact with metals. Metallic deposits were found beneath electric burns by Schrader (1920) in the dermal connective tissue in the area around hair roots and in the musculature. He judged these traces to be metal transport as a specific effect of the electric current. Koeppen (1928, 1935, 1955) detected more superficial deposits and regarded them as evidence of a lesion caused by electricity.

Visualization of the metallization is possible in many different ways. The acroreaction test (Adjutantis 1962) is carried out by dropping dilute nitric acid onto the lesion, thus bringing the metal into solution. The solution is absorbed by a strip of filter paper impregnated with benzoin-oxine. In this way, a distinct staining reaction takes place. The sensitivity of the acroreaction can be increased by dithiooxamide for evidence of copper and by potassium ferricyanide for evidence of iron (Schäffner 1965). The metal reagents can also be sprayed onto the sites to be investigated (Böhm 1967). Dithiooxamide has only proven useful in the histochemical detection of copper in cryostat sections (Pearse 1961; Schäffner 1965). It should be borne in mind that copper can also make its way into the connective tissue from the skin surface by diffusion (Böhm 1966).

In the histochemical test for iron with the Berlin blue reaction, it should also be taken into consideration that in the formalin fixation of the tissue samples the blue stain can diffuse into the musculature. It is, therefore, recommended that the fixation be done in alcohol or by using cryostat sections (Schäffner 1965). Comparative studies of burns caused by electricity and heat showed that in the case of electric lesions the spreading of the iron metallization was deeper. The findings are not constant, however, so it is not feasible to rely on this criterion (Schäffner 1965). It has not been possible for electric burns produced postmortem to be distinguished from those incurred intravitally (Lo Menzo 1975).

Recently, the possibilities for visualizing metallic traces have been extended by means of spray-on reagents and electrographic methods (Pierucci and Danesino 1980; Marcinkowski and Pankowski 1980).

The sulfide method of silver staining according to Timm (1958, 1968) is very well suited to detecting unspecific metals in histological sections and visualizing the form of deposition (Voigt 1959; Pioch 1967, 1968; Schwerd and Lautenbach 1960). Precipitation of the metal as a sulfide is achieved by means of fixation of the tissue samples in hydrogen sulfide-alcohol. By subsequent treatment of the sections with a photographic developer containing silver nitrate, this is deposited on the metal sulfide particles in the tissue. Using this method, even the smallest metallic traces in the tissue can be precisely visualized. In this manner, the metallic traces are evident in the peripheral areas of electric burns in the spaces of the integumentary appendages. Bandlike and striate metallization in the upper epidermal layers are also characteristic of electric burns; they can be distinguished from the more compact metallization on the surface of a burn produced by heat.

Quantitative determinations of copper in burns caused by heat and electricity gave roughly equal values (Sellier 1966). The surface impression of the metallization should be noted. The electric lesion is characterized by a non-uniform distribution of the metallic traces. Small fused cavities develop at the point of current passage within a lesion, in the vicinity of which the metal is more intensely deposited. The fused cavities are due to sparking. This finding on the surface resembles a target (Böhm 1967, 1968).

Thermal contact defects of the skin produced by metallic strips led to metallization with a negative impression of the surface of the metal strip but no punctiform metal deposition (cf. Bosch 1965). Nowadays, it can be assumed that metallization in the form of a target is characteristic of being caused by an electric current (Sellier 1975).

The electrophysical and micromorphological processes in the development of electric metallization were studied experimentally by Böhm and Milz (1975). The results can also be applied in the reconstructive assessment of death caused by the effects of electricity.

By means of scanning electron microscopy (SEM) and electron microprobes, various metallic properties can be determined in electric metallization. In this way, different metal electrode qualities could be assigned to the points of current passage (Böhm 1970). However, through uneven surface structure of the test samples with non-uniform absorption of the X-radiation, different concentrations can be simulated (Schneider and Hantsche 1973).

The present means of examination, particularly SEM combined with element analysis and transmission electron microscopy, permit a very extensive distinction to be made between burns produced by electricity and those caused by heat. The structural analysis of metallization especially allows a reliable etiological classification to be made in the majority of cases (Figs. 143, 144) (Böhm 1976).

Vital reactions with inflammatory reactions in the immediate environment following electric tissue lesions are slow to appear compared with other forms of injury (Jellinek 1932). Later, electric lesions undergo particularly good healing without local bacterial infection.

The electronecroses can be visualized with NAD-diaphorase. After the effects of an electric current that are survived for a short time or applied postmortem, the necroses are sharply demarcated against the undamaged tissue. In the case of electronecroses that are survived for longer periods of time, the demarcation is indistinct (Pioch 1966). With increasing survival times, histochemically detectable enzyme losses are evident in the cells outside the necrosis. After prolonged current flow of more than 10 s, there is, just as in normal thermal contact burns, a positive esterase reaction outside the negative vital reaction zone; this surrounds the necrosis in a wall-like manner.

In the first few hours after the effects of electricity, the lesion enlarges as a result of peripherally advancing necrobiosis. After a lapse of about 10 h, the initially unaffected marginal cell groups are no longer in evidence due to nuclear elongations and a faveolate structure caused by the heat (Pioch 1967). In animal experiments,

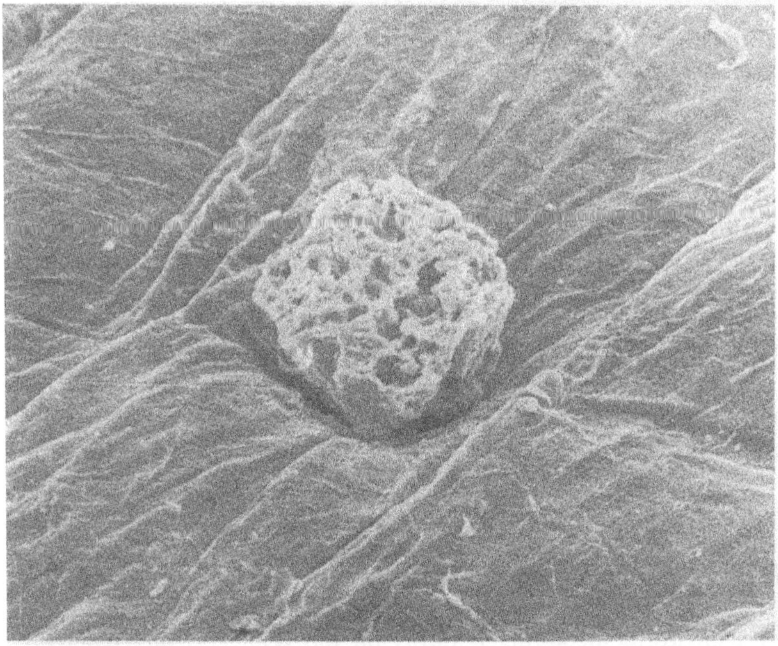

Fig. 143. Electric lesion with circumscribed papular metallization on the surface (Böhm 1976). Scanning electron microscope, × 500

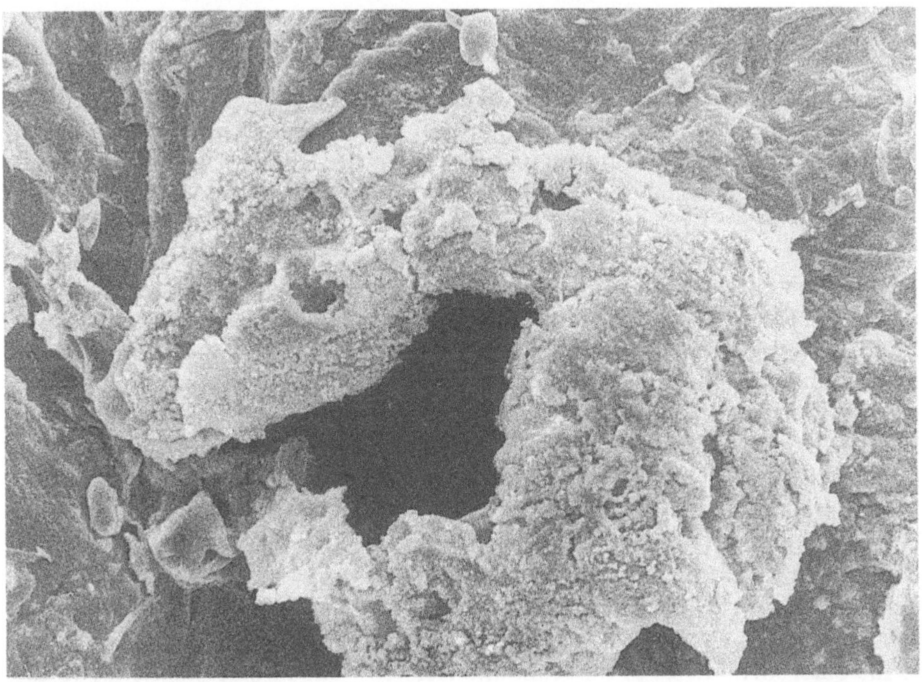

Fig. 144. Electric lesion with metallization papule and central perforation (Böhm 1976). Scanning electron microscope, × 500

Stichnoth (1961) observed parietal leukocytes in the vessels after a survival time of 2 h, and after 4 h the first leukocytic emigrations. An inflammatory demarcation wall can be detected after 8–14 h (Schrader 1920; Pioch 1967). An early vital reaction following the effects of electricity was observed by Böhm (1975) in the aortic intima. In SEM studies, he found thrombotic changes in the vascular endothelia of rabbits after a current flow lasting up to 1 min. These changes could be micromorphologically distinguished from traumatically incurred vascular lesions and thromboses.

A critical evaluation of the methods of investigation thus far applied indicates that in the case of dubious electric burns a combined procedure is recommended – histological evidence, evidence of metals, histochemical test for earlier vital reactions, SEM examination combined with ultimate analysis.

From a forensic point of view, there are only a few findings that can contribute toward establishing whether a skin lesion was caused by electricity:

a) A histologically-histochemically easily visualized irregular quality of the connective tissue necrosis, with an indistinct boundary and branch-like radiations into the surrounding unaffected tissue. A sharply demarcated necrosis does not, however, preclude electric injury.
b) Metallization in the integumentary appendages, when sharply bordered and not blurred.
c) Punctiform metal-tinged burns on the skin, i.e., target-shaped according to Böhm (1967, 1968).

3. Inner Organs

The histological findings in the inner organs of humans killed by the effects of electricity have, on the whole, no diagnostic significance without comprehensive knowledge of the circumstances and the presence of electric lesions. The following histological findings in the inner organs have frequently been observed in cases of acute death incurred by electricity. In the cardiac musculature, particularly following prolonged resuscitative measures, there are either no pathological changes at all or there is severe damage to the muscle fibers with plaquelike destruction, striate infarctions, hemorrhages, fine-droplet fatty infiltrations, and edema (Baur and Bissig 1962). It is debatable what the significance may be of fragmentation of cardiac muscle fibers after death from electric shock, since this finding probably develops postmortem and has also been found in fatal cases caused by many other agents. A conspicuous zigzag fragmentation has occasionally been observed following death from electricity (Tabbara 1962). We found a distinct wavelike arrangement of the cardiac muscle fibers (Fig. 145) in the case of death caused by lightning with marked lightning figures on the skin. Animal experimental studies concerning the question of the cause of death in lightning accidents revealed small necroses in the myocardium in cases where the accident had been survived for longer periods of time (Karobath et al. 1977). Electron microscopically, Bujdosó et al. (1969) found detachment of the outer membranes of mitochondria isolated from cardiac muscle tissue and sporadic total destruction of the mitochondrial structures in rabbits following shocks from alternating current.

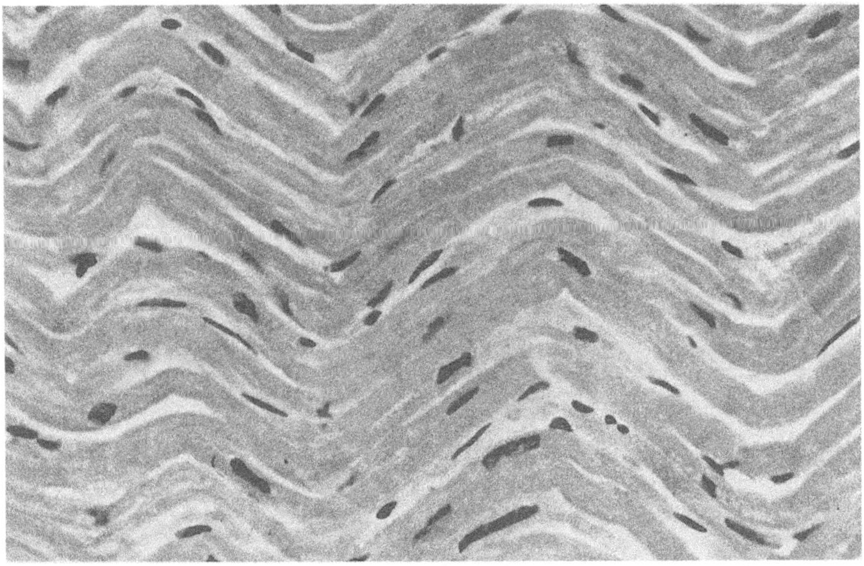

Fig. 145. Death through lightning stroke. Wave-like arrangement of myocardial cells. H and E, 1:400

Granulations have been detected in the bed of the electrodes of cardiac pacemakers that had extended to a depth of 4 mm into the myocardium. These local myocardial changes were thought to be due to the electric impulse of the pacemaker (Noeske and Knothe 1965).

Contractions of the muscle fibers and compaction of the Z bands have been found in the skeletal musculature of electric shock victims. The characteristic signs of a vital electropathological injury are hypercontraction bands in strange barklike patterns (Fig. 146) and intravascular thrombocytic aggregations. These findings have a close topographic connection with the path of the current (Püschel and Brinkmann 1979). Otherwise, findings include swellings of the mitochondria, loss of the filamentary structure of actin and myosin, hemorrhages, laceration of the muscle fibers, and normal thermal changes (Fig. 147) (Schmidt 1910; Viterbo and Pasetti 1965; Mazzucchelli and Andreuzzi 1966; Nevelös et al. 1967).

The elastic fibers in the region of electric burns showed a change in birefringence under the polarizing microscope and a reduction in their resistance to digestion by elastase (Somogyi et al. 1966 a, b).

Direct lesions by electric shock have occasionally been observed in the brain; these are seen as electrothermal coagulation necroses, which in isolated cases have been survived for up to several weeks (Descamps and Castan 1963). After a fatal stroke of lightning which was survived for 24 h, the findings comprised epidural hematoma, extensive subarachnoid hemorrhages, and multiple diapedetic hemorrhages, which were dispersed over the whole brain with no special histological features (Spaar 1955). The cerebral changes otherwise evident in connection with death from electric shock are explained as being unspecific general effects as a result of a large increase in blood pressure (Sellier 1975). Histologically, microhemorrhages

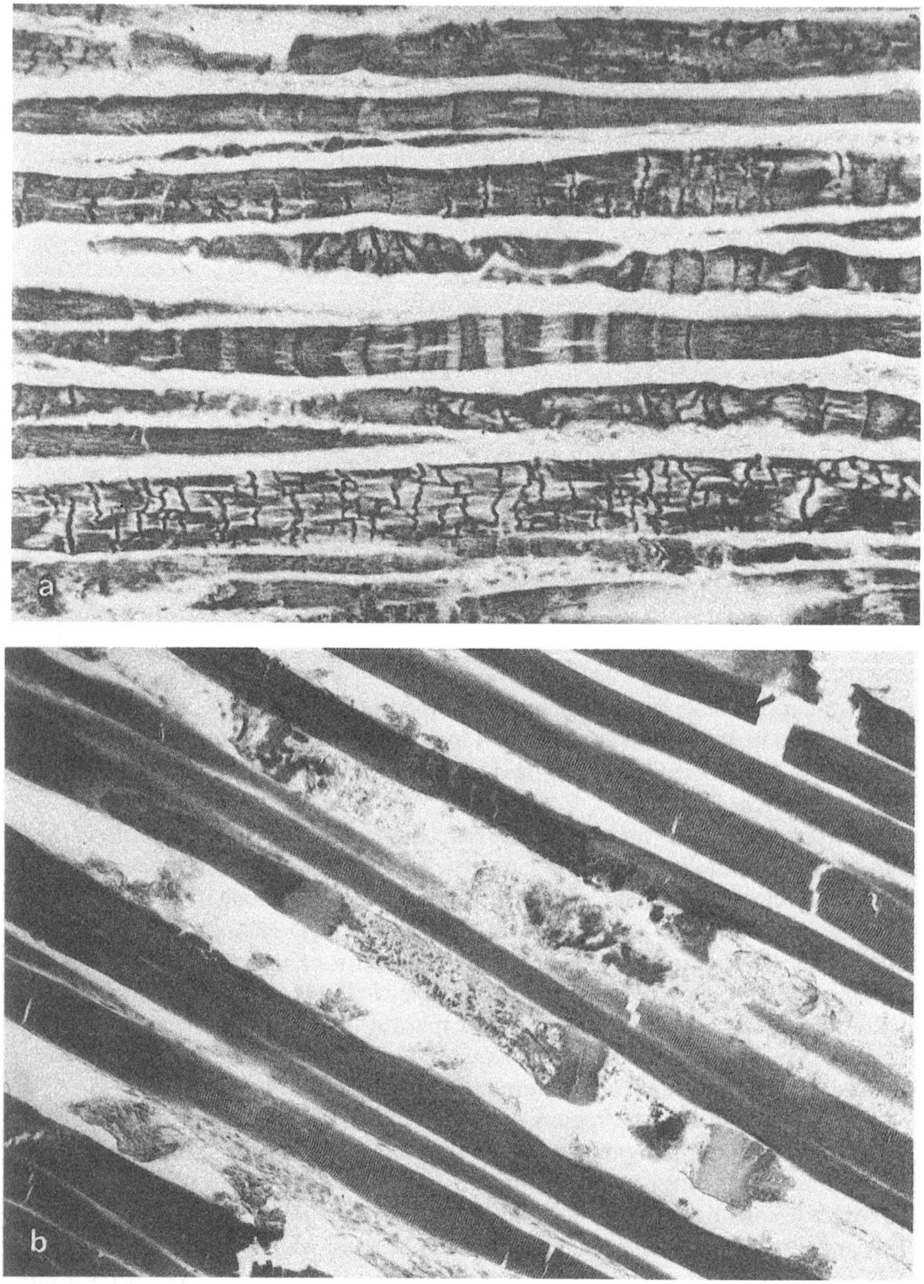

Fig. 146. a, b Rat skeletal muscle following effects of alternating current (220 V, 150 mA, 2 × 15 s) with hypercontraction bands, necroses, and empty sarcolemmic tubes. PTAH, 1:250

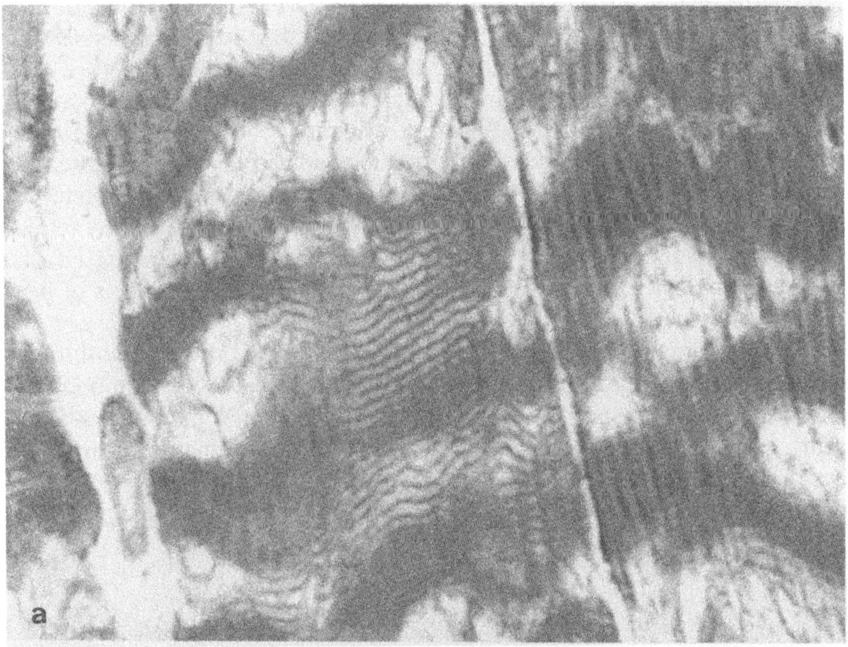

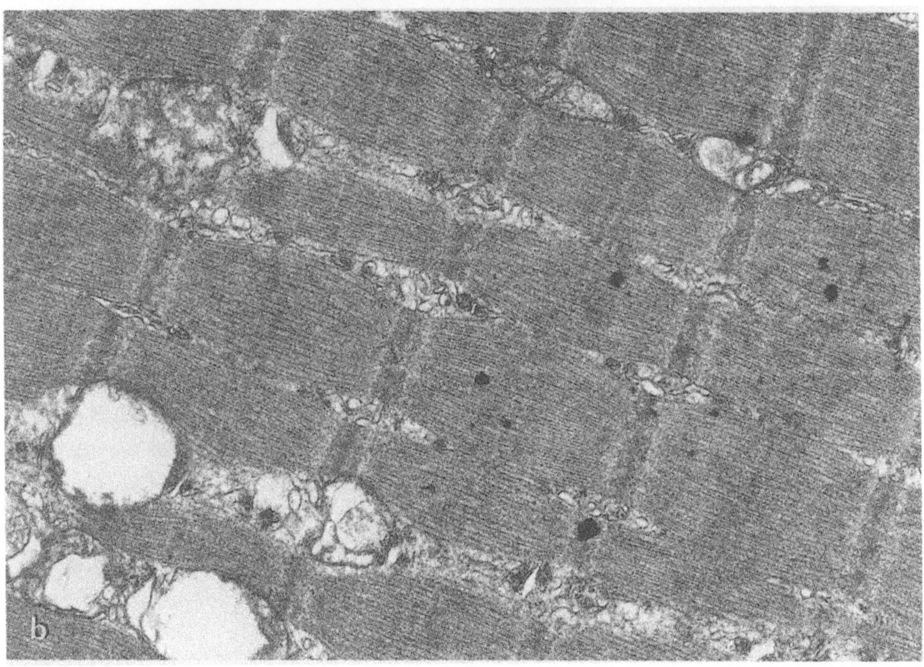

Fig. 147. a, b Rat muscle following effects of alternating current (270 V, 400 mA, 30 s) with contraction and detachment of the I bands, intratubular protein precipitation, hydropic dilation of the tubules, and partial translucence of the tubular sarcoplasma. Retention of the transverse striation. 1:800 semithin-section, EM × 23800

were found in the region of the third and fourth cerebral ventricles; after temporarily successful resuscitation there were circumscribed "anoxic-vascular" necroses in the cerebral medulla of both hemispheres of the brain (Gaszner 1969).

Histologically detectable changes in the nuclei of the medial layer can occur in the vascular walls of the current path. These are evident as corkscrew-like deformations, splitting, and fibrous degradation; the nuclei sometimes disaggregate into several, equal-sized fibrous fragments that are adjacent to each other and connected at one end. Cellular vacuoles and swellings of the endothelia were also found. These findings were interpreted by Jellinek (1961) as electric polarizing effects. However, it appears that all these findings can be explained by the effects of heat and circulatory disorders.

Unspecific liquefaction and tissue discontinuities may occur in bone through the effects of electric current (Kolár and Vrabec 1976; Harsányi 1979). In bony tissue, electrothermal effects and laser beams cause destruction of the bone collagen and melting of the inorganic material. By means of SEM examination, a bricklike pattern can be identified on the surface of the liquefied inorganic bony substance. This finding may be judged as indicative of the effects of electricity (Harsányi 1979).

VIII. Injuries Caused by Radiation and Ultrasound

1. General

Radiation injuries in humans can be caused by light rays, high-energy radiation, radar, ultrasound, and laser beams (Klein 1975). They also comprise the effects on the human organism of the detonation of nuclear weapons (König 1967). Numerous studies and observations over the last 7 decades have created the basis for a specific "radiopathology", which developed into a special branch of science bordering on medicine, physics, biology, and chemistry and is nowadays termed "radiobiology" and "biophysics of ionized rays." In the field of medicine, radiation injuries predominantly concern the effects of high-energy ionizing rays and the action of radioactive substances. Radiation injuries occur not only in therapeutic operations but also in diagnosis, accidents, and illegal procedures.

The action of ionizing rays on a biological system is the result of a series of reactions at the beginning of which are the physicochemical primary processes (Gössner 1972). The action of radiation on a cell leads to the absorption of energy in the plasma and nucleus. The transfer of energy involves changes to the molecules either directly or indirectly via radiochemical intermediates. In this manner, chemically corrosive free radicals and peroxides develop, which transfer their destructive influence to biologically important macromolecules. At the end of such a chain of reactions are the detectable biological effects and morphologically evident lesions. A schematic synopsis by Meissner (1974) clarifies this reaction principle (Table 8).

Toward an understanding of the histologically detectable radiation injuries, it should be pointed out that the biological action of all ionizing rays is principally due to the same primary processes. However, it must be taken into account with the various types of radiation that the same doses can have different biological effects. Here, reference is made to the relative biological effectiveness (RBE). In the slightly ionizing forms of radiation, e.g., electron rays, the individual packets of energy appear at relatively large intervals and are statistically dispersed in a cell. Conversely, the ionizations of other rays, e.g., proton and alpha rays, are very close to one another (Gössner 1972). The energy absorbed per micrometer wavelength of an ionizing particle is characteristic for the various forms of radiation (LET = linear energy transfer). The effect of radiation with a high LET, e.g., alpha or neutron rays, is basically greater than that of radiation with a lower LET, as for instance X- or gamma rays.

For the relationship between radiation dose and biological radiation effects, the "median lethal dose" (LD 50) is defined as that which leads to death in 50% of a group of irradiated animals after 30 days. The effect of radiation is dependent on

Table 8. Series of reactions in the effect of ionizing radiation on cell tissue. (After Meissner 1974)

Radiation exposure
↓
Energy absorption in the cells (nucleus and plasma)
↓
Effect on organic molecules

Direct | Indirect via radical formation from H_2O and O_2
↓
Structural changes to vital molecules in the cell
↓
Abnormal biochemical reactions
Damage to cell functions
↓
Morphological lesions
↓
Death of cell
↓
Damage to the tissue function through cumulative effect or intoxication

the temporal and spatial distribution of the dose. Repair and compensatory processes also play a part. When radioactive substances are incorporated, the situation is basically more complex than when radiation is external, since the spatial and temporal evidence of the dose distribution is determined by the chemical and physical nature of the substances and their dissemination in the organism.

The different sensitivity of the various cells, tissues, and organs is also a substantial contributory determinant in the occurrence of radiation injuries. The radioactive sensitivity of cells is directly proportional to their ability to divide and indirectly proportional to their degree of differentiation (Bergonie and Tribondeau 1906). The most sensitive to radiation are vegetative intermitotic cells, e.g., the stem cells of hematopoiesis, spermatogenic cells, cells of the intestinal crypts and stratum basale of the epidermis (Gössner 1972). The injuries that develop are, however, not only an expression of the radiosensitivity of the tissues concerned but also the result of the radioactive lesion and subsequent reactive and reparative processes.

Pathological findings following the action of ionizing rays include numerous localized and general changes: electron-microscopically detectable changes in the cells, histologically evident tissue and organ lesions, severe lesions in the irradiated zone with fatal complications, and severe injuries to the whole organism in the various acute radiation syndromes, e.g., bone-marrow syndrome, intestinal syndrome, central nervous syndrome, and radiation-incurred tumescence. This roughly demarcated radiopathological framework comprises all elements of general pathology. The results of radiopathological studies in humans and animals have, for example, been comprehensively presented by the following authors: Zollinger 1960; Scherer and Stender 1963; Cottier 1966; Berdjis 1971.

From the forensic point of view, examining victims for the effects of radiation or ultrasound must to a particular degree be oriented to the securing of all morphological means of evidence. This entails an examination of the local lesions and a complete histological general status including various sites in the bone marrow.

In the case of radiation injuries following therapeutic or diagnostic measures, histopathological examination of the ailment that occasioned those measures is of particular importance. With fatal hemorrhages or paralysis following tumor irradiation, it should as far as possible be clarified by extensive histological investigation whether the injury was caused by the primary disease, the radioactive therapy, or a combination of both. The forensic assessment is particularly difficult when inevitable, sometimes even intentional, therapeutic sequelae and side effects have to be distinguished from avoidable ones. Here it is necessary for there to be close cooperation with clinical radiotherapeutic experts, who should also take into account the results of a complete histological examination.

2. Early and Delayed Cell and Organ Damage

The forensic histopathology of specific cell and organ lesions through radiation and ultrasound will be confined to relevant findings and references under various headings. The type of radiation will largely not be taken into account. In the following section, cell and organ changes will be given primary consideration.

Cell. The first reactions of the cell to ionizing rays are manifest electron microscopically as detachment of the outer lamellae of the nuclear membrane and localized vacuolar expansion of the intermembranous space. Light microscopically, these changes are evident as juxtanuclear vacuoles. The nuclear plasma is initially changed very little; the chromosomal substance thickens and becomes positioned at the inner nuclear membrane. Chromatin depletion occurs. The further phases of cell damage are nuclear swelling, giant-cell formation, pyknosis, crenulation of the nuclear membrane, karyolysis, and karyorrhexis. The nucleoli enlarge as a result of the effects of radiation within the tissue; the ribonucleic acid synthesis is initially undisturbed. Specific microirradiation led to fragmentation, disturbance of mitosis, and inhibition of RNA and protein synthesis (Bergeder et al. 1963).

Vessels. The first morphologically detectable reaction to radiation is dilation of the capillaries (Zollinger 1960). A few hours after irradiation, swelling of the nuclei and cytoplasm in the endothelial cells occurs. Perinuclear vacuoles develop and indentation of the nuclei and detachment of whole sections of endothelium are observed, such that the basal membrane borders directly onto the bloodstream. As a counterregulatory reaction, circumscribed endothelial proliferation with bizarre pyknotic nuclei, reminiscent of those in tumors, develop in the capillaries, arterioles, and venules. It is supposed that the endothelial damage is not caused by the action of radiation alone but also by a disorder in the circulation as a result of shrinking of the perivascular tissue. In the larger vessels, there is fibrinoid precipitation between the intima and media and the formation of foam cells, which can also be observed in the vessels of the uterine musculature in the vicinity of irradiated carcinomas. According to Thurner (1970), this is a typical actinic disorder. With stronger effects of radiation on the abdominal wall, obliterative vasculitis develops in the superficial tissue layers of arteries and veins. In the deeper tissue layers, on the other hand, only the veins are affected, which are probably more sensitive to radiation than the arteries (Windholz 1933).

In the capillaries, early thickening of the basal membrane occurs; it is destroyed if connective tissue proliferations occlude the vascular lumen. In larger vessels, the media is occluded in the initial stages of radiation damage; later it appears hyalinized. The smooth muscle fibers contain accumulations of pyknotic nuclei. The elastic medial fibers are relatively resistant.

In medium-sized arteries, "productive actinic entarteritis" can develop, which has a progressive character for years after the termination of irradiation (Thurner 1970). Circumscribed marginal necroses can develop in the aorta after intense irradiation (Thomas and Forbus 1959). Following implantation of radiogold into the pituitary, localized parietal lesions were observed in the arteria carotis interna (Kricke 1961). Radiation lesions of the arterial walls can also lead to severe and fatal hemorrhages. Following irradiation of the cervical lymph nodes, which was performed because of lymphogranulomatosis with deep-seated defects in the soft parts of the irradiated area, we observed a fatal hemorrhage in a 25-year-old woman as a result of erosion of the arteria thyreocervicalis. Histologically, the lymphogranulomatosis in the cervical area was no longer evident. In the pathological assessment, we affirmed a causal connection between irradiation and death of the young woman.

Skin. Following UV irradiation with a sixfold threshold erythema dose, vacuoles developed in the keratinocytes, fibrocytes, and endothelial cells of the capillaries. After 24 h, the findings were at their most pronounced. These changes led to intercellular edema via an increase in permeability (Itscher et al. 1979). X-ray dermatitis is one of the early acute radiation injuries to skin; in its severest form it is accompanied by bullous-gangrenous dermititis. In this condition, hydropic swellings of the epithelia, pigment displacement, hyper- and parakeratosis, and atrophy are found histologically in the epidermis and stratum papillare. The delayed lesions lead to neoplasm of the tightly packed silver-stainable fibrils in the corium. The areas affected are, after a long period of time, poorly vascularized and tend to form radiation ulcers. These ulcers are difficult to heal and histologically present an ulcerous base layer, relatively poor in cells and vessels. After prolonged irradiation with very low radiation doses, there is high-grade epidermal atrophy with disturbed keratinization. The development of carcinomas or sarcomas in skin damaged by radiation is well known.

Skeleton. Osteoradionecrosis develops by damage to the osteocytes and blood vascular system in the haversian canals. Formation of atypical bony tissue also occurs with disordered primitive trabeculae, which are to some extent fibrously transformed. Histologically, the bone concerned contains empty marrow cavities as a result of necrosis of the osteocytes. Depending on the radiation dosage, necrosis of the bone with spontaneous fractures can still occur after a period of years (Thurner 1970 – references).

Bone Marrow. Here the distinction has to be made between topical radiation lesions after localized irradiation and general radiation injuries following whole-body irradiation. However, pathological changes can also develop in nonirradiated bone marrow after localized irradiation, just as in whole-body exposure. Independent of the kind of irradiation, the bone marrow shows hyperemia with extensive sinus hemorrhages and serous inflammation at the beginning of the injury. There then follow mitotic disorders, signs of necrosis in erythropoietic and later in granulocytopoietic cells, mucoid swellings of the ground substance, and regressive nuclear polymorphism, which subsequently also affects thrombocytopoiesis.

In advanced stages of local radiation damage, bones and sections of marrow situated in the path of rays, e.g., ribs and intravertebral bodies, contain an empty gelatinous, fibrous marrow, which is edematous and later transformed to a pure fat or fibrous marrow.

After intensive whole-body irradiation, panmyelopathy practically always develops, sometimes not until after a latency of several years. It is a moot point whether this severe bone-marrow damage is caused by a direct radiation effect alone or is also affected by decomposition brought about by substances from other irradiated tissues. The extent of the bone marrow lesion is thought to be approximately proportional to the radiation dose absorbed (Rajewsky 1956; Zollinger 1960; Bergeder 1962; Fliedner et al. 1964).

Cardiac and Skeletal Musculature. The human heart can be directly injured by therapeutic doses of ionizing rays. This is usually seen as exudative pericarditis, which can appear about 1 year after the beginning of treatment (Fajardo 1977). Additionally in a few cases, diffuse myocardial fibrosis develops, which is caused by a microcirculatory disorder owing to damage to the capillary endothelial cells. The connection between irradiation and coronary arteriosclerosis is difficult to assess. In animal experiments, the development of arteriosclerosis only occurred under radiation stress when the animals received a cholesterol-rich diet. Histomorphologically, it is difficult to distinguish true coronary arteriosclerosis from vascular disease induced by radiation (Fajardo 1977). Studies investigating “actinic myocardiopathy” in animals revealed opaque swelling of the cardiac muscle cells, loss of transverse striation, fine-grained to coarse-fragmentary ceraceous degeneration, nuclear depletion, and atrophy of the muscle fibers leading to the development of empty sarcolemmic tubes (Werthemann 1930).

The delayed reactions of the myocardium occurring a long time after irradiation are probably due to primary vascular lesions according to the animal experimental studies of Morgenroth et al. (1967).

Following higher radiation doses, ceraceous degeneration, fragmentary disintegration, nucleosis, myogenic giant cells, and extensive atrophy in the skeletal musculature occur (Windholz 1933).

Joints. The epiphyseal growth zones, which show high radiosensitivity, in the vicinity of joints are particularly endangered in juveniles (Günsel 1953). Impediment of endochondral ossification occurs through damage to the cells in the cartilage development zone (Melanotte and Follis 1961). The result is a disorder in the ossification process. Exostosis and sarcomata also develop in these regions (Becker 1937).

Central Nervous System and Peripheral Nerves. Radiation lesions of the brain (encephalopathia actinica) and spinal cord are expressed first of all in the vessels. Hypopermeability occurs, allowing the passage of highmolecularweight protein complexes, which coagulate in the vascular wall. This leads to impaired oxygen diffusion and "asphyxiation" of the cerebral matter (Thurner 1970). This is referred to as "plasma infiltration necrosis." The further consequences are decomposition of the medullary sheaths and axis cylinders, necroses with fat-granule cells, demyelination, and coarse fibrous gliosis or cystic transformations of the damaged cerebral areas. "Amyloid" substances, which accumulate outside the vessels in a crescent-shaped fashion, also develop in the primary vascular lesion (Zeman 1955; Zülch 1960). With van Gieson's stain, the injured vessels of the brain and spinal cord display a yellow-brown shade in their swollen walls. The surrounding fibrinous plasmatic necroses are similarly stained.

Delayed radiation necrosis of the brain is a notable development and behaves like an autonomous process, extending over a long period of time. It can also appear after normal therapeutic doses. Histologically, it is a radionecrosis that tends to affect the white matter; it emanates from a focus, advances peripherally, and becomes cicatrized in central regions (Fig. 148) (Zülch 1960). Delayed radiation necrosis is probably an autoimmune process, induced by myelin from the damaged medullary sheaths, leading to the development of antigenic properties and antibody formation.

Actinic damage to the spinal cord tends to affect the white matter; the ganglion cells, on the other hand, are only slightly impaired. Otherwise, the same changes oc-

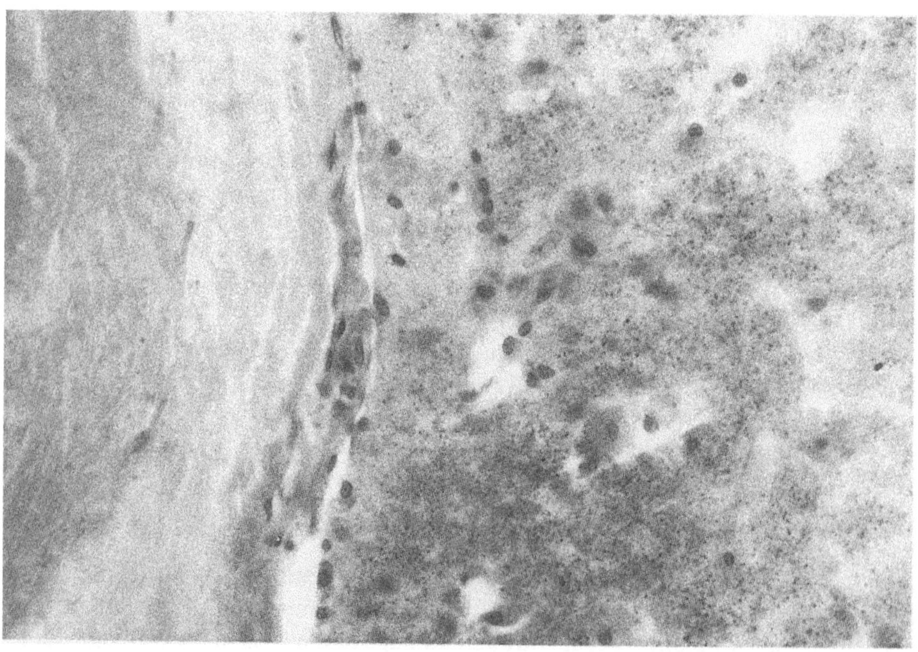

Fig. 148. Radiation necrosis of the brain. Marginal area with macrophages and fine-granule calcification. H and E, 1:250

cur as in the brain. High radiation doses bring about direct necrosis. Low radiation doses lead after about 3 months to the previously described vascular changes with hypopermeability, influx of plasma into the surrounding tissue, and development of edematous necrosis of the spinal cord (Franke 1963; Girgensohn and Witzel 1965). Opinions concerning the pathogenesis of radiation myelopathy are divided: There is a vascular or mesenchymal theory, a parenchymal theory, a combination of the two, and the autoimmune hypothesis (Fröscher 1976).

"Radiogenic peripheral neuropathy" is probably due, according to histological findings, to actinically induced connective tissue proliferation with cicatrization and embedding of the nervous filaments, which atrophy and perish. Direct destruction of the medullary sheaths or axis cylinders through the effects of radiation in therapeutic measures is still disputed.

Liver. Therapeutic irradiation of the human liver causes pronounced hyperemia with temporary stasis in the small hepatic veins and isolated necroses of the central acinar epithelia (Reed and Cox 1966). Subsequently, partial fibroses and regeneration nodules develop, sporadically also biliary proliferation and hepatogenous giant cells (Frýdl 1962). Occasionally, slow progressive connective tissue obliteration of small hepatic veins also occurs. Here, all stages from the formation of very fine fuchsinophilic collagen fibers in the vascular lumen to complete vascular occlusion through acellular collagenous tissue may be observed. This vascular process is interpreted as a variation of an obliterative venous disorder of the liver (veno-occlusive disease) and is compared with Budd-Chiari syndrome. After injection of radioactive substances, liver fibrosis and fatty atrophy are seen. Similar changes, which developed under the symptoms of hepatitis, have been observed following injuries caused by atomic explosions, e.g., among the Bikini fishermen.

Oehlert and Wenig (1975) made the important experimentally confirmed finding that no possibility whatsoever exists of recognizing whether latent radiation injury is present from the hepatic tissue of an individual. Almost every effect of ionizing rays on the liver can lead to conditioning, with the altered course of many disorders. Increased regenerative power of the liver can cause such latent radiation lesions to become manifest.

In animal experiments, reduction in the cytoplasmic granules occurred 3 days after irradiation. After 1 week, indistinct protoplasmic structures and nuclear damage developed, and after 3 weeks vacuoles appeared in the liver epithelia. These changes receded after about 6 weeks (Mignard et al. 1965). Following whole-body irradiation on rats, an increase in cytochrome oxidase activity was observed (Krompecher 1971).

Kidney. "Radiation kidney" involves glomerulotubular nephrosis (Zollinger 1966); the term "radionephritis" is insuitable for this disease since basically it does not have an inflammatory character. The sparse inflammatory interstitial cell infiltrates that occur in all cases are to be judged as concomitant nephritis.

Opinions differ with regard to the site of attack of the primary radiation lesion in the kidneys. It is only certain that ionizing rays tend to cause damage to the glomeruli, tubular system, and vascular connective tissue. In rats, hyaline drops and granular transformations of the mitochondria were seen in the proximal tubules 8 h after irradiation. A few days later, thickening of the basal membrane in the glomeruli occurs; this change spreads to the intertubular membranes. After about 2 weeks, nuclear pyknoses develop in the distal limb of Henle's loops. Subsequently, focal epithelial necroses and the formation of giant cells are observed. After 3 weeks, interstitial fibroses and round-cell infiltrates develop in the peritubular stroma. The glomerular loops are then highly swollen. Intraglomerular capillary lesions also lead to the formation of regular aneurysms (Bianchi 1961 a, b). A few months later, the organs are shrivelled and the glomeruli show collapsed loops, thickened basal membranes, nuclear changes, and complete obliteration. In humans, a radiation kidney almost always leads to hypertension and the corresponding changes to the arterioles; they can be differentiated from purely actinic vascular lesions, which are characterized by anuclear connective tissue proliferations in the vascular lumina (Thurner 1970).

The renal tissue of juveniles is more sensitive to radiation damage. The latent period prior to the appearance of morphological changes is shorter than in adults. The latent period is often very variable; it has led to the distinction between acute and chronic radiation kidneys (Campanacci et al. 1968).

Radiation injuries to the efferent urinary tracts do not induce any characteristic histological findings (Zollinger 1966 – references).

Lung. The reactions of human pulmonary tissue to ionizing rays are dose-dependent and proceed in phases. They do not begin immediately after irradiation but after a latent period of variable duration. In animal experiments, immediate reactions have also been observed which were histologically detectable after a few hours: Hyperemia, serous inflammation, mucosal secretion, escape of leukocytes, degeneration of the mucosal epithelia and lymphatic follicles (Villiers and Gross 1967; Jennings and Arden 1962). A differentiation can basically be made between an early stage I with predominantly exudative changes and a later stage II with fibrosis and shrinking. If the radiation dose is not too high, the exudative changes can be reversible. They begin as proteinaceous acellular edema in the perivascular and peribronchial connective tissue sheaths, spread onto the intra-alveolar septa, and appear lastly in the alveoli as a ligamentous parietal lining, which bears a certain similarity to hyaline membranes. This radiation effect is probably due to an early lesion of the vascular walls and a dysoric effect (Zollinger 1960). These findings have to be distinguished from secondary pneumonic or bronchopneumonic processes, which are more similar to virus pneumonitis and are thus designated "radiopneumonitis" by Eger and Gregl (1965). With higher radiation doses, the exudative pulmonary changes are not so pronounced. The lung tissue loses the ability to develop an inflammatory reaction as a result of the stronger irradiation, and it becomes directly atrophic.

The phaselike process of the pulmonary tissue reaction to a single radiation injury progresses without any sharp divisions. The first acute stage, which can also be accompanied by intense serous-cellular inflammations and the occurrence of alveolar macrophages and epithelial giant cells, subsides in the course of 2–6 months and passes into increasing connective tissue proliferation (Engelstad 1934). These proliferative processes also include proliferations of the bronchial epithelium and pleural mesothelium and terminate in cicatrized induration of the lung tissue. Degenerative cellular and nuclear polymorphs and hyaline alveolar membranes can still be detected for a long time in the proliferations. The fibrous sections contain coarse, fragmented and undulate fibers, which can stain in a similar manner to elastic fibers. However, this is probably due to collagenous material.

In the case of general amyloidosis, after irradiation an increased accumulation of amyloid was observed with fibrosis of the pulmonary tissue in the affected areas of the lungs (Spath 1963). A reduction in ATPase and alkaline phosphatase and an increase in acid phosphatase, attributable to a rise in the number of phagocytes, were enzyme-histochemically detected in the lungs in animal-experiments after whole-body irradiation (Kosmider and Jonek 1963).

Radioembryopathy. In the first half of pregnancy, the periods of preimplantation, organogenesis, and fetal development are particularly susceptible to radiation damage (Fritz-Niggli 1960). In the preimplantation period, even a slight radiation dose can have a lethal effect. Mortality is lower during the formation of the germ layers; there are however numerous malformations. In the second half of pregnancy, on the other hand, radiolesions are less common. The damage involved here is inhibition of growth, microcephaly, hydrocephalus, encephalocoele, etc. (Thalhammer 1967, refs.). Following attempts at abortion using irradiation, cases of nanism and microcephaly have been observed (Zollinger 1960).

Thorotrast Lesions. Thorotrast is a colloidal solution of thorium dioxide which has not been used in radiodiagnostics for some time because of its hazardous nature. However, owing to the latent period, which can sometimes be a matter of decades, tissue Thorotrast lesions must even nowadays be expected (Thurner 1970; Abbatt 1979). After intravascular application, an accumulation of Thorotrast in the liver, spleen, and bone marrow occurs within 1 h. Histologically, the thorium dioxide it contains may be easily detected. With H and E stain, it has a granular brownish, sometimes also a slightly lustrous quality. Best's glycogen stain and dark-field examination are also suitable (Staemmler 1955). The accumulation of thorium dioxide occurs chiefly in the reticuloendothelia and histiocytes. The cytoplasm of the cells affected contains so many irregularly formed granules that the nucleus is concealed.

Even if in the injection only negligible quantities of Thorotrast enter the tissue perivascularly, the development of granulomas occurs; they are termed "Thorotrastomas." Their histomorphology is marked by a foreign-body stimulus and a radiation effect, largely alpha radiation from thorium X. The radiation induces damage to reticulohistiocytary cells, producing nuclear pyknosis and cytolysis. Thorotrast thus becomes liberated again and is either taken up by other macrophages or transported into regional lymph nodes via the lymph tract. Dystrophic tissue changes with necroses, collagenization, and hyalinization then occur at these sites.

The liver is a main area of deposition, where Thorotrast forms fixed depots, particularly in the periportal areas in the vicinity of the biliary ducts (Gehrmann et al. 1963; Hennekeuser et al. 1970). The right lobe of the liver is thought to be more frequently affected than the left (Hieronymi 1957). The sequelae of hepatic Thorotrastosis are broadened and fibrotic portal areas. After several years, a particular form of cirrhosis of the liver develops with fibrous choking of the hepatic lobules and nodular hepatic cell regeneration products. Pseudotuberculous granulomas have also been observed (Rotter 1951). The reticulocytic proliferations and regeneration in a Thorotrast-damaged liver are probably also the starting point of tumors, particularly hemangioendothelial sarcomas.

In the spleen, Thorotrast is deposited on the margins of trabeculae and follicles and in the perivascular connective tissue. Removal from the liver and spleen via the lymph tract becomes increasingly blocked by fibrous obstructions of the lymph vessels such that the main mass of Thorotrast persists in these organs.

In the bone marrow, Thorotrast is especially deposited in the reticular cells and endothelia of the venous sinus. There it leads to diffuse and focal neoplasms of connective tissue and keloidal cornification.

A synopsis of Thorotrast lesions comprises the following findings, which can occur individually or together:

a) Granulamatous pseudotumors, "Thorotrastomas", in the region of perivascular injections
b) Lesions of the hematopoietic system and the development of fatal panmyelopathy or leukemia
c) Progressive dystrophy in the liver, spleen, and kidneys
d) Development of malign mesenchymal and epithelial tumors at various sites of the body after latent periods of years or decades (comprehensive references in Thurner 1970)
e) Radiopneumonitis after hot lymphography and transport of Thorotrast via the ductus thoracicus into the lung (Oehlert 1970).

3. Injuries Caused by Ultrasound

Tissue lesions as a result of the effects of ultrasound are known predominantly through animal experiments. A survey by Cowden and Abell (1963) shows that exposure to ultrasonic waves gives rise to three different changes, thermal, mechanical, and chemical, although allocating the observed findings into these groups can prove difficult. The effect of ultrasound is largely mechanical. The sound waves probably attack the vasomotor system and lead to effects via the circulation. Depending on the strength of the ultrasonic source, hyperemia, anemia, or necrosis develop. In animal experiments, ruptures and lacerations of tissue structures have been established as specific for the mechanical effect of sound waves (Brettschneider 1952). In the area affected, the plasma of the cells had burst into individual particles. Considerable differences in resistance were also conspicuous among the individual tissues.

A summary of ultrasound lesions in individual organs and tissues cited in the literature is as follows.

In the *skin,* edema and inflammation developed depending on the intensity of the sonic effect; in the *skeletal musculature,* destruction of muscle fibers, lacerations of the sarcolemma, and nuclear degeneration; in the *testes,* giant-cell reactions and necroses. In the *intestine,* ulcers, inflammations, and hemorrhages developed. In the *skeletal system* there were circumscribed bony necroses. In the *kidneys,* hyaline-droplet degenerations of the tubular epithelia were observed. In the *lungs,* anemic cuneate areas with hemorrhagic marginal zones were present. In the *cardiac muscu-*

lature, hemorrhages, circumscribed necroses, and myocardial fibrosis developed. In the *liver,* focused ultrasound waves gave rise to circumscribed necroses when locally applied. Ultrasonic treatment of a removed liver led to lacunal formation, which was probably due to an accumulation of gas bubbles. In the *brain and spinal cord,* after a short latent period, "sonic foci" developed with diapedetic hemorrhages, necroses, ganglion cell shrinking, and vacuolar cell degeneration (Höpker and Heyck 1951; Peters 1955). In the *adrenal glands,* after direct exposure to ultrasonic waves or after the effects of ultrasound on the brain, there were high-grade hyperemia, diapedetic hemorrhages, cortical infarctions, and reduction in the fuchsinophilic granules in the epithelial cytoplasm of the zona glomerulosa. The adrenal changes following cerebral exposure to ultrasonic waves are explained by a disorder in the adrenocorticopituitary system (Jankowiak et al. 1963).

IX. Histological Findings in Starvation

1. General Remarks on Cause and Definition

The morphologically detectable sequelae of lack of food (inanition) can develop in various ways: Morbid impairment of digestion with a sufficient supply of food (maldigestion), inadequate resorption of a properly degraded and sufficient food supply (malabsorption), or external food shortage, the consequences of which are termed exogenous inanition. The latter form, in which deficiency of food leads to inanition, is of prime forensic interest. A basic understanding of the causes of pathological inanition is an important prerequisite for the identification and forensic assessment of metatrophia of exogenous origin. A comprehensive summary of the pathogenesis and pathomorphology of the most important diseases that can lead to inanition in adults and children is provided in the studies by Becker (1970) and Harms (1973). It should be stressed that the causes of a number of these morbid disorders cannot be detected by morphological methods. These diseases bring about general inanition, the cause of which cannot be clarified without knowledge of the course of the disease and complex clinical examinations.

The numerous possibilities in natural morbid inanition require, particularly when there is the suspicion of death through external food deficiency, comprehensive anamnestic inquiries; in a fatal case, a very thorough histological status examination, including the endocrine system, is necessary. If need be, an appropriately experienced pathologist should be consulted (Mueller 1975).

Clinical and morphological investigation findings of exogenously caused inanition, including metatrophia with fatal consequences, have already been widely reported (Mueller 1975). Detailed metabolic and circulatory studies and biochemical investigations concerning reduced food intake under clinical conditions stem from Voigt et al. (1967), Baumann et al. (1966), Voigt and Apostolakis (1969), Houtrouw (1973), and Lüdtke (1973).

Evidence of the guilt of another person in cases of fatal starvation in infants is particularly difficult. Problems arise, for instance, in precisely differentiating deliberate malnutrition from enteropathic reactions or injuries through nonculpable errors in diet. These problems cannot be solved without consulting an experienced pediatrician. A further difficulty in the assessment is brought about by the fact that the death of infants is not directly induced by starvation but by general weakness with the development of respiratory tract infections, bronchopneumonia, aspirations, and infections of the gastrointestinal tract.

2. Organ and Tissue Findings

From the outset, it should be stressed that the histomorphologically detectable effects of metatrophia in the inner organs do not usually permit a differentiation to be made as to whether the condition was due to disease or exogenous denutrition. The findings can only be utilized in connection with other results of the investigation, including the judicial enquiries.

The findings produced hitherto are based largely on animal experiments and isolated observations in humans.

In *fatty tissue,* which is macroscopically particularly conspicuous under the epicardium and marrow of long bones through gelatinoid atrophy, shrinking of the individual fat cells can be microscopically observed. The size of the fat cells is proportional to the nutritional state. In the case of sufficiently fed people, the cell diameter is on average 70–120 µm (Reh 1953). In emaciated people, the fat cells have a diameter of less than 70 µm. In obese people and in lipomas, the fat cells have an average diameter of over 120 µm.

Electron microscopically, the fat cells in a state of hunger show an indented cell surface, numerous pinocytic vesicles, cytoplasmic vesicles, membrane-bound dense vesicular bodies, and areas with flocculent material. The mitochondria and the nuclear structure remain comparatively unaltered (Napolitano and Gagne 1963). It is assumed that the intracellular structural changes are connected with adaptation and alteration of the cell metabolism. In neonates and infants, brown adipose tissue is affected by a high-grade cyanochrome-granular transformation in states of hunger. Similar findings have been observed in the adipose tissue of adults in cases of pheochromocytomas (Feyrter 1973). These changes are probably based on a disorder in the thermoregulation of brown adipose tissue. Interestingly, the lipoma fat cells are spared from all damage caused by metatrophia.

The histological changes in the *liver* in exogenous food deficiency have thus far been investigated the most extensively. In the initial period of hunger, the fat content increases in the liver epithelia. The centrolobular sections are predominantly affected. After about 2 days, the fat content then dramatically decreases to such an extent that histologically intracellular fat becomes barely detectable (Schlicht 1955). Fat assimilation occurs, just as in oxygen deficiency, by pinocytic incorporation of fat particles via Disse's spaces into the ergastoplasm and Golgi area of the epithelial cells. Primary fatty infiltration of the liver following denutrition involves "transportational" fat assimilation, in which the fat is derived from mobilized depots (Bade and Schuhmacher 1964). Centrolobular epithelial necroses were observed in absolute denutrition in animal experiments. The liver loses a considerable proportion of its weight. In the course of hunger, a larger number of liver epithelial cells die, about 40 per 1000 cells; however, the normal cell death rate, about 25 per 1000 cells, should also be taken into account (Zaletaeva 1963).

In the case of long-term protein deficiency, depletion of the endoplasmic reticulum, reduction in the swollen mitochondria, vacuolar lipid accumulation, and an increase in glycogen occurred in the liver epithelia (Svoboda et al. 1966). Pigment increases in the hepatic epithelia have also been detected. The pigment granules can be visualized with the silver reduction method according to Masson; they are found in various quantities and distribution patterns. Electron microscopically, the pigment granules are seen to be surrounded by a simple membrane (Lamotte et al. 1965); ferritin granules are sometimes located in the immediate vicinity. The pigment granules also contain vacuolar translucent areas with bile pigment inclusions. The chemical nature of these "hunger pigments" is largely unclarified.

Histochemically, a distinct increase in succinodehydrogenase activity was evident in all hepatic lobule sections after the 4th day of starvation; in contrast, a loss in alkaline phosphatase was detected. Glycogen was no longer evident after the 2nd day of starvation. The rise in succinodehydrogenase activity in a state of hunger is explained by increased substrate dehydration via the succinooxidase system (Tessmann 1963).

Histological evaluations of over 200 liver biopsies after non-fatal starvation dystrophy revealed morphologically a restitutio ad integrum of the liver parenchyma (Otto and Würstlein 1964). Specific histomorphological symptoms of "delayed hepatic lesions after starvation dystrophy" do not occur according to these results.

Histological changes in the *skeletal musculature* in metatrophia largely correspond to the findings in progressive spinal muscle atrophy. Electron microscopically, the loss of substance is seen to affect the myofibrils and sarcoplasm with its organelles. The surface of the muscle cells forms festoonlike protrusions. At particular sites, fragmentation of the myofibrils occurs, and the fragments shift toward one another. This finding corresponds to the symptoms of fibrous homogenization and fragmentary destruction of muscle fibers. These pathological changes are developed to varying degree in muscle fibers. All transitional stages are found from normal undamaged muscle fibers to advanced stages of disintegration (Gieseking 1962).

In a prolonged state of hunger, multiple cuneate hemorrhagic erosions develop in the gastric mucous membrane of the fundus and in the pyloric region. The mucous membrane concerned is to some extent necrotic. The neighboring unaffected mucosal epithelia contain vacuoles (Tarasitano 1939). In the mucosa of the jejenum, the formation of PAS-positive granules, showing local connections with lysosomes, can occur (Baker 1964). In the large intestine, edema of the mucosa and fibrinous membranes may form. It is uncommon for severe colitis ulcerus to develop.

In the pancreas, animal experiments and isolated observations in humans indicate a decrease in the nuclear size in the exocrine gland cells and a reduction in the zymogen granules. In the centroacinar cells, shrinking of the cytoplasm and thickening of the fine elements develop (Paradisi 1965; Svoboda et al. 1966). In cardiac muscle, only minor degenerative changes in the muscle fibers were detected. Similar unspecific signs of degeneration were also found in the ganglion cells of the diencephalon. In the adrenal glands, distinct broadening of the cortex and simultaneous lipoid depletion in the epithelia develop. The thyroid loses 50%–70% of its weight in chronic states of hunger. Colloidal condensation, collapse of the follicle, and atrophy of the follicular epithelium occur. Any colloidal nodules that may be present are not involved in the changes (Gerhartz 1955). The kidneys of neonates who died from primary malnutrition showed very heterogeneous histopathological findings – calcinosis, fat embolisms, metastatic abscesses, dilation of the tubules, and papillary fibroses (Stirling 1962).

X. Histological Contribution to the Investigation of Gunshot Wounds

Forensic-histological examination can contribute to the clarification of the following questions with regard to gunshot wounds: signs of close-range shots, direction of shot, point of entry and exit of projectile, identification of a gunshot wound, vital reactions, age determination of wound.

In practice, there is sometimes competition in the investigation of gunshot wounds between the interests of the medical examiner and those of the criminologist. This particularly concerns the investigation of close-range shots and the determination of range. Unfortunately, what often happens is that the soft parts in the vicinity of the entry and exit wounds are removed for investigation in criminological laboratories. Thus, a division occurs between the autopsy and histological examination, which is then usually made impossible. Efforts should be made wherever possible to carry out the medicolegal and criminological investigations together at the same institute.

For the histological investigation, the external shot perforations should be cut in a circular fashion at least 1–2 cm apart and removed together with the subcutaneous tissue. On the skull, the soft parts should be removed with the epidermis down as far as the outer surface of the bone. The cylindrical piece of tissue removed, with the path of the projectile in the center, then has to be carefully mounted and fixed for a few hours in formalin solution. Then, by sectioning parallel to the axis of the projectile track, the appropriate tissue segments can be taken and embedded for histological examination. The removal technique is similar with inner organs and muscle sections that have been shot.

A frequent histological finding is *basophilia* of the connective tissue in the peripheral areas of the projectile path. This "lesion metachromasia" was detected by Orsós using Mallory's stain (1935) following mechanical injuries or the effects of heat. Metachromasia in gunshot wounds was systematically investigated by Krauland (1938) and Mueller (1942); it is seen as a very dark blue discoloration, particularly of the connective tissue fibers close to the projectile track. The blue discoloration is best visualized with H and E stain. It is probably caused by the direct effects of the gunpowder flash and heat of the projectile. The basophilia can also be utilized as an indication of a shot from close range and in determining the point of entry. Around the exit wound, basophilia of the connective tissue is mostly absent or only slightly developed. However, one drawback must be stressed, namely that minor basophilia can also arise as a result of later desiccation; thus, according to Mueller (1942), basophilia in gunshot wounds ought not to be taken as a determining factor in the assessment. Similar findings involving basophilia of the connective tissue have also been detected in bomb and shell fragment injuries, also in the region of the exit wound (Mueller 1941). On the palms of the hands and soles of the feet, a typical abrasional limbus can fail to develop in the case of gunshot wounds. The corneum is raised and radially lacerated around the opening of the entry wound (Pollak 1980). Histologically, signs of burning can be determined on the epidermis and hair as a consequence of the effects of the gunpowder flash in shots fired from close range; however, this is assuming that the areas under inspection have not been altered by blood or other liquids. In a positive case, the findings include heat reticulation in the epidermis, homogenization and liquefaction of the stratum corneum and also of the deeper epithelial layers. Thermal changes to the hair are usually best seen by examination under a magnifying glass.

Smoke stain and *interspersions of gunpowder* are important histological findings. The smoke stains are found as a thin black film on the surface of the epidermis. The gunpowder interspersions can be of various size and shape, but are usually amorphous black or blue-black forms. They can be detected in all layers of the epidermis, in the upper parts of the corium, and in the wall of the channel created by the projectile. They are the partly burnt components of the propelling charge, which can, particularly with close-range shots from a weapon touching the skin, also be driven into the deep sections of the projectile path. Where a smoke-lined cavity develops, it is usually the case that the wall is only superficially impregnated with these particles. Gunpowder interspersions and smoke particles can be visualized quite well in histological section by their own coloration without special treatment. In our expe-

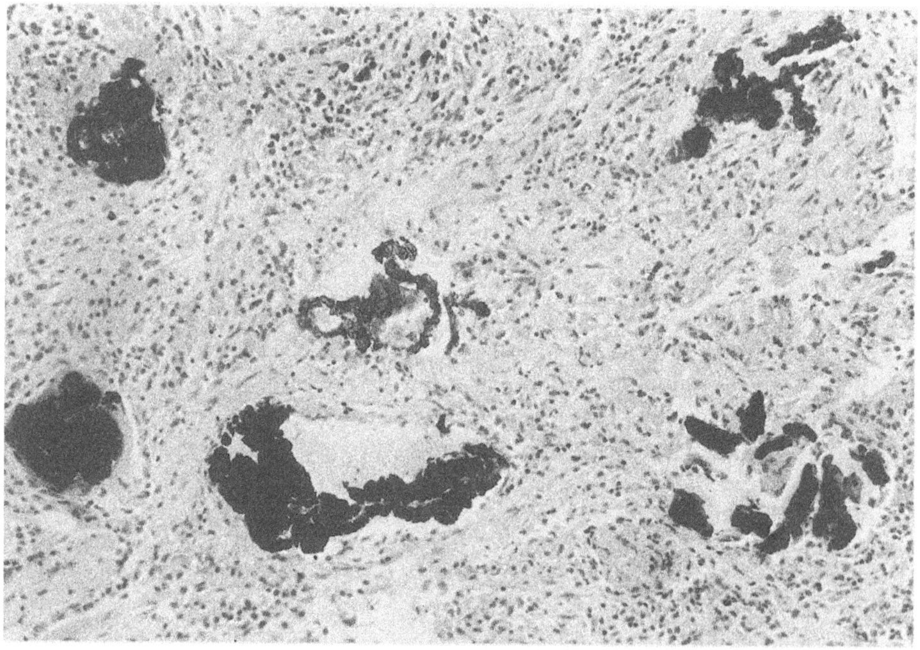

Fig. 149. Old shell-splinter wound of the lung. Scar and granular tissue with inclusion of small splinters. Berlin blue reaction positive, 1:150

rience, we have found that there is no danger of mistaking these for natural skin pigments (cf. Francisco 1980).

Systematic histological studies on the outer margins of the projectile entry wound have revealed in the region of the stretched limbus a torn raised corneum, which is usually folded over to the outside, away from the wound (Krauland 1938). On the inner border of this region, there is a zone with fissured epithelium, which passes into an epithelial inner ring toward the edge of the entry wound. This part of the exposed corium falls away like a funnel toward the opening of the wound. Such a gradation of the stretched limbus toward the projectile channel was not evident round the exit wound. In our experience, this useful distinction between the exit and entry wounds is only clear in material that is in good condition and unaltered by the effects of liquid.

In gunshot wounds, foreign bodies and parts of the tissue layers, perforated on their upper surface, can be transported deep into the channel by the projectile. Such foreign bodies and tissue fragments can be identified by histological examination of the walls of this channel (Fig. 149). A comparison of the findings in the projectile channel around the external perforations can thus indicate the entry or exit wound.

The skeletal musculature near the projectile channel can be changed in various unspecific ways by the blunt violence of the projectile. Animal experimental studies have shown hyalinization, fragmentation, vacuolization, sporadic contraction bands, and pyknotic nuclei in an area of up to 15 mm around the wound in the skeletal muscle fibers (Hopkinson and Watts 1963, 1964). With Giemsa stain, the damaged muscle fibers were selectively stained blue.

Nonfatal gunshot wounds in the musculature of sheep produced vigorous proliferation of vascularized connective tissue and filling of the projectile channel within 3 weeks. After 5 months, necrotic material was no longer evident. The discontinuity in the muscular tissue had been replaced by a collagenous scar.

For clarification in a doubtful case whether a penetrating wound is in fact a gunshot wound, the histochemical test for nitrite and nitrate radicals according to Rolfe et al. (1971) is recommended. These radicals are released by the projectile in the area of the projectile channel and are reported to be in the form of blue-stained particles. This test, which we are unable to assess from personal experience, is reported to be possible for a shooting range of up to about 3 m.

Gunshot wounds in the brain almost always give rise to hemorrhages outside the projectile channel in the cerebral tissue. Usually, numerous punctiform, partly confluent hemorrhages develop, even at some distance from the projectile channel and debris zone, especially on the apices of the gyri cerebri (Henn and Liebhardt 1969). Histologically, they are evident as fresh perivascular erythrocytic accumulations, predominantly located in basal parts of the cerebrum and cerebellum.

In scanning electron-microscopic studies, Speeter and Ohnsorge (1973) found traces of abrasion and lamellar flexions following the direction of the projectile in gunshot wounds in bones, particularly in the compact substance of the femur. There was evidence of ruptures in the substantia spongiosa ossium following the missile direction and secondary flexion breaks on the exit wound side of the spongiosa trabecular walls.

The early vascular reactions in the region of gunshot wounds have been investigated in rabbits by Russian authors (Venglinskaya et al. 1967, 1970) using various methods. As early as a few minutes after the production of the gunshot wound, distinct edematic development was evident; this reached a peak after about 1½ h. After 30 min, sporadic leukocytes could be detected in the wall of the projectile channel; after 60 min, normal infiltrates were found. After 24 h, mononuclear cells were evident.

Finally, it should be stressed that the histological examination of penetrating injuries is wholly recommended if their identity has not been conclusively demonstrated by other means.

XI. Histological Findings in Poisoning

1. Preliminary Note

Histologically detectable lesions in poisoning belong in a broad sense to forensic toxicology, which we understand to signify the study of poisons and poisoning as applied in the administration of justice (Weinig 1957). As a form of "applied toxicology," it comprises clinical symptomatology, pharmacology, pathoanatomy, and pathophysiology, as well as the evidence of poison using chemical, pharmacological, and pharmacognostic methods. In the definition according to Reuter (1938), poisons are inorganic or organic substances that impair health by chemical or physical interactions with the organism. The toxic effect is dependent on quantity, concentration, form of exposure, condition, and individual type of reaction of the organism concerned. Poisoning is a morbid condition directly caused by toxins (Clarmann 1971). The mode of action and speed of the toxic effect are important in the development of morphological changes. Quick-acting poisons giving rise to acute dysfunctions do not usually induce any changes that can be detected in the corpse and utilized. There is often an apparent contradiction between the acute course of a disease developing from a condition of perfect health, suggestive of poisoning, and the absence of morphological findings in the autopsy and histological examination. On the other hand, chronic poisoning, which can resemble natural clinical symptoms, leads to tissue and organ lesions that are relatively easy to identify.

It should be particularly emphasized that all histological changes occurring in association with poisoning are unspecific. It is only seldom that poisoning can be proven from the histological findings alone. Where the anamnesis is unknown, histological findings can provide the impetus toward specific toxicological investigations. Equally, autopsy and histological examination can be fruitless in the search for signs of poisoning. Histologically detectable lesions from natural pathological conditions that either singly or in combination with the toxic action can be fatal have a similar unspecific character. A complete histological organ status should therefore be included in the investigation of every case of poisoning.

In the assessment of toxic damage to tissues, it should be taken into account that frequently it cannot be proven whether a direct toxic action is involved or an indirectly caused lesion is responsible, e.g., by toxic cytolytic products, disorders in the circulation, disturbances in permeability. The majority of histological findings that have been described in connection with poisoning have to be judged with this proviso in mind. A systematic etiological-pathogenetic presentation is impeded for the same reason. It is necessary therefore to restrict the assessment to essential and reliable histological findings. In the following sections, the divisions of specific toxicology have been adhered to. Many toxic substances and their effects on the tissues could only be incompletely discussed or mentioned as examples. The literature is only quoted in part. The following remarks are based particularly on the summaries of morphological findings of Petri (1930), H. Leithoff and T. Leithoff (1969) and the papers on toxicology by Reuter (1938), Weinig (1957), v. Clarmann (1971), Moeschlin (1972), Kuschinsky (1972), and Geldmacher v. Mallinckrodt (1975). Mention should also be made of the summaries by Schreiner and Maher (1965), Rouiller et al. (1965), Aragona (1965), Altmann and Klinge (1972), Klinge (1973), and Altmann (1980).

2. Specific Histomorphology in Poisoning

Inorganic Toxins

Lead. A great many unspecific changes are known in the gastrointestinal tract, bone marrow, and brain (encephalitis saturnina). The histological findings in the kidney and liver deserve emphasis. Typical round, intensely eosinophilic inclusions are found in the nuclei of the epithelia of the renal proximal tubules after chronic lead poisoning (Zollinger 1953; Müller and v. Ramin 1963; and v. Dallenbach 1965). These nuclear inclusions are mainly restricted to the proximal sections of the renal tubules. In animal experiments, the eosinophilic inclusion bodies developed after chronic lead poisoning of 10–13 months' duration (Horn 1970). After isolation by density gradient centrifugation and analysis by means of atomic absorption the inclusion bodies had a lead content of up to 38 mg/g dry weight, which corresponds to more than 70 times the lead concentration of the whole kidney. Electron microscopically, two types of nuclear inclusion could be determined (Totović 1964): a) corpuscular structures with uniformly distributed fine-granular and mycelium-like filamentous components; b) inclusions of cytoplasmic components that were displaced into the nucleus post-mitotically – these are not specific for chronic lead poisoning since they can also be observed in colchicine poisoning. In patients with chronic lead poisoning, the nuclear inclusion bodies are almost a regular finding in kidney biopsies, usually together with tubular degenerations and interstitial fibroses (Galle and Morel-Maroger 1965; Morgan et al. 1966). The nuclear inclusions can remain in the kidneys for up to 10 years after the end of exposure to lead.

Similar nuclear inclusions have also been detected in the liver epithelia of rats after chronic lead poisoning (Lesch 1968); autoradiographic evidence shows this to be incorporation of lead. Identification of nuclear inclusion bodies in liver biopsy material could thus be indicative of chronic lead poisoning.

In Kupffer's cells, large plaque-like ferruginous nuclear inclusions and PAS- and diastase-positive deposits may appear. In animal experiments, hyperplasia is initially observed in the bone marrow; it then develops into osteomyelitic fibrosis and osteomyelitic sclerosis. The multiple occurrence of so-called nephradenomas can in connection with high blood pressure indicate lead poisoning (Zollinger 1953). These "lead tumors" are explained as excessive regeneration following lesions of the tubules in areas of the kidney receiving deficient blood supply (Franke and Kyrieleis 1976). Histochemical and histological changes induced by lead to the livers and kidneys of dogs are predominantly seen as a dose-dependent depletion of enzymes (White 1977).

Mercury. The findings most indicative of mercury poisoning can be detected in the proximal renal tubules: nuclear pyknosis, vacuolar formation, cytoclasis, and early changes in the mitochondria (Dejung 1963; Taylor 1965). The alcian-blue-phloxine stain after Sanfelice fixation is recommended for the visualization of changes in the kidney. In rats acutely poisoned with mercuric chloride, the first changes were evident electron microscopically after 5–6 h; light microscopically this did not occur until after 24 h. These changes involved spherical bodies with homogeneous contents in the apical cell pole of the epithelia of the proximal tubules and fusiform distension and translucency of the microvilli in the region of the cuticular border, which after 4 days was completely destroyed (Mölbert et al. 1964). There are extensive calcium deposits in the region of the damaged renal sections and in the interstitium of the medullary pyramid, which after the exclusion of other causes can indicate a "sublimate kidney."

Enzyme-histochemical studies of the kidneys, liver, and cardiac muscle have led to varying results; there was usually a drop in the activity of adenosine triphosphate and unspecific esterases; on the other hand, there are reports of an increase in the reactivity of 5-nucleotidase and acid phosphatase (Jonek and Kosmider 1964; Jonek et al. 1964a, b; Taylor 1965).

Experimental poisoning of guinea pigs by subcutaneous injection of methyl mercury hydroxide caused, in addition to the known renal changes and fatty infiltration of centrolobular liver cells, multiple calcified necroses in the cerebral cortex and nuclear pyknosis in the inner granular layer of the cerebellum (Falk et al. 1974).

For histological evidence of chronic mercury poisoning, specifically of mercuric chloride, the sulfite-silver method of Timm (1961, 1962) is recommended: Unmodified tissue sections are fixed with H_2S gas and cut; H_2S sections are immersed in potassium ferrocyanide with hydrochloric acid or perchloric acid; then, immersion in potassium cyanide solution; finally, sections are developed in gum arabic solution and silver nitrate solution with hydroquinone and citric acid. In sublimate poisoning, the mercury circulates in the body bound to albumin. It makes its way into the kidneys and is deposited at the basal membranes of the proximal tubules. Here the familiar necrosis is induced. In this manner, argyrophilic, sulfur-containing metabolic products develop in the proximal tubules and in their basal membranes. With this method by Timm, acute sublimate poisoning is characterized by the occurrence of argyrophilic reaction products in the kidney. The sulfide-silver pattern shows the reactive site of the mercury in the kidney, where it initiates the morphologically recognizable organ lesions by binding to the mitochondria of the cells of the proximal tubules.

Clinical studies also report apallic syndrome and peripheral polyneuropathy through chronic mercury poisoning after the consumption of sprayed corn in Iraq (Gerstenbrand et al. 1977).

Thallium. The generally unspecific, predominantly inflammatory changes effect the gastrointestinal tract and degenerative fatty infiltration in the liver (Weinig and

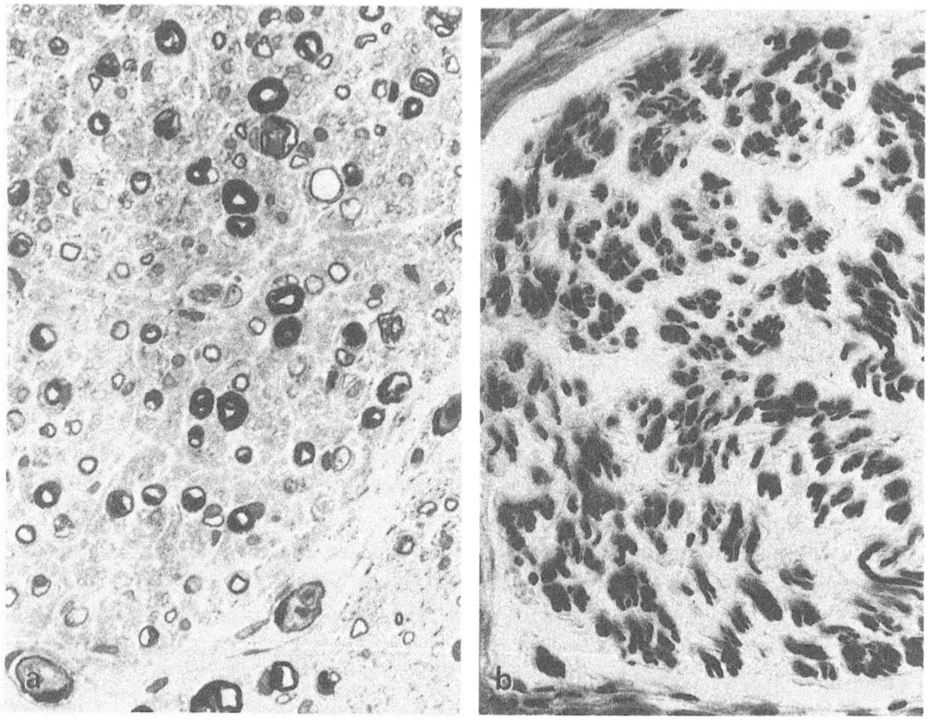

Fig. 150. a Nervus suralis in thallium poisoning. Pronounced myelinic degeneration. Woelcke's, 1:220. **b** Nervus suralis in thallium poisoning. Massive axon regeneration. Bielschowsky's, 1:250

Schmidt 1966). The findings in the central nervous system are of prime interest: In the region of the peripheral nerves there is extensive polyneuritis with myelinic degeneration, leading to complete demyelinization (Fig. 150); vascular changes occur, with swelling of the endothelium, disaggregation of the media, and proliferation of the adventitial cells. In the region of the anterior and posterior roots, pericytes and glial cell reproduction in the spinal ganglia and degeneration of the posterior white column of the spinal cord and vegetative cell groups of the nucleus intermediolateralis are found. The nerve cell changes correspond to the clinical symptoms of "primary stimulation." Depletion and pyknosis of the Nissl substance are also observed. In the brain, regressive changes in the nucleus dentatus and olivae and regressive nerve cell changes in the corpus mamillare and nucleus paraventricularis are found. Occasionally, vessel-dependent pale foci in adventitial fibroses of the accompanying arterioles and capillary budding are evident in the region of the cerebral cortex (references in Bredemann 1954; Prick et al. 1955). Outside the CNS, necroses of muscle fibers, increases in the muscle nuclei, and perivascular inflammatory infiltrates have been detected in the skeletal musculature.

The microscopically detectable changes in the hairs of the head have diagnostic significance (Widy 1956; Rauschke 1963). In the acute toxic stage, there is migration of thallium into the nonkeratinized sections of hair, close to the roots. It is still unclear in what form and to which elements of hair the thallium binds and what determines the microscopically recognizable opacity of the affected sections of hair. It has, however, been demonstrated that thallium is contained in the dark band-like zones. By means of experiments with freshly plucked papillary hairs, the development of opaque inclusions could also be reproduced using water and dye solutions in vitro. Even after a single administration of thallium, layered inclusions could be detected in the hairs; after fractional doses, however, they may be absent. The number of inclusion zones in head hairs thus does not permit reliable inferences to be made as to the frequency of previous thallium intake. Animal experiments have shown that similar inclusions in hair can also occur as a result of the acute action of other metallic compounds. Nonetheless, the morphologically detectable changes in hair are to a high degree an excellent indication of thallium poisoning.

The sulfide-silver method of Timm (1958) is also recommended for the histological detection of thallium, which counts as an accumulating toxin. It can be carried out just as well in material fixed in H_2S-alcohol and embedded in paraffin as in cryostat sections, e.g., renal tissue treated with H_2S gas prior to freezing. The cryostat sections are briefly fixed in alcohol and treated for 10 min with aqueous 10% hydrogen peroxide solution prior to physical development and subsequent rinsing. The thallium sulfide that forms in the treating of the pieces of tissue with H_2S is exceptionally easily oxidized. It can, however, be transformed into thallium selenide, which is resistant even to hydrogen peroxide (Voigt 1971).

Cadmium. Cadmium pneumonopathy is generally known; it develops through the inhalation of cadmium vapor over a long period of time. In animal experiments, the clinical symptoms were evident in albino rats over a period of 55 days (Fruscella 1963). Histologically, an extensive mesenchymal cell reaction is evident in the interalveolar septa. A connective tissue proliferation follows, with occlusion of the alveoli and complete disappearance of the normal pulmonary structure. After the inhalation of a $CdCl_2$ aerosol by rats, acute lesions and reactions were produced in the alveolar cells and respiratory tracts (Strauss et al. 1976; Asvadi and Hayes 1978). Histological and electron-microscopic studies have revealed focal epithelial lesions in the centrilobular sections of the bronchioli respiratorii. Initially, there was edema and destruction of type I alveolar cells. Within 3 days of exposure to a $CdCl_2$ aerosol, this were replaced by proliferating granular type II alveolar cells. The micromorphological changes and symptoms can be compared with the findings following inhalation of nitrous gases. The damage to the type I alveolar cells is due to inhibition of oxidative phosphorylation. It is possible that the cadmium inhaled in the smoking of cigarettes also promotes the centrilobular localization of pulmonary emphysema.

In cases of acute cadmium poisoning, there has been evidence of severe gastroenteritis, necrotizing tracheobronchitis, and small hemorrhagic pulmonary infarctions. In a 73-year-old man, acute diffuse leukocytic myocarditis, centrolobular necroses of the liver, and calcium nephrosis were found 12 days after inhaling cadmium vapor (Peter 1955). In animal experiments, desquamations of the epithelia, vacuolar formation and granulation of the cytoplasm, and destruction of the nuclei were produced in the kidneys in the region of the proximal tubules by $CdCl_2$ injections (Axelsson and Piscator 1966). Hyaline thickenings of the basal membranes of the glomeruli have only rarely been observed in this connection. Opaque swellings in myocardial cells and vacuolization in the cells of the conduction system have sometimes been found in animal experiments.

Poisoning through other metals and metalloids, e.g., manganese, beryllium, silver nitrate, gives rise to unspecific changes that can also be produced by many other substances. In principle, the same also applies to acute and chronic arsenic poisoning (Maresch 1978). Mention should be made of the questions that occasionally arise in assessing cirrhoses of the liver and epithelioma of the skin after long exposure to arsenic (Lüchtrath and Krüger 1971; Fritsch et al. 1971).

Phosphorus. Poisoning with elementary white phosphorus is scarcely observed in European countries nowadays and is thus usually only discussed in passing, if at all. Observations and specific studies of fatal cases of poisoning in humans, where the course of the disease can be from a few hours to about 10 days, and in animal experiments permit a relatively precise insight into the histomorphological pathogenesis of this classic liver toxin.

In the initial stages, swelling of the liver parenchymal cells occurs with a uniform diffuse fatty infiltration of a fine-droplet kind. There is also sporadic hyaline-droplet degeneration of the liver cells, and the sinus becomes engorged with blood. In the second phase, increase in fatty infiltration is observed, spreading variably within the hepatic lobules; in centrolobular sections the droplets are fine, in intermediary zones they are medium to coarse. In addition, liver cell necroses and the beginnings of regeneration in the periportal area are evident, with proliferation in the bile duct and cell infiltrates, predominantly composed of lymphocytes and plasma cells. Kupffer's cells are involved to different degrees and are in parts highly fatty or necrotically altered. The further course is variable; either a postnecrotic liver cirrhosis develops with numerous cell infiltrates, or the fatty infiltration and necrosis advance rapidly, essentially without granulations and fibroses, until there is total collapse of the hepatic tissue (Caroff et al. 1968). Despite advanced destruction of the liver, in isolated cases it is possible for peripheral lobule sections to remain unchanged and establish early proliferations in the bile ducts of the periportal region (Salfelder and Seelkopf 1963). Experimental phosphorus poisoning in rats led to the occurrence of extracellular droplets and plaque-like fatty deposition in the liver within 24 h. The postmortem histological findings in the liver are probably also determined by supravital effects of the phosphorus. In humans, a fine-droplet fatty infiltration of the tubular epithelia in the kidneys and cardiac muscle cells has been observed in addition to a general hemorrhagic diathesis. Basically similar histological findings have been determined after poisoning with phosphine (Hallermann and Pribilla 1959).

The histological findings in the liver are typical where poisoning by phosphorus is definite. Without a reliable poisoning anamnesis, however, even fully developed histological findings do not have a specific significance in the liver since they can also occur in many other kinds of intoxication (solvents, fungi, etc.) and diseases (acute hepatosis, eclampsia, shock, etc.).

Prussic Acid. With this enzymatic toxin, which after appropriate dosage and uptake usually leads very rapidly to death, virtually no histological findings whatsever can be detected that provide an indication of the cause of death. The rapid course of intoxication hinders the development of the appropriate tissue reactions. It is only from isolated observations with a protracted toxic course, e.g., after percutaneous uptake, that unspecific histological dermal changes, in the form of cauterization or circumscribed pale areas and necroses of the liver and brain, have become known (Raestrup 1926; Ule and Pribilla 1962; Patscheider and Dirnhofer 1973; Brettel et al. 1968). Myocarditis (Janssen and Burger 1968) and a myocardial infarct (Salomone and Scorsone 1961) have been described as rare complications of prussic acid poisoning. Electron-microscopic studies of the cardiac muscle of rats that had been poisoned with KCN revealed unspecific changes in the mitochondria: septal formation, cristolysis, and dilation of the tubular apparatus (Balogh and Rubanyi 1978).

Carbon Monoxide. Comprehensive reports on histomorphological findings as a result of CO poisoning are found in Mosinger et al. (1953), Adebahr (1954), Letterer (1957), Dalgaard (1962), and Finck (1966).

As a rule, histological lesions can only be detected after CO poisoning with a survival time of days or weeks. Thus far, it has not been possible to prove that carbon monoxide has a direct toxic action on tissue. Lesions that occur particularly after protracted CO poisoning are attributed to CO-incurred hypoxia or associated circulatory disorders and shock conditions, i.e., they are lesions that can develop through other hypoxic conditions.

In the case of fatal CO poisoning, histological changes could usually not be detected in the central nervous system. Death occurs before alterations become evident in cerebral tissue or nerve cells. In cardiac muscle, on the other hand, Korb (1962) and Korb and David (1962) were able to identify small circumscribed necrobioses and necroses of the cardiac muscle fibers even after acute CO poisoning by means of fluorescence and electron microscopy. The findings were influenced by postmortem breakdown processes. Electron microscopically, the first lesions appeared in the mitochondria. These findings could not be confirmed in rats by other authors (Frommhold 1964). Fuchsinophilic substances in the sarcoplasm of cardiac muscle cells and regular myocardial infarctions were observed in apes after acute CO poisoning (Marek and Piejko 1972; Prochnicka and Marek 1973; De Bias et al. 1973). Histochemically, Nanikawa et al. (1960) found a quantitative reduction of SDH in cardiac muscle. In the older literature (in Korb 1962), there are also reports of hemorrhages, fatty infiltration, and necroses of the cardiac muscle, which did not appear until after a latent period of at least 24 h.

The development of a myocardial infarction through CO poisoning has been debated for some time (Klavis and Schulz 1966). In the case of previous damage to the coronary arterial system and after an appropriate survival time, histomorphological detection of a myocardial infarction is possible. In demonstrating a causal connection, proof of CO intoxication then becomes significant. Following sublethal CO poisoning, with CO-hemoglobin levels in blood of about 40%, and simultaneous stenosing coronary sclerosis, we registered an accidental death in terms of insurance regulations (toxically induced coronary insufficiency). Papillary muscle necroses have also been observed in the intact coronary system after longer periods of CO exposure (Balogh and Sótonyi 1977). The connections between CO poisoning and arteriosclerotic development in the coronary arteries have also been debated (Cucu 1978).

Necroses in the pallidum of the brain following CO poisoning were described as early as the middle of the nineteenth century. These findings appear after cerebral oxygen deficiency, chiefly in the area of the lenticular nucleus and deeper layers of the cerebral cortex, when the oxygen deficiency is survived for a relatively long time. They are usually seen as bilateral pale areas and necroses with round-cell infiltrates and glial reactions in the peripheral areas. Small necroses, destruction of ganglion cells in various sections of the brain, perivascular edema, myelinic swelling, hyperemia of various vascular regions, fresh and older hemorrhages with hemosiderin deposits, and destruction of myelin sheaths have also been observed (Adebahr 1954; Gerstenbrand et al. 1976). Together with an appropriate CO exposure, such findings in the brain can be judged as evidence of a CO lesion.

With fatal CO poisoning, an increase in the consistency of the brain has also been determined in the region of the white matter (Krug 1965).

In liver cells, fat-free vacuoles could be determined as a result of acute CO intoxication (Meier 1962). Older experiments led to diffuse and focal fatty liver cell degeneration, mainly in periportal areas; this "hepatitis oxycarbonica" tends to give rise to cirrhosis (Mosinger 1953).

Chronic myositis, atrophy, and wax-like degeneration of the musculature were observed by Hedinger after CO poisoning that was survived for a long time. The tissue destruction of the muscular lesion caused findings in the kidney that were comparable with a crush syndrome.

Further histological studies following CO poisoning have concerned acute renal insufficiency (Burck and Portwich 1964), changes in the hematopoietic system (Schmidtmann 1934; Mosinger et al. 1953), and findings following prenatal CO poisoning (Müller and Graham 1955; Colmant and Wever 1963).

Animal experimental and histochemical studies of the respiratory enzymes in cardiac muscle tissue have led to the conclusion that it is possible for CO to exert a direct histotoxic effect (Lo Menzo 1966; Petelenz et al. 1972).

Fluorine. The histomorphologically detectable effects of intoxication with fluorine compounds and other halogens are essentially of an unspecific nature (Waldbott 1963; Pribilla 1966). According to the route of intake, peroral or by inhalation, the organs directly affected are characterized by cauterization. Subsequently, within a short period of time, the findings include hemorrhagic gastritis, severe ulcerating mucosal lesions in the respiratory tracts, pronounced hemorrhagic pulmonary edemas, and the onset of pneumonia (Milana and Fichera 1962; Greendyke and Hodge 1964). Occasionally, parenchymal lesions in the liver, kidneys, and heart also develop. It has not been clarified here whether these changes involve direct effects of the fluorine compounds or the sequelae of severe mucosal lesions in the respiratory system or gastrointestinal tract. In hepatic cells, fat-free vacuoles and fatty degeneration were evident; in one case, extensive liver necroses also occurred. Sporadically, swellings of the glomerular loops, were seen in the kidneys. In the heart, pancarditis (Calderón and Cualla 1962), extensive cardiac muscle necroses (Fasske 1962), and interstitial edema of the cardiac musculature with isolated necroses of the fibers were detected (Pribilla 1966).

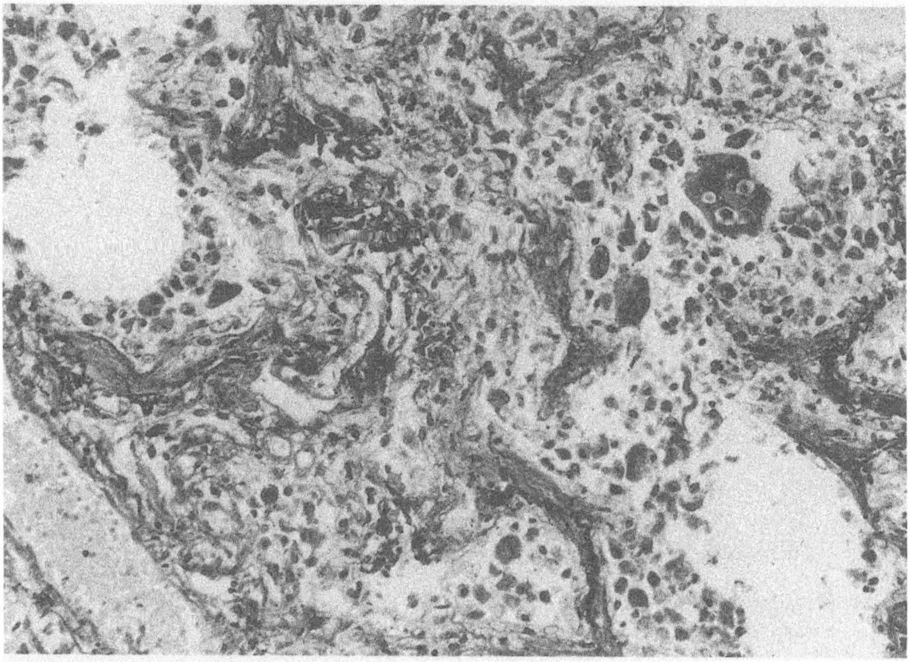

Fig. 151. Lung following 3 weeks' intensive artificial respiration. Pronounced alveolar cell reaction, partly involving giant cells; proliferation of the interstitial connective tissue. Subject 15 years old, ♀, automobile accident. PTAH, 1:320

Oxygen. The damaging effects of hyperbaric oxygen have thus far only been observed in connection with therapeutic measures or presented in animal experiments. The phases in the course of oxygen intoxication are: first, an acceleration of oxidative processes and the formation of free radicals; second, disorders in the cell metabolism with oxidation of sulfhydryl groups and peroxidation; and third, organ changes that may be indicative of the cause (Walther 1972). Of prime importance are the changes in the lungs. The term "respirator lung" is familiar, referring to the state following prolonged respiration. In neonates, it leads to "bronchopulmonary dysplasia." In premature newborns, after about the 10th day of artificial respiration, the following histological changes occur: dedifferentiation of the ciliated epithelial cells in the bronchial tree, constriction of the bronchial mucosal glands, hypertrophy of the bronchial musculature, necroses, and desquamation of the alveolar cells. Particular note should be made of the changes in the pulmonary interstitium; it is the most important site of attack in oxygen intoxication. Here, widening of the alveolar septa, increase in the fibers of the local connective tissue (Fig. 151), and swelling and necrosis in the endothelial cells of the septal vessels occur. An increase in the distance between the alveolar lumen and accompanying capillaries causes the gas exchange disorder to become histomorphologically distinct. The morphological evidence may also be affected by the primary disease and concomitant disorders in addition to the "oxygen toxicity" of the inspired air (Reineke 1977). The histological

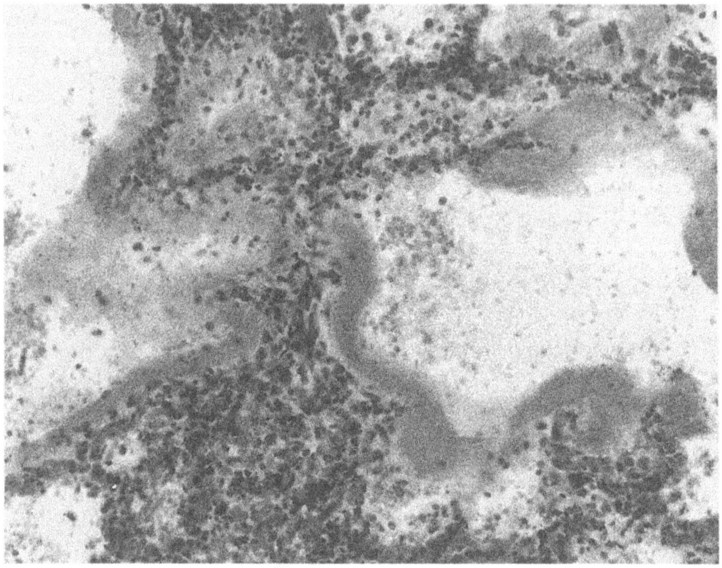

Fig. 152. Hyaline membranes of the lung following 10 days' artificial respiration. Subject 40 years old, ♀, barbiturate poisoning, PTAH, 1:180

findings of the oxygen lung in animal experiments resembles those of the shock lung in humans (Büsing 1978).

Further complications involve the formation of regular hyaline membranes (Fig. 152) (Cederberg et al. 1965; Kleinschmidt 1972; Giusti and Gentile 1974), pulmonary fibroses, disaggregation of the arterial walls (Nasseri et al. 1966), and generalized microthrombi. Outside the lungs, the following have been observed: disaggregation and widening of the interstitium in the myocardium, cardiac muscle necroses, necroses in the brain, retrolental fibroplasia in premature neonates (Purschke 1972; Podlesch 1972; Somogy 1972).

Predominantly animal experimental studies have shown that artificial respiration of pure oxygen leads in the lungs to swelling, dissolution, and mobilization of the pneumonocytes and nuclear and mitochondrial changes (Kapanci et al. 1967). In the liver, there was loss of glycogen, enlargement and deformation of the mitochondria, increase in the number of cristae mitochondriales, and vacuolar formation and accumulation of ribosomes (Schaffner and Felig 1965). Histochemical examination of the liver and cardiac muscle of rats revealed an increase in the enzyme reactions following oxygen intoxication (Walther and Lieven 1971). In addition there was clear damage to Leydig's cells (Brandt et al. 1972).

The toxic action of ozone should be considered. The triatomic oxygen molecule binds as a strong oxidant to lipids and proteins and can damage the cell membranes by reaction with sulfhydryl groups (Schlipköter and Bruch 1973). In animal experiments, severe changes were detected in the alveolar tissue following ozone exposure of 10 months' duration. These findings occurred focally and usually did not extend beyond the area of the terminal bronchioles. The pneumonocytes were particularly affected; they showed swellings and mitochondrial changes as well as detachment from the conspicuously thickened basal membrane (Bruch and Schlipköter 1973).

Boric acid. Intracytoplasmic inclusions in the epithelia of the exocrine part of the pancreas were described in children following boric acid poisoning (Fisher 1951). These inclusions are rounded structures surrounded by vacuoles and easily stainable with H and E; they are mostly located in the peripheral areas of the acinar cells and have a diameter of 2–10 μm. They are thought to be proof of the effects of boric acid.

Organic Toxins

Carbon Tetrachloride (CCl_4). This important solvent toxin is known for its pronounced hepatotoxic effects (Browning 1965). The hepatic lesions can be histologically determined 1–2 days after the toxic action. They begin as droplike fatty infiltration of the liver epithelia in the central lobule sections, which soon become necrotic. After a few days, the complete symptoms of acute hepatosis, with collapse of large parts of the hepatic tissue, are present in the majority of fatal cases of poisoning. Hemorrhages occur in the necrotic areas of tissue as well as inflammatory reactions, particularly in the region of Glisson's tissue. Electron-microscopic and histochemical investigations in animals revealed vacuolization in the granular endoplasmic reticulum, detachment of the membrane-bound ribosomes, a large increase in the number of free ribosomes, and a decrease in glucose 6-phosphatase activity 1 h after the toxic action. The mitochondria in the liver epithelia and Kupffer's cells were split and became tubular (Reynolds 1963; Huebner 1965). Even prior to necrosis, vacuolar degeneration can appear in the intermediary liver epithelia and proximal renal tubules (Aizawa 1962). In the case of intoxication survived for longer periods of time, the occurrence of hyaline bodies was observed in the liver epithelia after about 10 weeks. They are evident as eosinophilic cytoplasmic inclusions composed of lamellar bodies, which are layered in the fashion of onion skins, and located mainly within or at the periphery of glycogen-poor zones. Electron microscopically, they correspond to circumscribed accumulations of the endoplasmic reticulum, which according to histochemical studies show a powerful reaction with the nuceloside-di-phosphatase method (Braunstein and Stenger 1966; Stenger 1966).

Effects on the other organs can usually not be detected until after a survival time of several days. In the lungs, hemorrhagic edema, chronic bronchopneumonia, interlobular hemorrhages, proliferations of pneumonocytes, and fibrinous casts of the alveoli with eosinophilic cells are found. With longer periods of survival, the findings in the lungs increase in intensity. They are interpreted as the consequence of exhalation of the toxin (Umiker and Pearce 1953). In the kidneys, partially necrotic tubular nephroses of varying severity develop. Sporadically, the occurrence of fat embolisms has also been observed in the lungs and vessels of the systemic circulation (Lahl 1973).

The CCl_4 lesions are intensified and accelerated by the simultaneous administration of barbiturates or steroids and by a long-term state of hunger (Tsinronis and

Papacharalampous 1973; Reynolds et al. 1972; Tessmann 1964; Krishnan and Stenger 1966). In animal experiments, a delay and reduction in the tissue lesions can be achieved by hypothermia of the animals and spinal severance (Kurstak et al. 1973; Larson et al. 1964). It is assumed that the liver toxicity of CCl_4 is basically in the initial period due to a direct effect on the liver parenchyma, whereas the later damage is attributed to a dysfunction of the autonomic nervous system.

The CCl_4 delayed hepatic lesions are expressed as a postnecrotic liver cirrhosis, which about 7–8 weeks after the toxic action proceeds from the central hepatic veins and initially has no connection with the periportal tissue (Altermann 1954; Kaufmann 1953). In the advanced phase, the development of large nodal liver cell regeneration products occurs (Caulet 1972). The hepatic sinusoids are probably transformed into capillaries and vessels and portovenous connections occur (Stenger 1966).

Diffuse purulent myocarditis (Janssen 1962) and leukoencephalopathy (Korenke and Pribilla 1969) have been observed as special, probably secondary, organ lesions. In the case of juvenile toxicomania, in which CCl_4, trichloroethylene, and benzine were inhaled or drunk, usually severe arteriosclerotic changes were detected in the coronary arteries, such that a causal connection has been suggested (Sorgo 1976).

Trichloroethylene. This solvent frequently used in industry causes histologically pronounced acute pseudomembranous gastroenteritis following oral intake. In other inner organs, the changes are sparse. In the liver, a diffuse, fine-droplet fatty infiltration of the epithelia is found. In the kidneys, there is an opaque swelling of the epithelia in the proximal tubules (Stahl et al. 1969; Woźniak and Kosicki 1973). After longer exposure, chronic ischemic and toxic damage to the ganglion cells in the ganglion gasseri and cerebellum can occur. At the same time, the activity of acid phosphatases increases (Bartoníćek and Brun 1970). In a 33-year-old woman who died within a few hours of oral intake of trichloroethylene, we found massive damage to the kidneys with collapse and necroses of the vascular loops in the glomeruli (Fig. 153).

After fatal intoxication by inhalation, no particular histological findings can usually be detected other than general vascular congestion and pulmonary and cerebral edema.

Benzine. In acute fatal poisoning from benzine or similar chemical compounds, there are no special histologial findings other than general vascular congestion and cerebral and pulmonary edema.

Chronic intoxication following an exposure of several years leads to characteristic lesions in the hematogenic areas of bone marrow and to the development of leukemia (references in Seidel 1978). The question is whether all leukemias develop from such bone marrow lesions after benzine exposure. Clinically and histologically, the lesions are manifest as a panmyelopathy, with the corresponding signs of insufficiency in the form of agranulocytosis and hemorrhagic diathesis. In animal experiments, after 3 weeks' benzine treatment, the myeloid parenchymal proportion was observed to fall from 80% to 40%. At the same time there was an increase in the fatty tissue and in the number of reticular cells in the bone marrow, sometimes with

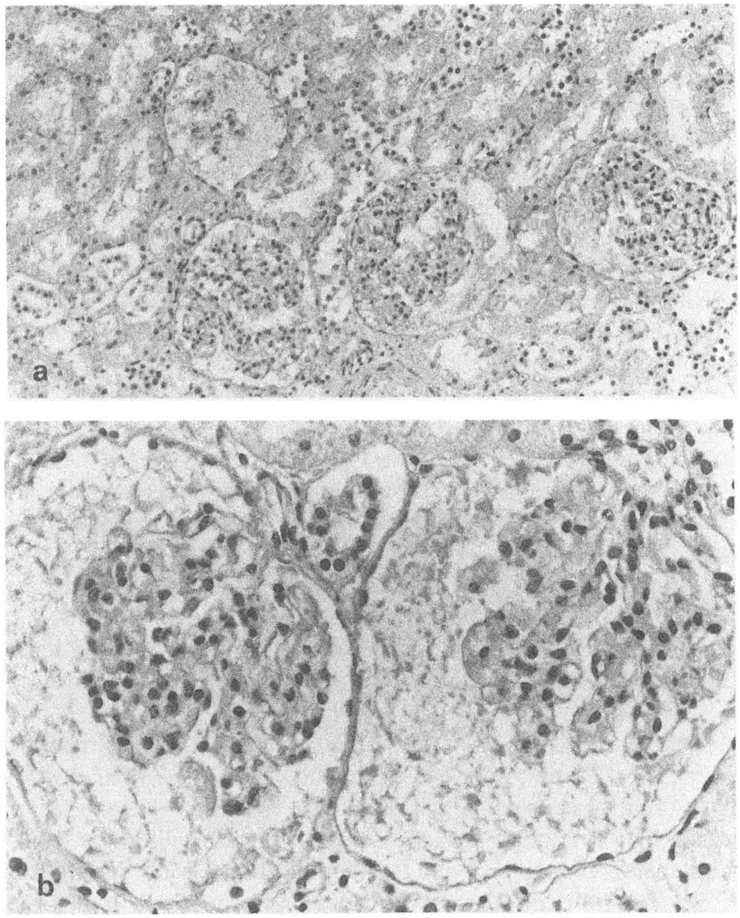

Fig. 153. a, b Severe renal damage with collapse and necroses of the glomerular loops. Trichloroethylene poisoning. Subject 33 years old, ♀, H and E, 1:180, 1:320

the transition into a partial osteomyelofibrosis. The bone marrow sinus was expanded. Lesions occurred in the sinus walls with hemorrhages and edema. Disorders in mitosis, DNA-synthesis defects, and lesions to the various enzymal systems developed parallel with the parenchymal lesions (Noeske and Martens 1972).

The regenerative medullary and reticular cell proliferations after benzine and toluene lesions can develop into real myeloid leukemias (Janssen 1958; Ludwig and Werthemann 1962; Seidel 1978). Clinical studies of alkaline leukocytic phosphatase in workers exposed to benzine and toluine revealed a distinct reduction in enzyme activity (Girard et al. 1970). Individual sensitivity to hemocyte-damaging toxins is variable as is the intensity of the histologically detectable medullary lesions in the different skeletal sections.

Outside the bone marrow, severe permeability disorders, edemas, and hemorrhages were observed in the lungs following narcotic inhalation of benzine and toluine (Kenyeres et al. 1978). After the injection of petroleum, Maresch and Probst

(1962) found miliary infarction like necroses and phlegmonous inflammations. Interesting case reports concern the development of Goodpasture's syndrome following exposure to various hydrocarbons (Reichel et al. 1973). This syndrome is a combination of pulmonary hemosiderosis and progressive glomerulonephritis. It is probable that immunological factors are important here; certain individuals are genetically capable of forming antibodies directed against the basement membrane damaged by hydrocarbons.

One particular clinical condition involves vinyl chloride sickness, which has been observed particularly in workers involved in the production of PVC after injury through halogen-hydrocarbons (Szadkowski 1976; Friedel 1976; Heusermann and Stutte 1977). The chronic vinyl chloride intoxication is characterized by hepatic lesions, splenomegaly with Banit's syndrome, acro-osteolysis, Raynaud's disease, thrombocytopenia, and facultative scleroderma-like changes. The extent of the hepatic lesion is decisive in the course of the disease and the fate of the patient. Histologically focal hydropic swellings in the hepatocytes, toxic fatty infiltration, paracrystalline inclusions in enlarged mitochondria, fibroses of the sinusoid walls, and isolated necroses are found in the liver. In addition, the development of angiosarcomas has been observed.

After fatal intoxication through drinking benzine, there is a severe hemorrhagic interstitial and intra-alveolar edema of the lungs as well as a pronounced fatty degeneration in the ganglion and glial cells in the brain (Klein 1950). Following benzine poisoning, delayed lesions in the brain can be expected.

Alcohol. The histomorphology of alcohol lesions comprises numerous findings which are difficult to present systematically. In acute fatal alcohol poisoning, there are no findings that can be diagnostically assessed. In a large series of 68 fatal cases, a fine-droplet fatty infiltration of cardiac muscle cells and a focal release of lipoids from the adrenal cortex were frequently found (Bschor and Keilbach 1968).

In chronic alcohol lesions, the histological findings in the liver are of prime importance. The diagnosis of an alcoholic hepatic lesion can nowadays only be accomplished with sufficient reliability with the aid of histological examination. Intravitally, the bioptic–histological examination enables definitive statements to be made regarding the extent and activity of alcohol-induced hepatic processes. Nevertheless, it should be taken into account that individual histological findings are unspecific. Only a large spectrum of histomorphological changes in the liver and the clinical findings permit the determination and assessment of an alcoholic hepatic lesion (Lieber 1975).

Large serial tests on chronic alcoholics show that about 20%–30% present a normal finding in liver biopsy (Lelbach 1972). Constitutional individual factors have been postulated as being responsible for the negative finding (Lorenz 1978). Of 3165 cases, adiposis hepatica was detected in 66.7%; in 879 cases (43.7%), alcoholic fatty infiltration of the liver was present. Different forms of this disorder can be distinguished. Adiposis hepatica alone without complications can either be moderately pronounced in the form of fine droplets or be highly diffuse and in the form of large droplets (Fig. 154) (Broicher et al. 1962). Small fatty cysts can form in fatty hepatocytes through ruptures in the cell membranes. Such changes are reversible. Enzyme-histochemical studies of alcoholic adiposis hepatica have shown no con-

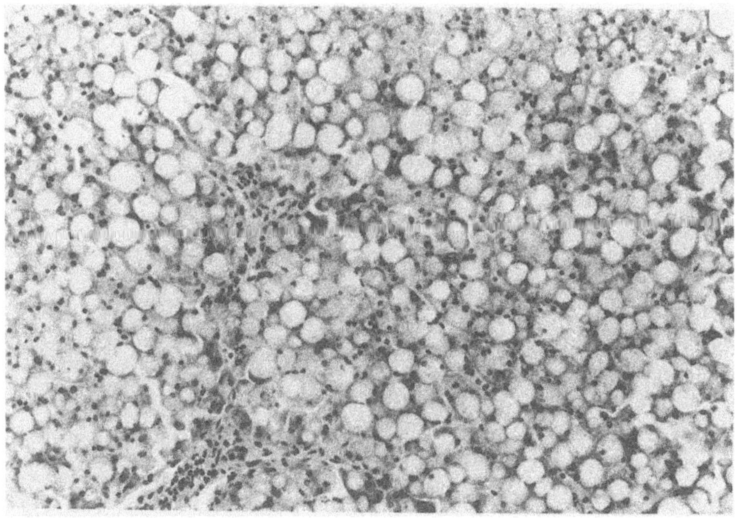

Fig. 154. Diffuse coarse-droplet fatty infiltration of liver cells after chronic alcohol abuse. Subject 26 years old, ♂. Sudan, 1:150

nection between this and the occurrence of atypical ADH (Ryvarden 1973). Conversely, focal loss of LDH activity appears to be more frequent in alcoholics than nonalcoholics. In rats, acute ethanol poisoning led to increased storage of triglycerides in liver cells (Ashworth et al. 1965). From this, the inference is made that the fatty deposition cannot be the result of cell destruction or reduced protein synthesis but a metabolic disturbance of fat utilization. Through analysis of the fat, the pattern of fatty acids, and the enzyme activities in the human liver, a differentiation of adiposis hepatica between alcoholics and nonalcoholics is possible (Miyabe 1976; Berghaus 1978).

Alcohol-induced lesions of the liver can also occur independent of hepatic cell fatty infiltration. These are chronically or acutely developed infiltrates which occur in the portal areas and central parts of the liver lobules, predominantly in the vicinity of necroses. This clinical pattern is still reversible in the initial stages. In German-speaking countries, it is termed "alcoholic fat-liver hepatitis" or "toxic hepatosis" (Fig. 155) (Altmann 1973). In English-speaking countries it is referred to as "acute alcoholic hepatitis."

Characteristic features of alcoholic lesions are intracytoplasmic hyaline deposits which predominantly develop in the centrolobular hepatocytes. These structures, termed "alcoholic hyalin" or Mallory bodies, are condensed cytoplasm close to the nucleus. They are rounded or oval and have an acidophilic character, blurred borders, and a cloudy appearance Fig. 156) (Reppart et al. 1963; Schaffner et al. 1963; Biava 1964; Flax and Tisdale 1964; Iturraiaga et al. 1966; Stötzner et al. 1973; Lesch 1974). The liver epithelia affected are degenerated to varying degrees. In the surrounding areas, leukocytic infiltrations are occasionally found. The hyaline deposits are seen in the electron microscope as drop-shaped, striate material of moderate electron density; with stronger magnification the material can be identified as hav-

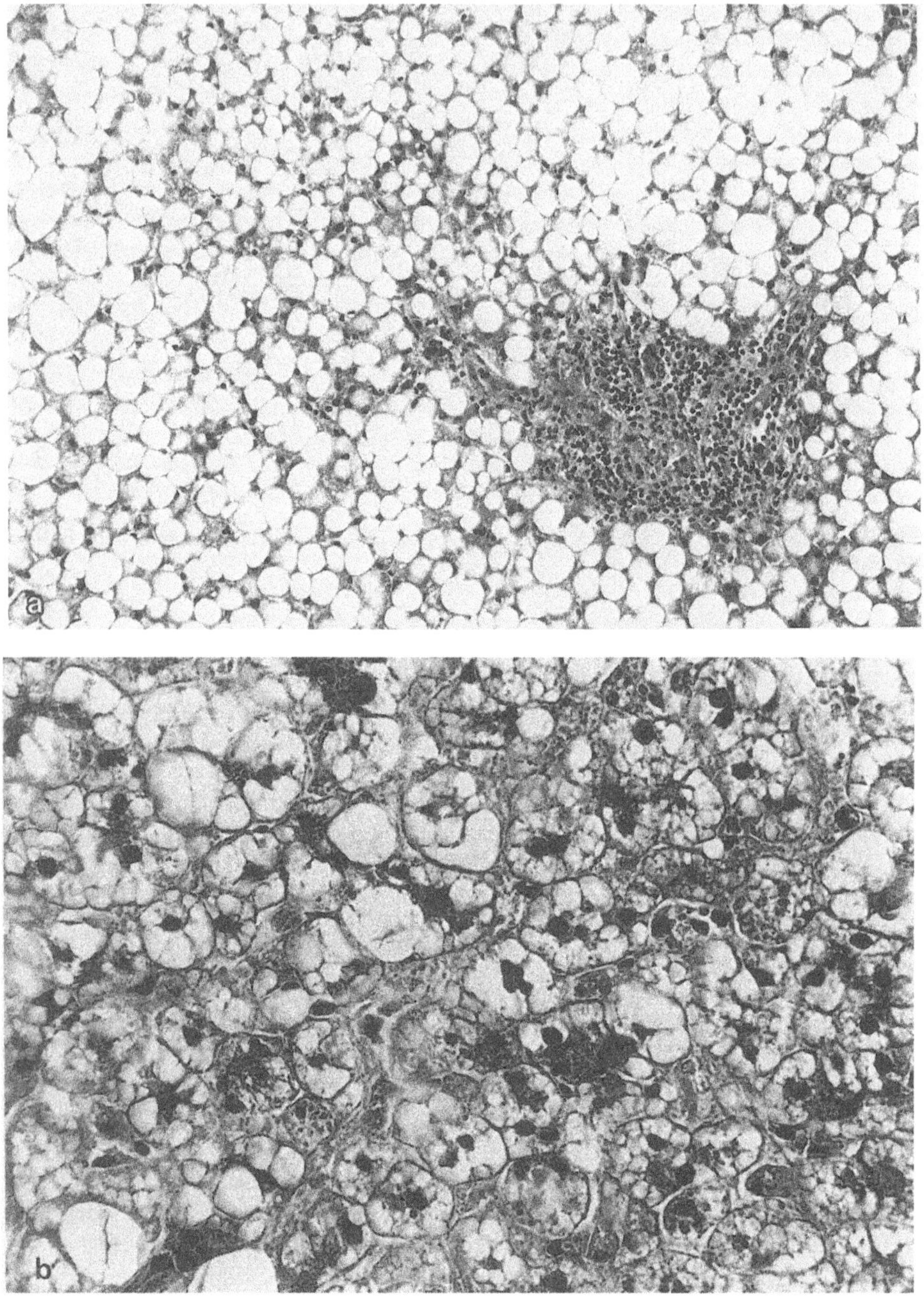

Fig. 155. a, b "Alcoholic fat-liver hepatitis." Subject 64 years old, ♀. Sudan, 1:150, 1:350

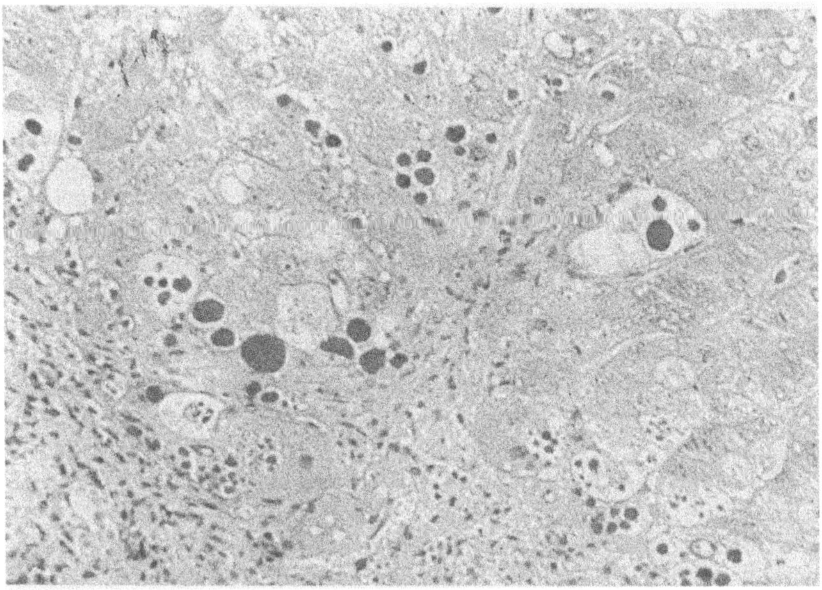

Fig. 156. "Alcoholic hyalin" of the liver epithelia (strongly acidophilic). PAS, 1:400

ing a three-layered membrane structure and granular areas. An external membranous border could not be detected around the bodies. The nature of these hyaline bodies, which do not occur exclusively in alcohol-damaged hepatic epithelia, is not uniformly assessed. Origins in the endoplasmic reticulum, degenerated or clumped mitochondria, or development through a change in the ergastoplasm have all been considered. They are complexes of various proteins which are also present in normal hepatocytes (Okamura 1976). These Mallory bodies are probably important in autoimmune and regenerative processes (Petersen 1977; Chomette 1978).

Giant mitochondria (Lesch 1974) have to be distinguished from alcoholic hyalin (Mallory bodies). Giant mitochondria are basically much more uncommon; they are found as small, homogeneous, sharply bordered cytoplasmic inclusions in the hepatocytes and usually have a rounded or cigar-shaped outline. These mitochondrial structures are possibly a compensatory attempt for a weakness in the performance of the mitochondria. In large serial tests in Japan, alcoholic hyalin was practically never detected (Ichida 1970; Kagawa 1970). The discrepancy between these results and those in Europe and America is explained by a different alcoholic tolerance of the central nervous system and differences in the type of nutrition. In Germany, on the other hand, about 40% of cases of alcoholic adiposis hepatica showed Mallory bodies. The bodies are almost always present if at the time of biopsy, the patient is under alcoholic strain.

In alcoholic liver lesions, Kupffer's cells are usually enlarged, increased in number, and contain inclusions of iron pigment, so-called drunkard's iron (Lesch 1974). In the central lobule, it is also possible in reversible adiposis hepatica for there to be an increase in the number of reticulin and collagen fibers, with a reticular structure forming around individual or groups of liver epithelia. This finding of a "mesh fibrosis" is, together with Mallory bodies, an important sign for the presence of alcoholic liver damage. Phosphorus poisoning, Wilson's disease, or primary biliary liver cirrhosis should also be considered in differential diagnosis.

The transition of alcoholic adiposis hepatica to a chronic form is marked by histiocytic cell infiltrates and activated stellate cells becoming more prominent. Proceeding from the lobule centers, fibrosis and sclerosis of the liver parenchyma occur, with encroachment on to the intermediary and periportal areas. The liver cirrhoses that result have variable forms; they are either uniformly nodular, or heterogeneous with parenchymal islands of various size, as in the case of postnecrotic cirrhoses of the liver (Roschlau 1977; Balázs et al. 1977; Hawkins 1978; Thaler 1979). A cirrhosis develops in about 10%–20% of all alcoholics. The development takes about 10–15 years in chronic alcoholism.

In rabbits, the elimination of alcohol from the blood was not affected by experimentally produced liver necroses, even though the liver was extensively damaged by CCl_4.

Alcoholic lesions of the central nervous system include clinical symptoms with variable histomorphological findings. Hitherto, it has not been clarified whether these diseases are due to direct damage incurred by the alcohol or secondary lesions by means of a metabolic disturbance. However, direct alcoholic damage to the brain is thought to exist, whereby certain areas tend to be particularly affected (Sattes 1973). Chronic atrophy of nerve cells has been described in the cerebrum, cerebellum, hypothalamus, corpora mamillaria, and end plates of the hippocampus (Miyakawa et al. 1977).

The lesions thus far established in the CNS in connection with alcoholic effects are all unspecific (Colmant 1968). It is important that the sum of all the findings be assessed, as far as possible in conjunction with the clinical course of the disease. One of the best-known alcohol-induced morbid conditions is Wernicke's encephalopathy, which is clinically accompanied by Korsakoff's psychosis, opthalmoplegia, and ataxia. Histomorphologically, this condition is evident as characteristic changes around the third and fourth ventricles and aqueductus. These changes comprise proliferations of the glia, particularly of the astroglia and microglia, together with a proliferation of the capillaries, which are increased in number and have thickened walls (Fig. 157). The nerve cells located in the surrounding area are unaffected for a long time. The findings and course of disease are complicated by pseudomalacia and hemorrhages. The corpora mamillaria also tend to be affected.

Further neuropathological clinical pictures induced by alcoholic damage are: central pontine myelinolysis; Marchiafava-Bignami disease, which is largely observed in red-wine drinkers in the Mediterranean region; pontocerebellar dystrophy; primary degenerative disorder of the cerebellar cortex, with a tendency to affect the superior vermiform process; chronic alcoholic amblyopia, which occasionally leads to total blindness (references in Colmant 1968). In animal experiments, an increased transendothelial pinocytotic transport of peroxidase through the blood-brain barrier has been observed in alcohol-poisoned rats (Persson et al. 1979).

Alcoholic polyneuropathy is widespread. The disease can commence acutely, tends to affect the distal sections of the extremities, and leads to severe muscular atrophy. Histologically, often only the medullary sheaths of individual internodal segments are affected, while the axon is preserved. Biochemically, the enzyme activities

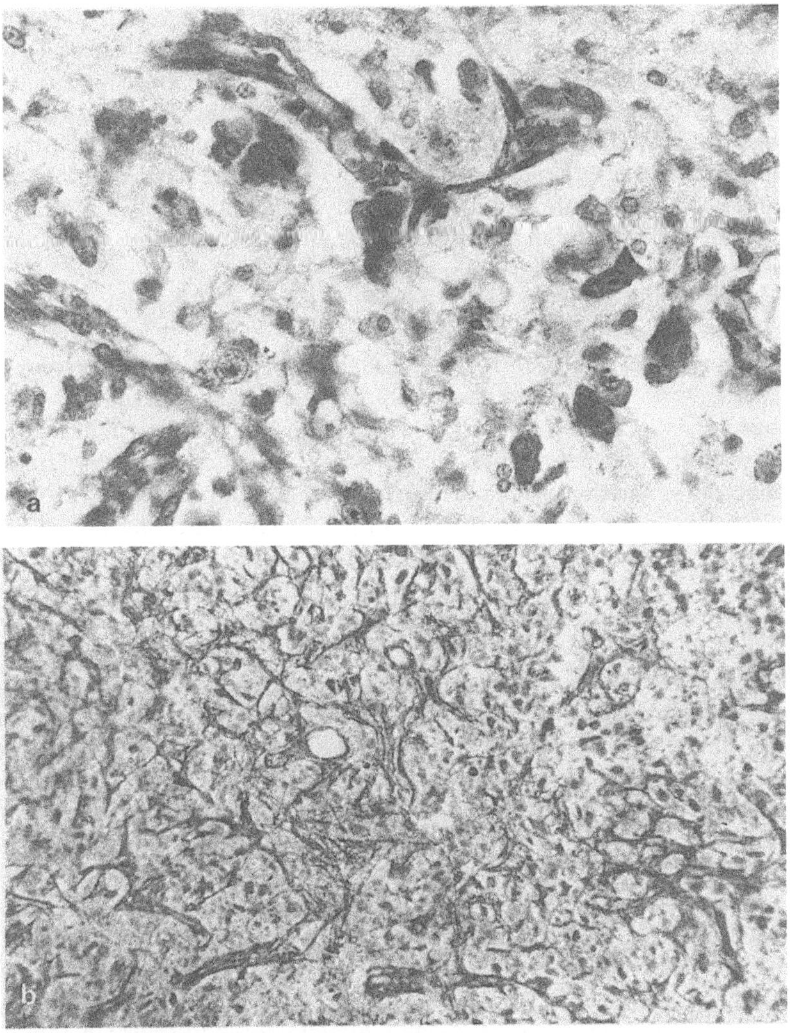

Fig. 157. a Wernicke's encephalopathy with thickened capillary walls, spongy changes in the neuropil, and fatty granule cells; the ganglion cells are preserved. Nissl, 1:400. **b** Wernicke's encephalopathy with pronounced capillary budding. Tibor-Pap, 1:280

of glycogenolysis and glycolysis were significantly reduced in the case of pronounced polyneuropathy in the skeletal musculature (Langohr et al. 1977). Circumscribed fiber necroses, variable strengths of the fibers, acute and chronic inflammatory reactions, and interstitial fibroses have been histologically observed (Rubin 1979). The occurrence of independent myopathy as a result of chronic alcohol abuse has not been conclusively proven. A rare myopathic disturbance following excessive alcohol consumption, with myoglobin casts in the collecting tubules of the kidneys, was reported by Poisson (1969).

The connections between alcoholism and hemorrhagic internal pachymeningitis are disputed and unclarified. Similarly unclear is whether the connective tissue thickenings of the pia mater, which are particularly localized in the anterior areas of the cerebellum, and atrophy of the brain, specifically the cerebral cortex, can be caused by chronic alcoholism (Sattes 1975). In a 13-year-old alcoholic, who died in status epilepticus following severe alcohol poisoning, ischemic cell degenerations were detected in the cerebral cortex and nucleus dentatus and there was a distinct mesenchymal reaction (Schéda 1960). In the rhombencephalon following acute alcohol poisoning with a fatal outcome, dystrophic changes of the ganglion cells in the motor nuclei and in the region of the nucleus vestibularis were found by Bereźnoy (1973).

Alcoholic pancreatitis is an organic disorder that histomorphologically can be easily distinguished. Böcker and Seifert (1972) found 171 cases (1.8%) of pancreatitis among 9703 autopsies; in 20%, alcohol pancreatits was present. This illness chiefly occurs in men, often in combination with cirrhosis of the liver, occasionally together with cholelithiasis. Chronic sclerosing pancreatitis, induced in over 30% of cases by alcoholism, presents, with two-thirds of all cases, the most frequent form of pancreatitis and thus also the prototype of alcoholic pancreatitis. Histologically, it is a peri- and intralobular sclerosis with parenchymal atrophy, but without basically interstitial inflammatory infiltrations. In addition, there is dilation and secretory inspissation in the acinic lumina, ectasis of the efferent ducts, epithelial flattening, and marked parietal sclerosis of the pancreatic vessels. A moderate periinsular and intrainsular fibrosis is found in the region of the islets of Langerhans. In chronic relapsing forms of alcoholic pancreatitis, there are necroses, inflammatory infiltrates, minor hemorrhages, and sometimes also rapidly fatal total necrosis of the whole organ (Dürr 1977). Sporadic hyaline bodies, similar to Mallory bodies, have also been observed in the exocrine pancreatic cells of alcoholics (Kojima 1973). According to Liem (1970), chronic alcoholic pancreatitis rarely leads to death, frequently, however, to invalidity. Alcoholic injury to the heart affects the myocardium; it is nonuniform and diagnostically difficult to detect. More from the clinical point of view, two forms of alcoholic cardiopathy can be distinguished: (1) the beriberi type; (2) chronic myocardiopathy as an irreversible, metabolically dependent, direct cardiac muscle lesion. Histologically, the cardiac musculature contains hypertrophied and partly degenerated muscle fibers, interstitial fibroses, thickening of the endocardium, isolated focal necroses, and inflammatory infiltrates; in addition there are mural thrombi and inflammatory foci in the endocardium and epicardium (Ferrans 1965 et al.). Fat and glycogen concentration are typical; histochemically, the reaction of mitochondrial oxidation enzymes is reduced (Wink 1978). Electron microscopically, an increase in the number of mitochondria, with swelling and cristolysis, was found; at the same time, numerous lipid vacuoles and pigment deposits were present (Riesner and Janssen 1978). The changes to the myofibrils extend as far as total loss of transverse striation and dissolution of the myofilaments (Hibbs et al. 1965). In patients with alcoholic cardiac muscle lesions, histological damage and fragmentation, dissociations of the contractile elements, and giant mitochondria could be detected by biopsy (Alexander 1966). Fragmentation of the myofibrils, swellings in the mitochondria, dissolution of the membranes and cristae, dilution of the sarcoplasm, and disintegration of the sarcoplasmic reticulum were seen in the electron-microscopic examination of the myocardium of alcohol-poisoned rabbits (Ito et al. 1966; Alexander et al. 1977). These partially reversible findings have been

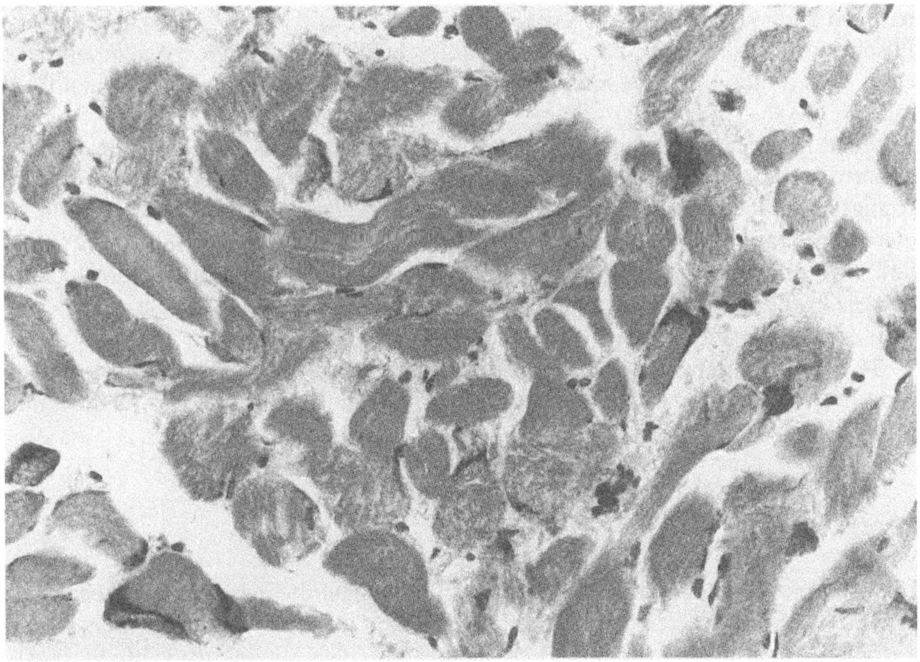

Fig. 158. Alcoholic cardiomyopathy. Interweaving (brush-like appearance) of muscle fibers in the ventricular septum. H and E, 1:300

interpreted as the result of a myocardial ischemia. Histological studies of the small myocardial vessels in patients who died of alcoholism or its sequelae revealed vascular wall edema, perivascular fibroses, sclerosis of the vascular wall, inflammatory parietal infiltrates, and protusions of the endothelium (Factor 1976).

The clinical and morphological findings in alcoholic cardiomyopathy were synoptically presented by Shanoff (1972) (Fig. 158).

In the lungs, the behavior of type II alveolar cells is negatively affected by alcohol, as a result of which a reduction in dipalmitoyl phosphatidylcholine is found (Heinemann 1977). Morphometric studies of the mucosa of rat stomachs under the chronic effects of alcohol showed a significant enlargement of the border cell surfaces in histological and cytological preparations (Al-Abadi et al. 1977). In a fatal Antabus–alcohol reaction, which was probably induced by the action of acetaldehydemia on the terminal vascular system, histological examination revealed peracute serous glomerulitis and acute nephrosis in the kidneys (Illchmann-Christ 1954).

Investigation of the bone marrow of chronic alcoholics yielded vacuole-containing medullary cells in the immature forms of erythropoiesis and thrombocytopenia with hemorrhagic symptoms (Pribilla et al. 1966; Paraf et al. 1971).

Fazekás (1964) pointed out a connection between histologically detectable adrenal hypoplasia and reduced alcohol tolerance on the basis of observations on humans and experimental studies.

Alcoholic embryopathy and alcohol lesions in infants have been variously summarized and systematically investigated (Hanson et al. 1976; Majewski et al. 1976; Püschel and Seifert 1979; Püschel and Mätzsch 1981). Histological examination of cases with a fatal outcome have produced general indications but no special findings.

Fatal intoxication through methanol and other alcohols such as ether, glycols, and trivalent alcohols rarely lead to appropriate histological findings. The following changes are worth pointing out: vacuolar degeneration in cardiac muscle cells in methanol poisoning (Prokop 1950); renal and cerebral lesions following intoxication with ethylene glycol, in which the microscopic evidence of calcium oxalate crystals in the renal tubules and walls of cerebral vessels should be observed (Patscheider and Hetzel 1961).

In rhesus monkeys, methanol produced thickening and clumping of the mitochondria, destruction of the neurotubuli, and vesicles in the axons of the optic nerve.

Pesticides

The active substances comprising this group differ mainly in their chemical composition, physical characteristics, and mode of action. Many of these substances have a strong toxic effect on humans; they include convulsive, respiratory, blood, metabolic, and corrosive toxins. These qualities also permit a toxicological grouping to be made (Geldmacher v. Mallinckrodt 1975). The presentation of histologically detectable toxic effects will follow the toxicological division. The toxins involved here are quick-acting and, with an appropriate dose and intake, lead to death within a short period of time, usually less than an hour. Accordingly, the histomorphological findings are mainly restricted to the signs of acute death. The sparse histological findings are unspecific and can only be determined after a special examination. They are, however, suitable in supplementing the general finding of acute death from pesticide, even through negative assertions and the exclusion of other possibly fatal factors and illnesses.

E 605 (Parathion). Histologically detectable lesions that can be ascribed to the direct effect of E 605 have thus far not been proven. In short survival times, up to 35 min after intake of E 605, Adebahr (1960) was able to determine epithelial necroses in the straight sections of the renal tubules. In the epithelia of the remaining renal cortical sections, pronounced plasma granulation, nuclear wall hyperchromatosis and clumping and reduction in the chromatin and marginal nucleoli were found. The epithelia in Henle's loops and collecting tubules were severely swollen. Adebahr regards the cause of the particularly short time until the appearance of epithelial necroses as due to an interplay of massive toxic influx in the kidneys with toxically incurred hypoxia and hypotonia.

Studies of the hepatic parenchyma in 178 cases of E 605 poisoning showed in part the typical symptoms of opaque swelling and glycogen depletion (Adebahr 1963). The liver apparently shows resistance to E 605 or its oxidation product. This property is explained by the capability of the liver to inactivate cholinesterase-inhibiting substances and to be able itself to form serum cholinesterase. Clinically, transitory hepatic lesions have been observed in very severe cases of nonfatal E 605 poisoning, the patients being saved by Toxogonin treatment (Barkow et al. 1969; Boelke and Gaaz 1970). In the histological examination of 30 cases of Wofatox intoxication (methyl parathion) destructive changes in the liver cell strands, detached epithelia, and perivascular edemas were found (Fazekas 1971). Fine-maculate perivascular hemorrhages were detected in the myocardium, medulla oblongata, and vagal nucleus area of the brain. Multiple circumscribed necroses could be produced in the skeletal musculature of rats within 2 weeks of intraperitoneal administration of E 605 (Kibler 1973). In the lungs of rats that had been poisoned with an "organic phosphorous substance", Astolfi et al. (1970) found lesions of the epithelium and basement membrane in the terminal bronchial sections. Clefts were light-microscopically evident in the zona pellucida of the ripe, nonovulated human ovum following E 605 poisoning. The oolemma was damaged, in parts to the extent of necrosis (Fig. 159) (Adebahr 1966, 1970, 1971). Contrary to earlier observations, necroses did not occur in the tubular epithelia of the kidneys until after a matter of days in the case of simultaneous barbiturate poisoning, which leads to a depression of tissue respiration. Investigations of the glomus caroticum in humans in 23 cases of E 605 poisoning revealed interesting cytological changes, including an increase in the number of dark-cell nuclei (Täschner 1973). This is probably the consequence of increased nuclear metabolism owing to augmented demand, which, after the exhaustion of the glomus caroticum as a regulatory system, leads to pyknosis and hyperchromasia of the nuclei.

A phosphororganic pesticide used in Poland which has the designation "Naled" gave rise to cytoplasmic changes and circumscribed necroses in the central nervous system and liver in animal experiments (Sosnierz et al. 1970).

Nicotine. A histological examination of 48 cases of acute nicotine poisoning, including three cases of murder, revealed indications of a general shock, which was interpreted as the result of increased activity of the sympathoadrenal system (Fazekas and Kósa 1964, 1970). Additional findings were: dissociation of liver cells, high-grade hemorrhagic pulmonary edema, detachment of the alveolar epithelia, necroses and detachment of the epithelia in the straight and convoluted renal tubules. These lesions were attributed by the authors to a direct, cytolytic toxic effect of the nicotine. The findings presented in the reports are not, however, convincing as specific consequences of the effects of nicotine.

In acute fatal nicotine poisoning in humans and experimentally in rats, Adebahr and Voigt (1963) found plaque-like granulations in the cytoplasm of centrolobular and intermediary liver cells, aqueous impregnation and vacuolization of the arterial wall with lacerations of the elastica interna, and intrapulmonary hemorrhages. The lesions of the arterial walls are connected with the extreme fluctuations in blood pressure from the effects of nicotine. Interesting experiments on rabbits, in which a 1% nicotine solution was injected daily for up to 60 days, were concerned with chronic changes to the aorta wall. The observations included the development of a subendothelial edema, with subsequent fibrosis and the formation of abundant elastic fibers until about day 20 of the experiment. After this, there were changes to the aortic media with degeneration of the smooth musculature and elastic fibers, which formed fusiform fragments, disintegrated, became necrotic, and showed ear-

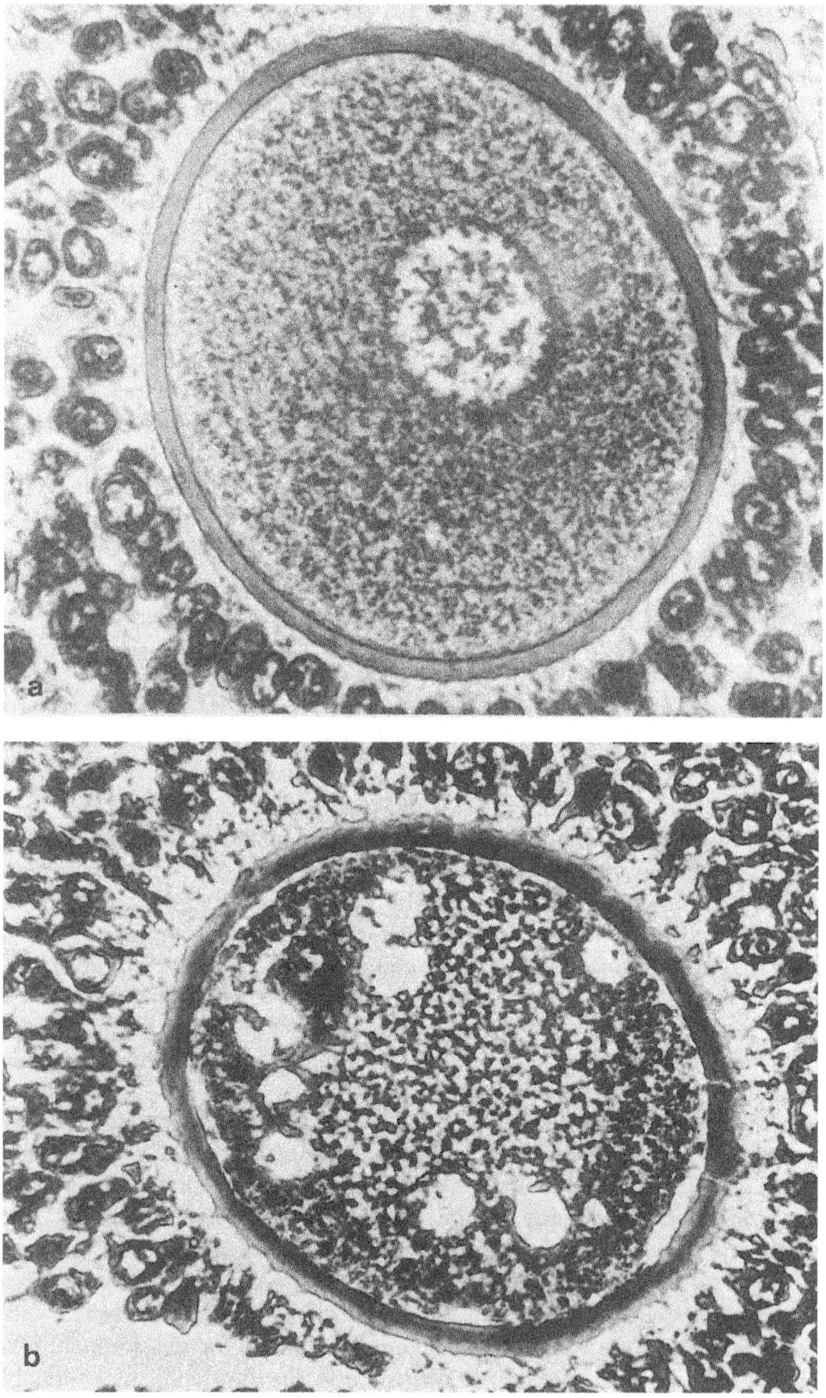
a
b

ly calcification (Grosgogeat and Roubelakis 1965). With good reason, these changes following nicotine administration have been compared with those after the effects of adrenaline. It is assumed that nicotine acts via the mechanism of catecholamine release.

Paraquat. This preparation is used as a herbicide in agriculture. In acute poisoning, it leads to local cauterization, states of agitation, and oliguria. Several days after intake of the toxin, distinctive symptoms develop which in their pneumotropism are characteristic for paraquat (dimethyl dipyridilium). These symptoms are changes in the lungs, with the development of a pulmonary edema, hyaline membranes, and capillary hemorrhages. In protracted intoxication, the pulmonary changes are not dominant until about 1 week after the beginning of toxin intake. This form of poisoning, which has become more frequent in recent years and which, because of its particular pathological course and histological findings, has often been reported, has been extensively observed and researched in numerous reports and some animal experimental studies (Tilling 1968; Lanzinger et al. 1969; Iff et al. 1971; Grabensee et al. 1971; Kimbrough and Linder 1971; Kodagoda et al. 1973; Eisenmenger et al. 1974; Borchard et al. 1974; Okonek 1976; Grabinski 1975; Neoral et al. 1977).

Histologically, the following findings in pulmonary tissue should be particularly emphasized. At the beginning of the toxic process, severe degenerative changes develop in the pneumonocytes with fatty infiltration, desquamation, necrosis, and detachment. Subsequently, there is splintering of the basement membranes, fragmentation, aneurysmal formation, multiple ruptures with hemorrhages, and escape of fibrinous edematous fluid into the interstitium and alveoli. Regular hyaline membranes develop in places. Of particular significance is then the onset of extensive mesenchymal interstitial and epithelial proliferations, which lead to a filling of the alveoli and large-scale dissolution of the pulmonary structure (Fig. 160). Intra-alveolar hematoxylin bodies could also be produced in animal experiments along with paraquat-induced respiratory distress syndrome (Hundsdörfer and Röse 1980). Similar findings in the lungs also occur in cadmium intoxication, advanced Hamman-Rich syndrome, and in animal experiments with nitrosomethylurethane (Grabinski 1975). The development of peroxides and oxidation of cell membranes has been identified in animal experiment as being the cause of pulmonary lesions from paraquat poisoning. In humans, the formation of hydrogen peroxide is similarly regarded as the probable damaging mechanism. Such a mode of action would also explain why the toxicity and lethality of paraquat is enhanced in intoxicated humans by oxygen-rich respiratory air (Neoral et al. 1977).

In the liver, centrolobular necroses, cholestasis, and giant mitochondria with paracrystalline inclusion bodies were found. Histological findings in the kidneys were mainly confined to opaque swellings and sporadic epithelial necroses. An extensive renal cortical necrosis was observed by Kodagoda et al. (1973). Edematous disaggregation of the sarcoplasm and sporadic fragmentation of the myofibrils were observed in the cardiac musculature. In all, it can be seen from the histomorphological findings that paraquat affects the lungs in an almost specific manner and leads to direct toxic lesions in other organs (Borchard et al. 1974).

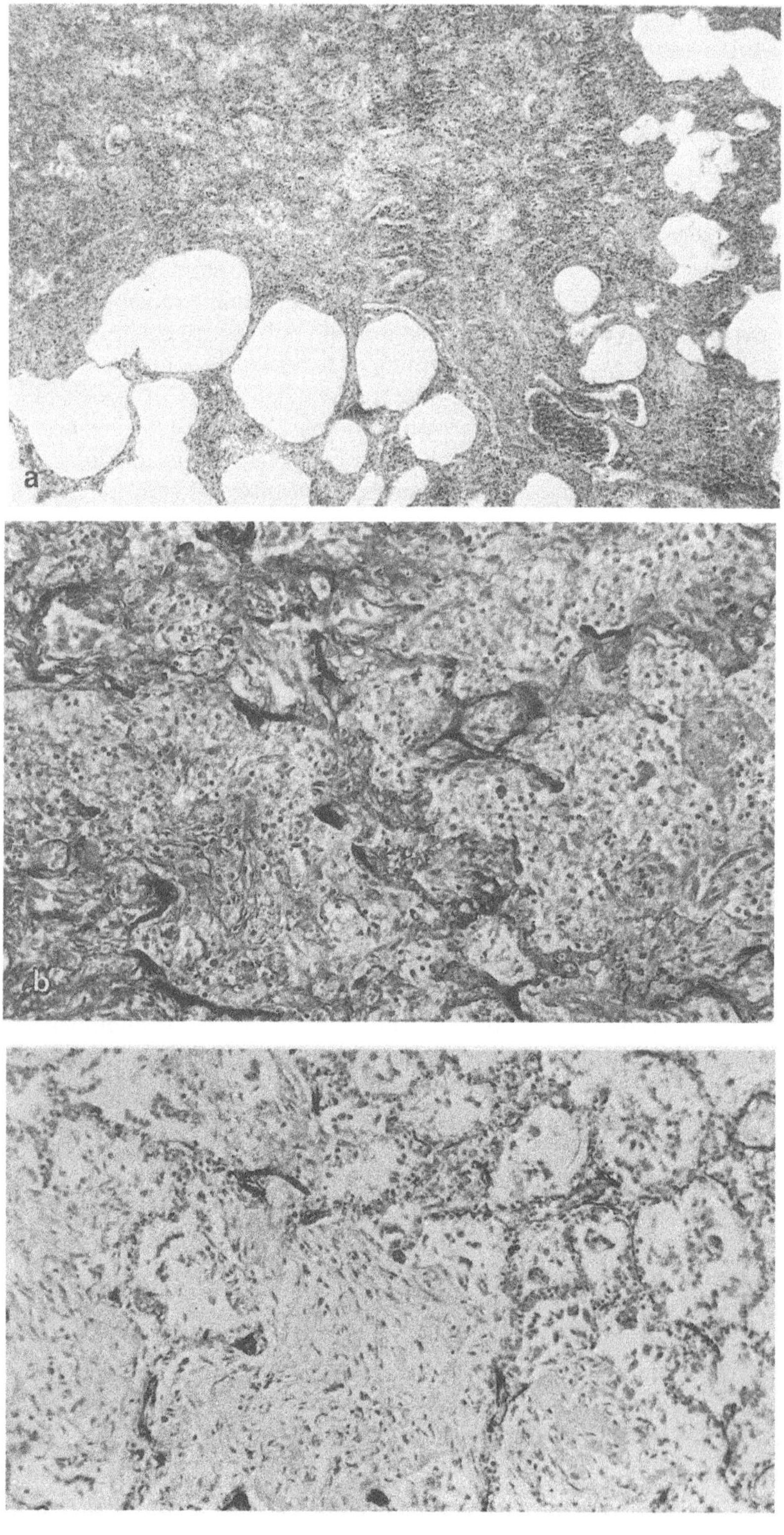

Fig. 160 a–c

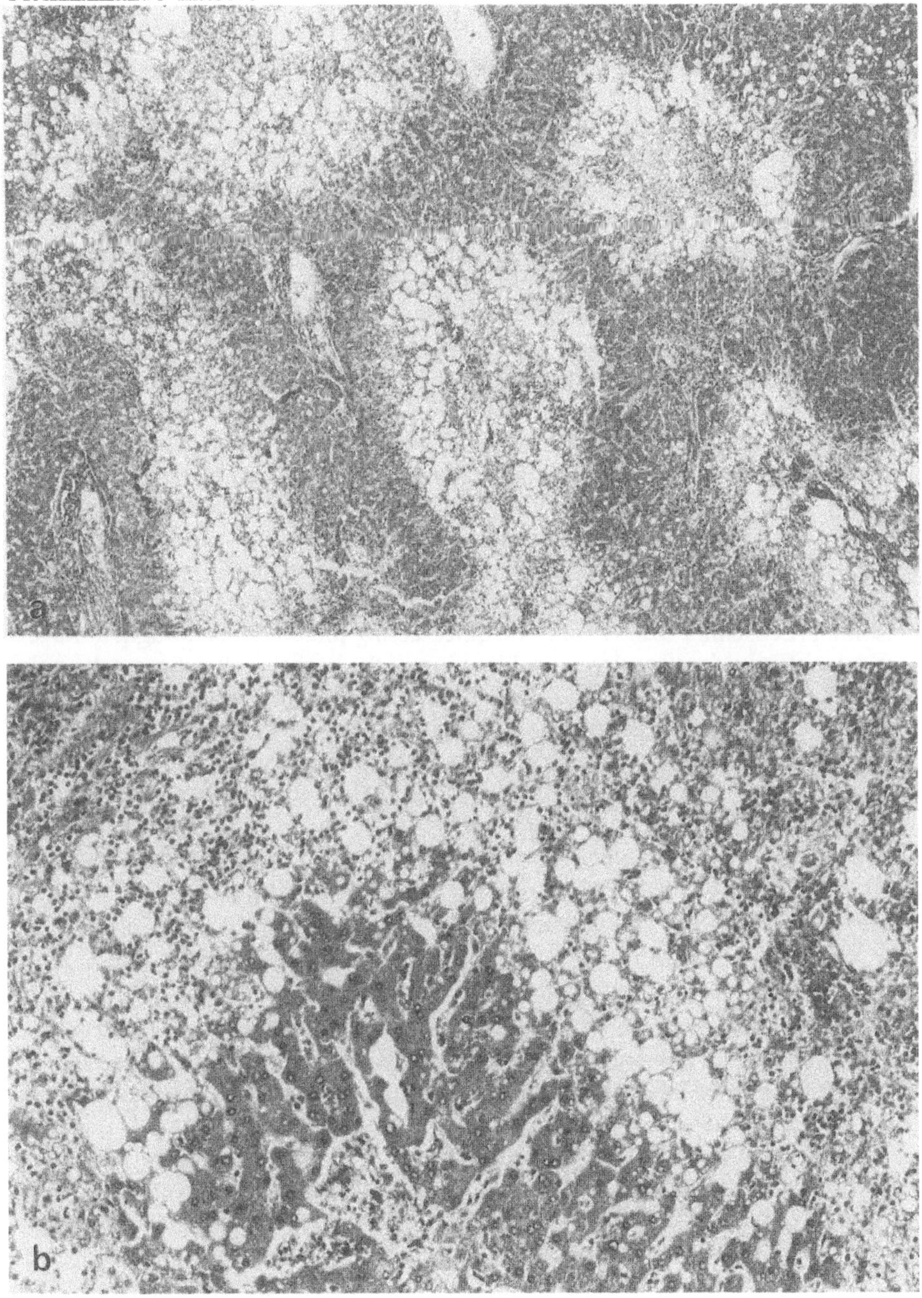

Fig. 161 a, b. Mycetismus *(Amanita phalloides)* with severe acute yellow atrophy. Subject 72 years old, ♀. H and E, 1:80, 1:250

◁ **Fig. 160 a–c.** Paraquat poisoning in the stage of mesenchymal and epithelial proliferations with extensive dissolution of the normal lung structure. Subject 56 years old, ♂. H and E and PTAH

Fungi

Mycetismus. Phalloidin from the destroying angel and death cap *(Amanita phalloides)* and its effects are the commonest cause of all forms of fatal mushroom poisoning. Phalloidin is a distinctly hepatic toxin, which leads to striking histological changes in this organ. On about the 3rd–5th day after eating *A.phalloides,* a severe acute hepatosis develops in the liver, which as a histological finding is analogous to typical acute yellow atrophy. In the initial stages, fatty infiltration of the liver epithelia is prominent. In many cases, this fatty infiltration is divided into three zones within the hepatic lobules. In centrolobular and peripheral areas, the droplets tend to be fine; in the intermediate zone they are coarser (Raszeja 1960). Later, single and grouped necroses, hemorrhages, necroses of Kupffer's cells, and leukocytic infiltrates on the border with undamaged lobules are observed. The necrotic breakdown mainly affects central areas of the lobules (Fig. 161). The portal connective tissue is, on the whole, only moderately infiltrated by inflammation. In experimental phalloid poisoning in rats, basically similar findings were produced in the liver (Koch et al. 1978; Schimassek and Jeckel 1978). In some cases, wholly necrotic hepatic lobules were found adjacent to relatively well preserved sections within the same organ. Electron microscopically, changes were evident in the nuclei, endoplasmic reticulum, and mitochondria in the liver tissue of patients suffering from *A.phalloides* poisoning (Leuschner et al. 1976). The quick-acting phalloidin is thought to have a particular affinity for the microsomal fraction of the hepatic cell, whereas the point of attack of the slower-working α-amanitine is believed to be in the nucleus. Outside the liver, general hemorrhagic diathesis and severe brain edema often exist (Moeschlin 1972; Krienke 1975). Isolated studies of mushroom poisoning in pregnant women have given rise to variable findings in the livers of the mother and fetus (Kaufmann et al. 1978; Slodkowska et al. 1980).

Contributory determinants in the extent and course of mycetismus are probably general factors such as age, sex, previous damage and function of the liver, and individual toxic qualities of the fungi ingested.

Drugs

The histologically detectable tissue changes caused by drugs cover a large area which extends from poisoning to therapeutically induced reactions or consciously accepted side effects. Lesions from drugs are found in accidental, suicidal, premeditated, and medicinal poisoning, e.g., as a result of a mistake or apparently false dosage. An area that can give rise to difficulties in differentiation concerns lesions connected with diagnostic and therapeutic measures. These injuries caused by false therapy have been scientifically studied as "pathology of therapy" or "iatrogenic pathology" (Thurner 1970).

There are direct or obligate toxic substances, which in appropriately high doses lead to injuries in all humans. In addition, there are, however, also substances that are "indirect" or "facultatively or potentially toxic" and lead to considerable, under certain circumstances fatal, injuries only in a small number of people (Altmann and Klinge 1972). The occurrence of hypersensitive reactions should also be considered in therapeutic dosage.

In the forensic assessment of drug-therapy lesions, the effects of the primary disease and therapeutic indication should themselves be given particular consideration. Owing to the mainly unspecific lesions, a list of morphological principal signs or differential diagnostic tables of poisoning, as could be applied clinically and pathologically, are of little practical use. A restriction to a summary presentation of a few forms of medicinal intoxication inducing specific tissue injury is thus more expedient.

Soporific Agents. This group of medicaments is still the commonest cause of all forms of poisoning. The main representatives of this group are the barbituric acid derivatives. The toxic effect is largely dependent on the dose administered. The toxic, excessive narcotic action proceeds via damage to central nervous regulation of respiration and circulation to circulatory disorders and hypoxic tissue lesions. Focal pneumonia, as a consequence of aspirations or bronchogenic infection, develops in the patients affected, who go into a deep state of unconsciousness with dysphagia and impaired ventilation of the lungs. These complications are still the most frequent direct cause of death in narcotic intoxication since cases often do not receive medical treatment in time. Histologically, these effects on the respiratory system do not show any specific characteristics. From the point of view of forensic medicine, however, bronchopneumonia should be considered, which appears under uncertain circumstances of death in young, otherwise healthy individuals. The finding in the lungs should then occasion specific toxicological investigation.

The behavior of mast cells was histologically examined in the lungs of guinea pigs following peroral high-dose narcotic poisoning (Rüdell et al. 1978). The release of mast cells and the reduction in their cell density in pulmonary tissue were significantly more pronounced after administration of bromine carbamide than after barbiturate intoxication.

In about 4%–7% of acute cases of barbiturate poisoning, blistering develops in the region of pressure sores on the skin within 24 h of intake, when the subject is in a state of unconsciousness (cf. p. 234). The dermal finding here is typical for this kind of intoxication. Histologically, the blistering is analogous to an acute serous inflammation, in which the epidermis including the upper basal cell layer becomes detached. Histological examination cannot be dispensed with in differentiating heat blisters from putrefactive vesicles.

Numerous uncharacteristic, mostly degenerative changes can occur in the skin and inner organs in acute and chronic soporific intoxication. They are not so much due to a direct toxic action as to the effects of circulatory disorders and hypoxia. These lesions occasionally develop as a result of shock or allergy.

In a few cases, necroses of the sweat glands and skeletal musculature have been observed in acute barbiturate poisoning (references in Geldmacher v. Mallinckrodt 1975). Following Adalin (carbromal) administration, punctiform and diffuse hemorrhages developed in the skin in the form of purpura pigmentosa progressiva via a delayed reaction allergy (Illig 1976). Histologically, the changes in this "Adalin purpura" are limited to the epidermis and upper corium. The hemorrhages and perivascular infiltrates are located in the papillary ridges; they are predominantly composed of mononuclear and eosinophilic cells. In older lesions, hemosiderin becomes deposited.

The findings in the brain, particularly after the use of narcotics, include symmetrical necroses in the pallidum, vacuolar formation and ischemic necroses of the Purkinje cells, pronounced edema, and changes resembling intermittent CO poisoning (Holczabek 1953; Meyer 1961; Peiffer 1963; Schweikert and Kapfhammer 1965).

In the vascular system, particularly in the capillaries of the lungs, liver, and kidneys, necroses and endothelial lesions were found together with desquamation, vacuolization, and high-grade fatty infiltration, at times as early as 10–12 h after the beginning of poisoning. Similar changes have also been detected in animal experiments in cardiac muscle and the aortic media (Schollmeyer 1961; Schweikert and Kopfhammer 1965; Hagedorn et al. 1975). Following an intra-arterially injected overdose of short-term narcotics, connective tissue thickening of the intima, with increasing secondary thrombosis, and necroses, with inflammatory reactions of the skeletal musculature in the associated circulatory area, were observed (Liebegott 1967). In experiments on bats, arterial obstruction could be produced in the same manner by blood platelets in the large wing arteries (Wiedemann et al. 1977).

The frequent pulmonary edema and degenerative lesions of the renal tubules do not have any indicative value with regard to poisoning, owing to their unspecific mode of origin (Kühn and Arnold 1963; Balzereit and Arnold 1965; Adebahr 1961).

The liver is a central target organ for soporific intoxication and the effects of many other drugs. The changes and lesions associated with drugs have been particularly extensively investigated in recent years (Altmann and Klinge 1972; Altmann 1980). Generally speaking, the connections between drugs and their effects in the liver are only clear in a few cases; they are usually complex and difficult to fathom. The condition of the particular hepatic cell affected and the individual as a whole, with regard to genetic constitution and specific enzyme supply, are just as significant as the type of drug.

The metabolism of barbiturates and many other substances in the liver is seen electron microscopically to effect an increase in the smooth endoplasmic reticulum and cytochrome P45, in the epithelia. Cytochrome P45 extensively participates in the degradation of lipophilic substances (Fouts and Rogers 1965; Altmann and Klinge 1972). Light microscopically, such metabolically strained liver epithelia show a pale-eosinophilic, sometimes fine-vacuolar cytoplasm. In addition, there is a displacement of basophilic plaques into the marginal areas of the cell, particularly into the region of the biliary pole. Electron microscopically, the plaques correspond to rough endoplasmic reticulum. Previous chronic inflammatory disorders and alcohol stress evidently have an adverse effect on tolerance to narcotics (Force and Miller 1974). A specific hepatotoxic effect could not be demonstrated for halothane (Scholler 1968; Kessler et al. 1975).

Reactions of the liver induced by drugs are less common in children than in adults. In principle, however, there is no difference in the form of the liver reaction (Klinge 1979). The danger of the combined effects of alcohol and drugs, leading rapidly to central death, is generally known (Geldmacher v. Mallinckrodt et al. 1976).

Pain-killers. Fatal poisoning with pyrazolic and salicylic acid derivatives and drugs of the phenacetin group does not offer any characteristic histological findings from which the kind of intoxication may be inferred. In pyrazol poisoning, the early acute inflammatory and degenerative changes in the proximal sections of the nephrons should be noted, where there is edema, swelling of the basal membrane in the glomeruli, fatty infiltration and necroses of the tubular epithelia, and protein precipitation in the glomerular capsules (Fazekas 1957, 1962). Conditions of shock also occasionally develop which histologically tend to involve the liver and adrenal glands (Okumura 1969). In poisoning with salicylic acid derivatives, a general hemorrhagic diathesis of the mucosa in the region of the gastrointestinal tract and serous coats is evident macroscopically and histologically. Ceraceous contractions and ruptures of the muscle fibers have been observed in the diaphragm after aspirin intoxication (Szabó 1940). Phenacetin poisoning similarly leads to hemorrhagic, inflammatory changes in the gastrointestinal tract and sporadically also to centrolobular liver necroses and necrobiotic changes of the epithelia in the distal renal tubules. Combined treatment with phenacetin and acetylsalicylic acid led after 12 months in animal experiments to flattening and atrophy of the epithelia and pronounced peritubular connective tissue proliferation in the renal tubules. In addition, intratubular calcium deposition was found. The glomeruli and proximal tubules, on the other hand, were not damaged (Clausen 1964). Marked fibroses of the papillary apices in the kidneys could be produced in rabbits by administration of phenacetin alone. In humans after phenacetin abuse of several years' duration severe renal damage gradually develops, which has become known as "phenacetin kidney" (Zollinger 1966; Gsell 1974). Histologically, this renal damage corresponds to a chronic interstitial nephritis, with shrinking of the entire renal parenchyma and formation of necroses in the papillary apices.

The chronic effects of phenacetin or aminophenazone lead to a macroscopically and histologically particularly striking lipofuscinosis in the liver, kidneys, and cardiac musculature. The formation of lipofuscin is due to peroxidation of unsaturated lipids caused by free radicals. As a result, polymeral residual products remain which are difficult or impossible to break down (Altmann and Klinge 1972; Hübner 1976). The stimulating effect of phenacetin could be due to a disturbance in the normal degradation of lipids. An abnormally increased level of lipofuscin is a histological basis for suspecting phenacetin abuse. Lipofuscinosis has proof value in this regard if the granules are of particular size and are present not only at the biliary pole of the liver epithelia, but also in the whole cell and in the epithelia of the lobule periphery. The individual granules are, relative to their structure and maturity, of variable size; they are either pale and rounded, have an almost droplet-form, or have a more polymorphic character with a bright or dark individual shade. A change in liver function is not connected with the increase in pigment. Occasionally, however, solitary hepatic cell necroses and secondary pigment desposits are found in the phagocytotic stellate cells.

Hallucinogens, Opiates, Psychopharmacological Agents, and Stimulants. Fatal poisoning by the groups of drugs in this section rarely leads to histologically detectable organ lesions capable of providing a good diagnostic indication of the cause of death. Careful determination and analysis of these lesions together with toxicological investigations is an essential part of the often difficult clarification and objectification of "drug death." These substances are basically capable, under certain circumstances, of producing dependence and addiction. Clarification of death incurred as a result, either through fatal intoxication or auxiliary fatal complications, becomes very difficult if the case history and the known details do not provide unequivocal indications and if toxicologically the "drug" cannot be detected with certainty in the body of the deceased. In such a situation, the histologically reliable exclusion of natural causes of death or evidence of indirect sequelae or concomitant diseases connected with drug administration can be useful.

A great many isolated findings have already been described concerning consumers of narcotics (Gerber 1976; Gerlach 1978; Gerlach et al. 1978; Montalto et al. 1978; Metter 1978). They mainly concern lesions connected with the form of drug administration and contamination and accompanying infections. Thus far, it has not been clarified with certainty whether these lesions are caused directly by the effects of the drugs.

The findings in the liver, lungs, and heart are of prime importance in fatal cases of drug abuse. In the liver, inflammatory disorders are dominant. Of 80 fatal cases of drug abuse, Beckmann and Püschel (1982) found unspecific reactive hepatitis in 17 cases (21.2%), chronic persistent hepatitis in 25 cases (31.2%), drug or "hippy" hepatitis in 6 cases (7.5%), chronic active hepatitis in 9 cases (11.1%), transition to cirrhosis of the liver in 6 cases (7.5%), and acute yellow atrophy in one case. The histologically detectable effects of viral infections should be taken into account; they can be observed comparatively often predominantly in intravenous drug consumption (Heilmann et al. 1970; Eknoyan et al. 1973; Aenishänslin et al. 1975). By means of biopsy case control studies in drug addicts, clinical case controls, and determination of hepatitis antigen status, it has become clear in recent years that inflammatory hepatic changes in drug addicts are due to a viral etiology in the vast majority of cases (Beckmann and Püschel 1982). The inoculation of hepatitis viruses is chiefly accounted for by the use of contaminated syringes.

The effects on the lungs are largely chronic, unspecific changes such as edema, bronchitis, bronchiectasis, emphysema, and sclerotic changes to the pulmonary vessels. Numerous intra-alveolar macrophages are commonly found. Pulmonary foreign-body granulomas, which are largely perivascular, should be particularly observed. They contain material that entered the bloodstream during intravenous administration and which then spread as a granuloma-inducing effect in the lungs. Püschel (1982) found such pulmonary granulomas in 50% of 50 fatal cases of drug abuse. In one case, talcum was identified in the granulomas. Combined with the evidence of foreign-body granulomas near injection sites, the detection of similar foreign-body granulomas in the lungs signifies a distinct indication of previous intravenous drug consumption (Fig. 162).

Histological investigation of other inner organs, particularly the cardiac muscle, kidneys, and brain, usually provides findings that point to a general infection (Möllhoff and Schmidt 1976).

One special feature concerns fatal cases after the nasal application of heroin (Püschel et al. 1980). Chronic inflammations of the nasal mucosa and squamous metaplasias were histologically identified in such cases.

Fig. 162. a Foreign-body granuloma with talcum inclusions in the wall of an elbow vein following drug injection. H and E, 1:200. **b, c** Granuloma in the pulmonary circulation following drug administration. Foam cells and foreign-body inclusions in the walls of small arterioles. H and E, 1:550, 1:280

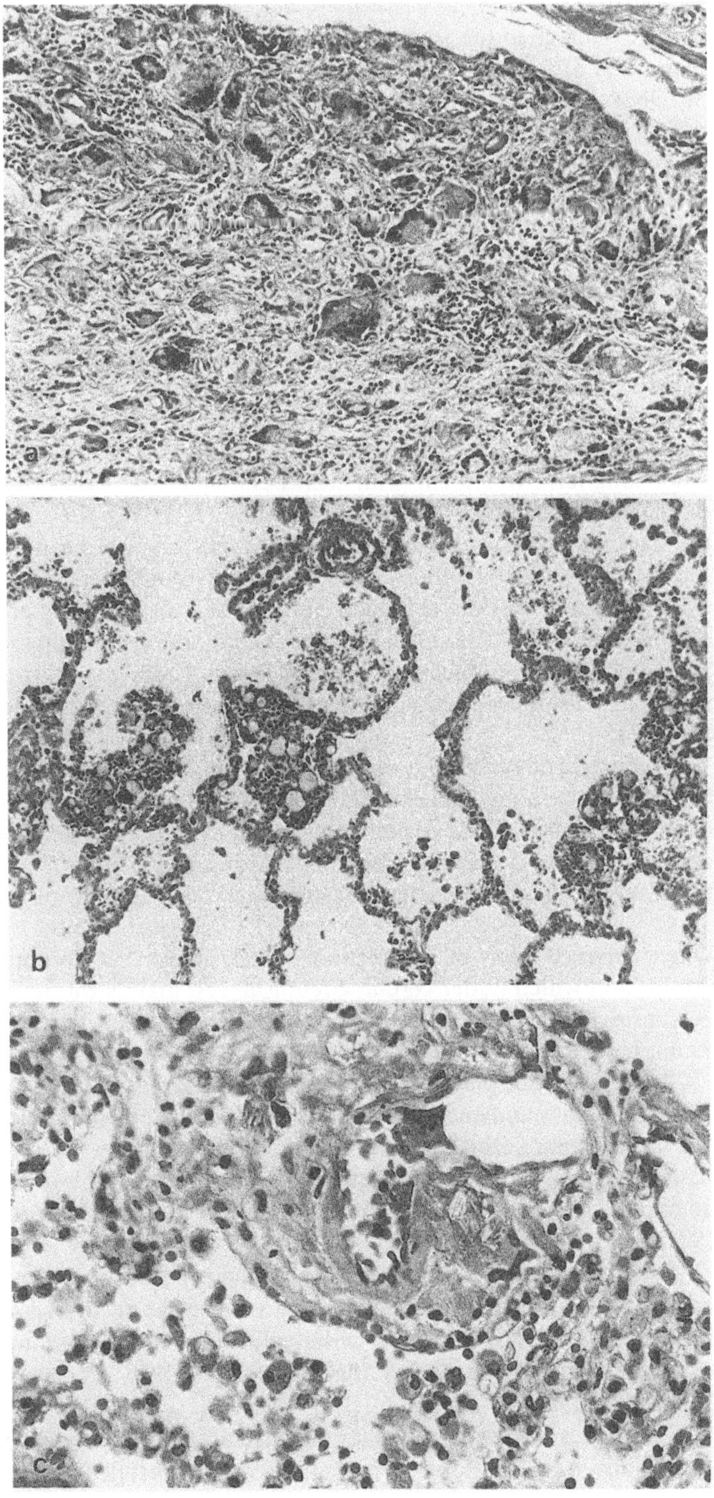

Fig. 162 a–c

Some phenothiazine derivatives, e.g., chlorpromazine, can also directly cause hepatic damage in the form of typical cholestatic hepatosis (Moeschlin 1972; Altmann and Klinge 1972; Altmann 1980). This "chlorpromazine icterus" clinically develops with the symptoms of an extrahepatic obstructive jaundice. Other histological findings in the liver are typical mechanical jaundice, biliary thrombi in the bile capillaries, bile pigment inclusions in hepatic and swollen Kupffer's cells, sporadic cell infiltrates in the portal connective tissue, and liver cell necroses.

In the case of inadvertent intra-arterial injection of phenothiazines, gangrene of the hand and lower arm developed. Histoligically, necrotizing inflammations of the arterioles could be detected in this region (Heber and Helmig 1976).

A pathogenetically still unclarified organic tropism has been observed in connection with the consumption of amphetamine derivatives. Following abuse of appetite depressants, e.g., menocil, over a period of many years, lethal pulmonary hypertension resulted. Histologically, this fatal pulmonary disease resembled severe diffuse pulmonary arteriosclerosis (Moeschlin 1972; Kaindl 1971; Lang et al. 1969). After long-term treatment with dextroamphetamine because of depression, cardiomegaly developed in a 45-year-old man, which with the signs of a severe biventricular cardiac insufficiency led to death. Histological examination revealed cardiomyopathy with diffuse necroses of the individual fibers, lymphocytic and histiocytic infiltrates, and disseminated fibrotic foci; the coronary arteries were delicate (Smith et al. 1976). There is a hypothesis that high amphetamine doses over a long period of time can induce a myocardial lesion. Panmyelophthisis was also once observed in a 28-year-old patient after 8 years' abuse of appetite depressants (Lisch et al. 1977).

Hypoxic delayed lesions of the brain as an indirect result of the chronic effect of heroin were found by Strassmann et al. (1969) in postmortem examinations of death from drug abuse. These lesions comprised symmetrical necroses in the pallidum and glial, cell, and vascular reactions. According to our own histological investigations, severe disorders in spermiogenesis and testicular atrophy can also occur.

Other Drugs. By way of completion, several drugs that do not fall into particular groups and which under certain circumstances, mainly through overdosage or hypersensitivity, can lead to histologically detectable tissue lesions are described with examples below.

Anticoagulants, particularly coumarin derivatives, which cause a reduced coagulative tendency and an increase in vascular permeability, can in the case of overdosage or particular pathological concomitant circumstances lead to a general hemorrhagic diathesis. Cholestatic hepatoses, central liver cell necroses, stomatitis, and dermal necroses have also been described in this connection (Geipel 1969; Linke 1971).

Cytostatic drugs lead occasionally to fatal complications through damage to the hematogenic bone marrow; they also lead to hepatic necroses, glomerular necroses, and severe pulmonary changes, with hyaline membranes and intra-alveolar and interstitial fibroses (Rizzi 1962; Lange and Dippell 1970; Cochran and Watson 1969; Gebbers et al. 1975).

Antibiotics and tuberculostatic agents can lead to severe conditions of shock and lesions in the case of hypersensitivity or uncontrolled administration. It is well known, for instance, that chloramphenicol has a cytostatic effect on the bone marrow, involving the development of aplastic anemia. In the liver, "toxic cellular swellings" are found with abnormal glycogen accumulation and distended, vesiculose liver epithelia, which also present a peribiliary basophilia (Klinge 1973). Sometimes there are also individual and lobule necroses in the liver. Other antibiotics, e.g., cephalothin, prove to be exceptionally nephrotoxic and lead to acute renal failure with histological signs of severe damage to the tubules and epithelial necroses (Müller et al. 1973). The development of fatal ulcerative enteropathy indirectly through antibiotic disturbance of the normal intestinal flora has also been reported.

Further lesions develop, for example through purgatives with phenolisatin; "laxative hepatitis" is familiar. This involves cholestatic partly necrotizing hepatitis, which can also develop into cirrhosis (Lindner et al. 1975). Chloroquine and atebrine cause vacuolar muscular degeneration, hemolysis, and liver necroses (Rewcastle and Humphrey 1965; Bonciu et al. 1962). Acute liver atrophy developed through the inhalation of a barium-sulfur salt (Tovo 1962). Strychnine gives rise to degeneration of the anterior motor horn cells (C. Yates and D. Yates 1964), and camphor can lead to hypoxic cerebral lesions (Illchmann-Christ 1952).

Hormones. According to the general definition of poisoning, certain hormones must also be taken into account here, since when externally introduced they can also lead to diseases with tissue lesions and fatal complications.

Insulin. Experience in postmortem diagnosis of death through insulin overdosage has predominantly been obtained in cases of suicide and sporadically also in cases of murder (Pioch 1960; Zschiesche 1962). The possibilities for making a conclusive morphological diagnosis of acute death from hypoglycemia are limited. Only after a survival time of a few hours can disseminated necroses in the liver, cardiac muscle, and medulla of the cerebral hemispheres be found. Such findings are accompanied by uncharacteristic fine-droplet fatty infiltration of the liver and cardiac muscle.

Cortisone and Cortisone Derivatives. Following long-term treatment with high doses of corticosteroids, hypercortisonism, steroid pseudorheumatism, and degenerative and inflammatory lesions come into consideration here. The consequences to the liver, skeletal system, skeletal musculature, mucosa of the gastrointestinal tract, and arterial vascular system deserve attention (Jansen 1977). Steroid cardiomyopathy and steroid nephropathy also occur. In the following section, the essential histological findings are summarized.

Liver: In humans and in animal experiments centrolobular epithelial necroses and fatty infiltration (Fleischer and Riedel 1964; Simon et al. 1964; Bässler 1961).

Skeletal System: Aseptic osteonecroses in the form of bone infarcts, particularly in the heads of the femur and humerus. Direct causes are probably inflammatory and edematous vascular occlusions (Uehlinger 1964; Janssen 1967).

Skeletal Musculature: Coagulation necroses with resorptive inflammations and cicatrization, particularly in the musculature of the extremities (Janssen 1962; Smith 1964).

Arteries: Proliferating endarteritis and periarteritis nodosa, generalized or with the tendency to affect individual organs (Janssen and Michot 1960; Wunderer and Schuch 1963).

Gastrointestinal Tract: "Steroid ulcerations" similar to shock ulcers, without penetration, mainly restricted to the mucosa with sparse inflammatory reaction (Robert and Nezamis 1964; Hoffmeister 1967).

Kidneys: Nodular glomerulosclerosis, necrotizing nephrosis, renal cortical necroses, fibrinous casts of the renal arterioles and glomerular capillaries (Klima and Ort 1966; Wilson et al. 1962; Nienhaus et al. 1963).

Brain: After intrathecal methotrexate therapy and irradiation in the case of lymphoblastic leukemia, a necrotizing encephalopathy developed in three cases (Liu et al. 1978).

Contraceptives, Ovulation Inhibitors. The thromboses and embolisms observed after long-term therapy do not show histologically any particular characteristics. Primary disorders of the vein walls cannot be histologically excluded in the region of thromboses (Müller 1965; Pesendorfer and Platthy 1973; Radford and Oliver 1973). Thromboses of the cerebral arteries with apoplexy in young women histologically revealed intimal edema and endothelial and intimal proliferations, which are directly linked with the effect of ovulation inhibition (Goertchen 1973; Wohlfeil et al. 1973; Voit and Dorndorf 1971; Kühne and Götze 1978). Occasionally, fatal hepatic vein thromboses have also been detected that histomorphologically corresponded to a Budd-Chiari syndrome (Asbeck et al. 1972). Cases of "steroid hepatitis" deserve emphasis; they are histologically striking as a typical cholestatic hepatitis and are accompanied by pronounced lipofuscinosis (Stoll et al. 1966; Altmann and Klinge 1972). Recently, a great deal has been reported about the occurrence of tumors in the liver following the use of oral contraceptives (Dammermann et al. 1979; Lesch et al. 1980; Eisenburg 1981). Histologically, these are evident as hepatocellular adenomas and carcinomas.

D. References

References to A–B I: Introduction, Postmortem Changes

Adebahr G (1963) Zur Genese traumatischer Pallidum-, Balken- und Marknekrosen. Dtsch Med Wochenschr 88: 2097

Adler CP (1969) Verändert sich der DNS-Gehalt des Myokards postmortal? Experimentelle Untersuchungen am Bullenherzen. Autumn meeting of German pathologists, Wiesbaden, 10 Oct 1969

Althoff H (1974) Bei welchen Fragestellungen kann man aussagefähige pathomorphologische Befunde nach Exhumierung erwarten? Z Rechtsmed 75: 1

Altmann HW (1955) Allgemeine morphologische Pathologie des Zytoplasmas. Die Pathobiosen. Springer, Berlin Göttingen Heidelberg, p 427 (Handbuch der Allgemeinen Pathologie, vol 2/1)

Andersen H (1960) Post-mortem autolysis in human fetuses and its influence in some histochemical reactions. Acta Pathol microbiol Scand 50: 225

Ardenne M v, Reitnauer PG, Rohde K (1970) Messungen des pH-Verlaufs im Großhirn der Ratte bei Eintritt des Todes aus verschiedener Ursache. Dtsch Gesundheitswesen 25: 1677

Arnoldt F (1937) Über die Einwirkung von sauren und alkalischen Lösungen auf Organschnitte und ihre Beziehungen zur Karyolyse. Virchows Arch 229: 710

Aschoff L (1925) Über die Bedeutung der pathologischen Anatomie für Medizin und Naturwissenschaften. In: Vorträge über Pathologie. Gustav Fischer, Jena

Bakulev SN (1966) Blood changes in the area of the liversspots in violent and sudden death. Sud Med Ekspert (Mosk.) 9: 3 (1966) Ref Z Gerichtl Med 60: 330

Bandmann H (1977) Exhumierungen im Auftrag von Berufsgenossenschaften. – Fragestellungen, Ergebnisse, Aussagewert. Dissertation Hamburg

Beek van C, Haex AJCh (1943) Der Anteil der postmortalen Autolyse an der Nekrose des Leberparenchyms bei subakuter Leberatrophie. Ned Tijdschr Geneeskd 26: 6

Beneke G (1970) Veränderungen der Leber im Schock. In: Horatz K, Leber- und Pankreasschäden durch Schock und Narkose. Hrsg.: Thieme, Stuttgart, p 2

Beneke G (1972) Altersbestimmungen von Verletzungen innerer Organe. Z Rechtsmed 71: 1

Berg S (1957) Beiträge zur Gewinnung und Bewertung von Befunden in der forensischen Haaruntersuchung. Dtsch Z Ges Gerichtl Med 46: 531

Berg S (1963) Zur Todeszeitbestimmung bei Skelettbefunden. Beitr Gerichtl Med 12: 18

Berg S (1964) Die Altersbestimmung von Skelettbefunden als forensische und archäologische Aufgabe. Münch Med Wochenschr 21: 989

Berg S (1972) Die Altersbestimmung von Hautverletzungen. Z Rechtsmed 70: 121

Berg S, Specht W (1958) Untersuchungen zur Bestimmung der Liegezeit von Skeletten. Dtsch Z Gerichtl Med 47: 209

Berg S, Döring G, Suchenwirth H, Weiner K-L (1969) Beobachtungen über das Verhalten von Fettwachsleichen in größerer Wassertiefe. Arch Kriminol 143: 148

Bernardi DeA, Gatti R (1963) Di una nuova tecnica microfluoroscopica per la dimonstratione delle architettura dei parenchimi putrefatti e per il loro riconoscimento. Minerva Med 83: 126

Bernardi DeA, Tappero P (1964) Gli aspetti microfluoroscopici dell' edema polmonare. II. Possibilità di una diagnose differenziale con il liquame putrefattivo. Minerva Med 84: 14

Bernheim P, Willot M, Muller P (1966) Quelques aspects de l'autolyse du muscle strié humain aux microscopes optique et électronique. Ann Med Leg 46: 447

Born E (1959) Über natürliche Mumifizierungen. Zentrbl Allg Pathol 99: 490

Borra G (1966) Possibilitá di diagnosi istopatologia delle neoplasie in cadaveri esumati. A. proposito di una osservazione di carcinoma gastrico con metastasi epatiche. Arch Soc Lombarda Med Leg 2: 30
Bradley HC (1938) Autolysis and atrophy. Physiol Rev 18: 173
Braun-Falco O, Winter W (1964) Untersuchungen über die Autolyse der Haut. Histochemische Veränderungen: Morphologische Veränderungen Arch Klin Exp Dermatol 220: 344 u. 417
Bryc R, Tomaszewska Z, Sawa J (1972) A histological study to determine aeration of the lungs of newborn infants in cases of mummification. Forensic Sci Int 1: 189
Büchner F (1959) Die Veränderungen der Ultrastruktur der Herzmuskelzelle bei Störungen der Aerobiose. Aerztl Forsch 131: 307
Burck H-C (1966) Histologische Techniken. Leitfaden für die Herstellung mikroskopischer Präparate in Unterricht und Praxis. Thieme, Stuttgart
Buss H (1970) Histochemische Frühdiagnose des experimentellen Herzinfarktes unter Berücksichtigung der Autolyse. Beitr Pathol Anat 140: 257
Caesar R (1962) Elektronenmikroskopische Untersuchungen bei der Autolyse in vivo. Zentralbl Allg Pathol 103: 154
Carvalho HV, de (1964) Ultra vital reactions. Acta Med Leg Soc (Liege) 17: 65
Colmant H (1965) Cerebrale Hypoxie. Thieme, Stuttgart
Cook M, Osvaldo L, Jackson JD, Latta H (1965) Changes in renal glomeruli during autolysis. Electron microscopic observations. Lab Invest 14: 623
Cossel L (1966) Elektronenmikroskopische Befunde beim intravitalen Untergang von Leberepithelzellen. Beitrag zur Kenntnis von Kolliquations- und Koagulationsnekrose. Beitr Pathol Anat 133: 156
Daldrup T (1979) Postmortaler Eiweißzerfall in menschlichen Organen. – Reaktionen und zeitliche Zusammenhänge. Dissertation, Triltsch, Düsseldorf
David E, Marx I, David H (1970) Das ultrastrukturelle Bild der Nervenzellen in verschiedenen Regionen des Meerschweinchengehirns im Verlauf der postmortalen Autolyse. Exp Pathol (Jena) 5: 98
Derbarge A, Wiliot M, Muller P (1966) Etude histologique de l'autolyse expérimentale du muscle strié du cobaye. Ann Med Leg 46: 440
Dietrich A (1904) Die an aseptisch aufbewahrten Organen auftretenden morphologischen Veränderungen in ihren Beziehungen zur „Autolyse". Verh Dtsch Ges Pathol 6: 81
Eder M (1969) Histochemische Fermentnachweise – ihre Bedeutung in der Pathologie. Verh Dtsch Ges Pathol 42: 374
Evans E (1962) Some histological findings in spontaneously preserved bodies. Med Sci Law 2: 155
Fallani M (1961) Contributo allo studio della circolazione ematica postmortale. Minerva Med Leg (Torino) 81: 108
Fasske E (1964) Lehrbuch der histologischen Technik. Urban & Schwarzenberg, München Berlin
Fitting W (1950) Über die Bedeutung histologischer Knochenmarksuntersuchung. Klin Wochenschr 28: 783
Fornari A, Pierucci G (1965) Le possibilità di diagnosi istopatologica sui polmoni putrefatti. Arch Soc Lombarda Med Leg Assicuraz 1: 7
Frank KH (1971) Konservierende Leichenerscheinungen in der Umgebung von Metallgegenständen. 3. Tagung der Gesellschaft für gerichtliche Medizin der DDR, 1.10. 1971 Berlin
Fukita K, Sugimoto M (1966) The effect of vinyl on postmortem changes. Acta Crim Med Leg Jap 32: 184
Gallagher CH, Judah JD, Rees KR (1956) Enzyme changes during liver autolysis. J Pathol 72: 247
Gallos P (1960) Biochemical significance of myocardial tissue changes associated with rigor mortis, under normal conditions and in experimental poisoning with gammahexane. Cardiology [Suppl I] 37: 1
Gerin C (1965) Les méthodes histologiques en médecine légale. 30. Inter Kongr Gerichtl Soz Med Coimbra 3.–7.5. 1965
Giesler E (1927) Über die Möglichkeit, bei exhumierten Leichen exakte pathologisch-anatomische Diagnosen zu stellen. Zentralbl Allg Pathol 40: 139
Gilli R, De Bernardi A, Baima-Bollone PL (1967) Degli aspetti cito-morfologici dell'edema delle fibre cardiache e della possobilità di una loro sicura differenziazione dagli aspetti indotti in tali fibre dai fenomeni transformativi postmortali. Arch Soc Lombarda Med Leg 3: 400

Glanzmann E (1941) Physiologie der Leukozyten nach den Arbeiten von 1929–1940. Rev Physiol Biochem Pharmacol 44: 473
Goebel A (1955) Die Pathologie des Mineralstoffwechsels der Zelle. Springer, Berlin Göttingen Heidelberg (Handbuch der Allgemeinen Pathologie, Bd. II/1, p 398)
Gössner W (1955) Untersuchungen über das Verhalten der Phosphatasen und Esterasen während der Autolyse. Virchows Arch 327: 304
Gössner W (1960) Studien zur Nekrose und Autolyse in vivo. Verh Dtsch Ges Pathol 44: 204
Goffin Y, Beeckmans Y (1973) Histochemistry of succinate dehydrogenase, glucose-6-phosphate dehydrogenase and NADPH tetrazolium reductase in human skin. I. Postmortem variations and effects of autolysis, and histotopography. II. Regional differences in histochemical activity. Forensic Sci 2: 221 u. 223
Gresham GA, Leithoff H (1977) Farbatlas der gerichtlichen Medizin. Schattauer, Stuttgart New York
Greuer W, Hess E, Rosteck I (1956) Ednogene proteolytische Fermente und ihre Bedeutung. Arzneim Forsch 6: 269
Griffin ChC, Waravdekar VS, Trumpf BF (1965) Studies on necrosis of mouse liver in vitro. Alterations in activities of succinoxidase, succinic dehydrogenase, glutamic dehydrogenase, acid phosphatase, uricase, glucose-6-phosphatase and NAD-pyrophosphorylase. Am J Pathol 47: 833
Grohme S, Schneider H, Masshoff W (1969) Encephalopathien bei Vita reducta. Internist 10: 430
Gropp A (1963) Morphologie und Verhalten lebender Zellen. Med Welt 20
Hadjioloff A (1929) A propos des phénoménes de fluorescence déterminés par la lumière de Wood au niveau des organes de l'homme et des animaux, à l'état frais, après autolyse et putréfaction et après calcination. C R Soc Biol (Paris) 102: 779
Harms D (1972) Über Thrombocytenzahl und Thrombocytenfunktion im Leichenblut. Med Welt 23: 975
Harraszti A, Korb G (1964) Fluoreszenzmikroskopische Untersuchungen an Leberzellnekrosen. Z Gesamt Inn Med 19: 129
Hecht A (1962) Untersuchungen über den Einfluß der Autolyse auf histochemische Veränderungen beim experimentellen Herzinfarkt der Ratte. Acta Biol Med German 8: 617
Helmer R (1970) Möglichkeiten und Methoden der zellkernmorphologischen Geschlechtserkennung an Körpergeweben und Sekretspuren. Schmidt-Römhild, Lübeck
Henn R (1971) Elektive Körnerzellnekrosen nach Trauma. 50. Jahrestag. Dtsch Ges Rechtsmed 3.–7. 10., Köln
Hilgermann R (1971) Neuere histochemische Erkenntnisse über die sog. Diffusionstotenflecken (keine perivasale Imbibition, sondern intravasale Hämokonzentration). 50. Jahrestag. Dtsch Ges Rechtsmed 3.–7. 10. 1971 Köln
Hilgermann R (1973 a) Histochemische Untersuchungen zur Frage der sogenannten Diffusions-Totenflecke. Habil Schrift, Marburg
Hilgermann R (1973 b) Neuere histochemische Erkenntnisse über die sogenannten Diffusions-Totenflecke. Leitz Mitteil f Wissenschf u Techn 4: 45
Hofmann ER v (1898) Lehrbuch der gerichtlichen Medizin, 8 edn Urban & Schwarzenberg, Wien, Leipzig
Hofmann ER v, Haberda A (1927) Lehrbuch der gerichtlichen Medizin 11 edn Urban & Schwarzenberg, Berlin, Wien
Holczabek W (1970) Über die chromotropen Lipoide (Lipoproteide) des Herzfleisches. Z Rechtsmed 67: 99
Holzner JH, Kaufmann F (1962) Der Einfluß der postmortalen Autolyse auf die histochemisch darstellbare Adenosintriphosphatase-(ATP-ase-)Aktivität. Pathol et Microbiol (Basel) 25: 193
Ikuta F, Hirano A, Zimmermann HM (1963) An experimental study of post-mortem alterations in the granular layer of the cerebellar cortex. J Neuropathol Exp Neurol 22: 581
Jannoni-Sebastianini G (1930) Ulteriori ricerche sull'influenza del dongelamento nel l'autolisi asettica postmortale. Arch di Antropol Criminol 50: 1515
Janssen W (1958) Morphologie und Pathogenese der Leukaemien. Habilitationsschrift, Leipzig 1958
Janssen W (1963) Riesenzellenbildung bei Erstickung. Dtsch Z Gerichtl Med 54: 200
Janssen W (1967) Zur Beurteilung von Blutungen der Leichenhaut, unter besonderer Berücksichtigung von Haematomen der Orbita. Dtsch Z Gerichtl Med 59: 69

Janssen W, Bärtschi G (1964) Vitale und supravitale Reaktionen der Alveolarzellen nach protrahiertem Sauerstoffmangel. Dtsch Z Gerichtl Med 55: 47
Kasianow P (1954) Abrisse der gerichtlich medizinischen Histologie. Medgiz, Moscow
Kent SP (1957) Effect of post-mortem autolysis on certain histochemical reactions. Arch Pathol 64: 17
Kernbach M (1962/63) Karyologische Befunde bei menschlicher perakuter Hypoxie. Zentralbl Allg Pathol 104: 477
Kernbach M, Fisi V, Bernariu D (1927) Recherches histochemiques sur les substances graisseuses pendant la putréfaction. Ann Med Leg 7: 598
Kimura Y (1961) Unusual findings of the exhumed body. Acta Crim Med Leg Jpn 27: 142
Kitaev Yu (1962) On postmortem changes of the fibrillar apparatus of the skeletal muscles. Sud Med Ekspert 5: 34
Klages U, Wilhelmi F (1974) Eisenwanderung in faulenden Geweben. Z Rechtsmed 74: 63
Klauer H, Walcher H (1937) Über postmortale Knötchenbildung an der Haut einer Wasserleiche. Dtsch Z Gerichtl Med 28: 464
Koslowski L (1959) Autolyse-Krankheiten in der Chirurgie. Thieme, Stuttgart
Krause C (1927) Über die Bestimmung des Alters von Organveränderungen bei Mensch und Tier aufgrund histologischer Merkmale. Fischer, Jena
Krefft S (1969) Über postmortale Struktur- und Farbveränderungen der Haare und weiterer keratinhaltiger Hautanhangsgebilde. Arch Kriminol 60: 76
Krejci J, Hradil J (1962) Ein Fall weitgehender postmortaler Verwesung nach 12 Stunden. Soud Lek 7: 10
Lake BD, Ellis RB (1976) What do you think you are quantifying? An appraisal of histochemical methods in the measurement of the activities of lysosomal enzymes. Histochem J 8: 357
Lambertini G (1930) Alterazione cadaveriche della neurotete del Donaggio negli elementi nervosi spinali di feti umani, ed alterazioni sperimentali della neurotete negli elementi nervosi spinali di feti di mammiferi. Arch di Antropol Criminol 50: 1189
Lancker JL van, Holtzer RL (1959) The release of acid phosphatase and beta-glucuronidase from cytoplasmic granules in the early course of autolysis. Am J Pathol 35: 563
Latka H, Adam W (1953) Hyaluronidase als Ursache früher postmortaler Veränderungen der Hypophyse. Dtsch Z Ges Gerichtl Med 42: 31
Latta H, Osvaldo L, Jackson J, Cook ML (1965) Changes in renal cortical tubules during autolysis. Electron microscopic observations. Lab Invest 14:635
Laves W (1931 a) Über den histologischen Nachweis postmortaler physikochemischer Frühveränderungen der Leberzellen. Dtsch Z Gerichtl Med 16: 61
Laves W (1931 b) Histologische Untersuchungen mit gepufferten Farblösungen zum postmortalen Abbau der Kernchromatine und des Plasmas der Leberzellen. Virchows Arch 279: 618
Laves W (1932) Über regressive Zellveränderungen. – Vergleichende morphologische, physikalisch-chemische und chemische Untersuchungen an Leberepithelien. Frankf Z Pathol 43: 283
Leder LD (1964) Über die selektive fermentcytochemische Darstellung von neutrophilen myeloischen Zellen und Gewebsmastzellen im Paraffinschnitt. Klin Wochenschr 42: 553
Lee, MMC (1961) Postmortem changes in glycogen content of human eccrine sweat glands. J Invest Dermatol 37: 207
Lennert K (1952) Zur Praxis der pathologisch-anatomischen Knochenmarkuntersuchungen. Frankf Z Pathol 63: 267
Letterer E (1959) Allgemeine Pathologie, Grundlagen und Probleme. Allgemeiner und geweblicher Tod. S.147, Thieme, Stuttgart
Liebhardt E, Spann W (1968) Todeszeitbestimmung durch Vitalfärbung der Nebenhodenspermatozoen. Dtsch Z Gerichtl Med 62: 176
Lindlar F (1962) Das Auftreten von Lysophosphatiden bei der Autolyse. Naturwissenschaften 49: 543
Lison L (1960) Histochimie et cytochimie animales. Principes et methodes. Gauthier-Villar, Paris
Lochte Th (1938) Atlas der menschlichen und tierischen Haare. Dr. Paul Schöps, Leipzig
Loehry CA, Creamer B (1969) Post-mortem study of small-intestinal mucosa. Br Med J 1: 827
Lojda Z, Gossrau R, Schiebler TH (1976) Enzym-histochemische Methoden. Springer, Berlin Heidelberg New York

Lorke D (1953) Die post-mortale Wasserstoffionenkonzentration an der Oberfläche tierischer Organe. Dtsch Z Gerichtl Med 42: 167
Lorke D, Schmidt O (1952) Fäulnis und Verwesung im Experiment. Dtsch Z Gerichtl Med 41: 236
Mackie FP (1929) The microscopical changes occurring in organs after death. Indian J Med Res 16: 827
Magee PN (1966) Toxic liver necrosis. Lab Invest 15: 111
Marczinkowski T (1963) Patomorfologia ośrodkowego ukladu nerwowego plodów i noworodków w zespole niedodmowym. Poznán, Akademia Medyczna Posnaniu
Marozzi E, Lodi F (1961) Cromatografia su carta di estratti di organi: studio della putrefazione e delle sue possibili interferenze sui risultati delle indagini tossicologico-forensi. II. Riv Med Leg 3: 497
Martines G (1964) Autolisi postmortale del tubulo nefronico sperimentalmente provocata. Riv Patol Clin Sper 5, 263
Melnikov YuL (1969) Post-mortem changes in the liver: an indication of death time. Sud Ekspert (Mosk) 12: 20
Merkel H (1937) Leichen- und Fäulniserscheinungen an menschlichen Leichen. Ergeb Pathol 33: 1
Miam EU, Palagi U (1968) Studio sulle modificationi itotopochimiche della cute ai fini tanato cronologici. Comportamento delle stationi deidrogenasiche. Scritti in onore prof. Folco Domenici 209
Minovici N, Kernbach M, Cotutiu C (1930) Kritische Untersuchungen über histologische und histochemische Veränderungen bei der Leichenfäulnis in Beziehung zur Todeszeitbestimmung. Dtsch Z Gerichtl Med 14: 383
Mitsuki K (1962) Histologische und histochemische Untersuchungen über das Leichenwachs. Tohoku J Exp Med 76: 74
Mönninghoff H (1939) Untersuchungen über die Autolyse der Zellen bei „trüber Schwellung" und „postmortaler kadaveröser Trübung". Beitr Pathol Anat 102: 87
Moloney WC, McPherson K, Fliegelman L (1960) Esterase activity in leucocytes demonstrated by the use of naphthol ASD chloracetate substrate. J Histochem Cytochem 8: 200
Monacelli M (1929) Über die Autolyse der Haut. Arch Dermatol Syph (Berl) 157: 31
Monacelli M (1943) Beitrag zum Studium der autolytischen Prozesse der Haut. Arch Dermatol Syph (Berl) 170: 285
Morrison JH, Kronheim S (1962) The cytochemical demonstration of succinic dehydrogenase in mouse leucocytes. J Histochem Cytochem 10: 402
Mueller B (1951) Untersuchungen über die Histologie der Totenflecke. Dtsch Z Gerichtl Med 40: 499
Mueller B (1961) Zur Frage des Beginnes einer umfangreichen Fettwachsbildung an der Leiche und zur Schätzung der Todeszeit. Arch Kriminol 127: 35
Mueller B (1975) Gerichtliche Medizin. Springer, Berlin Heidelberg New York
Mueller B, Walcher K (1938) Gerichtliche und soziale Medizin einschl. Ärzterecht. J. F. Lehmanns, München Berlin
Müller E (1955) Der Zelltod. Springer, Berlin Göttingen Heidelberg (Handbuch Allg. Pathologie, Bd II/1, p 613
Müller R (1938) Über feinere, gewebliche Veränderungen bei der Gerinnungsnekrose und Autolyse, untersucht am Niereninfarkt. Frankf Z Pathol 52: 433
Müller M (1967) Über den chemischen und morphologischen Nachweis von freien höheren Fettsäuren im autolysierenden Pankreas. Inaugural-Dissertation, Kiel 1967
Muller M, Debarge A, Willot M, Oliveira de SA FM (1965) L'apport de colorations spéciales à l'étude morphologique de l'autopsie du foie. Acta Med Leg Soc (Liège) 18: 231
Muller PH, Willot M, Oliveira de SA FM, Debarge A (1965) Aspects histologiques de l'autolyse hépatique. Acta Med Leg Soc (Liège) 18: 243
Mukai S (1955) Determination of post-mortem interval by histological examination of pancreas. Jap Z Legal Med 9: 19
Naeve W (1971) Zum histologischen Nachweis einer akuten Malaria tropica an fäulnisveränderten Organen. Z Rechtsmed 69: 210
Nanikawa R, Janssen W (1965) Über das postmortale Verhalten der Succinodehydrogenease-Aktivität in Geweben und Leukozyten. Dtsch Z Gerichtl Med 56: 44

Nanikawa R, Tawa N (1960) A colorimetric method of determination of succinic dehydrogenase activity in animal tissues by neotetrazolium. Nagoya Med J 6: 13
Neubauer O (1928) Abbau von Gewebseiweißen (einschl. der Autolyse) Springer, Berlin, (Handbuch der normalen und pathologischen Physiologie, vol 5, p 72)
Neureiter F v, Pietrusky F, Schütt E (1940) Handwörterbuch der gerichtlichen Medizin und naturwissenschaftlichen Kriminalistik. Springer, Berlin
Nicolas G, Leroux M-J, Bouhour JB (1969) Etude de l'autolyse du myocarde humain. Med Leg Dommage Corp 2: 120
Nippe P (1913) Studien über Leichenzersetzung. Vjschr Gerichtl Med 3: 46
Oehmichen M, Gencic M (1980) Postmortal Diffusion of plasma albumin in rat brain. Z Rechtsmed 84: 113
Oehmichen M (1980) Enzyme alterations in brain tissue during the early postmortal interval with reference to the histomorphology: Review of the Literature. Z Rechtsmed 85: 81
Oliveira de SA FM, Debarge A, Muller PH (1964) A propos de l'aspect histologique de l'autolyse. Ann Med Leg 44: 403
Orsós F (1935) Die vitalen Reaktionen und ihre gerichtsmedizinische Bedeutung. Beitr Pathol Anat Allg Pathol 95: 163
Osvaldo L, Jackson JD, Cook ML, Latta H (1965) Reactions of kidney cells during autolysis. Light-microscopic observations. Lab Invest 14: 603
Paulsen A (1966) Untersuchungen über eine neue, elektronische Methode zur (postmortalen) Todeszeitbestimmung beim Menschen. Dissertation, Hamburg
Pearse AGE (1968) Histochemistry. Theoretical and applied, vol I. Churchill, London
Pearse AGE (1972) Histochemistry. Theoretical and applied, vol II. Churchill, London
Penttilä A (1971) Histochemische Darstellung der Katechinamine und von 5-Hydroxytryptamin in verschiedenen Rattenorganen in Beziehung zur Todeszeit. Beitr Pathol 142: 381
Penttilä A, Laiho K (1981) Autolytic changes in blood cells of human cadavers. II. Morphological studies. Forensic Sci Intern 17: 121
Penttilä A, Ohman J (1977) Transformation of rat blood cells postmortem. A scanning electron microscopic study. Zacchia 52: 451
Perper JA, Wecht CH (1980) Microscopic diagnosis in forensic pathology. C. Thomas, Springfield-Illinois
Petersohn F (1962) Postmortale Veränderungen am Gehirn und ihre Abgrenzung zu intravital entstandenen Gewebsreaktionen. Acta Med Leg Soc (Liege) 15: 23
Petersohn F (1963) Postmortale Veränderungen am Gehirn – Ein Beitrag zum Problem der Hirnschwellung und des Gehirnödems. Dtsch Z Gerichtl Med 54: 178
Pioch W (1963) Histochemische Untersuchungen über die Darstellbarkeit früher Zell- und Gewebsalterationen nach lokaler Hitzeeinwirkung auf die Haut von Mäusen und Meerschweinchen. Habilitationsschrift, Bonn
Pioch W (1966) Die histochemische Untersuchung thermischer Hautschäden und ihre Bedeutung für die forensische Praxis. Max-Schmidt-Römhild, Lübeck
Pierucci G, Garibaldi R, Catto AM (1965) Manifestations de „vie rèsiduelle" dans quelques cellules pulmonaires chez le noyé. Acta Med Leg Soc (Liège) 18: 287
Ponsold A (1967) Lehrbuch der gerichtlichen Medizin, 3. Aufl Thieme, Stuttgart
Popielski B, Kobiela J (1972) Medycyna Sadowa PZWL-Verlag Warschau
Preda I, Ander Z, Manolescu A, Belis V (1965) The value of the histological examination in forensic medicine. Prob Med Judic Crim (Bucuresti) 4: 13
Prokop O (1966) Forensische Medizin, 2nd edn VEB Verlag Volk und Gesundheit, Berlin
Raekallio J (1961) Histochemical studies on vital and postmortem skin wounds. Helsinki, p 8
Raekallio J (1965) Die Altersbestimmung mechanisch bedingter Hautwunden mit enzymhistochemischen Methoden. M. Schmidt-Römhild, Lübeck
Raekallio J (1970) Enzyme histochemistry of wound healing. Fischer, Stuttgart
Remagen W, Stolpmann HJ (1962) Zur Frage der postmortalen Veränderungen am Knochen und der Entkalkungsartefakte. Verh Dtsch Ges Pathol 46: 297
Reimer L (1967) Elektronenmikroskopische Untersuchungs- und Präparationsmethoden, 2nd exp edn Springer, Berlin Heidelberg New York
Ricci P (1957) Ulteriori osservazioni sulle modificazioni putrefattive degli elementi figurati del sangue periferico. Med Leg (Genova) 5: 63

Richterlich R (1958) Enzymopathologie. Enzyme in Klinik und Forschung. Springer, Berlin Göttingen Heidelberg, p 247
Rössle R (1933) Bemerkungen zu vorstehender Arbeit von Doljanski, V. Untersuchungen über die proteolytischen Fermente der Rana temporaria in verschiedenen Stadien der Metamorphose. Virchows Arch 291: 427
Romeis B (1968) Mikroskopische Technik, 16. Aufl. R. Oldenbourg, München Wien
Roulet F (1948) Methoden der pathologischen Histologie. Springer Wien
Rozsa Gy, Sotonyi P (1964) Histochemische Untersuchungen der Autolyse und Bewertung der Gomori-Takamatsuschen alkalischen Phosphatasereaktion. Acta Morph Acad Sci Hung 13: 35
Rudnew GP, Schurpe O (1931) Zur Frage über die morphologischen Veränderungen des Blutes nach dem Tode. Virchows Arch 279: 401
Satoh K (1955) Fluid blood and clotted blood in the cadaver. Jpn J Legal Med 9: 440
Schleyer F (1952) Die Fäulnisveränderungen am Lungenepithel des Neugeborenen. Beitr Gerichtl Med 19: 135
Schleyer F (1960) Über Beziehungen zwischen postmortaler Leukozytenvitalität und Leichenalter. Blut 6: 147
Schmeisser H (1926) Beitrag zur Frage der Zweckmäßigkeit gerichtlicher Exhumierungen unter besonderer Berücksichtigung histologischer Organbefunde bei exhumierten Leichen. Dtsch Z Gerichtl Med 8: 162
Schmid H (1965) Die Granula der Gewebsmastzellen der Ratte bei Autolyse. Virchows Arch [Path Anat] 339: 168
Schmidt O (1943) Potentiometrische Untersuchungen über die Reduktionsvorgänge in der Leiche und in Leichenorganen. Dtsch Z Gerichtl Med 37: 20
Schmidt O (1959) Studie über postmortale Abbauvorgänge. Dtsch Z Gerichtl Med 49: 206
Schrader G (1930) Experimentelle Untersuchungen zum Paralysenachweis an faulendem Gehirn. Dtsch Z Gerichtl Med 14: 401
Schröder J (1959) Über Gesetzmäßigkeiten bei der Nekrose und Autolyse von weißen Blutzellen und ihre biologische Bedeutung. Habilitationsschrift, Hamburg
Seifert G (1970) Das Pankreas als Schockorgan. In: Horatz K (ed) Leber- und Pankreasschäden durch Schock und Narkose. Thieme, Stuttgart, 17
Sellier K (1966) Schußentfernungsbestimmung. In: Weinig E, Berg S (eds) Arbeitsmethoden der medizinischen und naturwissenschaftlichen Kriminalistik. Schmidt-Römhild, Lübeck
Sellier K (1969) Schußwaffen und Schußwirkungen. Ballistik – Medizin – Kriminalistik. Schmidt-Römhild, Lübeck
Severinghaus EL, Koehler AE, Bradley HC (1923) Studies of autolysis. – IX. Hydrogen ion concentration in autolysis. J Biol Chem 57: 163
Sinapius D (1958) Die frühen Leichenerscheinungen des Gefäßendothels. Virchows Arch 331: 138
Sinapius D (1962) Autofermentative Basophilie. Quellung und Auflösung von Fetttropfen der fixierten Leber. Z Zellforsch [Abt. Histochem] 3: 150
Sinapius D (1963) Die Fette der Leichenleber bei spontaner und künstlicher Autolyse. Beitrag zur Topographie der Esteraseaktivität. Virchows Arch [Pathol Anat] 337: 215
Sinapius D, Kalbfleisch H (1963) Zur Morphologie und Histochemie der Lipide normaler Säugerlebern bei künstlicher Autolyse. Arch Pathol Anat 336: 311
Smekal v P, Chriske HW, Kübler W, Castrup HJ, Schramm G (1973) Postmortale Enzymaktivitäten im infarzierten und nichtinfarzierten menschlichen Herzmuskelgewebe. Med Welt 24: 1008
Specht W (1937) Chemische Abbaureaktionen bei der Leichenzersetzung. Ergeb Allg Pathol 33: 138
Stevens HM (1967) A rapid general screening method for drugs in post-mortem viscera. J Forensic Sci Soc 7: 184
Strassmann G (1924) Über Leichenveränderungen, autolytische Fäulnis- und Verwesungsvorgänge. Dtsch Z Gerichtl Med 3: 359
Strassmann G (1954) In: Gradwohl RBH (ed) Legal medicine. Mosby St. Louis, cited in J. Raekallio (1961) Histochemical studies on vital and postmortem skin wounds. p 8, Helsinki
Strassmann G, Schmidt O (1928) Fäulniseinwirkung und Einwirkung des elektrischen Stroms auf die Haut. Dtsch Z Gerichtl Med 11: 200
Suzuki T (1976) An ultramicroscopic study on rigor mortis. Forensic Sci 8: 207
Tappero P (1969) Contributo allo studio tanatologico della milza. Minerva Med Leg (Torino) 89: 12

Tedeschi CG, Eckert WG, Tedeschi LG (1977) Forensic Medicine – a study in trauma and environmental hazards. Saunders, Philadelphia London Toronto
Tovo W, De Bernardi A, Tappero P (1965) A proposito di alcune alterazioni post-mortali dell' alveolo polmonare. Minerva Med Leg (Torino) 85: 214
Uotila U (1970) Oikeuslääketiede (Forensic medicine). Werner Söderström Osakeyhtiö Porvoo, Helsinki
Volk P, Hartmann S (1970) Untersuchungen an 900 Jahre alten Haaren aus den Kaisergräbern von Speyer. Beitr Gerichtl Med 27: 245
Wagner H-J (1960) Die Bedeutung der Antibiotika und Sulfonamide für Todes- und Tatzeitbestimmungen in der gerichtlichen Medizin. Habilitationsschrift, Mainz
Walcher K (1927) Studien über die Leichenfäulnis mit besonderer Berücksichtigung der Histologie derselben. Zentralbl Allg Pathol 39: 1
Walcher K (1950) Leitfaden der gerichtlichen Medizin für Ärzte und Medizinstudierende. Urban & Schwarzenberg, Berlin
Werner W (1954) Zur Pathologie reaktiver und leukämischer Myeloblastosen. Frankf Z Pathol 65: 478
Winkelmann E, David H, Marx I (1965) Autolytische und submikroskopische Zellveränderungen im Cortex cerebelli der weißen Ratte. Hirnforsch 7: 453
Winter W, Braun-Falco O (1965) Untersuchungen über die Autolyse der Haut. Fluorescenzmikroskopische Veränderungen. Arch Klin Exp Dermatol 222: 192
Wolff EK (1924) Untersuchungen über autolytisches Ferment. Zentralbl Allg Pathol 35: 270
Zimmermann H, Platt D (1962) Über die Beeinflussung der histochemischen Darstellbarkeit oxydativer Enzyme durch Narkose. Frankf Z Pathol 71: 453
Zink P, Reinhardt G (1978) Zur histologischen Beurteilung faulender Organe. Beitr Gerichtl Med 36: 333
Zollinger HU (1948) Phasenmikroskopische Beobachtungen über Zelltod. Schweiz Z Pathol Bakteriol 11: 276

References to B II: Vital Reactions

Adebahr G (1949) Experimentelle Studien über Luftembolie und Berücksichtigung der cerebralen Form. Dissertation, Köln
Adebahr G (1953) Studien zum anatomischen Nachweis der Luftembolie unter besonderer Berücksichtigung der morphologischen Verhältnisse des Herzblutes. Virchows Arch [Pathol Anat] 323: 155
Adebahr G (1954) Beobachtungen und experimentelle Untersuchungen zum anatomischen Nachweis der Luftembolie. Zentralbl Allg Pathol 92: 53
Adebahr G (1960a) Anatomischer Nachweis der Luftembolie im Herzblut. Zentralbl Allg Pathol 101: 347
Adebahr G (1960b) Gehirnveränderungen nach wochenlanger posttraumatischer Bewußtlosigkeit. Dtsch Z Gerichtl Med 49: 680
Adebahr G (1963) Zur Genese traumatischer Pallidum-, Balken- und Marknekrosen. Dtsch Med Wochenschr 88: 2097
Adebahr G (1971) Über traumatische Nebennierenblutungen. Hefte Unfallheilkd 107: 90
Adebahr G (1979) Die Bedeutung von Sperrarterien für die Entstehung von Blutungen und kleinen hämorrhagischen Infarkten in der Lunge des Menschen bei Fettembolie. Z Rechtsmed 83: 291
Adebahr G, Kupffer A (1967) Morphologischer Nachweis der Luftembolie im Herzblut. Abwandlung des Befundes in der Barbituratvergiftung beim Kaninchen. Dtsch Z Gerichtl Med 61: 1
Adebahr G, Staak M (1969) Morphologischer Beitrag zur Frage der Verbrauchs-Koagulopathie bei Luftembolie. Virchows Arch [Pathol Anat] 346: 224
Adebahr G, Weiler G (1976) Blutverteilungsmuster in der Niere bei Tod durch Verbluten. Forensic Sci Int 7: 179
Adebahr G, Weiler G (1977) Blutverteilungsmuster in der Niere bei Tod durch Verbluten. Z Rechtsmed 80: 9
Adkins RB, Forster JH (1962) Experimental study of the genesis of fat embolism. Ann Surg 156: 515

Althoff H (1967) Fremdkörperembolie in das Gehirn nach Betriebsunfall. Monatsschr Unfallheilk 70: 124
Ander Z, Jung J (1976) Die Häufigkeit der Fettembolie nach tödlichen Verletzungen und ihre Bedeutung in der Thanatogenese. Forensic Sci Int 7: 179
Anderson WAD (1971) Pathology, vol 1. C. V. Mosby St. Louis, p 132
Andrew JH (1976) Pulmonary skin embolism: a case report. Pathology 8: 185
Apitz K (1934) Die Wirkung bakterieller Kulturinfiltrate nach Umstimmung des gesamten Endothels beim Kaninchen. Virchows Arch [Path Anat] 293: 51
Apitz K (1939) Zur Frage der postmortalen Fibrinolyse. Z Exp Med 105: 89
Apitz K (1942) Die Bedeutung der Gerinnung und Thrombose für die Blutstillung. Virchows Arch [Pathol Anat] 308: 540
Asbeck F, Joist H, Löhrs U (1972) Lebervenenthrombose und Ovulationshemmer. Ein weiterer Fall von Budd-Chiari-Syndrom nach Einnahme eines oralen Kontrazeptivums. Med Klin 67: 82
Attwood HD (1964) A histological study of experimental amnion fluid and meconium embolism in dogs. J Pathol 88: 285
Axhausen H (1930) Zur Frage der Häufung der Thrombosen und Embolien. Virchows Arch [Pathol Anat] 274: 188
Bang NU, Beller FK, Deutsch E, Mammen EF (1971) Thrombosis and blood disorders, theory and methods. Thieme, Stuttgart; Academic, New York
Barker: cited by Sandritter und Beneke 1966
Bassermann FJ (1960) Zum Problem der Bildung von Riesenzellen in der menschlichen Lunge. Acta Tuberculosa Scand 38: 267
Bauer G, Missliwetz J (1978) Fettembolie und Blutung. Beitr Gerichtl Med 36: 11
Bässler R (1959) Zur Pathologie und Symptomatologie der sogenannten metatraumatischen Hämobilie. Bruns Beitr Klin Chir 199: 208
Beau A, Prevot Collignon P (1963) Les thromboses veineuses chez l'enfant à propos de 4 cas. Ann Chir Infant 4: 191
Bednár B (1976) Skin wound healing (an electronoptic study). Csl Pat 12: 67
Beneke G (1972) Altersbestimmung von Verletzungen innerer Organe. Z Rechtsmed 71: 1
Beneke G (1976) Thrombogenese in Venen. Med Welt 27: 1222
Beneke G, Hey D (1965) Modelluntersuchungen zur fermentativen Löslichkeit von Fibrin im histologischen Schnitt. Histochemistry 5: 366
Berg S (1969) Der Beweiswert der Todeszeitbestimmung (Überlebenszeit). Beitr Gerichtl Med 25: 61
Berg S (1972) Die Altersbestimmung von Hautverletzungen. Z Rechtsmed 70: 121
Berg S, Bonte W (1971) Praktische Erfahrungen mit der biochemischen Wundaltersbestimmung. Beitr Gerichtl Med 28: 108
Berg S, Ebel R (1969) Altersbestimmung subkutaner Blutungen. Münch Med Wschr 111: 1185
Berg S, Ditt J, Friedrich R, Bonte W (1968) Möglichkeiten der biochemischen Wundaltersbestimmung. Dtsch Z Gerichtl Med 63: 183
Berg S, Ditt J, Kunze P, Garbe G (1971) Beziehungen zwischen Histamingehalt und Aktivität der Histidindecarboxylase im Bereich von Hautverletzungen. Z Rechtsmed 69: 26
Berg S, Friedberg KD, Garbe G (1974) Histaminspiegel und Lungenmastzellen bei Tod durch Verblutung. Z Rechtsmed 74: 245
Bergentz SE (1961) Studies on the genesis of posttraumatic fat embolism. Acta Chir Scan [Suppl] 282: 1
Bergström S, Gelin LE, Zederfeldt B (1959) The formation of vein thrombi following tissue injury: an experimental study in rabbits. Acta Chir Scand [Suppl] 247: 1
Bessis M (1962) L'hémosidérine et le mouvement du fers dans l'organisme. Exposé des différents points de vue. Nouv Rev Fr Hematol 2: 153
Blum H (1937) Zur Frage der Unterscheidbarkeit vitaler und postmortaler Gewebeveränderungen am Beispiel der Strangfurchen beim Erhängungstod. Virchows Arch 299: 754
Böhm E (1974a) Zur Ultrastruktur von Blutungen nach wiederholter Traumatisierung. Z Rechtsmed 74: 197
Böhm E (1974b) Zur Faser- und Netzstruktur des Fibrins bei intravasculärer Gerinnung. Z Rechtsmed 74: 217

Böhm E (1979) Zum morphologischen Nachweis der frühen lokalen Vitalreaktion mit kombinierter Untersuchungstechnik. Beitr Gerichtl Med 37: 127

Böhm N, Wybitul K (1980) Autotransplantation von Milzgewebe nach traumatischer Milzruptur (traumatische Splenose). Chirurg 51: 158

Böttger G, Strik W (1970) Fettembolie. Münch Med Wochenschr 112: 51

Bonte W, Herrmann V (1978) Aktivitätsveränderungen der unspezifischen Esterasen im Wundheilungsprozeß. Untersuchungen mit Hilfe der Elektrofokussierung. Z Rechtsmed 82: 179

Bosch K (1968) Über den forensischen Beweiswert histologischer und mikrochemischer Untersuchungen bei Stichverletzungen. Dtsch Z Gerichtl Med 62: 4

Brack E (1928) Arterienthrombosen als Ursache plötzlichen Todes. Dtsch Z Gerichtl Med 12: 440

Brack E (1933) Über die Begutachtung des Unfallspättodes. Dtsch Z Gerichtl Med 22: 178

Bratzke H (1979) Zur Kenntnis der zentralen Hirnverletzungen. Beitr Gerichtl Med 37: 189

Brettel HF, Lutz FU (1973) Die Knorpelembolie als Sonderform vitaler Reaktionen. Z Rechtsmed 72: 161

Brinkmann B (1975) Traumatische Aortenrupturen im Hamburger Sektionsmaterial der Jahre 1969 bis 1973. Monatsschr Unfallheilk 78: 117

Brinkmann B, Borgner M, v. Bülow M (1976) Die Fettembolie der Lungen als Todesursache. – Ätiologie, Pathogenese und Beweisführung. Z Rechtsmed 78: 255

Brüning E (1955) Über Entstehung und Bedeutung intraarterieller Fremdkörperembolien der kindlichen Lunge. Virchows Arch 327: 460

Brüning E (1955) Über Fremdkörpergranulome in den Lungenarterien eines weiblichen Scheinzwitters. Zentralbl Allg Pathol 93: 100

Brunner P, Schellmann B (1979) Gibt es eine Topographie der posttraumatischen Fettembolie? Histologische Untersuchungen an Lungengroßflächenschnitten. Beitr Gerichtl Med 37: 153

Bschor F: Zur Pathogenese und Morphologie der zentralen Fettembolie. In: Fette in der Medizin, part 5. Pallas-Verlag Lochham, München, p 27 (Med u Ernährung)

Bschor F (1962) Zum histologischen Nachweis intravasaler Fettstoffe. Fette, Seifen, Anstrichmittel. Die Ernährungsindustrie 64: 669

Bschor F (1963 a) Fettleber und Fettembolie. Dtsch Med Wochenschr 88: 1112

Bschor F (1963 b) Histologische Befunde bei Alkoholhyperlipämie. Acta Med Leg Soc (Liege) 16: 77

Bschor F (1963 c) Örtliche Kreislaufschäden durch partikuläres Blutfett. Histologische Beobachtungen. Med u Ernährg Sonderh. „Fett, Transport und Fettverwertung nach oraler und intravenöser Fettzufuhr“, Lochham, München

Bschor F (1963 d) Über Chylomikronenaggregate in Herzmuskelkapillaren bei alimentärer Lipämie. Med Welt 190

Bschor F, Deininger R (1964) Einfluß der Hyperlipämie auf die Thrombogenese im Coronarsystem des isolierten Katzenherzens. Klin Wschr 42: 435

Bschor F, Haasch K (1964) Fluoreszenzoptische Untersuchung zur Fettembolie. Hefte Unfallheilkd 78: 261

Buris L (1978) Untersuchungen über vitale und postmortale Verletzungen und über das Anfangsstadium der Wundheilung. Kriminal Forens Wiss 32: 55

Buris L, Poczkodi S, Gömöry A (1979) Embolism of heart tissue to the middle cerebral artery as a complication of heart surgery. Z Rechtsmed 83: 87

Burkhardt K (1970) Untersuchungen zur Pathogenese der Fettembolie. Med Welt 21: 1969

Busse-Grawitz P (1964) Hören beginnende Entzündungsprozesse mit dem Eintritt des Todes auf? Zentralbl Allg Pathol 105: 446

Büchner C (1964) Traumatische Knochenmarksembolie der Lungen, zugleich ein Beitrag zur Pathogenese der Fettembolie. Dtsch Med Wochenschr 89: 1390

Büchner Th (1971) Entzündungszellen im Blut und im Gewebe. Zellkinetische Studie über die experimentelle granulierende Entzündung durch Fremdkörper und bei der Wundheilung. G. Fischer Stuttgart

Cameron HM, Park WW (1965) Decidual tissue within the lung. J Obstet Gynecol Br Comm 72: 748

Cammermeyer J (1978) Is the solitary dark neuron a manifestation of postmortem trauma to the brain inadequately fixed by perfusion? Histochemistry 56: 97

Carstairs KC (1965) The identification of platelets and platelet antigens in histological actions. J Pathol 90: 225
Carvalho HV (1964) The vital reaction in the central nervous system. Med Sci Law 4: 111
Christeller E (1920) Über agonale Blutungen im Gebiet der oberen Hohlvene. Beitr Pathol Anat 67: 505
Dalal AR, Pitney WR (1972) Primary thrombosis of the axillary-subclavian veins. Med J Aust 59: 633
David H, Reimann W (1960) Lungenfettembolie und intravasales Fett nach lokaler postmortaler Verbrennung der Lungen. Dtsch Z Gerichtl Med 49: 382
David H, Marx I, Krastev E (1967) Elektronenmikroskopische Befunde bei der experimentellen Fettembolie der Kaninchenlunge mit arteigenem Fett. Exp Pathol 1: 185
Dell'Erba A, Vimercati F (1966) Inalacione di liquido anniotico e causa della morte dell prodotto di concedimento. G Med Leg Infortun Tossicol 12: 349
Dettori AG, Ponari O, Redenti L (1962) Contributo allo studio della coagulazione del sangue nel cadavere. Minerva Med Leg 82: 239
Dietrich A (1921) Die Entwicklung der Lehre von der Thrombose und Embolie seit Virchow. Virchows Arch [Pathol Anat] 235: 212
Dietrich A (1925) Thrombopathie mit parietaler Herzthrombose und paradoxer Embolie. Virchows Arch [Pathol Anat] 254: 230
Dietrich A (1930) Abstimmung des Gefäßendothels als Grundlage der Thrombenbildung. Virchows Arch [Pathol Anat] 274: 425
Dietrich A (1931) Wesen und Bedingungen der Thrombose und Embolie. Klin Wochenschr I: 54
Dietrich A (1932) Thrombose. Ihre Grundlagen und ihre Bedeutung. Julius Springer Berlin, Wien
Dietrich A (1941) Reaktive Thrombose im Tierversuch. Virchows Arch [Pathol Anat] 307: 281
Dohm G (1965) Die Nebennierenrinde im Kindesalter. Orthologie und Pathologie. Springer, Berlin Heidelberg New York
Dotzauer G, Adebahr G (1964) Trauma und Karotisthrombose. Dtsch Z Gerichtl Med 55: 237
Dotzauer G, Tamaska L (1968) Hautveränderungen an Leichen. In: Jadassohn J (ed) Anatomie der Haut. Springer, Berlin Heidelberg New York. Handbuch der Haut- und Geschlechtskrankheiten. Ergänzungswerk vol 1, Part 1, p 708
Duda E, Papilian VV (1962) Exitus post partum durch Fruchtwasserembolie. Zentralbl Gynäk 84: 690
Eidlin LM (1965) On the wrong interpretation of fat drops in tissues and blood vessels as of sure sign of intravital origin. Sud Med Ekspert 8: 10
Eisenmenger W, Gilg P, Diem G, Neuhann T (1978) Zur histologischen und histochemischen Altersbestimmung gedeckter Hirnrindenverletzungen. Beitr Gerichtl Med 36: 281
Emmrich P (1969) Zur Frage der Organisation von Coronarthrombosen. Z Gesamt Innere Med 24: 861
Ess T, Weiler G (1979) Histomorphologische Befunde am Chiasma opticum bei Schädel-Hirntrauma. Z Rechtsmed 82: 257
Falzi G, Henn R, Spann W (1964) Über pulmonale Fettembolien nach Traumen mit verschieden langer Überlebenszeit. Münch Med Wochenschr 106: 978
Fazekas JG (1967) Über den Gehalt der menschlichen Haut verschiedener Körperregionen an freiem und Gesamthistamin. Dtsch Z Gerichtl Med 61: 107
Fazekas JG (1970) Der Gehalt von Wunden an freiem Histamin als vitale Reaktion im Tierversuch. Zacchia 45: 626
Fazekas JG (1971) Der Gehalt verschiedener Verletzungen an freiem Hitamin als Vitalreaktion. Z Rechtsmed 68: 86
Filippov VV, Pashinyan GA (1971) Diagnosing intravital character of trauma by studying the inorganic composition of bone marrow. Sud Med Ekspert 14, 23
Fischer H (1963) Beitrag zur Frage der Fettembolie bei tödlicher Druckfallkrankheit. Monatsschr Unfallheilkd 66: 318
Foedisch HJ, Kloos K (1966) Thrombotische Verschlüsse im Stromgebiet der Arteria carotis nach stumpfen Schädelhalstraumen. Hefte Unfallheilkd 88: 1
Fonio A (1964) Über die Fibrinfibrillenbildung und Fibrinquerstreifung. Acta Haematol (Basel) 31: 262

Fromm H (1962) Zur Differentialdiagnose und Prognose der cerebralen Fettembolie. Nervenarzt 33: 430
Fuchs U (1965) Elektronenmikroskopische Befunde bei der Erythrocytendiapedese im Granulationsgewebe. Z Mikroskop Anat Forsch 73: 37
Furuta S (1924) Morbus Addisonii durch arterielle Embolien der Nebennieren. Nebst Bemerkungen über den embolischen anämischen Infarkt der Nebenniere. Virchows Arch [Pathol Anat] 251: 553
Gainter JR, Jackson BP, Conley CL (1962) Morphologic studies of clot retraction. Bull Johns Hopkins Hosp 111: 266
Gedigk P (1958) Die funktionelle Bedeutung des Eisenpigmentes. Erg Allg Pathol Anat 38: 1
Gedigk P, Strauss G (1954) Zur formalen Genese der Eisenpigmente. Virchows Arch 326: 172
Gee EJ (1967) Cerebral fat embolism. Its experimental production. J Forensic Med 14: 60
Geiler G (1965) Untersuchungen über die immunhistochemische Fibrindarstellung an Biopsie- und Obduktionsmaterial. Histochemistry 5: 361
Geppert M (1978) Spättodesfall nach Contusio cordis. Med Welt 29: 739
Gergen M (1966) Schwerer bleibender Hirnschaden nach Fettembolie. Monatsschr Unfallheilkd 69: 596
Gevers W (1975) Biochemical aspects of cell death. Forensic Sci Int 6: 25
Gherson G, Pierucci G (1968) Studio istologico ed istoenzimatico solla cronologia della lesioni traumatiche del fegato. Scritti in Onore Prof Folco Domenici 1968, p 133
Giese W (1960) Die Atemorgane. In: Staemmler M, Lehrbuch der speziellen pathologischen Anatomie, vol 2, part 3. de Gruyter, Berlin, pp 1605 and 1963
Gilbert P, Borchard F (1980) Hautembolie der Lunge. Pathologe 1: 161
Gilsa B v (1976) Die Altersbestimmung von Hautwunden. Med Dissertation, Würzburg
Glass JM, Zaki SA, Rivers RL (1980) Intracranial missile emboli. J Forensic Sci 25: 302
Goldstein MN (1954) Formation of giant cells from human monocytes cultivated on cellophane. Anat Rec 118: 577
Gordon I, Mansfield RA (1955) Subpleural, subpericardial and subendocardial haemorrhages; study of their incidence of necropsy and of the spontaneous development, after death, of subpericardial petechiae. J Forensic Med 2: 31
Gormsen H (1961) On air embolism. Acta Pathol Microbiol Scand [Suppl] 144: 97
Graev M, Fabroni F (1962) Sulla evoluzione dei focolai di aspirazione ematica polmonare. Minerva Med Leg 82: 255
Greendyke RM (1964) Fatembolism in fatal automobile accidents. J Forensic Sci 9: 201
Greifenstein A (1931) Pathologisch-anatomische Untersuchung über Entstehung und Ausbreitung thrombotisch-entzündlicher Vorgänge im Halsvenensystem unter besonderer Berücksichtigung der nach Graumenmandelentzündung entstehenden Formen. Virchows Arch [Pathol Anat] 281: 748
Gross R, Jahn D, Schölmerich P (1970) Lehrbuch der Inneren Medizin. Schattauer, Stuttgart New York, p 185
Gross R, Jahn D, Schölmerich P (1977) Lehrbuch der Inneren Medizin. Schattauer, Stuttgart
Gusek W (1958) Die Feinstruktur der einkernigen Makrophagen und der mehrkernigen Riesenzellen im Fremdkörpergranulationsgewebe. Frankf Z Pathol 69: 429
Gusek W, Uerlings I (1958) Feinstruktur von Makrophagen und mehrkernigen Riesenzellen im Fremdkörpergranulationsgewebe. Naturwissenschaften 45: 371
Haberda A (1898) Über das postmortale Entstehen von Ekchymosen. Gerichtl Med u. Öffentl Sanitätswesen 15: 248
Haberer K, Ellebrecht K, Walther G (1972) Tierexperimentelle Untersuchungen über die Schutzwirkung des Sauerstoffs bei der Druckfallkrankheit. Beitr Gerichtl Med 29: 303
Hardaway RM (1961) Disseminated intravascular coagulation syndromes. Arch Surg 83: 842
Hardaway RM (1966) Syndromes of disseminated intravascular coagulation. CC Thomas Springfield (Ill)
Hardaway RM, Elovitz MJ, Brewster WR, Houchin DN, Renzi NI, Jackson BR (1964) Influence of vasoconstrictures and vasodilators on disseminated intravascular coagulation in irreversible hemorrhagic shock. Surg Gynecol Obstet 119: 1053
Hardaway RM, Chun W, Rutherford RB (1965) Coagulation in shock in various species including man. Acta Chir Scand 130: 157

Hardaway RM, Brewster WR, Elovitz MJ (1966) The influence of vasoconstriction and acidosis on disseminated intravascular coagulation. Surgery 59: 804
Hardmeier T (1963) Schwere Fettembolie bei Erfrierungen an beiden unteren Extremitäten. Schweiz Med Wochenschr 93: 465
Harman JW, Ragaz FJ (1950) Experimental fat embolism. Am J Pathol 26: 551
Harms D (1971) Postmortale Fibrinolyse beim Menschen. G. Fischer Stuttgart
Harter L (1947) Über Zirkulationsstörungen des Zentralnervensystems bei experimenteller Fett- und Luftembolie. Virchows Arch [Pathol Anat] 314: 211
Hartmann H (1961) Druckfallkrankheit und intravasale Gasblasen. Int Z Angew Physiol 19: 67
Hausberger X (1976) Effects of lipemia and trauma on experimental fat embolism Am J Pathol 84: 515
Hausbrandt F (1938) Beitrag zur Frage der kombinierten Luftembolie des kleinen und großen Kreislaufs nach Abtreibungsversuchen. Dtsch Z Gerichtl Med 30: 19
Haymaker W (1957) Decompression sickness. In: Scholz W (ed) Nervensystem, Springer, Berlin: Handb d spez Pathol Anat u. Histol vol XIII, p 1600
Hecht A, Korb G (1960) Über Beziehungen zwischen rechtsseitigem intrakardialem Druck und dem Auftreten von Herzmuskelnekrosen sowie Fettdurchtritt durch die Lungenkapillaren bei der experimentellen Fettembolie. Beitr Pathol Anat 123: 383
Hegglin R (1965) Tierexperimentelle Untersuchungen über den Zusammenhang zwischen Fettembolie und Kreislaufversagen. Helvetica Chir Acta 32: 547
Helpap B, Cremer H (1970) Proliferationsvorgänge in der traumatisch geschädigten Leber. Virchows Arch [Cell Pathol] 6: 365
Helpap B, Cremer H (1972) Zellkinetische Untersuchungen zur Wundheilung der Mäuseleber. Virchows Arch [Cell Pathol] 10: 134
Helpap B (1973) Pathologisch-anatomische Folgen der Leberkeilexzision. Dtsch Med Wochenschr 98: 81
Helpap B, Grouls V, Johaentges F (1977 a) The wound healing of the liver after thermonecrosis. Autoradiographical investigations with 3 H-thymidine on rats. Res Exp Med (Berlin) 171: 1
Helpap B, Rodenbusch U, Grouls V (1977 b) Die Niere nach Thermonekrose. Zellkinetische Untersuchungen an Ratten. Virchows Arch [Pathol Anat] Abt A 375: 319
Henn RH, Spann W (1965) Untersuchungen über die Häufigkeit der cerebralen Fettembolie nach Trauma mit verschieden langer Überlebenszeit. Monatsschr Unfallheilkd 68: 513
Henn RH, Spann W (1968) Experimentelle Untersuchungen über das postmortale Verhalten embolischen Neutralfetts in den Lungen. Dtsch Z Gerichtl Med 62: 170
Henn RH, Spann W (1970) Mikroskopische Nierenbefunde bei der tödlichen Fettembolie des großen Kreislaufes. 49. Jahrestag. Dtsch Ges Rechtsmed 16.–19. 9. 1970 Bern
Henn RH, Kaiser R, Ulleweit S (1970) Serienschnittuntersuchungen an Blutungen bei der posttraumatischen Hirnpurpura. 49. Jahrestag. Dtsch Ges Rechtsmed 16.–19. 9. 1970, Bern
Herberg D, Braasch W, Meesmann W (1965) Veränderungen der Atmung und des Kreislaufs nach experimenteller Fettembolie. Arch Kreislaufforsch 47: 37
Hinz P, Tamaska L (1971) Die Beweiswerte der sog. vitalen Zeichen bei Toten im Straßenverkehr mit Halswirbelsäulenverletzung. Z Rechtsmed 68: 95
Hirst AE, Gore I (1976) Is cystic medionecrosis the cause of dissecting aortic aneurysm? Circulation 53: 915
Hirvonen J (1968) Histochemical studies in vital reaction and traumatic fat necrosis in the interscapular adipose tissue of adult guinea pigs. Ann Acad Sci Fenn [Med] 136: 7
Hoak JC (1964) Structure of thrombi produced by injections of fatty acids. Br J Exp Pathol 45: 44
Hobalek A (1951) Die Veränderungen am Fettgewebe in der Umgebung der Strangfurche bei dem Erhängungstod. Inaugural-Dissertation Heidelberg
Holczabek W (1964 a) Todesursachen bei frischen Thoraxverletzungen. Thorac Cardiovasc Surg 12: 89
Holczabek W (1964 b) Zur Frage der Entstehung der Lungenfettembolie aufgrund dünnschichtchromatographischer Untersuchungen. Klin Med 19: 483
Holczabek W (1964 c) Dünnschichtchromatographische Untersuchungen von Lipidextrakten aus der menschlichen Lunge unter besonderer Berücksichtigung der Fettembolie. Dtsch Z Gerichtl Med 55: 242

Holczabek W (1968a) Der Triglyzeridgehalt der normalen Lunge und bei Lungenfettembolie. Akt Fragen Gerichtl Med 3: 174
Holczabek W (1968b) Das Verhalten der arterio-venösen Anastomosen bei der Lungenfettembolie. Dtsch Z Gerichtl Med 62: 170
Holczabek W (1971) Dünnschichtchromatographische Untersuchungen an Gewebsschnitten. Acta Histochem [Suppl] 9: 507
Holczabek W, Machata G (1971) Gaschromatographische Untersuchungen zur Frage der Entstehung der Fettembolie beim Menschen. Beitr Gerichtl Med 28: 82
Holzer FJ (1965) Verschluß der Wirbelsäulenschlagader am Kopfgelenk mit nachfolgender Thrombose durch Seitwärtsdrehen des Kopfes. Dtsch Z Gerichtl Med 44: 422
Hou-Jensen K (1968) Histochemical demonstrations of some hydrolytic enzymes as vital reaction in medico-legal practise. J Forensic Med 15: 91
Hou-Jensen K (1969) Some enzyme conditioned vital reactions in the initial phase of wound healing. Med Bull 16: 305
Howard AN, Gresham GA (1964) The dietary induction of thrombosis and myocardial infarction. J Atherosclerosis Res 4: 40
Hueck W (1912) Pigmentstudien. Beitr Pathol Anat Allg Pathol 54: 68
Hueck W (1921) Die pathologische Pigmentierung. In: Krehl L, Marchand F (eds) Handbuch der Allgemeinen Pathologie III/2. Hirzel, Leipzig, p 298
Hupe K, Roeper R (1965) Tierexperimentelle Untersuchungen über die Wundheilung. Bruhns Beitr Klin Chir 211: 214
Huth K (1971) Die Fettembolie. Ärztl Fortbildung 21: 368
Illchmann-Christ A (1952) zitiert von Bässler 1959. Hefte Unfallheilkd 43: 234
Irniger W (1963) Histologische Altersbestimmung von Thrombosen und Embolien. Virch Arch [Pathol Anat] 336: 220
Jacques BE, Saini N (1962) A physiologic and anatomic study of experimental fat embolism in dogs. Exp Mol Pathol 1: 57
Jakoby F (1930) Chemische Untersuchungen am Leichenblut. Ein Beitrag zur Blutgerinnungs- und Thrombosefrage. Virchows Arch [Pathol Anat] 274: 392
Jannsen W (1962) Zur Bedeutung der perinatalen Nebennierenblutungen. Dtsch Z Gerichtl Med 52: 578
Janssen W (1967a) Zur Pathogenese und forensischen Bewertung von Hirnblutungen nach cerebraler Luftembolie. Dtsch Z Gerichtl Med 61: 62
Janssen W (1967b) Zur Beurteilung von Blutungen der Leichenhaut unter besonderer Berücksichtigung von Hämatomen der Orbita. Dtsch Z Gerichtl Med 59: 70
Janssen W, Jaecker O, Erbach A (1968) Zur Unterscheidung von Druck- und Stauungsblutungen in den Halsweichteilen. Dtsch Z Gerichtl Med 64: 147
Jarecki R, Arndt U, Schultz C, Klein H (1969) Zur Unterscheidung vitaler und postmortaler Wunden durch Bestimmung des Esterasemusters der Haut. Dtsch Z Gerichtl Med 66: 161
Jarecki R, Pogacar P, Günther G, Klein H (1970) Early enzyme changes in skin wounds demonstrated by isoelectric focusing in polyacrylamide gel. Z Rechtsmed 67: 313
Jellinger K (1976) Neuropathologie anhaltender Bewußtseinsstörungen. Ideggyóg Szle 29: 51
Jellinger K (1977) Pathology of intracerebral hemorrhage. Zentralbl Neurochir 38: 29
Johnson SA, Balboa RS, Pederson HJ, Buckley M (1965) The ultrastructure of platelet participation in hemostases. Thromb Haemost (Stuttgart) 13: 65
Jones JP Jr, Engleman EP, Najarian JS (1965) Systemic fat embolism after renal homotransplantation and treatment with corticosteroids. Engl J Med 273: 1453
Jorgensen L, Borchgrevnik CF (1963) The platelet plug in normal persons. I. The histological appearance of the plug. 15 to 30 min. and 24 hours after the blooding and its role in the capillary hemostases. Acta Pathol Microbiol Scand [A] 57: 40
Juhl O (1921) Beiträge zur pathologischen Anatomie der Grippe. Virchow Arch [Pathol Anat] 232: 58
Jurukova Z, Knieriem H-J (1970) Elektronenmikroskopische Untersuchungen über die Organisation arterieller Thromben. Virch Arch [Pathol Anat] 349: 368
Kaeser HE (1955) Einseitige Carotisthrombosen nach Strangulation. Confinia Neurol (Basel) 15: 369
Kampmann H, Garbe G, Ropp D, von der Berg S, Bode G (1978) Der Einfluß von Säure- und Lau-

geneinwirkung auf die Entwicklung der morphologischen und biochemischen Wundreaktionen. Z Rechtsmed 82: 71
Kampmann H, Garbe G, Armbrust H, Bode G (1980) Untersuchungen zur Morphologie und Biochemie der Wundheilung bei Leberschnittverletzungen. Z Rechtsmed 84: 291
Karkola K, Möttönen M (1971) Embolism of brain tissue to the pulmonary arteries after head injury. Med Sci Law 49
Kaufmann E (1970) Experimentelle Lungenembolie mit jodhaltigen Kontrastmitteln an der Ratte. Eine elektronenmikroskopische Untersuchung. Z Ges Exp Med 152: 201
Kaulbach W, Benninger K (1962) Experimentelle Fettembolie mit elektrokardiographischen und histologischen Untersuchungen. Langenbecks Arch Klin Chir 300: 48
Kelemen A (1962) Die Fettembolie. Acta Med Leg Soc (Liege) 15: 67
Kellner G (1964) Histochemische Methoden des Eisennachweises, ein neuer hochempfindlicher Eisennachweis. Wien Z Inn Med 45: 399
Kernbach M, Cotutiu C, Dahnovici V (1937) Contribution á l'étude de la reaction vitale après les blessures. Am Med Leg 17: 1039
Keyl W (1979) Wann reißt die Achillessehne? Münch Med Wochenschr 121: 1241
Kischer CW (1979) Fine structure of granulation tissues from deep injury. J Invest Dermatol 72: 147
Klages U (1970) Spontane oder traumatische tödliche Subarachnoidalblutung. Z Rechtsmed 67: 67
Klages U, Wilhelmi F (1974) Eisenwanderung in faulenden Geweben. Z Rechtsmed 74: 63
Kleiber M, Bause H-W (1976) Bilio-venöse Fistel als seltene Komplikation nach stumpfem Bauchtrauma. Z Unfallheilkd 79: 483
Klein H (1951) Leberriß mit posttraumatisch in die Bauchhöhle implantiertem Lebergewebe. Zentralbl Allg Pathol Pathol Anat 87: 349
Knoch HG, Lenser G (1963) Die Fettembolie aus klinischer Sicht. Zentralbl Chir 88: 385
Kovacs M, Harsanyi L (1971) Über histochemisch nachweisbare vitale Reaktionen am Knochengewebe. Acta Histochem [Suppl] 9
Köberle F (1956) Über die Dauer der Riesenzellenbildung. Zbl Pathol Allg [Pathol Anat] 95: 540
Köhn K (1952 a) Kritische Bemerkungen zur histologischen Diagnostik der arteriellen Luftembolie des Gehirns. Frankf Z Pathol 63: 360
Köhn K (1952 b) Grundsätzliche Fehlerquelle des makroskopischen und histologischen Nachweises der Luftembolie des Herzens und des Gehirns. Verhandlg Dtsch Ges Pathol 63: 247
Köhn G, Berg T (1965) Tierexperimentelle chronische pulmonale Hypertonie nach rezidivierender Mikrolungenembolie und ihre Rückwirkung auf Herz und Arterien. Beitr Pathol Anat 132: 86
Krauland W (1950) Über Hirnschäden durch stumpfe Gewalt. Dtsch Z Nervenheilkd 163: 265
Krauland W (1954) Histologische Untersuchungen zur traumatischen Genese der sogenannten Pachymeningitis haemorrhagica interna. Dtsch Z Gerichtl Med 43: 337
Krauland W (1955 a) Fluoreszenzmikroskopische Untersuchungen an Wunden und Abschürfungen. Dtsch Z Gerichtl Med 44: 442
Krauland W (1955 b) Verletzungen der A. carotis interna im Sinus cavernosus und Verletzungen der großen Hirnschlagadern mit Berücksichtigung der Aneurysmabildung. In: Henke F, Lubarsch O (eds) Handbuch der speziellen pathologischen Anatomie und Histologie, vol 13, part 3. Springer, Berlin Göttingen Heidelberg
Krauland W (1963) Die pathologische Anatomie des Schädel-Hirntraumas. Z Wiener Klin Wochenschr 75: 489
Krauland W (1973) Über die Zeitbestimmung von Schädelhirnverletzungen. Beitr Gerichtl Med 30: 226
Krauland W, Stögbauer R (1961) Zur Kenntnis der Schlagaderverletzungen am Hirngrund bei gedeckten stumpfen Gewalteinwirkungen. Beitr Gerichtl Med 21: 171
Krause C (1927) Über die Bestimmungen des Alters von Organveränderungen beim Mensch und Tier aufgrund histologischer Merkmale mit besonderer Berücksichtigung der Hämosiderinbildung bei Pferd, Rind und Hund. Fischer, Jena
Kraus KA (1955) Über Fettembolie des Gehirns nach Unfällen. Monatsschr Unfallheilkd 58: 353
Kraus R, Eisenbach J, Tebrügge JF, Strand F (1961) Tierexperimentelle Untersuchungen zur Frage des röntgenologischen Nachweises der Fettembolie der Lunge. Med Welt 46: 2406
Kunz W (1932) Die postoperativen Thrombosen und Lungenembolien an der chirurgischen Klinik des St. Marienkrankenhauses zu Frankfurt a. M. in den Jahren 1921–1929. Bruns' Beitr 155: 453

Kuske H (1965) Fremdkörpergranulome. In: Jadassohn J (ed) Entzündliche Dermatosen. Springer, Berlin Heidelberg New York (Handbuch der Haut und Geschlechtskrankheiten. Ergänzungswerk, vol 2, part 2, p 402)
Kühnau J (1962) Biochemie der Wundheilung. Langenbecks Arch u. Dtsch Z Chirur 301: 23
Laiho K (1967) Immunohistochemical studies on fibrin in vital and postmortem subcutaneous haemorrhages. Ann Acad Sci Fenn (Med) 128: 1
Laiho K (1975) Haemostatic plugs as a histological vital reaction in the skin wounds of guinea pigs. Z Rechtsmed 76: 41
La Torre de E, Meredith J, Netzky G (1962) Cerebral air embolism in the dog. Arch Neurol 6: 307
Lauterburg W (1923) Ein Epidermoid frei im Wirbelkanal und seine Kombination mit Hirnläsionen. Virchows Arch [Pathol Anat] 240: 328
Leder LD, Nicolas R (1965) Untersuchungen zur Genese der Fremdkörperriesenzellen mittels der Hautfenstermethode. Frankf Z Pathol 74: 620
Lesser A (1912) Über Folgeerscheinungen postmortaler mechanischer Gewalteinwirkungen. Vierteljahresschr Gerichtl Med u Öffentl Sanitätswesen 44: 203
Letterer E (1959) Allgemeine Pathologie. Thieme, Stuttgart
Lewis A, Pappas M (1969) Experimental fat embolism. A. Evaluation of treatment with low molecular weight dextran. J Trauma 9: 49
Lindner J (1967) Vitale Reaktionen. Dtsch Z Gerichtl Med 59: 312
Lindner J (1971) Vitale Reaktionen. Acta Histochemistry [Suppl] 9: 435
Lob A (1968) Handbuch der Unfallbegutachtung. Ferdinand Enke, Stuttgart
Lo Menzo G (1962) Indagini istologische riguardanti il compartomento del tissuto reticulare, il tissuto elastico, del sistema vasale e degli elementi morfologici del sangue, neu confronti delle läsioni vitali e postmortali. Minerva Med Legalis 82: 340
Mäkinen P-L, Raekallio J (1967) Effect of hydrocortisone on aminopeptidase activation in early wound healing. Naturwissenschaften 54: 202
Mäkinen P-L, Raekallio J (1973) Biochemical distinction between antemortem and post-mortem skin wounds by isoelectric focusing in polyacrylamide gel II. Experimental investigation on phosphatases. Zacchia 48: 284
Mallach H-J (1978) Die Luftembolie als primäre oder konkurrierende Todesursache. Hefte Unfallheilkd 132: 52
Marcinkowski T (1964) Das Auftreten von Hirnfettembolien nach einer vollständigen Abtrennung des Kopfes vom Rumpf durch Zugräder. Arch Med Sadowej 16: 91
Mason JK (1968) Pulmonary fat and bone marrow embolism as an indication of antemortem violence. Med Sci Law 8: 200
Mason RG, Sharp D, Chuang HYK, Mohammad SF (1977) The endothelium. Roles in thrombosis and hemostasis. Arch Pathol Lab Med 101: 61
Masshoff W (1946) Über den Blutabbau im Lichte der allgemeinen Pathologie. Dtsch Med Wochenschr 92
Mayer A (1932) Bemerkungen zur Frage der Thrombose und Embolie. Monatsschr Geburtsheilkd 91: 39
Meinel A, Nemetschek-Gansler H, Holz U, Jonak R, Krahl H, Nemetscheck T, Riedl T (1977) Fibrilläre Gefügestörung bei Sehnenruptur. Arch Orthop Unfallchirur 87: 89
Meixner K (1940) Fettembolie. In: v. Neureiter F, Pietrusky F, Schütt E (eds) Handwörterbuch der gerichtlichen Medizin. Julius Springer, Berlin, p 208
Merker HF (1968) Die Cytochemie der Blutzellen. In: Heilmeyer L (ed) Allgemeine Hämatologie und Physiopathologie des erythrocytären Systems. Springer, Berlin Heidelberg New York (Handbuch der inneren Medizin, edn 5, vol 2, part 1, p 207)
Miller L, Whitting HW (1965) Mast cells and wound healing of the skin in the rat. Zellforsch 65: 597
Millington PF (1974) Histological studies of skin carrying bite marks. J Forensic Sci Soc 14: 239
Miner ME, Handel SF (1978) Traumatic embolization of the intracranial internal carotid artery. Neuroradiology 15: 141
Mityaeva NA (1965) Some histological criteria of vital tissue reactions in mechanical injuries. Sud Med Ekspert 8: 20
Möttönen M, Isomäki AM (1971) Amniotic fluid embolism, diagnosed by a new method. Med Sci Law 1: 35

Motin J, Chadencun O, Bouletreau (1970) Etude clinique des embolies grasseuses posttraumatiques. Med Leg Domm Corpor (Paris) 3: 385
Moylan JA, Birnbaum M, Katz A, Everson MA (1976) Fat emboli syndrome. J Trauma 16: 341
Mueller B (1953) Gerichtliche Medizin. Springer, Göttingen-Heidelberg Berlin, p 247
Mueller B (1964) Zur Frage der Unterscheidung von vitalen bzw. agonalen und postmortalen Blutungen. Acta Med Leg Soc (Liege) 17: 43
Mueller B, Erbach A, Ottmar U (1960) Studien über das Schicksal von Blutaspirationsherden. Riv Med Leg Legislac Sanit 2: 7
Mueller B (1975) Gerichtliche Medizin, 2 edn. Springer, Heidelberg New York
Müller E (1955) Untersuchungen über Art und Bedeutung strömungsmechanischer Vorgänge bei der Coronarthrombose nach Coronarsklerose. Virchows Arch [Pathol Anat] 328: 353
Müller E (1956) Leitfähigkeitsmessungen bei Arteriosklerose und Thromboseproblem. Virchows Arch [Pathol Anat] 329: 363
Müller E, Hofmann V, De Chesne A (1971) Enzymhistochemische Untersuchungen an tierexperimentell gesetzten Schnitt-, Quetsch- und Schürfwunden. Krim Forens Wiss 5: 151
Müller P (1964) Akute und subakute Fruchtwasserembolien, ihre Häufigkeit, ihre Ausbreitung und ihre Folgen. Beitr Pathol Anat 132: 262
Müller P (1966) Schleimembolie der Lungen als tödliche Geburtskomplikation. Frankf Z Pathol 75: 78
Murtazaev CM (1969) Pathologische Morphologie des nicht offenen stumpfen Traumas der großen Arterien der unteren Gliedmaßen im akuten Stadium. Voen Med Zh 7
Nadvornik F, Pavelcova B (1968) The demonstration of fat embolism by thin-layer chromatography. Soudni lék 13: 20
Naeve W, Bause H-W (1974) Experimentelle postmortale Kopf- und Hirnverletzungen. Z Rechtsmed 74: 187
Naeve W, Brinkmann B (1971) Zur Begutachtung der Medionecrosis aortae idiopathica als Todesursache beim Sport. Z Rechtsmed 68: 101
Nejmark EZ (1975) Thrombosen intracranialer Gefäße und Venen. Medicina, Moskau. From Zentralbl Ges Rechtsmed Grenzgebiete 11: 341 (1976 Summary)
Neugebauer W (1959) Über cerebrale Spätfolgen nach Fettembolie. Med Welt 49: 638
Neugebauer W (1961) Cerebrale Dauerschädigung durch Fettembolie. Med Welt 704, 706, 709
Neumann R (1939) Ursprungszentren und Entwicklungsformen der Bein-Thrombose. Virchows Arch [Pathol Anat] 301: 708
Nordmann O (1927) Die Häufung der Thrombosen und Embolien in letzter Zeit. Zentralbl Chir 54: 1900
Nordmann O (1930) Thrombose und Embolie bei chirurgischen Erkrankungen. Chirurg 2: 913
Nunes A (1966) Embolie, aspiration et déglutition de tissue cerebral. Ann Med Leg 46: 329
Nunes A (1970) Les embolies pulmonaires de fragments d'organes. Atti 32, Congrès Intern Med Leg Soc Ling Franc Genova 1969, p 707
Nunes A (1971) Pulmonary embolism by hepatic tissue. J Forensic Sci 16: 57
Obersteg J (1956) Tod und Blutgerinnung. I. Teil. Dtsch Z ges Ger Med 43: 177 (1954) II. Teil Privatdruck Basel
Oehmichen M (1978) Mononuclear phagocytes in the central nervous system. Springer, Berlin, Heidelberg New York
Oehmichen M, Gencic M (1980) Postmortal diffusion of plasma albumin in rat brain. Z Rechtsmed 84: 113
Oehmichen M, Raff G (1980) Timing of cortical contusion. Correlation between histomorphologic alterations and post-traumatic interval. Z Rechtsmed 84: 79
Örkös S (1961) Imprägnationsmethode zur Differenzierung von prä- und postmortaler Verletzung der Herzmuskulatur. Beitr Gerichtl Med 21: 135
Oeser J (1977) Zur Coronarembolie im rechtsmedizinischen Sektionsgut. Z Rechtsmed 79: 311
Ojala K, Lempinen M (1968) Die Initialphase der Muskelnekrose nach Schnittverletzung und ihr Identifizieren als vital im quergestreiften menschlichen Muskel. Dtsch Z Gerichtl Med 64: 102
Ojala K, Lempinen M, Hirvonen J (1969) A comparative study of the character and rapidity of the vital reaction in the incised wounds of human skin and subcutaneous adipose tissue. J Forensic Med 16: 29

Ore GD, Gerstenbrand F, Lücking CH, Peters G, Peters UH (1977) The apallic syndrome. Springer, Berlin Heidleberg New York
Orsós F (1935) Die vitalen Reaktionen und ihre gerichtsmedizinische Bedeutung. Beitr Pathol Anat Allg Pathol 95: 163
Orsós F (1940) Vitale Reaktionen. In: v. Pietruski F, Neureiter F, Schütt E (eds) Handwörterbuch der gerichtlichen Medizin. Springer, Berlin, p 918
Palmovic V, McCarroll JR (1965) Fat embolism in trauma. Arch Pathol Lab Med 80: 630
Panning G (1940) Die vitale Reaktion an Knochen, Veröffentlichungen aus der Konstitutions- und Wehrpathologie. Fischer, Jena
Patzelt D, Lignitz E, Keil W, Takatsu A (1979) Zur Problematik der Diagnose Luftembolie an der Leiche. Beitr Gerichtl Med 37: 401
Pauwaa MC, Aguam AS, Wilder JR, Schweitzer DL (1979) Schußwunde des Herzens mit arterieller Embolie. Eine Sammel-Übersicht und ein Bericht über einen Fall. Vasc Surg 13: 136
Perjes K, Kadas L (1968) Nilblauprobe zum Nachweis der Lipämie und der Fettembolie. Orv Hetil 109: 2279
Peters G (1969) Pathologische Anatomie der Verletzungen des Gehirns und seiner Häute. – In: Kessel FK, Gutmann L, Maurer G (eds) Neurotraumatologie mit Einschluß der Grenzgebiete, vol 1, Urban & Schwarzenberg, München Berlin Wien, p 37
Peters G, Spatz H (1972) Die Rindenprellungsherde bei stumpfer Schädelverletzung, ihre Entwicklung und ihre differentialdiagnostische Bedeutung. (quoted in Unterharnscheidt 1972a)
Petersohn F (1968) Über die forensische Bedeutung der Fruchtwasserembolie als unerwarteter Tod. Beitr Gerichtl Med 24: 167
Pfeifer RA (1930) Grundlegende Untersuchungen für die Angioarchitektur des menschlichen Gehirns. Springer, Berlin
Pierucci G, Gherson G (1970) Sul significato di particolari quatri de „reazione vitale" in possimita di focolai di frattura. Arch Soc sambarda med leg 6: 69
Pierucci G, Gherson G (1971) Etude histo-encymologique de lésion traumatique du system nerveus central. Acta Med Leg Soc (Liege) 20: 179
Pioch W (1963) Histochemische Untersuchungen über die Darstellbarkeit früher Zell- und Gewebsalterationen nach lokaler Hitzeeinwirkung auf die Haut von Mäusen und Meerschweinchen. Habilitationsschrift, Bonn
Pioch W (1964) Demonstration zum Thema: Gewaltsamer Tod. Hirngewebsembolie in die Lungen als Folge von Schädelquetschung. Acta Med Leg Soc (Liege) 17: 95
Pioch W (1966a) Die histochemische Untersuchung thermischer Hautschäden und ihre Bedeutung für die forensische Praxis. Max Schmidt-Römhild, Lübeck
Pioch W (1966b) Histologisch-histochemische Untersuchung zur Identifizierung von Strommarken. Dtsch Z Gerichtl Med 57: 165
Pioch W (1969) Epidermale Esterase-Aktivität als Beweis der vitalen Einwirkung von stumpfer Gewalt. Beitr Gerichtl Med 25: 136
Pioch W (1971) Die Bewertung histochemischer Befunde nach thermischen und stumpfen Hautverletzungen unter forensischem Aspekt. Acta Histochem [Suppl] 9: 405
Plamenac P, Pikula P, Crnalic H, Tomic I (1977) Some histologic findings in newborn aortic media. Acta Med Iugosl 31: 425
Plueckhahn B, Cameron JM (1968) Traumatic "myocarditis" or "myocarditis" in trauma. Med Sci Law 8: 177
Popwassilew I, Kratschmarov I, Varro A (1971) Zum Nachweis der Fettembolie mit lumineszierenden polyzyclischen Kohlenwasserstoffen. Kriminal Forens Wiss 6: 121
Preda I, Moraru I, Manolescu A (1963) Mort rapide post-traumatique par embolie cerebrale dans le cadre dans puste hydatique myocardique avec echinococose secundaire. Ann Med Leg 43: 481
Prinz F (1958) Über den Nachweis von Fettstoffen im Gewebe mit Nilblausulfat. Virchows Arch [Pathol Anat] 331: 558
Prokop O (1968) Einige kritische Fragen der gerichtlichen Medizin und Krininologie. In: Kriminologische Aktualität III. Kriminalistik-Verlag Hamburg
Prokop O, Wabnitz R (1970) Vorkommen von Bindehautblutungen bei Lebenden und Toten, dargestellt in 10 Tabellen. Z Rechtsmed 67: 249
Puppe E (1896) Über Fettembolie bei Phosphorvergiftung. Vierteljahrsschr gerichtl Med u Öffentl Sanitätswesen 12: 95

Putnoky J (1932) Vergleichende pathologisch-histologische Untersuchungen des Herzmuskels bei 1009 Obduktionen unter besonderer Beobachtung der Fälle von Thrombosen und Embolien. Virchows Arch [Pathol Anat] 287: 400

Raekallio J (1965) Die Altersbestimmung mechanisch bedingter Hautwunden mit enzymhistochemischen Methoden. Schmidt-Römhild, Lübeck

Raekallio J (1972) Determination of the age of wounds by histochemical and biochemical methods. Forensic Sci Int 1: 3

Raekallio J (1976) Timing of wounds in forensic medicine. Jpn J Leg Med 30: 125

Raekallio J (1980) Histochemical and biochemical estimation of the age of injuries. In: Perper JA, Wecht CH (eds) Microscopic diagnosis in forensic pathology. C. Thomas, Springfield (Illinois), p 3

Raekallio J, Mäkinen PL (1967) Biochemical and histochemical observations on aminopeptidase activity in early wound healing. Nature 213: 1037

Raekallio J, Mäkinen PL (1969) Serotonin content as vital reaction. Zacchia 44: 587

Raekallio J, Mäkinen PL (1970) Serotonin and histamin countance as vital reactions. Zacchia 45: 403

Raekallio J, Mäkinen PL (1971 a) Biochemical distinction between ante mortem and post mortem skin wounds by isoelectric focusing in polyacrylamide gel. I. Experimental investigation on acrylaminopeptidasis. Zacchia 46: 281

Raekallio J, Mäkinen PL (1971 b) Fermente in der frühen Heilungsphase der Knochenbrüche. Acta Histochem [Suppl] 9: 433

Rajs J (1977) Left ventricular subendocardial haemorrhages. A study of their morphology, pathogenesis and prognosis. Forensic Sci Int 10: 87

Ratschow M (1959) Angiologie. Thieme, Stuttgart

Rauschke T (1956) Beitrag zur Erkennung von Scherenstichverletzungen. Dtsch Z Ges Gerichtl Med 45: 53

Reinhardt G, Zink P (1977) Der Beweiswert der Blutaspiration als vitales Zeichen. Beitr Gerichtl Med 35: 189

Reisner H, Reisner T (1976) Über traumatisch bedingte zerebrale Gefäßthrombosen. Wien Klin Wochenschr 88: 158

Reisner H, Profanter W, Reisner T (1976) Zerebrale Gefäßthrombosen nach stumpfen Schädeltraumen. Wien Klin Wochenschr 88: 162

Remsch R (1964) Zur Frage der intrapulmonalen Fibrinembolie nach Gewebstraumen. – Z Aerztl Fortbild (Jena) 4: 826

Reye (1923) Zur Klinik und Ätiologie der postanginösen septischen Erkrankungen. Virchows Arch [Pathol Anat] 246: 22

Ribbert H (1915) Die Histologie der Blutungen und die extra- und intravasculäre Thrombose. Virchows Arch [Pathol Anat] 220

Richter WG, Bessis MC (1965) Commentary on hemosiderin. Blood 25: 370

Robia FJ, Schulz H (1963) Elektronenmikroskopische Untersuchungen des Blut-Luft-Weges bei der experimentellen Fettembolie der Lunge. Beitr Pathol Anat 128: 78

Romeis B (1968) Mikroskopische Technik. Oldenbourg, München Wien

Rosenkranz KA (1971) Commotio und contusio cordis. Langenbecks Arch Chir 329: 163

Ross R (1968) The fibroblast and wound repair. Biol Rev 43: 51

Ross R, Benditt EP (1961) Wound healing and collagen formation. J Biophys Biochem Cytol 11: 677

Roudier R, Thuiller J, Marchadier J (1965) Mort expérimentale d'animaux soumis à un stress par accélération. Ann Med Leg 45: 372

Rozsahegyi I, Soos I (1956) Caissonkrankheit und Zentralnervensystem. Arb Med 30

Rössle R (1937) Über die Bedeutung und Entstehung der Wadenvenenthrombosen. Virchows Arch [Pathol Anat] 300: 180

Rössle R (1943) Über die serösen Entzündungen der Organe. Virchows Arch [Pathol Anat] 311: 252

Rössle R (1944) Über die Luftembolie der Kapillaren des großen und kleinen Kreislaufs. Virchows Arch [Pathol Anat] 313: 1

Rössle R (1947) Ursache und Folgen der arteriellen Luftembolie des großen Kreislaufs. Virchows Arch [Pathol Anat] 314: 511

Rössle R (1948) Über die ersten Veränderungen des menschlichen Gehirns nach arterieller Luftembolie. Virchows Arch [Pathol Anat] 315: 461
Rössle R (1959) Cited by Bässler 1959
Sandritter W, Bergerhof H (1954) Die Morphologie der fermentativen Auflösung von menschlichen Thromben. Frankf Z Pathol 65: 330
Sandritter W, Beneke C (1966) Thrombose – Formen, Entstehung und Folgen. Hippokrates (Stuttg) 37: 325
Satoh K (1955) Fluid blood and clotted blood in the cadaver. Jpn J Leg Med 9: 440
Satoh T, Sanaka A, Masumato K (1953/54) Studies on the liquid blood of the cadaver after sudden death. Arch Shinsho Univ 3 u. 4
Säker G (1955) Fettembolie bei Verkehrsunfällen. Münch Med Wochenschr 625
Scarborough DE (1971) The pathogenesis of thrombosis in artifical organs and vessels. Curr Top Pathol 54: 95
Schäfer V (1977) Altersbestimmung von Thrombosen und Embolien unter besonderer Berücksichtigung forensischer Gesichtspunkte. Med Diss, Hamburg
Schauwecker K (1930) Über Nierenvenenthrombose. Virchows Arch [Pathol Anat] 274: 197
Schenk RK, Willenegger HR (1977) Zur Histologie der primären Knochenheilung. Modifikation und Grenzen der Spaltheilung in Abhängigkeit von der Defektgröße. Unfallheilkd 80: 155
Schewe G (1968) Zur Differentialdiagnose der Purpura cerebri. Beitr Gerichtl Med 24: 178
Schlatmann JM, Becker AE (1977) Histologic changes on the normal aging aorta: implications for dissecting aortic aneurysm. Am J Cardiol 39: 13
Schmalbruch H (1976) The morphology of regeneration of skeletal muscles in the rat. Tissue Cell 8: 673
Schmidt MB (1940) Störungen des Eisenstoffwechsels und ihre Folgen. X. Die Hämochromatose (Eisenspeicherkrankheit) Ergebn Allg Pathol 35: 105
Schmidt MB (1943) Die Innenpigmentierung retinierter Foeten. Beitr path. Anat Allg Pathol 93: 441
Schmidt O (1929) Zum Nachweis cerebraler Fett- und Luftembolie. Dtsch Z Gerichtl Med 13: 231
Schmidt U, Hartmann G, Morschner E, Elke M (1970) Zur möglichen Rolle der Fettembolie in der Pathogenese der idiopathischen Femurkopfnekrose. Schweiz Med Wochenschr 100: 820
Schneider V (1974) Über rasterelektronenmikroskopische Untersuchungen an vital und postmortal entstandenen „Thromben“. Z Rechtsmed 74: 47
Schneider V, Klug E (1971) Fettembolie der Lungen nach äußerer Herzmassage. Beitr Gerichtl Med 28: 76
Schollmeyer W (1962) Zur Frage der Fettembolie des Lungengewebes bei postmortal Verbrannten. Acta Med Leg Soc (Liege) 15: 77
Schollmeyer W (1965) Über die Fettembolie des Lungengewebes nach Verbrennung. Forum Kriminalistik 5: 32
Schollmeyer W (1971) Zum histologischen Nachweis einer Lungenfettembolie im faulen Gewebe. Krim Forens Wiss 5: 175
Schubert EE, Krüger GA (1962) Morphologische Befunde nach parenteraler Zufuhr feintropfiger Fettemulsionen. Z Gesamte Exp Med 135: 505
Schubert W (1963) Erfahrungsbericht über Luft- und Gasembolien sowie experimentelle Druckfallkrankheit nach Anwendung von z. T. neuen Nachweismethoden. – Int Arch Gewerbepathol Gewerbehyg 20: 261
Schulte HJ (1932) Thrombose und Embolie (Statistische Betrachtungen über 2000 Fälle mit 8 Tabellen und 2 graphischen Darstellungen im Text). Z Klin Med 121: 380
Schulz E (1968) Gefäßleukocytose bei gewaltsamen Tod. Blut 17: 336
Schulz F, Hildebrand E (1977) Exzessive generalisierte Fettembolie bei akut dystrophischer Fettleber. Med Klin 72: 59
Schulz R (1896a) Über den Wert vitaler Zeichen bei mechanischen Verletzungen. Vierteljahresschr Gerichtl Med [Suppl] 12: 44
Schulz R (1896b) Über vitale und postmortale Strangulation. Vierteljahresschr Gerichtl Med 11: 211; 12: 44
Schwarz N, Feigl W, Neuwirth E, Holzner JH (1976) Venöse Thrombosen und Lungenembolien im Obduktionsgut. Wien Klin Wochenschr 88: 423

Schwerd W (1962) Der rote Blutfarbstoff und seine wichtigsten Derivate. Schmidt-Römhild, Lübeck
Seifert KE, Friedrich H (1965) Wundheilung und Psychopharmaka. Bruhns Beitr Klin Chir 211: 288
Seitz HD, Köhnlein HE, Ocker K, Tonn M (1978) Untersuchungen zur Wundheilung von Sekundär- und Tertiärwunden. Z Exp Chir 11: 121
Serck-Hanssen A (1965) Post traumatic fat embolism. Red cell aggregation, hyaline microthrombi and platelet aggregates in 5 fatal cases. Acta Pathol Microbiol Scand 65: 31
Sessner HH, Schütterle G, Remmolo W, Lehmann V, Lasch HG (1962) Allgemeine hämorrhagische Diathese und vaskuläre Fibrinabscheidungen im sekundären Stadium der experimentellen Fettembolie. Med Welt, p 2105
Sevitt S (1962) Fat embolism. Butterworth, London
Shapiro HA (1962) Death from fat embolism. Acta Med Leg Soc (Liege) 15: 81
Silverman L, Shorter RG (1963) Histogenesis of the multinucleated giant cell. Lab Invest 12: 985
Sinapius D (1967) Zur Morphologie und Histochemie der Fette in Coronarthromben. Virchows Arch [Pathol Anat] 342: 144
Singur NA (1970) Mechanismen der Entstehung, pathologische Anatomie und gerichtsmedizinische Diagnostik (in Russian). Vgl. Medizinia, Moscow
Sloder MH, Lock FR (1952) Sudden maternal death associated with amniotic fluid embolism. Am J Obstet Gynecol 64: 118
Slunsky R, Mirejovsky P (1963) Fruchtwasserembolie als Ursache einer Blutgerinnungsstörung. Zentralbl Gynecol 85: 1396
Smith S (1945) Forensic medicine. Churchill, London
Soloway HB, Robinson EF, Sleeman HK et al (1970) Resolutions of experimental fat embolism. Arch Pathol 90: 230
Spann W, Henn R (1970) Posttraumatische Hirnpurpura und cerebrale Fettembolie. Lebensvers Med 22: 16
Staak M (1968) Das Coma dépassé. Ein Beitrag zur Problematik des klinischen Todes. In: Dürwald W (ed) Aktuelle Fragen der gerichtlichen Medizin (III), Wissenschaftl. Beiträge der Martin-Luther-Universität Halle-Wittenberg, 1968/12 (R8), p 238
Stelzig HH, Kössling FK (1969) Lungenfettembolie bei Leberverfettung. Med Welt 20: 401, 405
Stöhr W, Kazda F (1928) Über die Bedeutung der Infektion für die postoperative Thrombose und Thrombembolie. Dtsch Z Chir 208: 105
Struck H, Engelhardt GH (1971) Altersabhängigkeit der Wundheilung? Z Gerontol 4: 356
Struck H (1976) Morphologische und biochemische Grundlagen der Wundheilung. Unfallheilkunde 79: 449
Suppan A (1963) Experimentelle Untersuchungen zum Problem Cytostatica und Wundheilungsstörungen. Z Krebsforschg 65: 547
Szabo G (1971) Die Fettembolie. Akad Kiadò, Budapest
Tapfer S (1933) Thrombose und tödliche Embolie an der Innsbrucker Frauenklinik in den Jahren 1919 bis 1929. Zentralbl Gynaekol 796
Tendeloo N (1933) Plötzlicher Tod durch Embolie. Nederl Tijdschr Geneesk 2282
Thomas E (1977) In: Graumann W, Neumann K (eds) Histochemie der Enzyme im peripheren Nervensystem. Fischer New York (Handbuch der Histochemie, vol 7/5)
Timm F (1958) Zur Histochemie der Schwermetalle. Das Sulfidsilberverfahren. Dtsch Z Gerichtl Med 46: 706
Timm F (1960) Der histochemische Eisennachweis. Histochemistry 2: 143
Unterharnscheidt FJ (1972a) Mechanogenese und Pathomorphologie der traumatischen Hirnschäden. Beitr Gerichtl Med 29: 73
Unterharnscheidt FJ (1972b) Die traumatischen Hirnschäden. Mechanogenese, Pathomorphologie und Klinik. Z Rechtsmed 71: 153
Uta K (1924) Die isolierte Thrombose des Sinus cavernosus bei Ohrerkrankungen. Virchows Arch [Pathol Anat] 249: 131
Vadasz G, Földes G, Kiraly M, Vajda J (1973) Ein Fall von juveniler Thrombosis Arteriae carotis internae. Münch Med Wochenschr 115: 561
Veit B (1922) Ein Beitrag zur pathologischen Anatomie des Morbus Addisonii (Agenesie der linken

Nebenniere, Verödung der Marksubstanz infolge Blutung durch Venenthrombose der kompensatorisch hypertrophischen rechten Nebenniere). Virchows Arch [Pathol Anat] 238: 269
Vesterby A, Gregersen M (1980) Atrial fibrillation resulting from cardiac trauma. Z Rechtsmed 85: 153
Voigt GE (1962) Experimentelle pulmonale Gewebstrümmerembolie. Dtsch Z Gerichtl Med 52: 558
Voigt GE (1971) Metallnachweis. Acta Histochem [Suppl] 9: 489
Wagner HJ (1959) Das Erkennen und Verhalten von fettfärbbaren Substanzen in den Lungen vor und nach Brandeinwirkung mittels histochemischer und papierchromatographischer Untersuchungen. Dtsch Z Gerichtl Med 49: 130
Walcher K (1930) Über vitale Reaktionen. Dtsch Z Gerichtl Med 15: 16
Walcher K (1935) Zur Differentialdiagnose einiger Zeichen vitaler Reaktionen. Dtsch Z Gerichtl Med 24: 16
Walcher K (1936) Die vitale Reaktion bei der Beurteilung des gewaltsamen Todes. Dtsch Z Gerichtl Med 26: 193
Walther G (1972) Spättodesfall nach Contusio cordis. Monatsschr Unfallheilkd 75: 38
Walther G, Lieven T (1971) Histochemische Organveränderungen in Leber und Herzmuskel der Ratte nach Sauerstoffintoxikation. Beitr Gerichtl Med 28: 50
Warniez C, Loffredo V (1977) Le risque thrombotique sous oestro-progestatifs anticonceptionnels: éléments de pathogénie. Rev Fr Gynecol 72: 141
Wegener F, Sack K (1967) Artefizielle postmortale Fettembolie. Tag Nordd u Westdtsch Pathol 27.–29.10. 1967 Lüneburg
Wegmann R, Petrescu F, Marcy R, Eymard P (1970) Modifications histo-enzymologiques du système nerveux central au cours de l'épilepsie et du traumatisme. Approche expérimentale. Rev Neurol 123: 153
Weiler F, Reinhardt V, Nau H-E, Gerhard L (1980) Beitrag zum intracraniellen „traumatischen Aneurysma". Z Rechtsmed 85: 225
Weimann W (1929) Über die Hirnveränderungen bei cerebraler Fettembolie. Dtsch Z Gerichtl Med 13: 95
Weinig E, Schwerd W (1951) Histochemische Beobachtungen nach Seifenwassereinspritzung in die schwangere Gebärmutter. Dtsch Z Ges Gerichtl Med 40: 649
Weitbrecht W-U, Nuber B, Sandritter W (1976) Atraumatische Rhabdomyolyse. Med Welt 27: 1261
Werkgartner A (1926) Postmortale, nicht agonale Blutungen im Halsgebiet (eine Nachprüfung der Arbeit Christeller's: Über agonale Blutungen im Gebiet der oberen Hohlvene). Dtsch Z Gerichtl Med 6: 630
Whitenack SH, Hausberger FX (1971) Intravasation of fat from the bone marrow cavity. Am J Pathol 65: 335
Wilhelmi F, Hildebrandt E (1972) Tödliche Lungenembolie nach Aortenaneurysma-Ruptur in die Vena cava caudalis. Z Rechtsmed 71: 246
Wille R, Ebert M, Cornely M (1969) Zeitstudien über Hämosiderin. Arch Kriminol 144: 28
Winter R (1931) Über die Entstehung von Thromben im rechten Herzen (Endocarditis thrombotica parietalis carcinomatosa) und in den Ästen der Lungenschlagader (Thrombarteriitis pulmonalis carcinomatosa) auf dem Boden von Krebszellenembolien. Virchows Arch [Pathol Anat] 282: 99
Wohlgemuth B (1962) Riesenzellen. Dtsch Med Wochenschr 87: 489
Wojtek E (1955) Entzügelungshochdruck durch Fettembolie. Medizinische (Berlin) 544
Wurm E (1956) Über die Entstehung der Fremdkörperriesenzellen. Beitr path Anat Beitr Pathol Anat 116: 149
Zagryadskaya AP (1965) Histological study of cuts and step wounds. Sud Med Ekspert 8: 3
Zahir M (1964) Contraction of wounds. Br J Surg 51: 456
Ziegler H-K (1977) Lungenembolie aus der Sicht des Pathologen. Med Klin 72: 1063
Zollinger H (1966) Niere und ableitende Harnwege. In: Doerr W, Uehlinger E (eds) Spezielle Pathologische Anatomie, vol 3. Springer, Berlin Heidelberg New York
Zollinger HU (1962) Die Wundheilung vom Standpunkt der pathologischen Anatomie. Helvet Chir Acta 29: 181
Zülch KJ (1955) Gedanken zur Entstehung und Behandlung der Schlaganfälle. Wien Med Wochenschr 105: 1035

References to B III: Oxygen Deficiency

Adebahr G (1960) Gehirnveränderungen nach wochenlanger posttraumatischer Bewußtlosigkeit. Dtsch Z Gerichtl Med 49: 680

Altmann HW (1944) Über das Auftreten von Vakuolen, Einschlußkörperchen und hyalinen Tropfen in den Leberzellen beim experimentellen Sauerstoffmangel. Verh Dtsch Ges Pathol 60

Altmann HW (1960) Über das Cytozentrum in Epitheloid- und Riesenzellen. Berl Med 11: 27

Angstwurm H, Kugler J (1978) Ärztliche Aspekte des Hirntodes und Feststellung des Todeszeitpunktes. Fortschr Neurol Psychiat 46: 297

Bade GE, Schumacher A (1964) Veränderungen der submikroskopischen Struktur der Leberzellen der Maus nach temporärer Ischämie. Frankf Z Pathol 74: 29

Bajusz E, Jasmin G (1964) Histochemically demonstrable phosphorylase as an early index of anoxic myocardial damage. Experientia (Basel) 20: 373

Bargmann W (1935) Zur vergleichenden Histologie der Lungenalveole. Z Zellforsch 23: 335

Beneke G, Scomazzoni G (1962) Beziehung zwischen Erythrophagozytose epithelialer Zellen und hyalintropfigen Ablagerungen. Verh Dtsch Ges Pathol 46: 194

Bertalanffy FD, Lieblund CP (1953) The continous renewal of the two types of alveolar cells in the lung of the rat. Anat Rec 115: 515

Biavia C (1964) Mallory alcoholic hyalin: A heretofore unique lesion of hepatocellular ergastoplasm. Lab Invest 13: 301

Bowden DH (1971) The alveolar macrophage. Curr Top Pathol 55: 1

Burdette WJ, Ashfort TP (1965) Structural changes in the human myocardium following hypoxia. J Thorac Cardiovasc Surg 50: 210

Büchner F (1937) Die pathogenetische Bedeutung der Hypoxämie. Klin Wochenschr 1409

Büchner F (1942) Die pathogenetische Wirkung des allgemeinen Sauerstoffmangels, insbesondere bei der Höhenkrankheit und dem Höhentod. Klin Wochenschr 721

Büchner F (1944) Die pathogenetische Bedeutung des allgemeinen Sauerstoffmangels. Verh Dtsch Ges Pathol p 20

Büchner F (1950) Allgemeine Pathologie. Urban & Schwarzenberg, München, p 111

Büchner F (1957) Die Pathologie der zellulären und geweblichen Oxidationen. Die Hypoxidosen. In: Der Stoffwechsel II. Springer, Berlin Göttingen Heidelberg (Handbuch der allgemeinen Pathologie, vol 4, part 2, p 569)

Büchner F (1970) Hypoxämische Verfettung und Nekrosen der Herz-Muskelzellen im lichtmikroskopischen Bild. Beitr Pathol Anat 140: 142

Büchner F, Onishi S (1968) Der Herzmuskel bei akuter Coronarinsuffizienz im elektronenmikroskopischen Bild. Urban & Schwarzenberg, München Berlin Wien (Fortschritte der morphologischen Pathologie, Hrsg. v. Büchner, F.)

Cain H (1962) Histologische und histochemische Befunde bei hypoxidotischen Schäden des Herzmuskels. (Forum Cardiologicum) C. F. Boehringer und Söhne, Mannheim-Waldhof p 49

Colmant H (1965) Cerebrale Hypoxie. Thieme, Stuttgart

Cooper DKC (1977) Versuch zur Feststellung der Lebensfähigkeit wiederbelebter und funktionsfähig gehaltener Herzen mittels Anfärbung des Herzmuskels durch Hämatoxylin - basisches Fuchsin - Pikrinsäure. Histochem J 9: 285

Eisenmenger W, Beckmann G, Tröger H-D, Wilske J (1976) Hirnveränderungen nach passagerer erfolgreicher Reanimation. Beitr Gerichtl Med 34: 35

Eppinger H (1935) Die seröse Entzündung. Springer, Wien

Erich WE (1956) Reaktionen. Springer, Berlin Göttingen Heidelberg (Handbuch der allgemeinen Pathologie. vol VII, part 1)

Evans M, Dekker NP, Cabral-Anderson LJ, Freeman G (1978) Quantitation of damage to the alveolar epithelium by means of type 2 cell proliferation. Am Rev Respir Dis 118: 787

Flax MH, Tisdale WA (1964) An electron microscopic study of alcoholic hyalin. Am J Pathol 44: 441

Gebbers JO, Tetzner C, Burkhardt A (1979) Alveolitis due to hairspray. Ultrastructural observations in two patients and the results of experimental investigations. Virchows Arch [Pathol Anat] 382: 323

Gieseking R (1958) Aufnahme und Ablagerung von Fremdstoffen in der Lunge nach elektronenoptischen Untersuchungen. Ergeb Allg Pathol Pathol Anat 38: 92

Gieseking R (1959) Das experimentelle Lungenödem im elektronenoptischen Bild. Verh Dtsch Ges Pathol 43: 344
Hambach R (1958) Ein Beitrag zur exakten morphologischen Diagnose der Erstickung. Soud lek 3: 182
Hasper B (1964) Ultramikroskopische Herzmuskelveränderungen nach wiederholter Hypoxie. Beitr Pathol Anat 130: 321
Holle G, Burghardt R, Arndt S, Blödorn M (1955) Über manometrische, histochemische, histologische und phasenoptische Befunde bei ischämischer Hypoxidose. – Beitrag zur Morphogenese und zur Frage des örtlichen Gewebstodes. Virchows Arch 327: 150
Janssen W (1963) Riesenzellenbildung bei Erstickung. Dtsch Z Gerichtl Med 54: 200
Janssen W (1969) Der forensische Beweiswert histologischer Untersuchungen. Beitr Gerichtl Med 25: 51
Janssen W, Bärtschi G (1964) Vitale und supravitale Reaktionen der Alveolarzellen nach protrahiertem Sauerstoffmangel. Dtsch Z Gerichtl Med 55: 47
Jetter WW (1959) Post mortem biochemical changes. J Forensic Sci 4: 330
Kalimo H, Garcia JH, Kamijyo Y, Tanaka J, Trump BF (1977) The ultrastructure of "brain death". II. Electron microscopy of feline cortex after complete ischemia. Virchows Arch (Cell Pathol) 25: 207
Kernbach M (1963) Karyologische Befunde bei menschlicher perakuter Hypoxie. Zentralbl Allg Pathol Pathol Anat 104: 477
Köberle F (1956) Über die Dauer der Riesenzellenbildung. Zentralbl Allg Pathol Pathol Anat 95: 540
Lance JS, Latta H (1963) Hypoxia, atelectasis and pulmonary edema. The role of hypoxia in the production of pulmonary edema, atelectasis and hyaline membranes Arch Pathol Lab Med 75: 373
Lange F (1909) Untersuchungen über das Epithel der Lungenalveolen. Frankf Z Pathol 3: 170
Letterer E (1959) Allgemeine Pathologie. Thieme, Stuttgart, p 520
Löblich HJ (1962) Quantitative Untersuchungen über das Verhalten der alveokapillären Membran bei experimentellem Sauerstoffmangel. Verh Dtsch Ges Pathol 46: 278
Lucas BGB, Strangeways DH (1956) Experimental cerebral anoxia. J Pathol Anat 95: 540
Montaldo G, Serreli A (1964) Bläschenabgabe aus dem Glomerulus-Endothel in normalen und experimentell anoxämischen Kaninchennieren. Mikroskopie 19: 204
Mueller B (1961) Tierexperimentelle Studien über den Erstickungstod, insbesondere über Erdrosseln und Erwürgen. Dtsch Z Gerichtl Med 51: 377
Oliver WJ, Brody GL (1965) Effect of prolonged hypoxia upon granularity of renal juxtaglomerular cells. Circ Res 16: 83
Oudea PR (1963) Anoxic changes of liver cells. Electron microscopic study after injection of colloidal mercury. Lab Invest 12: 386
Peschropka J (1942) Tierexperimentelle Untersuchungen zur pathologischen Histologie des akuten Höhentodes. Beitr Pathol Anat 107: 117
Poche R (1965) Über die Bedeutung der Blutkapillaren für die herdförmige Anordnung von sog. hypoxischen Herzmuskelveränderungen. Verh Dtsch Ges Path 49: 219
Policard A (1955) Le poumon. Masson, Paris
Ponsold A (1961) Erstickung. Dtsch Z Gerichtl Med 51: 333
Prokop O, Göhler W (1975) Forensische Medizin. VEB Volk und Gesundheit, Berlin
Reh H (1969) Diagnostik des Ertrinkungstodes und Bestimmung der Wasserzeit. Michael Triltsch, Düsseldorf
Reppart JT, Peters RL, Edmundson HA, Baker RF (1963) Electron and light microscopy of sclerosing hyaline necrosis of the liver. The development of alcoholic hyaline bodies. Lab Invest 12: 1138
Rössle R (1944) Seröse Entzündung. Verh Dtsch Ges Pathol, 1
Saathoff J (1950) Medulläre und extramedulläre Blutbildung unter Sauerstoffmangel. Virchows Arch 319: 116
Sachs HW (1954/55) Die Deutung der Fettverteilung in der Leber in einem forensischen Sektionsgut. Dtsch Z Ges Gerichtl Med 43: 103
Sawaguchi A, Yoshinari K (1971) Studies on the activity of lactate dehydrogenase and its isozymes in acute suffocation. Jpn J Leg Med 25: 409

Schlicht I (1963) Experimentelle Untersuchungen über die hyalintropfige Eiweißspeicherung der Leber. Virchows Arch [Pathol Anat] 336: 342
Schlicht I (1955) Experimentelle Untersuchungen über den Ablauf der Leberverfettung bei Hunger und Sauerstoffmangel. Virchows Arch 326: 568
Schlütz GO (1954) Zum Problem der Vakuolenbildung in den zentralen Leberläppchen, zugleich ein neues Verfahren der Leberdurchströmung. Aerztl Forsch 8: 78
Schneider M (1959) Überlebens- und Wiederbelebungszeit von Gehirn, Herz, Leber, Niere nach Ischämie und Anoxie (Forschungsbericht des Landes Nordrhein-Westfalen, ed. v. Leo Brandt, Nr. 1369). Westdeutscher Verlag, Köln-Opladen
Schürmann P, McMahon HE (1933) Die maligne Nephrosklerose, zugleich ein Beitrag zur Frage der Bedeutung der Blutgewebsschranke. Virchows Arch [Pathol Anat] 291: 47
Sedláček J, Mráz J (1978) Postmortal activity of reticuloendothelial cells in the lungs. Sb ved Pr Lek Fak Univ Karlovy 21: 105
Seller MJ, Spector RG (1964) The effects of anoxia on the new born and adult rat lung. J Pathol 88: 309
Spector WG (1974) The macrophage: Its origin and role in pathology. Pathobiol Ann 4: 33
Swann HE (1964) The development of pulmonary edema during the agonal period of sudden asphyxial death. J Forensic Sci 9: 360
Sykes BI, Penny E, Purchase IFH (1976) Hepatocyte vacuolation and increased liver weight occurring in anoxic rats. Toxicol Appl Pharmacol 36: 31
Szabó G (1940) Zwerchfellveränderungen bei langsamer Erstickung. Dtsch Z Gerichtl Med 33: 1
Tausch D, Möller M (1973) Tierexperimentelle Untersuchungen über Sauerstoffmangelzustände im Hinblick auf den „plötzlichen Kindstod". Beitr Gerichtl Med 31: 130
Vogell W, Voss R, Schön HR, Becker WH (1964) Elektronenmikroskopische und cytochemische Befunde am Papillarmuskel des Kaninchenherzens nach Sauerstoffentzug. Acta Histochem (Jena) 19: 234
Wagner HJ (1966) Concerning the relationship between the histological findings in the lung and the capacity to function after attempts at suffocation. Acta Med Leg Soc (Liege) 19: 335
Wegmann R, Biget PL, Senela A, Loubiere R, Tordet-Caribroit C (1959) Effect de l'anoxy agu sur le succinodehydrogenasis. Ann Histochem (Paris) 4: 245
Wohlgemuth B (1962) Riesenzellen. Dtsch Med Wochenschr 87: 489
Wurm E (1956) Über die Entstehung der Fremdkörperriesenzellen. Beitr Pathol Anat 116: 149

References to B IV: Shock

Adebahr G (1971) Die Bedeutung des Schocks für die Entstehung der Gasbrandbazillensepsis nach Abtreibung. Beitr Gerichtl Med 28: 117
Ambrosi L, Vimercati F, D'nunno (1968) Aspetti istologici delle reazioni immunitarie nella morte da shock allergico. Minerva Medicoleg 88: 105
Archer RK (1965) On the functions of eosinophils in the antigen-antibody reaction. Br J Heamatol 11: 123
Baer DM, Osborn JJ (1960) The postperfusion pulmonary congestion syndrome. Am J Clin Pathol 34: 442
Balslov JT, Jorgensen HE (1963) A survey of 499 patients with acute anuric renal insufficiency. Causes, treatment, complications and mortality. Am J Med 34: 753
Bankl H, Jellinger K (1968) Schocktod nach oraler Penicillineinnahme. Wien Klin Wochenschr 80: 43
Beneke G (1970) Veränderungen der Leber im Schock. In: Horatz K (ed) Leber- und Pankreasschäden durch Schock und Narkose. G. Thieme, Stuttgart, pp 2–17
Benzer H, Lembert J, Regele H (1969) Oberflächenspannung in der Lunge und hyaline Membranen-Krankheit. Wien Klin Wochenschr 81: 145
Berndt V, Götz E, Schönleben K, Langhans P (1978) Das Streßulkus: derzeitiger Stand von Pathogenese, Klinik, Prophylaxe und Therapie. Prakt Anaesth 13: 108
Bleyl U (1970) Vergleichende Untersuchungen an Erwachsenen und Neugeborenen zur Entstehung pulmonaler hyaliner Membranen. Verh Dtsch Ges Pathol 54: 340

Bleyl U (1971a) Morphologische Untersuchungen zur Pathogenese pulmonaler hyaliner Membranen. Zentralbl Pathol Pathol Anat 114: 104
Bleyl U (1971b) Pathomorphologie und Pathogenese des Atemnotsyndroms. Verh Dtsch Ges Pathol 55: 39
Bleyl U, Büsing CM (1969) Disseminierte intravasale Gerinnung und perinataler Schock. Verh Dtsch Ges Pathol 53: 495
Bleyl U, Büsing CM (1970) Kreislaufschock und disseminierte intravasale Gerinnung bei intrauterinem und perinatalem Fruchttod. Klin Wochenschr 48: 13
Bleyl U, Büsing CM, Krempien B (1969) Pulmonale hyaline Membranen und perinataler Kreislaufschock. – Virchows Arch [Pathol Anat] 348: 187
Bleyl U, Heilmann K, Adler D (1971) Generalisierte plasmatische Hypercoagulabilität und pulmonale hyaline Membranen beim Erwachsenen. Klin Wochenschr 49: 71
Bohler RK, Bibighaus AJ (1967) Ultrastructural alterations of dog livers during endotoxin shock. Lab Invest 17: 537
Boyd JF (1967) Disseminated fibrin thromboembolism among neonates dying within 48 hours of birth. Arch Dis Child 42: 401
Bywaters EG (1948) Anatomical changes in the liver after trauma. Clin Sci 6: 19
Campiche MA (1963) L'ultrastructure pulmonaire chez le foetus et le nouveau-né. Thèse méd, Lausanne
Congdon CC (1964) The early histologic effects of antigenic stimulation. Arch Pathol Lab Med 78: 83
Dawes GS (1961) Change in the circulation at birth. Br Med Bull 17: 148
Dawes GS (1966) Pulmonary circulation in the foetus and newborn. Br Med Bull 22: 61
Day JM (1962) Death due to cerebral infarction after wasp stings. Arch Neurol (Chicago) 7: 184
De Palma RG, Levy S, Holden WD (1970) Ultrastructure and oxidative phosphorylation of liver mitochondria in experimental haemorrhagic shock. J Trauma 10: 122
Dirnhofer R, Sonnabend W, Sigrist T (1978) Zur erweiterten Diagnostik des tödlichen Penicillin-Zwischenfalles, immunhistologischer Nachweis der Antigen-Antikörper-Komplexe sowie von Antikörpern gegen die tubuläre Basalmembran nach Gabe von Depotpenicillin. Schweiz Med Wochenschr 108: 750
Doenicke A, Holle F (1962) Das Verhalten der Leberfunktion im postoperativen Schock. Fortschr Med 80: 253
Ellenberg M, Osserman KE (1951) Role of shock in production of central liver cell necrosis. Am J Med 11: 170
Fajers CM, Gelin LE (1959) Kidney-liver- and heartdamages from trauma and from induced intravascular aggregation of blood cells. Acta Pathol Microbiol Scand 46: 97
Faria JL, de (1962a) Histopathological changes in the coronary arteries of rabbits after orthostasis with arteriosclerotic features. Pathol Microbiol (Basel) 25: 1
Faria JL de (1962b) Histopathological changes in the coronary arteries following shock or hypotension in man. Their relation to thrombosis and atherogenesis, I. Pathol Microbiol (Basel) 25: 1
Faria JL de (1963) Histopathological changes in the coronary arteries following shock or hypotension in man. Their relation to thrombosis and atherogenesis, II. Pathol Microbiol (Basel) 26: 385
Faria JL de, Oliveira RB de (1962) Hypophysennekrose nach Schockzuständen. Zum Mechanismus der Nekrose bei Sheehan'schem Syndrom und zum Problem der Hypophysenvorderlappennekrosen bzw. – Atrophien und Hypopituitarismen unbekannter Ursachen. Beitr Pathol Anat 127: 213
Fazekas IG (1965) Altérations microscopiques dans des cas de mort par choc, d'origines différentes. Ann Méd Lég (Paris) 45: 145
Franklin KJ, McGee LE, Ullmann E (1949) Anoxic diversion of the renal cortical blood flow. Proc Soc Exp Biol 71: 339
Freudenberg N (1977) Untersuchungen des Endothels von Blutgefäßen bei Schock. Habilitationsschrift, Freiburg i. Br.
Freudenberg N (1978) Endothelium and shock. Pathol Res Pract 162: 105
Freytag G, Mitschke H, Klöppel G (1970) Immunpathologische Untersuchungen zur experimentellen Insulitis. Verh Dtsch Ges Pathol 54: 290
Gelin LE, Shoemaker WC (1961) Hepatic blood flow and microcirculatory alterations induced by dextran of high and low viscosity. Surgery 49: 713

Gruenwald P (1963) Normal and abnormal expansion of lungs of newborn infants obtained at autopsy. II. Opening pressure, maximal volume and stability of expansion. Lab Invest 12: 563
Guyton AG, Crowell JW (1961) Dynamics of the heart in shock. Fed Proc [Suppl 9] 20: 51
Halperin L (1936) Über die tödliche Wirkung der Bienen- und Wespenstiche. Dissertation Basel
Hardaway RM (1961) Disseminated intravascular coagulation syndromes. Arch Surg 83: 842
Hardaway RM (1966) Syndromes of disseminated intravascular coagulation. C. C Thomas, Springfield/Ill
Hardaway RM, Chun B, Rutherford B (1965) Histologic evidence of disseminated intravascular coagulation. A clinical shock report of a new finding. Angiology 2: 254
Hardaway RM, James PM, Anderson RW, Bredenberg CE, West RL (1967) Intensive study and treatment of shock in men. J Am Med Ass 199: 779
Harms D (1971 a) Postmortale Fibrinolyse beim Menschen. G. Fischer, Stuttgart
Harms D (1971 b) Grundlagen einer pathologisch-anatomischen Diagnostik der Verbrauchskoagulopathie. Blut 23: 261
Harms D, Lehmann H (1969) Untersuchungen über die periphere Mikrothrombose in einem ausgewählten Sektionsgut. Virchows Arch [Pathol Anat] 347: 57
Hassenstein J, Riede UN, Mittermayer C, Sandritter W (1980) Zur Frage der Reversibilität der schockinduzierten Lungenfibrose. Anaesth Intensivther Notfallmed 15: 340
Heene DL, Lasch HG (1977) Klinische Aspekte der Mikrozirkulationsstörungen unter besonderer Berücksichtigung des Schocks. In: Mikrozirkulation/Microcirculation. Springer, Berlin Heidelberg New York (Handbuch der Allgemeinen Pathologie, vol 3/part 7, pp 889–995)
Heymer R, Fischer R (1980) Gibt es eine Schocktrachea? Pathologe 1: 232
Janssen W (1966) Plötzliche Todesfälle durch Insektenstiche. Morphologie, Toxikologie und forensische Bedeutung. Dtsch Z Gerichtl Med 58: 3
Jensen OM (1962) Sudden death due to stings from bees and wasp. Report of 4 new cases, 3 with autopsy. Acta Pathol Microbiol Scand 54: 9
Joachim H, Riede UN, Mittermayer Ch (1978) The weight of human lungs as a diagnostic criterion (Distinction of normal lungs from shock lungs by histologic, morphometric and biochemical investigations). Pathol Res Pract 162: 24
Kent SG, Ekker EE (1965) The role of intravascular pulmonary occlusions in fatal anaphylaxis in the guinea pig. Am J Pathol 6: 959
Kief H, Vitak V (1971) Befunde an der Rattenleber bei verschiedenen Schockformen. Med Welt 22: 1183
Killip T, Payne MA (1960) High serum transaminase activity in heart disease. Circulatory failure and hepatic necrosis. Circulation 27: 646
Klein HJ, Gheorghiu T, Hübner G, Eder M (1971) Zur Pathogenese streßbedingter Magenulcera. Virch Arch (Pathol Anat) 352: 195
Knisely MH: zit. v. H. O. Zollinger 1966
Kolin A, Johanovsky J, Pekarek J (1965) Histological manifestations of cellular (delayed) hypersensitivity. I. Alterative component in tuberculin skin reaction in guinea-pigs. Z Immunol Allergieforsch 128: 117
Korb G, Müller R, Gedigk P (1968) Tierexperimentelle Untersuchungen über die Schockleber. Tag. Nord. u. Westdtsch Pathologen 11.–13. 10. 1968 Bielefeld
Korb G, Müller R, Gedigk P, Hellwig K (1969 a) Über die Entstehung und Abheilung von Lebernekrosen nach einem einmaligen Schock. Virchows Arch [Pathol Anat] 348: 374
Korb G, Gedigk P, Müller R, Müller U (1969 b) Tierexperimentelle Untersuchungen über die Netznekrose in der Leber. Virchows Arch [Pathol Anat] 347: 357
Koslowski L (1960) Angiographische Untersuchungen der Nierendurchblutung nach Trauma bei der Ratte. Beitr Pathol Anat 122: 443
Kovats TG, Reok A, Lazar G, Takats S, Vegh P (1961) Changes in fat metabolism during the Shwartzman phenomenon and its clinical significance. Z Gesamt Inn Med 16: 15
Kringsholm B, Thomsen JL, Lejers J, Jensen T, Hansen JPH, und Voigt J (1979) Acute oesophagogastroduodenal ulceration in forensic pathology. Ugeskr Laeger 141: 1074
Lange HP, Kornhuber B (1970) Obduktionsbefunde bei zwei Fällen immunologisch behandelter akuter Leukosen im Kindesalter. Verh Dtsch Ges Pathol 54: 322
Lapp H (1971) Elektronenmikroskopische Befunde an der terminalen Strombahn von Lunge und Niere bei Schock. Med Welt 22: 1180

Lasch HG (1959) Über latente Gerinnung in der Blutbahn. Habilitationsschrift, Heidelberg
Lasch HG, Heene DL, Huth K, et al. (1967) Pathophysiology, clinical manifestations, and therapy of consumptioncoagulopathy („Verbrauchskoagulopathie"). Am J Cardiol 20: 381
Lasch HG, Huth K, Heene DL, Müller-Berghaus G, Hörder MH, Zanzarik H, Mittermayer C und Sandritter W (1971) Die Klinik der Verbrauchskoagulopathie. Dtsch Med Wochenschr 96: 715
Lasch HG, Michelke K, Nusser E, Daoud F (1961) Der Einfluß der Fibrinolyse auf den Verlauf der hämorrhagischen Schocks. Klin Wochenschr 39: 1137
Lasch HG, Roka L, Heene D (1966) The defibrination syndrome. Thromb Haemost [Suppl] 20: 97
Leber HW, Schütterle G (1971) Zur Pathophysiologie der Schockniere. Med Welt 22: 1169
Lederer B, Mittermayer Ch (1967) Zur pathologisch-anatomischen Diagnose des Schocks. Zentralbl allg Pathol Pathol Anat 110: 167
Letterer E (1962) Morphologische Folgen der Antigen-Antikörperreaktion. Verh Dtsch Ges Pathol 46: 83
Loew B, Wiedemann R, Remmele W (1971) Gerinnungsanalytische und pathologisch-anatomische Untersuchungen beim traumatischen Schock. Klin Wochenschr 49: 1101
Lutz H (1972) Formen des Schocks. Dtsch Med Wochenschr 97: 287
Martin AM Jr, Hackel DB (1963) The myocardium of the dog in hemorrhagic shock. A histochemical study. Lab Invest 12: 77
Martin AM Jr, Hackel DB (1966) An electron microscopic study of the progression of myocardial lesions in the dog after hemorrhagic shock. Lab Invest 15: 243
Martin AM Jr, Hackel DB, Kurtz SM (1964) The ultrastructure of zonal lesions of the myocardium in hemorrhagic shock. Am J Pathol 44: 127
Marx R, Evertz K, Jahrmärker H, Georgii A (1966) Thrombozytenagglomeration als Teilkomponente der Muskelfrühgifttoxikation bzw. des Muskelfrühgiftschocks. Klin Wochenschr 44: 340
Mittermayer C, Vogel W, Burchardi H, Birzie H, Wiemers K, Sandritter W (1970) Pulmonale Mikrothrombosierung als Ursache der respiratorischen Insuffizienz bei Verbrauchskoagulopathie (Schock-Lunge). Dtsch Med Wochenschr 95: 1999
Mittermayer C, Hagedorn M, Böttcher D, Vogel W, Neuhof H, Mittermayer U (1972) Bromcarbamidvergiftung, ein Modell der Schocklunge. Klin Wochenschr 50: 467
Mittermayer C, Thomas C, Rengholt R, Schäfer H, Vogel W, Martinez G, Sandritter W (1973) Über den Gestaltwandel des Schocksyndroms innerhalb zweier Jahrzehnte. Klin Wochenschr 51: 37
Morgenroth K (1970) Immunologische Reaktionen der Meerschweinchenlunge nach wiederholten Injektionen von komplettem Freudschem Adjuvans. Verh Dtsch Ges Pathol 54: 284
Müller R, Korb G, Gedigk P (1970) Über zentrale Nekrosen in der Leber nach einem Schock. Verh Dtsch Ges Pathol 54: 511
Nayak NC, Roy S, Narayanan TK (1964) Pathologic features of altitude sickness. Am J Pathol 45: 381
Nick WV (1968) DNA antibodies in primate sera during hemorrhagic and endotoxic shock. Am J Surg 115: 769
Nick WV, Dodd MC (1967) DNA antibody in the serum of patients in shock. Ann Surg 166: 357
Nolte H (1968) Histologische Aspekte zum Problem der Sauerstoffintoxikation. In: Überleben auf See, 2. Marinemedizinisches Symposium in Kiel, p 139
Northway WH Jr, Rosan RC, Porter DY (1967) Pulmonary disease following respirator therapy of hyaline membrane disease. Bronchopulmonary dysplasia. N Engl J Med 276: 357
Oehlert W, Dischler W, Henke M, Strauch M (1978) Die akute Erosion der Magenschleimhaut im Biopsiematerial. Med Welt 29: 1149
Okumura T (1969) Studies on the human drug-shock cases (mainly by the histological studies on the liver and adrenals). Jpn J Leg Med 23: 450
Pokk LR (1963) Die Entwicklung des orthostatischen Kollapses und morphologischer Veränderungen in Kaninchenorganen bei Einwirkung auf das Zentralnervensystem. Arch Pathol (Mosk) 25: 26
Prose PH, Lee L, Balk SD (1965) Electron microscopic study of the phagocytic fibrin clearing mechanism. Am J Pathol 47: 403
Rajka E (1959) Insekten- und Würmerallergie. In: Allergie und allergische Erkrankungen, vol 2, p 664. Akadémiai Kiado, Budapest
Randerath P, Bohle A (1959) Die Pathomorphologie der Nierenausscheidung. In: Büchner-Lette-

rer-Roulet: Hilfsmechanismen des Stoffwechsels. Springer, Berlin Göttingen Heidelberg (Handbuch der allgemeinen Pathologie V/2, p 222)
Remmele W (1971) Zur Morphologie des Kreislaufschocks. 50. Jahrestag. Dtsch Ges Rechtsmed 3.–7. 10. 1971 Köln
Remmele W (1975) Kreislaufschock. In: Mueller B (ed) Gerichtliche Medizin, Springer, Heidelberg Göttingen New York
Remmele W, Goebel U (1973) Zur pathologischen Anatomie des Kreislaufschocks beim Menschen. V. Pathomorphologie der Schock-Lunge. Klin Wochenschr 51: 25
Remmele W, Harms D (1968) Zur pathologischen Anatomie des Kreislaufschocks beim Menschen. I. Mikrothrombose der peripheren Blutgefäße. Klin Wochenschr 46: 352
Remmele W, Loeper H (1973) Zur pathologischen Anatomie des Kreislaufschocks beim Menschen. IV. Pathomorphologie der Schock-Leber. Klin Wochenschr 51: 10
Remmele W, Leder LD, Graul W (1964) Herkunft und Bedeutung der intravasalen Zellansammlungen in der sog. Schockniere. Verh Dtsch Ges Pathol 48: 179
Rennert M, Thierot M, Höer PW, Görsch H (1964) Morphologische Veränderungen an den inneren Organen der Ratte im standardisierten, reversiblen und irreversiblen Schock. Virchows Arch [Pathol Anat] 338:21
Reynolds EO, Strang LB (1966) Alveolar surface properties of the lung in the newborn. Br Med Bull 22: 79
Robb HJ (1965) Microembolism in the pathophysiology of shock. Angiology 16: 405
Rösch W: Erosionen des Magens. In: Demling L (ed) Magen. Springer, Berlin Heidelberg New York (Handbuch der Inneren Medizin, vol 3/2)
Rolffs J, Prieme B, Schönbach R, Huth K, Sandritter W (1972) Intravitale und pathologisch-anatomische Beobachtungen beim generalisierten Sanarelli-Shwartzman-Phänomen des Kaninchens. Beitr Pathol 145: 149
Rollhäuser H, Vogell W (1960) Die tubuläre Phenolrotausscheidung und die Feinstrukturveränderungen der Glomerula bei der Rattenniere im traumatischen Schock. Z Zellforsch 52: 549
Rotter H (1959) Pathologie der Schockniere. 3. Deutsches Elektrolytsymposiun. Melsunger Med Pharmacol Mitt 91: 1754
Rotter W (1971) Das morphologische Substrat des Schocks. Med Welt 22: 1175
Ryvarden G (1973) Tod post partum unter dem allgemeinen klinischen Erscheinungsbild der Verbrauchskoagulopathie (Eclampsia sine eclampsia). Z Rechtsmed 72: 174
Saeger W, Hanke D (1978) Nekrosen der Hypophyse und ihre Beziehung zum Schock. Verh Dtsch Ges Pathol 62: 301
Saldeen T (1972) The microembolism syndrome. Forensic Sci Int 1: 179
Sandritter W (1966) Neuere Aspekte in der pathologischen Anatomie des Schocks. Zentralbl Allg Pathol Anat 109: 554
Sandritter W (1967) Pathologische Anatomie des Schocks. Dtsch Med J 18: 408
Sandritter W (1973) Zur pathologischen Anatomie des Schocks. Klin Wochenschr 51: 1
Sandritter W, Lasch HG (1967) Pathologic aspects of shock. Methol Archiev Exp Pathol 3: 86
Scheuer BJ (1968) Liver biopsy interpretation. Baillière, Tindall & Cassel, London
Schlag G, Voigt W, Schnells G, Glatzl A (1977) Vergleichende Untersuchungen der Ultrastruktur von menschlicher Lunge und Skelettmuskulatur im Schock. II. Anaesthesist 26: 612
Schlag G, Voigt W-H, Redl H, Glatzl A (1980) Vergleichende Morphologie des posttraumatischen Lungenversagens. Anaesth Intensivther Notfallmed 15: 315
Schmidt K, Potthoff PC (1976) Neurogener Schock. Forensic Neuropathol. Schattauer, Stuttgart, New York
Schneider M (1963) Zur Pathophysiologie der verschiedenen Schockformen. Bibl Haematol 16: 10
Schneider M (1964) Zur Pathologie des Schocks. Symposium Schock und Plasma-Expander. Springer, Berlin Göttingen Heidelberg New York, pp 1–22
Schneider M (1967) Die periphere Strombahn im Schock. Dtsch Med J 18: 401
Schultz H (1968) Thrombozyten und Thrombose im elektronenmikroskopischen Bild. Springer, Berlin Heidelberg New York
Schulz E, Albert K (1976) Streßläsionen des Magens und Zwölffingerdarms unter Intensivtherapie. Beitr Gerichtl Med 34: 19
Seifert G (1970) Das Pankreas als Schockorgan. In: Horatz K (ed) Leber- und Pankreasschäden durch Schock und Narkose. Thieme, Stuttgart

Sherlock S (1965) Krankheiten der Leber und Gallenwege. J. F. Lehmann, München, p 504
Spaet TH (1962) Studies on the in vivo behavior of blood coagulation products in rats. Thromb Haemost 8: 276
Spühler O, Zollinger HO (1941) Kreislaufkollaps, temporäre Anurie und extrarenale Azotämie. Schweiz Med Wochenschr 71: 1017
Staemmler M (1957) Die Harnorgane. In: Kaufmann E, Staemmler M (eds) Lehrbuch der speziellen Pathologie 11./12. 2. edn. de Gruyter, Berlin, p 644
Störmer S (1961) Tod durch einen Bienenstich. Ein Gutachten. Münch. Med Wochenschr 103: 606
Suda Y (1962) Acute renal failure. Histochemical and experimental investigations of factors causing oliguria. Tohoku J Exp. Med 76: 278
Szam I (1967) Schock und Lungenödem. Acta Med Acad Sci Hung 23: 309
Thaler H (1969) Leberbiopsie. Springer, Berlin Heidelberg New York
Umbach W (1971) Zentrale Faktoren bei der Schockauslösung. Med Welt 22: 1171
Veith FJ, Hagstrom JWC, Panossian A (1968) Pulmonary microcirculatory response to shock, transfusion, and pump-oxygenator procedures: a unified mechanism underlying pulmonary damage. Surgery 64: 95
Voigt J (1966) Eosinophils in the spleen in cases of the lethal anaphylactic shock. Med Sci Law 6: 162
Waisbren BA, Arena J (1965) Shock associated with bacteremia due to gram-negative bacili. Autopsy findings. Arch Intern Med 116: 336
Walther G, Lieven T (1971) Histochemische Organveränderungen in Leber und Herzmuskel der Ratte nach Sauerstoffintoxikation. Beitr Gerichtl Med 28: 50
Webster I, Blum LJ (1972) Traumatic Lung. Forens Sci Int 1: 167
Wegelin C (1933) Tod durch Bienenstich. Schweiz Med Wochenschr 63: 786
Wegelin C (1948) Anatomische Befunde bei tödlichem Bienen- und Wespenstich. Schweiz Med Wochenschr 78: 1253
Wichert v P, Riesner K (1977) Die sogenannte Schocklunge, ein Krankheitsbild des Lungenparenchyms. Langenbecks Arch Chir 344: 157
004106 WC, Mac Gregor AR, Stewart CP (1938) Clinical course and pathology of burns and scalds under modern methods of treatment. Br J Surg 25: 826
Witte I (1978) Proliferationsverhalten der Gefäßendothelien von Lunge, Leber und Niere der Ratte nach Endotoxinschock. Dissertation, Würzburg
Wollheim G (1952) Über die tubulären Funktionsstörungen der Niere. Verh Dtsch Ges Inn Med 58: 211
Zollinger HO (1952) Die hämatogenen interstitiellen Nephritiden. Ursache, Erscheinungsformen und Folgen. Verh Dtsch Ges Inn Med 58: 153
Zollinger HO (1966) Niere und ableitende Harnwege. In: Doerr W, Uehlinger E (eds) Spezielle pathologische Anatomie, vol 3. Springer, Berlin Heidelberg New York, p 155
Zühlke V, Quellhorst E, Hierholzer E, Mietzsch G (1972) Disseminierte intravasculäre Gerinnung nach allogener Nierentransplantation. Diagnostische Bedeutung und therapeutische Konsequenzen. Klin Wochenschr 50: 370

References to B V: Histological Contribution Toward Identification

Balthazard P, Lebrun R (1911) Les canaux de Havers de L'os humain aux différents ages. Ann Hyg Med Leg 15: 144
Berg S, Specht W (1958) Untersuchungen zur Bestimmung der Liegezeit von Skelett-Teilen. Dtsch Z Gerichtl Med 47: 209
Breitenecker L (1959) Historöntgenographische Untersuchungen bei Silikose. Dtsch Z Gerichtl Med 49: 194
Camba R (1958) Diagnosi di eta prenatalefondata sullo studio istologico della colonna vertebrale. Zacchia 33: 300
Camba R (1960) Diagnosi di eta prenatalefondata sullo studio istologico della colonna vertebrale. Minerva Med Leg 80: 43
Dechaume M, Derobert L, Payen J (1960) De la valeur de la termination de l'age par l'examen de dents en coupes minces. Ann Med Leg 40: 165

Degenhardt KH, Fränz J, Geisler M (1972) Kerngeschlechtsbestimmung an Haarwurzeln bei Sportlerinnen. Dtsch Ärztebl: 2079

Dobryak VI, Kirechinsky BR (1964) Some possibilities of microroentgenography in examination of bone tissue. SudMed Ekspert 7: 13

Frost: Cited by Knese 1970

Fuest H, Haas J, Schmitz GA (1965) Altersbedingte Veränderungen der Alveolen menschlicher Lungen. Zugleich ein Beitrag zum Problem von Form und Funktion. Med Welt: 2686 und 2791

Göring HD (1970) Bestimmung des Lebensalters an langen Röhrenknochen. Wiss Z Univ Halle, math-naturw Reihe 19: 177

Gustafson E (1950) Age determination on teeth. J Am Dent Ass 41: 45

Helmer R (1970) Möglichkeiten und Methoden der zellkernmorphologischen Geschlechtserkennung an Körpergeweben und Sekret-Spuren. In: Weinig E, Berg S (eds) Arbeitsmethoden der medizinischen und naturwissenschaftlichen Kriminalistik vol 9. Schmidt-Römhild, Lübeck

Hienz HA (1959) Die zellkernmorphologische Geschlechtserkennung in Theorie und Praxis. In: Schaeffer H (ed) Einzeldarstellungen aus Theorie und Klinik der Medizin. Hüthig, Heidelberg

Hienz HA (1971) Chromosomen-Fibel. – Einführung in die klinische Zytogenetik für Ärzte und Studenten. Thieme, Stuttgart

Janssen W (1957) Zur Frage der kindlichen Arteriosklerose, besonders der Herzkranzgefäße. Monatsschr Kinderheilkd 105: 361

Janssen W (1963) Arteriopathia calcificans infantum (Calcinose) und Kortikosteroid-Therapie. Zentralbl Allg Pathol 164: 182

Janssen W (1968) Arteriosklerose der Coronararterien jugendlicher Menschen. Dtsch Z Gerichtl Med 62: 39

Knese K-H (1970) Struktur und Ultrastruktur des Knochengewebes. In: Handbuch der Medizinischen Radiologie, vol 4, part 1, p 317. Springer, Berlin Heidelberg New York

Kovács M, Harsányi L, Sellyei M (1972) Y-body in cell nuclei of parenchymatous organs. Z Rechtsmed 71: 107

Leutert G, Rother P (1978) Schätzung des Lebensalters auf Grund histologischer Untersuchungen. In: Hunger H, Leopold D (eds) Identifikation. Johann Ambrosius Barth, Leipzig, p 183

Mueller B (1953) Gerichtliche Medizin. Springer, Berlin Heidelberg Göttingen

Rämsch R, Zerndt B (1963) Vergleichende Untersuchungen der Haversschen Kanäle zwischen Menschen und Haustieren. Arch Kriminol 131: 74

Rauchfuss R, Widmaier G (1971) Zur Bestimmung der fetalen Reife mit Hilfe der Fruchtwassercytologie. Zentralbl Gynaekol 93: 745

Saunders M (1965) Dental factors in age determination. Med Sci Law 5: 34

Shibata M, Hirota T (1962) Estimation of age of victims from pieces of their organs. I. The thickness of capsule of human spleen. J Nara Med Assoc 13: 189

Shibata M, Hirota T, Tsurozono M, Teranishi N, Naripa N, Yamamoto H, Kita H (1963) Estimation of age of victims from pieces of their organs. I. The spleen. 1. The thickness of capsule of human spleen. Jpn J Leg Med 17: 75

Shibata M, Naripa N, Hirota N, Tsurozono M, Teranishi N, Uehara M, Yamamoto H, Kita H (1963b) Estimation of age of victims from pieces of their organs. II. The lungs. 1. Anthracosis. Jpn J Leg Med 17: 83

Sperling U, Schwinger E (1973) Barr-Körperchen in Haarwurzelkernen nach Fluorescenz- und Diamantfuchsin-Färbung. Humangenetik 18: 181

Schröder HE (1971) Histologische Methoden in der forensischen Zahnheilkunde. Kriminalistik 25: 434

Schwartz Ph (1964) Morphologische und pathogenetische Untersuchungen über Veränderungen im Greisenalter. Zentralbl Allg Pathol Pathol Anat 106: 320

Slavik V, Meluzin F (1972) Bestimmung der Gruppenzugehörigkeit im System ABO aus histologischem Material. Z Rechtsmed 70: 79

Tröger HD, Jungwirth J (1975) Bestimmung der ABO-Gruppenzugehörigkeit an histologischen Präparaten. Beitr Gerichtl Med 33: 326

Watanabe T, Shimada H, Tanaka Y (1978) Human hepatocytes and aging: a cytophotometrical analysis in 35 sudden-death cases. Virchows Arch [Cell Pathol] 27: 307

Zanaldi L (1966) Reperto di villi coriali, a distanza ditreanni, in un catitere usato quele mezzo abortivo. Zacchia 41: 90

References to C I: Sudden Death from Natural Causes

Adebahr G (1966) Histologische Befunde am Herzmuskel bei Wiederbelebungsversuchen. Dtsch Z Ges Gerichtl Med 57: 205
Althoff H (1980) Zur morphologischen Diagnose Myokarditis. Z Rechtsmed 84: 305
Behrenhoff K (1966) Beitrag zur Problematik des stumpfen Herztraumas. Med Welt: 459
Böhm E (1981) Kardiorespiratorische Insuffizienz bei Schocktodesfällen. Beitr Gerichtl Med 39: 31
Bratzke H (1980) Contusio cordis nach Verkehrsunfall. Z Rechtsmed 84: 149
Büchner F, Onishi S (1968) Der Herzmuskel bei akuter Coronarinsuffizienz im elektronenmikroskopischen Bild. Urban & Schwarzenberg, München Berlin Wien
Doerr W (1979) Koronariitis. Dtsch. Aerztebl 32: 2033
Doerr W (1981) Sekundenherztod. Beitr Gerichtl Med 39: 1
Du Chesne A (1978) Unklare Todesfälle im gerichtsmedizinischen Sektionsgut. Kriminal Forens Wiss 32: 29
Ferris JAJ (1972) The heart in sudden infant death. J Forens Sci Soc 12: 591
Ferris JAJ (1974) Conducting tissue changes in sudden death. Med Sci Law 14: 36
Gregersen M (1979) Myocardiale Veränderungen beim plötzlichen unerwarteten Coronartod. Forensic Sci Int 13: 183
Hecht A (1964) Fermenthistochemische Frühveränderungen beim experimentellen Herzinfarkt. Virch Arch 337: 414
Heilmann K, Völkl A, Fölsch U (1972) Frühdiagnose des Myokardinfarkts. Vergleich histologischer, makro- und mikroskopischer, histochemischer und chemischer Untersuchungsmethoden am unausgewählten Sektionsgut. Aerztl Forsch 26: 207
Hirvonen J (1976) Practical approach to the diagnosis of sudden unexpected death of cardiac origin. Forensic Sci Int 8: 49
Holczabek W (1970) Über das histologische Bild der ischämischen Schädigung des Herzfleisches bei Anwendung der Weinsteinsäure-Kresylechtviolett-Einschlußfärbung. Beitr Gerichtl Med 27: 275
Holczabek W (1973) Nachweis von Isoproterenol-bedingten Herzmuskelschäden an der Ratte mittels der Weinsteinsäure-Kresylecht-Einschlußfärbung. Beitr Gerichtl Med 30: 175
Hort W (1964) Untersuchungen an Infarktherzen. Verhandl Dtsch Ges Pathol 169
Hort W (1965) Ventrikeldilatation und Muskelfaserdehnung als früheste morphologische Befunde beim Herzinfarkt. Virch Arch 339: 72
Hort W (1969) Herzinfarkt, Grundlagen und Probleme. Springer, Berlin Heidelberg New York
Jääskeläinen AJ (1968) Histochemical observations in phosphorylase, cytochrome oxidase, and succinic dehydrogenase in experimental and human fresh myocardial infarction. Kirjapaino Polytypos, Turku
Janssen W (1968) Zur Arteriosklerose der Coronararterien jugendlicher Menschen. Dtsch Z Gerichtl Med 62: 39
Janssen W, Naeve W (1975) Der plötzliche Tod aus natürlicher Ursache. In: Mueller B (ed) Gerichtliche Medizin. Springer, Berlin Heidelberg New York p 263
Klages U (1970) Spontane oder traumatische tödliche Subarachnoidalblutung. Z Rechtsmed 67: 67
Klages U, Gerken F (1972) Eine Methode zur Objektivierung fraglicher entzündlicher Zellvermehrung im Interstitium des Herzmuskels. Beitr Gerichtl Med 14: 429
Knieriem HJ, Mecking D, Seipel L (1980) 9. Pathomorphologie des Sinusknotens beim Sinusknotensyndrom und anderen Herzrhythmusstörungen. Pathologe 1: 233
Knight B (1979) Zur Frage der Zuverlässigkeit der HBFP-Färbung beim Nachweis von Myokardschäden. Forensic Sci Int 13: 179
Korb G (1964) Morphologische Untersuchungen an experimentellen Herzmuskelnekrosen. Habilitationsschrift, Marburg
Korb G, Knorr G (1962) Vergleichende licht- und fluoreszenzmikroskopische Untersuchungen frischer Herzmuskelschäden beim Menschen. Virch Arch 335: 159
Korb G, Totović V (1967) Elektronenmikroskopische Untersuchungen über Frühveränderungen im Zentrum und in der Peripherie experimenteller Herzinfarkte. Virch Arch 342: 85
Krauland W (1954) Zur tödlichen Commotio cordis. Dtsch Z Ges Gerichtl Med 43: 102
Krauland W (1966) Arteriosklerose im Tierversuch und beim Menschen. Ciba-Symposium 14: 15

Krauland W (1972) Forensische Aspekte zum plötzlichen Herztod. Verhandl Dtsch Ges Inn Med 78: 969
Lie JT, Holley KE, Kampa WR, Titus IL (1971) New histochemical method for morphologic diagnosis of early stages of myocardial ischemia. Mayo Clin Proc 46: 319–327
Liebegott G (1969) Über Organisationsvorgänge bei Coronarsklerose und Coronarthrombose. Arthur Weber z. 90. Geburtstag. 3.8. 1969 Bad Nauheim. Med Schriftenreihe Boehringer, Mannheim
Meessen H, Poche UR (1963) Pathomorphologie des Myokard. In: Bargmann W, Doerr W (eds) Das Herz des Menschen, vol 2. Thieme, Stuttgart, p 644
Müller E (1955) Pathologische Anatomie der Coronarthrombose unter besonderer Berücksichtigung der Coronarsklerose und Atheromatose. Verhandl Dtsch Ges Kreislaufforsch: 3
Neoral L, Kolin L, Kadousek B, Kvasnicka (1959) Beitrag zur Kenntnis der Frühstadien der experimentellen Myokardischämie. Zentralbl Allg Pathol Anat 99: 239
Noren GR, Staley NA, Bandt CM, Kaplan EL (1977) Occurrence of myocarditis in sudden death in children. J Forensic Sci 22: 188
Plueckhahn VD, Cameron JM (1968) Traumatic "myocarditis" or "myocarditis" in trauma. Med Sci Law 8: 177
Rajs J, Jakobsson S (1976a) Severe trauma and subsequent cardiac lesions causing heart failure and death. Forensic Sci Int 8: 13
Rajs J, Jakobsson S (1976b) Experiences with the hematoxylin basic fuxin picric acid staining method for morphologic diagnosis of myocardial ischemia – an experimental study in forensic pathology. Forensic Sci Int 8: 37
Reempts J van, Borgers M, Reneman RS (1976) Early myocardial ischaemia: evaluation of the histochemical haematoxylin-basic fuchsin-picric acid (HBFP) staining technique. Cardiovasc Res 10: 262
Sakurai I (1977) Pathology of acute ischemic myocardium. Special references to evaluation of morphological methods for detection of early myocardial infarcts, and lipid metabolism in infarcted myocardium. Acta Pathol Jpn 27: 587
Saukko P (1981) The reliability of the HBFP stain in detecting cases of sudden cardiac death. J Forensic Sci Soc 2: 138
Shnitka T-K, Nachlas MM (1963) Histochemical alterations in ischemic heart muscle and early myocardial infarction. Am J Pathol 42: 507
Staak M (1968) Eine atypische posttraumatische Herzmuskelnekrose bei einem vierjährigen Knaben. Dtsch Z Gerichtl Med 62: 14
Tausch D (1974) Experimentelle Untersuchungen über den histologischen Nachweis frischer ischämischer Herzmuskelschädigungen mit der Methode nach Lie und Mitarb. Beitr Gerichtl Med 32: 274
Thurner J (1977) Die Virusmyokarditis, am Beispiel einer erloschenen Coxsackie-Virus-Myokarditis-Endemie im Raum Salzburg. Med Welt 28: 1276
Voigt J (1976) Reflections on the value of histological examination of the cardiac conduction system in cases of natural unexpected death. Forensic Sci Int 8: 29
Voigt J, Steinmetz E (1977) Histopathology of the conduction system in patients with atriocentricular or intraventricular conduction disturbances. Acta Pathol Microbiol Scand [A] 85: 174
Walther G (1972) Spättodesfall nach Contusio cordis. Monatsschr Unfallheilkd 75: 38
Zebe H, Mall G (1979) Die Myokarditis. Dtsch Aerztebl 33: 2089

References to C II: Pregnancy – Abortion – Aborticide

Adebahr G (1964) Über das generalisierte Shwartzman-Phänomen bei Abtreibung. Dtsch Z Gerichtl Med 54: 124
Adebahr G (1967) Veränderungen der Niere bei Abtreibung. 1. Tag. Ges. Gerichtl Med DDR Halle, 10.–14. 10. 1967
Adelson L (1963) Maternal aspiration of amniotic fluid. Report of a case following criminal abortion. J Forensic Sci Int 8: 132
Althoff H (1980) Sudden infant death syndrome (SIDS). Fischer, Stuttgart New York

Bayer A, Zidova J, Dusek J, Hajsmanova T (1962) Zum Vorkommen der Haemotoxylinkörperchen in den Lungen der Neugeborenen. Zentralbl Allg Pathol Pathol Anat 104: 23

Bellinvia G, Aragona F (1963) Importanza clinica e medicolegale del fenomeno endometriale di Arias-Stella. G Med Leg 9: 391

Benirschke K (1962) A review of the pathologic anatomy of the human placenta [Symp]. Am J Obstet Gynecol 84: 1595

Bleyl U (1970) Vergleichende Untersuchungen an Erwachsenen und Neugeborenen zur Entstehung pulmonaler hyaliner Membranen. Verhandl Dtsch Ges Pathol 54: 340

Bleyl U (1971) Pathologie und Pathogenese des Atemnotsyndroms. Verhandl Dtsch Ges Pathol 55: 39

Bleyl U, Büsing CM (1970) Kreislaufschock und disseminierte intravasale Gerinnung bei intrauterinem und perinatalem Fruchttod. Klin Wochenschr 48: 13

Bleyl U, Büsing CM, Krempien B (1969) Pulmonale hyaline Membranen und perinataler Kreislaufschock. Virchows Arch [Pathol Anat] 348: 187

Bryc R, Tomaszewska Z, Sawa J (1972) A histological study to determine aeration of the lungs of newborn infants in cases of mummification. Forensic Sci Int 1: 189

Buris L, Töröcsik I, Poczkodi S (1979) Is the aeration of the lungs a reliable sign of live birth? Z Rechtsmed 83: 303

Caroff J, Celestin E (1973) Neonatal and still-birth problems: The forensic point of view. Forensic Sci Int 2: 459

Dallenbach F (1966) Experimentelle Untersuchungen zur Genese des Arias-Stella-Phänomens. Verh Dtsch Ges Pathol 50: 413

Dominok GW (1964) Beitrag zur Frage der geburtstraumatischen subependymären Blutungen. Zentralbl Allg Pathol Pathol Anat 106: 361

Dorfman SG, Dillaplain RP, Gambrell RD (1979) Antepartum pituitary infarction. Obstet Gynecol 53: [Suppl] 3: 21

Drese G (1967) Histologische Untersuchungsbefunde nach tödlichen kriminellen Aborten. 1. Tag. Ges Gerichtl Med DDR, Halle, 10.–14. 10. 1967

Essbach H (1961) Paido-Pathologie. Thieme, Leipzig

Esterly JR, Oppenheimer EH (1966) Massive pulmonary hemorrhage in the newborn. J Pediatr 69: 3

Fazekas IG, Kosa F (1970) Modellversuche zum Studium der Nabelringentstehung. Z Rechtsmed 67: 372

Fazekas IG, Kosa F, Fábrik E (1969) Untersuchungen über die periumbilikale Demarkationsentzündung im Hinblick auf die Lebendgeburt. Dtsch Z Ges Gerichtl Med 66: 35

Fazekas IG, Kosa F, Viragos Kis E, Jobba G (1973) Der Gehalt der Lungen Neugeborener an freiem und Gesamthistamin unter dem Gesichtspunkt des Lebendgeborenseins. Arch Kriminol 152: 164

Fritz E (1935) Die Bestimmung des Alters von Neugeborenen am Hautnabel. Beitr Gerichtl Med 8: 28

Glatthaar E (1962) Zur Frage der Beziehung zwischen geburtshilflicher Koagulopathie und postparturaler Hypophysenvorderlappen-Nekrose. Geburtshilfe Frauenheilkd 22: 1242

Goldbach H-J (1956) Die Entwicklung der elastischen Fasern in der menschlichen Lunge. Dtsch Z Gerichtl Med 45: 381

Grönert O (1954) Intracranial haemorrhage and blood-brain barrier problems in the new-born. Zentralbl Allg Pathol Pathol Anat 92: 235

Groniowski J (1963) Thrombotic arteriolar lesions in lungs of newborn. Arch Pathol Lab Med 75: 144

Grosser G (1962) Die gerichtsmedizinische Bedeutung der hyalinen Membranen in der Neugeborenenlunge. Acta Med Leg Soc (Liege) 15: 29

Hirvonen J, Tiisala R, Uotila U, Arko H, Tähti E, Laiho K, Marttila A, Tenhu M (1969) Roentgenological and autopsy studies on the gas content of the lungs and gastrointestinal tract in living and stillborn infants, and sources of error in resuscitation. Dtsch Z Ges Gerichtl Med 65: 73

Höpker WW, Ohlendorf B (1979) Placental insufficiency. Histomorphologic diagnosis and classification. Curr Top Pathol 66: 57

Hoppe E, Mildner G (1971) Untersuchungen der Zusammenhänge zwischen antepartaler maternaler Anamnese und Chorionzottenveränderungen bei lebenden Neugeborenen sowie Ver-

gleiche mit analogen Überprüfungen bei Totgeborenen und frühzeitig verstorbenen Neugeborenen. Zentralbl Gynaekol 93: 1593
Huth K, Müller-Berhaus G, Krecke H-J, Lasch HG (1964) Das Verhalten der Blutlipide beim generalisierten Sanarelli-Shwartzman-Phänomen. Verh Dtsch Inn Med 70: 437
Janssen W (1962) Zur Bedeutung der perinatalen Nebennierenblutungen. Dtsch Z Ges Gerichtl Med 52: 578
Janssen W, Naeve W (1975) Der plötzliche Tod aus natürlicher Ursache. In: Mueller B (ed) Gerichtliche Medizin. Springer, Berlin Heidelberg New York, p 248
Jobba G (1970) Lungenveränderungen bei maschineller Überdruckbeatmung asphyktischer Neugeborener. Z Rechtsmed 67: 364
Josey WE, Hoch W, Moon EC, Thompson JD (1966) Analysis of 21 septic abortion deaths with special reference to the Shwartzman phenomenon. Obstet Gynecol 28: 335
Klages U, Gehrken F (1972) Eine Methode zur Objektivierung fraglicher entzündlicher Zellvermehrung im Interstitium des Herzmuskels. Beitr Gerichtl Med 29: 429
Krecke H-J (1964) Zum generalisierten Shwartzman-Phänomen (Sanarelli Shwartzman-Phänomen) und seiner Bedeutung für die menschliche Pathologie. Veroeff Pathol. Fischer Stuttgart
Kuoda S, Namori H, Ebe M, Sasaki M (1965) Medico-legal studies on the fetus and the infant. Histological characteristics of the lungs of liveborn and stillborn infants. Jpn J Leg Med 19: 7
Kuoda S, Nagamori H, Ebe M, Sasaki M (1965b) Medico-legal studies on the fetus and infant: with special references to histological characteristics of the lungs of liveborn and stillborn infants. Tohoku J Exp Med 85: 40
Link M (1964) Über die sog. Hämatoxylinkörperchen in Neugeborenenlungen. Virchows Arch [Pathol Anat] 338: 1
Lo Menzo G (1969) Histochemical changes at base level of umbilical cord. I. Behaviour of alkaline and acid phosphatases. Dtsch Z Ges Gerichl Med 65: 1
Lo Menzo G, Chiara A (1966) In tema di goduta vita extrauterina. I. L'attività fosfatasica alcalina e acida. Med Leg (Genova) 14: 313
Lo Menzo G, Chiara A (1968a) Modificazioni istochimiche a livello della base d'impianto del funicolo ombelicale. III. Il comportamento dell'attività aminopeptidasica. Med Leg (Genova) 16: 323
Lo Menzo G, Chiara A (1968b) Modificazioni istochimiche a livello della base d'impianto del funicolo ombelicala. II. Ricerche micofluoroscopiche. Med Leg (Genova) 16: 129
Mahnke P (1973) Zwischenfälle bei der Geburt. Zentralbl Ges Rechtsmed Grenzgebiete 6: 41
Mascia D (1970) Sull'impiego dei fluorocromi nella diagnosi istologica di broncoaspirazione amniotica. Zacchia 45: 529
Meixner K (1926) Teilweise lufthaltige Lungen bei noch ungeboren abgestorbenem Kinde. Dtsch Z Ges Gerichtl Med 6: 5
Mityayeva NA (1970) Discriminating live- and stillborn infants according to histological features in the lungs. II. Sud Med Ekspert 13: 15
Müller G (1963) Der plötzliche Kindstod. Thieme, Stuttgart
Ogawa J, Imaeda S, Saito H (1962) Process of lung expansion. Autopsy findings of the lung of premature and mature newborn infants and of mammals. Nagoya Med J 8: 29
Pawlica F (1962) Erste Beobachtungen von angeborener Pneumozystenpneumonie bei einem reifen, ausgetragenen totgeborenen Kind. Zentralbl Allg Pathol Pathol Anat 103: 236
Perrin EVD, Kahn-Vander Bel J (1965) Degeneration and calcification of the umbilical cord. Obstet Gynecol 26: 371
Petersohn F (1964) Die Bedeutung des Stärkenachweises in den inneren Organen zur Beurteilung des Gelebthabens und der Todesursache des Neugeborenen. Dtsch Z Gerichtl Med 55: 215
Pisarski T, Breborowicz H, Przybora LA (1963) Leucocytic infiltration in the placenta and membranes. Biol Neonate 5: 129
Plank J (1965) Morphologische Befunde in nicht beatmeten, nicht retrahierten Lungen des Neugeborenen. Virchow Arch [Pathol Anat] 338: 245
Pliess G, Räntsch FE, Schäfer KH (1970) Interstitielle plasmazelluläre Säuglingspneumonie und Pneumozystosen. Ergeb Ges Tuberk Lung Forsch 19: 65
Potter EL (1953) Pathology of the fetus and the newborn. The Year Book Publishers, Chicago
Prokop O (1971) Zur Brauchbarkeit der elastischen Fasern der Lunge im Rahmen der Lebensproben. Z Rechtsmed 69: 177

Raubitschekt HV (1955) Die fetale Atelektase und die Lungenschwimmprobe. Virchow Arch 326: 692
Reiss KhI, Knolle Kh (1963) Congenital listeriosis. Arkh Patol 25: 29
Riemann H (1963) Kunstgerechte und gewaltsame Abnabelung. Arch Kriminol 132: 31
Robertson B, Sundelin P (1962) Cytomegalic inclusion disease. A report of two cases. Acta Paediat 51 [Suppl 135]: 178
Ross JJ, Dimmette RM (1965) Subependymal cerebral hemorrhage in infancy. Am J Dis Child 110: 531
Ruthig H-U (1973) Kindestötung. Kritische Untersuchungen zum histochemischen Phosphatase-Nachweis an Lungenschnitten Tot- und Lebendgeborener. Zentralbl Ges Rechtsmed 6: 368
Schwerd W (1959) Der gerichtsmedizinische Nachweis des Seifenaborts und der Seifenintoxikation. Dtsch Z Ges Gerichtl Med 48: 202
Schönfeld V, Dvorak V, Zrustova M (1964) Beitrag zum Wesen und diagnostischer Verwertbarkeit des sogenannten Arias-Stella-Phänomen. Zentralbl Gynaekol 86: 116
Scott JM (1961) Fatty change in the myocardium of the newborn. Br Med J II: 1746
Seifert G, Oehme J (1957) Pathologie und Klinik der Cytomegalie. Thieme, Leipzig
Sheehan HL (1957) Post-partum necrosis of the anterior pituitary. J Pathol 45: 189
Simonds M (1914) Über Hypophysisschwund mit tödlichem Ausgang. Dtsch Med Wochenschr 40: 322
Skogrand A, Harnaes Kr (1960) Causes of death in premature infants. Acta Pathol Microbiol Scand 49: 321
Spechter H-J (1953) Über die Deziduabildung ohne Schwangerschaft. Münch Med Wochenschr: 982
Tabbara W, Proteau J, Derobert L (1962) A propos de deux observations anatom cliniques de syndrome de Waterhouse-Friderichsen, dans les suites d'avortements criminels. Ann Med Leg 42: 177
Töndury G (1962) Embryopathien. Springer, Berlin Göttingen Heidelberg
Tomaszewska Z, Sawa J (1973) Demarcation reaction of umbilical cord's ring, its evidential evaluation. Arch Med Sadowej 23: 307. From Zentralbl Ges Rechtsmed 8: 214 (1974) (abstract)
Toshimitsu T (1972a) Medico-legal studies in breaking of umbilical cord. I. Medico-legal study on the location of breaking point of umbilical cord. Jpn J Leg Med 26: 171. From Zentralbl Ges Rechtsmed 6: 104 (1973)
Toshimitsu T (1972b) Medico-legal studies on breaking of umbilical cord. II. Medico-legal study on the nature of the breaking point of umbilical cord. Jpn J Leg Med 26, 184. From Zentralbl Ges Rechtsmed 6: 104 (1973)
Valdes-Dapena MA, Greene M, Basavanand N, Catherman R, Truex RC (1973) Das Herzmuskel-Reizleitungssystem beim plötzlichen Kindstod. N Engl J Med 289: 1179. From Zentralbl Ges Rechtsmed 9, 92 (1975) (abstract)
Volbert H, Schweitzer H (1954) Über Häufigkeit, Lokalisation und Ätiologie von Blutungen im Wirbelkanal bei unreifen Früchten und Frühgeburten. Geburtshilfe Frauenheilkd 14: 1041
Weiler G, Reinhardt V, Nau H-E, Gerhard L (1980) Beitrag zum intracraniellen „traumatischen Aneurysma". Z Rechtsmed 85: 225
Weinig E, Schwerd W (1951) Histochemische Beobachtungen nach Seifenwassereinspritzung in die schwangere Gebärmutter. Dtsch Z Ges Gerichtl Med 40: 649
Widder W (1978) Morphologische Plazentaveränderungen bei intrauterinem Fruchttod. Geburtshilfe Frauenheilkd 38: 389
Yamazaki M (1965) Light and electron microscopic studies of kidneys in toxemia of pregnancy by means of renal biopsy. Tohoku J Exp Med 87: 205

References to C III: Injuries Caused by Atmospheric Effects

Adebahr G (1972) Morphologische Schockäquivalente bei Luftembolie, Taucherunfall und Dekompressionskrankheiten. Beitr Gerichtl Med 29: 87
Adebahr G (1973) Über einen tödlichen Unfall beim Tauchen. Arbeitsmed Sozialmed Präventivmed 8: 213
Barres D, Neveux Y, Giry P, Durigon M, Drouet J (1978) Plongée sous-marine; étude expérimen-

tale des effects de la compression et de la décompression rapide sur la lignée plaquettaire. Bull Med Leg 21: 295
Fati S, Pennarola R (1972) Osservaziono anatomopathologiche sperimentali sull' embolia traumatica e sulla embolia gassosa. Folia Med (Napoli) 55: 231
Haberer K, Ellebrecht K, Walther G (1972) Tierexperimentelle Untersuchungen über die Schutzwirkung des Sauerstoffs bei der Druckfallkrankheit. Beitr Gerichtl Med 29: 303
Leithoff H, Gostomzyk JG, v. Daacke H (1972) Untersuchungen zur vitalen Reaktion bei explosiver Dekompression. Beitr Gerichtl Med 29: 113
Möttönen M, Karkola K (1971) The first fatal case of decompression sickness in Finland. Med Sci Law 11: 39
Mueller B (1975) Schädigungen und Tod durch Veränderungen des Atmosphärendrucks. In: Mueller B (ed) Gerichtliche Medizin. Springer, Berlin-Heidelberg-New York, p 493
Nikolaeva VI (1959) Morphological changes produced by sudden change of the atmospheric pressure in experimental conditions. Arkh Patol 21: 28
Peters G (1970) Klinische Neuropathologie. Thieme, Stuttgart, p 148
Pioch W (1961) Beobachtungen bei Unterdruck-Höhentod. Dtsch Z Ges Gerichtl Med 51: 420
Richter K, Löblich H (1978) Letale Dekompressionskrankheit nach therapeutischer Überdruckbehandlung. Z Rechtsmed 81: 54
Schneider V, Fien H (1978) Rasterelektronenmikroskopische Untersuchungen an den korpuskulären Bestandteilen des Blutes nach Dekompression aus Überdruck (Tauchversuche). Beitr Gerichtl Med 36: 373
Unterdorfer H (1979) Zur Morphologie des tödlichen Tauchzwischenfalles als Folge eines akuten positiven Barotraumas der Lungen. Beitr Gerichtl Med 37: 75
Wünsche O, Scheele G (1976) Frühformen von Skelettveränderungen nach Überdruckexposition im Tierexperiment und Röntgenkontrollen bei Druckluftarbeitern. Zentralbl Arbeitsmed 26: 108

References to C IV: Strangulation: Hanging – Choking – Throttling

Aguiar FA, Nunes MA (1962) Muskelblutungen beim Erhängungstod. Gaz Med Port 15: 365
Aguiar FA, Nunes MA (1963) Sur un signe de rèaction vitale dans la pendaison. Ann Med Leg 43: 33
Andrä F (1981) Untersuchungen zum sogenannten Luftemboliezeichen beim Erhängen. Med Dissertation, Hamburg
Bedrin LM, Levin VN, Rumyantsef YA YA (1979) Studies on microcirculation. Medico-legal practical aspects. Sud Med Ekspert (Mosk.) 16: 3; Zentralbl Ges Rechtsmed Grenzgeb 8: 89 (1974)
Berg S (1966) Adrenalin- und Noradrenalinwerte im Blut bei gewaltsamer Todesursache. Dtsch Z Ges Gerichtl Med 57: 179
Berg S, Bonte R (1973) Catecholaminwerte im Leichenblut und -liquor bei verschiedenen Agonieformen. Z Rechtsmed 72: 56
Blum H (1937) Zur Frage der Unterscheidbarkeit vitaler und postmortaler Gewebsveränderungen am Beispiel der Strangfurchen beim Erhängungstod. Virchows Arch 299: 754
Bonnet EFP, Pedace EA (1972) Ein gerichtsärztliches panoramisches Histodiagnosticum des Halses. Seine Anwendung bei Fällen von Ersticken durch Erhängen oder Erwürgen mit einer Schlinge. Zacchia 47: 594
Brinkmann B (1978a) Vitale Reaktionen in der Lungenstrombahn bei Tod durch Strangulation. Z Rechtsmed 81: 133
Brinkmann B (1978b) Zur Pathophysiologie und Pathomorphologie bei Tod durch Druckstauung. Z Rechtsmed 81: 79
Brinkmann B, Püschel K (1981) Die Lunge als Erfolgsorgan der Strangulationsagonie. Z Rechtsmed 86: 175
Brinkmann B, Koops E, Wischhusen F, Kleiber M (1981a) Halskompression und arterielle Obstruktion. Z Rechtsmed 87: 59
Brinkmann B, Püschel K, Bause H-W, Doehn M (1981b) Zur Pathophysiologie der Atmung und des Kreislaufs bei Tod durch obstruktive Asphyxie. Z Rechtsmed 87: 103
Bschor F (1964) Zum Mechanismus von Strangulationsblutungen aus Nase und Ohr. Dtsch Z Gerichtl Med 55: 284

Geserick G, Lignitz E, Patzelt P (1976a) Zum Aussagewert der ventralen Bandscheibenblutungen. Beitr Gerichtl Med 34: 259
Geserick G, Lignitz E, Dahse B (1976b) Zum Beweiswert der Simonschen Blutungen als vitales Erhängungszeichen. Kriminal Forens Wiss 26: 78
Hambeck W, Püschel K (1981) Death by railway accident: Incidence of traumatic asphyxie. J Trauma 21: 28
Henn RHE, Liebhardt E, Haug W (1973) Serienschnittuntersuchungen an Stauungsblutungen. Beitr Gerichtl Med 30: 146
Jankovich L, Incze J (1933) Blutungen in den Lymphknoten des Halses beim Erhängungstod. Dtsch Z Ges Gerichtl Med 20: 122
Janssen W (1967) Zur Beurteilung von Blutungen der Leichenhaut unter besonderer Berücksichtigung von Hämatomen der Orbita. Dtsch Z Gerichtl Med 59: 69
Janssen W, Jaecker O, Erbach A (1968) Zur Unterscheidung von Druck- und Stauungsblutungen in den Halsweichteilen. Dtsch Z Gerichtl Med 64: 147
Kaeser HE (1955) Einseitige Carotisthrombosen nach Strangulation. Confin Neurol 15: 369
Kleiber M, Koops E, Püschel K, Gottberg J, Brinkmann B (1982) Zur Pathologie des Erhängens unter besonderer Berücksichtigung vitaler Reaktionen. Beitr Gerichtl Med 40: 117
Klein H (1956) Mikroskopische Beobachtungen an Würgemalen. Dtsch Z Gerichtl Med 45: 17
Koops E, Kleiber M, Brinkmann B (1982a) Über Befundmuster und besondere Befunde bei homicidalem und suicidalem Erdrosseln. Beitr Gerichtl Med 40: 129
Koops E, Brinkmann B (1982b) Selbsterdrosselung. Z Rechtsmed 88: 221
Laiho K, Isokoski M, Hirvonen J, Ojala K, Marttila A, Tenhu M (1968) Über Obduktionsbefunde bei Selbstmord durch Erhängen. Dtsch Z Ges Gerichtl Med 63: 63
Marcinkowski T, Krzymanska M, Przybylski Z (1972) Punktförmige Blutungen auf der Vorderfläche der Zwischenwirbelscheiben als Zeichen für den Tod durch Erhängen. Zacchia 47: 260. From Zentralbl Ges Rechtsmed 5: 188 (1972) (abstract)
Mueller B (1975) Gerichtliche Medizin, Springer, Berlin Heidelberg New York, p 466
Nanetti L (1972) Über den Nachweis interkolloidaler Kristalle in der Schilddrüse von infolge Erhängens verstorbener Personen. Zacchia 47: 241. From Zentralbl Ges Rechtsmed 5: 188 (1972) (abstract)
Nasemann J, Brinkmann B (1982) Tierexperimentelle Untersuchungen zur Frage des akuten Emphysems bei Strangulation. Beitr Gerichtl Med 40: 123
Niedorf HR (1970) Die normale und pathologische Anatomie des Glomus caroticum. Med Welt 21: 251
Orsós F (1935) Die vitalen Reaktionen und ihre gerichtsmedizinische Bedeutung. Beitr Pathol Anat Allg Pathol 95: 163
Permyakov AV (1968) Histological findings: an aid to the diagnosing of death from strangulation. Sud Med Ekspert 11: 12
Pioch W (1969) Epidermale Esterase-Aktivität als Beweis der vitalen Einwirkung von stumpfer Gewalt. Beitr Gerichtl Med 25: 136
Pollak St (1975) Über die Häufigkeit des Lungenödems beim Erhängungstod. Beitr Gerichtl Med 33: 134
Prokop O, Wabnitz R (1970) Vorkommen von Bindehautblutungen bei Lebenden und Toten, dargestellt in 10 Tabellen. Z Rechtsmed 67: 249
Reh H, Haarhoff K (1975) Zum Beweiswert der Stauungs- und Weichteilblutungen beim Erdrosseln und Erwürgen. Z Rechtsmed 77: 47
Roer H, Koopmann H (1938) Ein Beitrag zur Histologie der Strangmarke. Dtsch Z Ges Gerichtl Med 30: 1
Simon A (1968) Weitere Beobachtungen vitaler Reaktionen im Bereich der Lendenwirbelsäule beim Erhängen. Aus: Aktuelle Fragen der Gerichtl Med (III), Wissenschaftl Beitr d Martin-Luther-Universität, Halle-Wittenberg
Simon A, Müller E (1976a) Ergebnisse histologischer Untersuchungen zur Entstehung der Strangmarke. Zacchia 51: 161
Simon A, Müller E (1976b) Ergebnisse histologischer Untersuchungen zur Entstehung der Strangmarke. Kriminal Forens Wiss 26: 77
Schollmeyer W (1961) Führte eine Blutung im Paraganglion caroticum den Tod herbei? Dtsch Z Gerichtl Med 51: 190

Schulz R (1896) Über vitale und postmortale Strangulation. Vierteljahrsschr Gerichtl Med 11: 211; 12: 44
Schulz R (1936) Blutungen in den Halslymphknoten bei Erhängten. Nieft C, Bleicherode a H
Stichnoth E (1954) Über Trommelfellblutungen beim Erhängungstod. Monatsschr Ohrenheilkd 88: 259
Wünscher W, Möbius G (1960) Über Gehirnveränderungen beim Spättod nach Strangulation. Dtsch Z Gerichtl Med 50: 235

References to C V: Drowning – Changes to Corpses Found in Water

Baragna M, Selvaggio G (1963) Sulla utilita di alcune indagini istologiche nello studie delle lesioni vitali e post-mortali nel cadavere sommerso. G Med Leg 9: 367
Berg S (1975) Leichenzersetzung und Leichenzerstörung. In: Mueller B (ed) Gerichtliche Medizin. Springer, Berlin Heidelberg New York, p 62
Böhm E (1973) Rasterelektronenmikroskopische Untersuchungen an Lungenalveolen. – Demonstration am Beispiel der Ertrinkungslunge. Beitr Gerichtl Med 30: 24
Brinkmann B, Butenuth W (1982) Zur Histologie und Ultrastrukturpathologie der Lungen beim experimentellen Ertrinken. Beitr Gerichtl Med 40: 95
Caroff J, Breton J, Hadengue A, Derobert L (1968) Chronologie des lésions pulmonaires de la submersion vitale en eau douce étude histologique. Med Leg Dommage Corp 1: 160
Cherkavsky NB, Stukochenko AG (1965) The findings of struvite crystals in serous cavities of seawater corpses. Sud Ekspert 8 (1): 18. Dtsch Z Gerichtl Med 59: 129 (1967)
De Bernardi A, Purini T, Tappero P (1965) Di alcuni aspetti microscopici del polmone nell' annegamento. Minerva Med Leg 85: 146
Dierkes K (1938) Über die Histologie der Waschhaut. Dtsch Z Ges Gerichtl Med 30: 262
Fazzari C (1963) Modificazioni stromali del polmone nell' annagamento sperimentale. Minerva Med 83: 147
Fukui Y, Hata M, Takahashi S, Matsubara K (1980) A new method for detecting diatoms in human organs. Forensic Sci Int 16: 67
Gatti F (1963) Sull' anemia splenica nell' annagamento. I. Indagini sperimentali. Minerva Med 83: 128
Goldbach H-J, Hinüber H (1956) Lassen sich aus dem Zustand der elastischen Fasern der menschlichen Fußsohlenhaut Rückschlüsse auf eine eventuelle Liegezeit im Wasser ziehen? Zentralbl Pathol 95: 105
Heinen M, Dotzauer G (1973) Problemfall: „Ertrinkungslunge". Beitr Gerichtl Med 30: 133
Hughes JMB (1977) Pulmonary oedema. Herz 2: 443
Janssen W (1969) Der forensische Beweiswert histologischer Untersuchungen. Beitr Gerichtl Med 25: 51
Klauer H, Walcher K (1937) Über postmortale Knötchenbildung an der Haut einer Wasserleiche. Dtsch Z Gerichtl Med 28: 464
Kunz J (1960) Über die Verwertbarkeit des Zustandes der Lungenelastica zur Bestimmung der Liegezeit von Wasserleichen. Dtsch Z Gerichtl Med 50: 559
Madert J, Bause H-W, Püschel K, Brinkmann B (1982) Hämodynamische Dysregulation beim Ertrinken in verschieden-osmolaren Flüssigkeiten. Beitr Gerichtl Med 40: 109
Montaldo S (1963) Reperti epatici ultrastrutturali nell' asfissia sperimentale da annegamento. Zacchia 38: 420
Montaldo S (1964) Reperti renali ultrastrutturali nell' asfissia sperimentale da annegamento. Zacchia 39: 145
Mueller M (1975) Ertrinken und Veränderungen an Wasserleichen, In: Mueller B (ed) Gerichtliche Medizin. Springer, Berlin Heidelberg New York, p 469
Nippe (1913) Studien über Leichenzersetzung. Vjschr Gerichtl Med 3: 46
Ökrös S (1938) Annähernde Bestimmung der Todeszeit aus dem Hautzustand. Dtsch Z Ges Gerichtl Med 29: 497
Patti M (1954) L'insufficienza cortico-surrenale acuta come causa di shock e di morte rapida nelle immersioni improvvise, quale grave fenomeno di disadattameto delle strutture endocrine allo stress trauma-freddo. Minerva Med II: 1353

Peters K, Glotz HJ (1968) Kristalline Substanzen als Folge fortgeschrittener Leichenveränderungen. Dtsch Z Ges Gerichtl Med 63: 142
Püschel K, Madert J, Bause H-W, Brinkmann B (1982) Zur Agonochemie des Ertrinkens. Beitr Gerichtl Med 40: 99
Recine H, Falchi Q (1963) Ricerche sperimentali sulla distribuzione dei liquidi radiopachi nell' annegamento rapido e lento. Minerva Med Leg 83: 168
Recine H, Filauro F (1963) Reperti istologici ed istochimici distintivi nella morte per annegamento rapido e lento. Med Leg (Genova) 11: 239
Reh H (1970) Diagnostik des Ertrinkungstodes und Bestimmung der Wasserzeit. Triltsch M, Düsseldorf
Reidbord HE, Spitz WU (1966) Ultrastructural alterations in rat lungs. Changes after intratracheal perfusion with fresh water and seawater. Arch Pathol Lab Med 81: 103
Santini M (1966) La microscopia di fluorescenza nella diagnosi differenziale tra annegamento in acque di fonte ed annegamento in acqua di mare. Ricerche sperimentali. Minerva Med Leg 86: 245
Spitz WU, Silverman BA, Michaelis M (1969) Histochemical changes in experimental drowning, pulmonary edema and asphyxia. J Forensic Med 16: 79
Schellmann B, Sperl W (1979) Diatomeen-Nachweis im Knochenmark (Femur) Nichtertrunkener. Z Rechtsmed 83: 319
Schleyer F (1951) Zur Histologie der Waschhaut. Dtsch Z Ges Gerichtl Med 40: 680
Terazawa K, Takatori T (1980) Isolation of intact plankton from drowning lung tissue by centrifugation in a colloidal silica gradient. Forensic Sci Int 16: 63
Timperman J, Thomas F (1980) Diatom identification and the diagnosis of drowning in microscopic diagnosis in forensic pathology. CC Thomas, Springfield
Udermann H, Schuhmann G (1975) Eine verbesserte Methode zum Diatomeen Nachweis. Z Rechtsmed 76: 119
Vimercati F, Colonna M, Altamura M, di Nunno C, Gagliano-Candela R (1976) Aspetti istoenzimatici del miocardio nell' annegamento sperimentale. Zacchia 51: 433
Wachholz L (1907) Die Diagnose des Ertrinkungstodes. Vjschr Gerichtl Med 33: 25

References to C VI: Injuries Caused by Heat and Cold

Bass H (1978) Lethality in mammalian cells due to hyperthermia under oxic and hypoxic conditions. Int J Radiat Biol 33: 57
Bellieni A (1959) Effetti del colpo di calore sulle capsule surrenali. Med Leg 7: 401
Breining H, Helpapa B, Cappel S, Sturm KW, Lymberopoulos S (1977) Morphologische Befunde am Rattengehirn nach lokaler Vereisung. Acta Neuropathol (Berl) 37: 137
Brinkmann B, Püschel K (1977) Zur Histomorphologie der Herz- und Skelettmuskulatur bei maligner Hyperthermie. Z Rechtsmed 80: 117
Brinkmann B, Kleiber M, Koops E, Püschel K (1979) Vitale Reaktionen bei akutem Verbrühungstod. Z Rechtsmed 83: 1
Cameron IL, Smith RE (1964) Cytological responses of fat tissue in cold-exposed rats. J Cell Biol 23: 89
Cotutiu C, Belis V, Streja D, Ceapraz-Drugescu N (1965) Histopathological and histochemical aspects of the skin in burns. Prob Med Judic Crim (Bucuresti) 3: 89
David H, Uerlings I, Grupe M (1971) Strukturveränderungen von Leberzellen bei supranormalen Temperaturen. Exp Pathol (Jena) 5: 2
Delarne J, Chomette G, Pinaudeau Y, Abelanet R, Monsaingeon A (1962) Les lésions viscérales des grands brulés. Etude anatomo-pathologique de 50 cas de brulures mortelles. Ann Anat Pathol 7: 53
Dirnhofer R, Sigrist T (1979) Muskelblutungen im Körperkern – ein Zeichen vitaler Reaktion beim Tod durch Unterkühlung? Beitr Gerichtl Med 37: 159
Dotzauer G, Jacob H (1952) Über Hirnschäden unter akutem Verbrennungstod. Dtsch Z Gerichtl Med 41: 129
Drüner HU, Grözinger K-H (1972) Streß-Ulzera nach Verbrennungen. Med Welt 23: 707

Eidlin LM (1965) On the wrong interpretation of fat drops in tissues and blood vessels as of a sure sign of intravital burning. Sud Med Ekspert 8/1: 10

Fain MA (1964) Suprarenal glands reaction in burn injury. Sud Med Ekspert 7/4: 22

Fazekas IG, Kósa F, Virágos-Kis E, Basch A (1973) Freier und Gesamthistamingehalt der Haut nach experimentell hervorgerufenen Verbrennungen. Z Rechtsmed 72: 203

Fazekas IG, Kósa F, Virágos-Kis E, Basch A (1973) Der freie und Gesamthistamingehalt von postmortalen Verbrennungen im Tierexperiment. Z Rechtsmed 72: 213

Feldmann H, Unger RR, David H, Marx I, Schulze HAF, Brauer Ch, Regling G (1976) Die Reaktion des Kaninchengehirns auf lokal angewandte tiefe Temperaturen; licht- und elektronenmikroskopische Befunde. Z Exp Chir 9: 10

Fineberg C, Miller BJ, Allbritten Jr FF (1954) Thermal burns of the respiratory tract. Surg Gynecol Obstet 98: 318

Fischer H (1965) Der Hitzschlag. Münch Med Wochenschr 107: 1049

Fischer H, Müller R (1971) Stauungsdermatose nach Erfrierung. Berufsdermatosen 19: 152

Gans O, Steigleder GK (1955) Entzündungen aus physikalischer Ursache. In: Histologie der Hautkrankheiten. Springer, Berlin, p 196

Goldbach H-J (1956) Gibt es vitale Reaktionen der Lunge nach Heißlufteinatmung? Dtsch Z Gerichtl Med 45: 394

Goodyear JE (1979) Heat hyperpyrexia in an infant. A case report. Med Sci Law 19: 208

Graev M (1964) Su talune espressioni istologische – allungamento delle cellule epidermiche – nelle ustioni sperimentali. Minerva Med Leg 84: 116

Haferkamp O (1962) Experimentelle immunohistologische Untersuchungen bei der Verbrennungskrankheit. Langenbecks Arch Chir 301: 118

Haferkamp O, Schäfer H, Henriquez M, Finger G, Martinez F, Yoshida M, Wegner H (1963) Untersuchungen zur pathogenen Bedeutung von spezifischen Iso- und Auto-Antikörpern nach Verbrennung. Arch Pathol Anat 337: 65

Hagedorn M, Perieme B, Mittermayer Ch, Sandritter W (1975) Intravitale und pathologisch-anatomische Beobachtungen beim Verbrennungsschock des Kaninchens. Beitr Pathol 155: 398

Hardmeier T (1963) Schwere Fettembolie bei Erfrierungen an beiden unteren Extremitäten. Schweiz Med Wochenschr 93: 465

Harsányi L (1977) Rasterelektronenmikroskopische Untersuchung hitzegeschädigter Knochen. Morphol Igazsogugyi Orv Sz 17: 26

Hering W, Dietz G (1960) Kindestötung durch Unterkühlung. Z Aerztl Fortbild 54: 1397

Herrmann B (1973) Möglichkeiten histologischer Untersuchungen bei Leichenbränden. Mitteilg Berl Ges Anthrop Ethnolog Urgeschr 2: 164

Herrmann B (1976) Neuere Ergebnisse zur Beurteilung menschlicher Brandknochen. Z Rechtsmed 77: 191

Hermann M, Goslar HG, Fetzer S (1965) Histochemische Untersuchungen an der Leber nach Verbrennung. Histochemie (Berl) 4: 541

Hirvonen J (1976) Necropsy findings in fatal hypothermia cases. Forensic Sci Int 8: 155

Hirvonen J, Elfving E (1973) Depletion of fats from the brown adipose tissue cells of rats dead from cold exposure. Z Rechtsmed 72: 50

Jacob H (1955) Wärme- und Kälteschäden des Gehirns. In: Scholz W (ed) Erkrankungen des zentralen Nervensystems. Springer, Berlin Heidelberg (Handbuch der speziellen pathologischen Anatomie und Histologie, vol 13/3)

Janezig-Jelacic O (1954) Les particularités histologiques des brulures post mortem. Ann Med Leg Soc (Liege) 34: 63

Keith Mant A (1964) Some post-mortem observations in accidental hypothermia. Med Sci Law 4: 44

Keith Mant A, Path FC (1969) Autopsy diagnosis of accidental hypothermia. J Forensic Med 16: 126

Klein H (1975) Körperschäden und Tod durch Hitze. In: Mueller B (ed) Gerichtliche Medizin. Springer, Berlin Heidelberg New York, p 504

Klein H, Mueller D (1964) Tod durch Hyperthermie im Säuglingsalter. Zwei Todesfälle mit elektrischem Heizkissen im Kinderbett. Med Welt 1958–1960

Könn G, Brandt J (1974) Über die Todesursachen bei der Verbrennungskrankheit. Monatsschr Unfallheilkd 77: 530

Koslowski L (1965) Verbrennungen bei Kindern. Z Kinderchir 2: 3
Kremer B, Schölmerich J, Schmidt K, Allgöwer M, Schweitzer GA, Schoeneberger GA (1979) Wirkung von Verbrennungstoxin auf Lebergewebe in vivo und in vitro. Therapiewoche 29: 800
Kuwabara S (1954) Nebennierenveränderungen unter künstlichem Winterschlaf im Verbrennungsschock (tierexperimentelle Untersuchung). Langenbecks Arch Chir 278: 61
Laiho K, Hirvonen J (1971) Reactions of the guinea pig's skin and adipose tissue to experimental frostbite. Acta Pathol Microbiol Scand [A] 79: 91
Lindlar F, Berger H (1962) Auffallende Aminosäureanreicherung und Verfettung der Leber nach schwerer Verbrennung. Schweiz Med Wochenschr 92: 110
Löfgren L (1963) Reaction of the adrenal cortex during controlled experimental hypothermia. Ann Med Exp Fenn 41: 319
Masshoff W (1957) Vitale Reaktion. In: Ponsold A (ed) Lehrbuch der Gerichtlichen Medizin. Thieme, Stuttgart
Maulhardt K (1975) Wärmetod. Kriminalistik 2: 69
McCaninch J, Matter P, Lynch JB, Lewis SR, Blocker Jr TG (1964) Renal pathophysiology in severe burns: five year review of kidney pathology in fatal burns. Tex Rep Biol Med 22: 348
Metter D, Schulz E (1978) Tödliche Verbrühung oder Lyell-Syndrom? Z Rechtsmed 81: 329
Moritz AR (1954) The pathology of trauma. Kimpton, London
Moritz AR, Henriques FC (1947) Studies of thermal injury. Relative importance of time and surface temperature in causation of cutaneous burns. Am J Pathol 23: 695
Mueller B (1975) Schädigungen und Tod durch Einwirkung von Kälte. In: Mueller B (ed) Gerichtliche Medizin. Springer, Berlin Heidelberg New York, p 500
Müller H (1971) Schädigungen durch Kälteeinwirkung. Münch Med Wochenschr 113: 1678
Naeve I (1981) Postmortale Hitzeschäden der Haut. Histomorphologische Differentialdiagnose und forensische Bedeutung. Dissertation, Hamburg
Nedwich A, Sokolic IH, Foreman J, Howard JM (1964) Histochemical observations of second-degree burns. J Trauma 4: 269
Olbrycht J (1927) Mikroskopische Untersuchungen von Lungen verbrannter Neugeborener zum Nachweis ihres Gelebthabens, nebst Bemerkungen über die forensische Bedeutung der histologischen Lungenprobe. Dtsch Z Ges Gerichtl Med 9: 529
Olbrycht J, Ramult M (1924) Der Einfluß der Verbrühung, des anaphylaktischen Schockes und der parenteralen Zufuhr verschiedener Eiweißstoffe auf das histologische Bild der Nebennieren. Dtsch Z Ges Gerichtl Med 3: 401
Pearson RW (1965) Response of human epidermis to graded thermal stress. A morphologic comparison of burns, cold-induced blisters, and pemphigus vulgaris. Arch Environm Health 11: 498
Petersohn F (1959) Ist das Vorhandensein von Kohlepartikeln in den Luftwegen von Brandleichen als Zeichen der vitalen Reaktion zu werten? Dtsch Z Gerichtl Med 49: 147
Pinchuk VM (1964) Morphological changes of the kidneys during the first period of burn. Arkh Patol 26/6: 40
Pioch W (1966a) L'image histologique des lésions vitales et post-mortem causées par brulures. Acta Med Leg Soc (Liege) 19: 327
Pioch W (1966b) Die histochemische Untersuchung thermischer Hautschäden und ihre Bedeutung für die forensische Praxis. Schmidt-Römhild, Lübeck
Pioch W (1966c) Histologisch-histochemische Untersuchungen zur Identifizierung von Strommarken. Dtsch Z Ges Gerichtl Med 57: 165
Pioch W (1971) Die Bewertung histochemischer Befunde nach thermischen und stumpfen Hautverletzungen unter forensischem Aspekt. Acta Histochem (Jena) 9: 405
Price PB, Call DE, Hansen FL, Zerwick CJ (1953) Penetration of heat in thermal burns. Surg Forum 4: 433
Püschel K, Mätzsch T, Brinkmann B (1980) Klinischer Verlauf und morphologische Befunde bei inhalatorischer Verbrühung. Unfallheilkunde 83: 592
Reh H (1960) Spättod nach Einwirkung von Kontaktwärme (55–60 °C) auf die Haut in einem Heißluftbad, zugleich ein Beitrag zur pathologischen Anatomie der Verbrennungskrankheit. Dtsch Z Gerichtl Med 49: 703
Remmele W (1975) Kreislaufschock. In: Mueller B (ed) Gerichtliche Medizin. Springer, Berlin Heidelberg New York, p 341

Rittenbury MS (1970) The response of the reticuloendothelial system to thermal injury. Surg Clin North Am 50: 1227
Sarajas HSS (1964) Myocardial damage induced by immersion hypothermia. Am J Cardiol 13: 355
Schickedanz H, Schickedanz E, Adam G, Wagner W (1975) Zur Morbiditäts- und Letalitätsentwicklung thermischer Verletzungen bei Kindern, eine 30-Jahres-Analyse. Z Aerztl Fortb 69: 613
Schmitt W, Schröter P (1962) Die Hyperpyrexie als Todesursache bei Verbrennungen im Säuglings- und Kleinkindesalter. Bruns Beitr Klin Chir 205: 240
Schneider G, Klug E (1980) Tod durch Unterkühlung. Gibt es neue Gesichtspunkte zur Diagnostik? Z Rechtsmed 86: 59
Schoenenberger GA, Allgöwer M, Kremer B, Städtler K (1976) Neue Gesichtspunkte zur Verbrennungskrankheit. Chirurg 47: 582
Schollmeyer W (1961) Zur histologischen Differentialdiagnose der Hautblasen nach Hitzeeinwirkung und nach Barbituratvergiftung. Dtsch Z Gerichtl Med 51: 180
Schollmeyer W (1962) Zur Frage der Fettembolie des Lungengewebes bei postmortal Verbrannten. Acta Med Leg Soc (Liege) 15: 77
Schubothe H, Gross F (1953) Wärmeveränderungen roter Blutkörperchen. Schweiz Med Wochenschr 1048
Sellès MM (1965) El "schock" de los quemados. Aspectos clinicos y mèdico-forense. An Med Forens Asoc Esp Med Forens 1965: 288
Senger IF (1955) Die Rolle des Nervensystems in der Entwicklung der pathologischen Veränderungen in den Lungen bei Abkühlung eines Tieres. Arkh Patol 17/H3: 41
Sevitt S (1979) A review of the complications of burns, their origin and importance for illness and death. J Trauma 19: 358
Shafer JC, Thompson AW (1955) Local cold injury. A report of sequelae. Arch Dermatol 72: 335
Shuda Y (1964a) Studies on vital reaction to the systemic hypothermia. Histopathological changes of the heart, I. Bull Yamaguchi Med Sch 11: 29
Shuda Y (1964b) Studies on vital reaction to the systemic hypothermia. Histopathological changes of the heart, II. Bull Yamaguchi Med Sch 11:77
Simon A, Müller E (1971) Einige Aspekte zur Physiologie und Morphologie des Kältetodes unter besonderer Berücksichtigung der sogenannten Kälteschilddrüse. Kriminal Forens Wiss 6: 131
Sochor FM, Mallory G (1963) Lung lesions in patients dying of burns. Arch Pathol Lab Med 75: 303
Thorban W (1963) Experimentelle und histologische Studien über die Entstehung organischer Früh- und Spät-Veränderungen an den Gefäßen nach Erfrierungen. Bruns Beitr Klin Chir 207: 87
Trube-Becker E (1967) Zur Begutachtung beim Tod durch Unterkühlung. Dtsch Z Ges Gerichtl Med 59: 211
Truss F (1968) Nierenstoffwechselveränderungen bei Hautverbrennungen. Langenbecks Arch Chir 322: 949
Wada T (1909) Über die Unterscheidung der Menschen- und Tierknochen. Vjschr Gerichtl Med Oeffl Sanitätswesen 37: 265
Zinck KH (1940) Pathologische Anatomie der Verbrennung. Veröffentlichungen aus der Konstitutions- und Wehrpathologie. Fischer, Jena
Zipper AJ, Ferrando GR, Guiloff EF, Sáez GR, Tchernitchin AV (1965) The response to in vivo freezing of the uterus and ovaries in rats. Am J Obstet Gynecol 93: 510

References to C VII: Injuries Caused by Electricity

Adjutantis G (1962) The identification of the electrical burn in cases of electrocution by the acroreaction test. J Forensic Med 9: 102
Baur E, Bissig H (1962) Tödliche Elektrounfälle an Hochspannungsanlagen. Elektromedizin 7: 150
Böhm E (1966) Untersuchungen über das Verhalten von Kupfer in und auf der Haut nach zufälliger und elektrischer Metallisation. Z Gerichtl Med 58: 166
Böhm E (1967) Untersuchungen über die Gestalt oberflächlicher Metallisationen der Haut. Dtsch Z Gerichtl Med 59: 26

Böhm E (1968) Zur Frage der Differentialdiagnose zwischen thermischen und elektrischen Verbrennungen. Dtsch Z Gerichtl Med 63: 149

Böhm E (1970) Untersuchungen an experimentellen Stromverletzungen mit Elektronenstrahlen. Z Rechtsmedizin 67: 293

Böhm E (1975) Zum Nachweis des Stromtodes. Beitr Gerichtl Med 33: 154

Böhm E (1976) Morphologische Befunde zur Differenzierung thermischer und elektrischer Hautverletzungen und ihre Bedeutung für die forensische Praxis. Habilitationsschrift, Aachen

Böhm E, Milz U (1975) Elektrische und morphologische Grundprozesse bei Verletzungen mit niedergespanntem Wechselstrom. Beitr Gerichtl Med 33: 308

Bosch K (1965) Makroskopische und lupenmikroskopische Untersuchungen zur Oberflächenbeschaffenheit an Strommarken. Dtsch Z Gerichtl Med 56: 318

Bujdosó G, Fonyó A, Somogyi E (1969) Structure and biochemical function of mitochondria isolated from heart tissue after electric injury. Zacchia 44: 3

Canale M, Bandini T, La Cavera A (1966) Sulla patogenesi della lesioni cutance da elettricità. Osservazione istologiche in fluorescenza ed in contrasto die fase. Med Leg (Genova) 14: 123

Descamps L, Castan P (1963) Nécrose encéphalique par électrocution. Etude anatomiclinique. Acta Neurol Belg 63: 739

Gaszner P (1969) Durch elektrischen Strom verursachte histopathologische Veränderungen des Nervensystems. Arch Psychiatr Nervenkr 212; 309

Harsányi I (1979) Knochenschäden durch elektrothermische Wirkung und Laserstrahlen. Kriminal Forens Wiss 35: 31

Heinlein G (1962) Modellversuche zur Deutung der morphologischen Veränderungen im Bereich der Strommarke. Elektromedizin 7: 175

Jellinek S (1932) Elektrische Verletzungen. Johann Ambrosius Barth, Leipzig

Jellinek S (1935) Die Sonderstellung der elektrischen Verletzung in Klinik und Histopathologie. In: Festschrift H. Zangger. Rascher, Zürich p 314

Jellinek S (1953) Klinische und histologische Bilder als poldifferenzierte Stromeffekte. Wien Klin Wochenschr: 774

Jellinek S (1955) Anschauliche Feststellungen zum Problem der Strommarke. Beitr Gerichtl Med 20: 56

Jellinek S (1961) Skizzen zur elektrogenen Vasopathie. Beitr Gerichtl Med 21: 133

Jellinek S (1964) Der elektrische Strom und die lebende Substanz; ein neues Kapitel der Heilkunde und der Naturforschung. Wien Klin Wochenschr 76: 637–645

Karobath H, Redtenbacher M, Hofecker G, Walde I, Syré G (1977) Zur Frage der Todesursache beim Blitzunfall. Münch Med Wochenschr 119: 29

Kawamura I (1921) Elektropathologische Histologie. Virchows Arch 231: 570

Koeppen S (1928) Die Anatomie der elektrischen Verletzungen. Dtsch Med Wochenschr 1928:2127

Koeppen S, Gerstner H (1935) Untersuchungen über elektrische Strommarken im Vergleich zu experimentell erzeugten Wärmeverletzungen der Haut. Virchows Arch 295: 679

Koeppen S, Panse F (1955) Klinische Elektropathologie. Thieme, Stuttgart

Kolár J, Vrabec R (1976) Knochenschäden bei Stromverletzungen. In: Handbuch der medizinischen Radiologie. Springer, Berlin Heidelberg New York, p 345

Lo Menzo G (1965) Le modificazioni dell' attivita' fosfatasica nelle lesioni cutanee da marchio elettrico. Tossicoligica XI: 4

Lo Menzo G (1975) Sulla metallizzazione del marcho elettrico; ricerche sperimentali. Med Leg (Genova) 23: 171

Marcinkowski T, Pankowski M (1980) Significance of skin metallization in the diagnosis of electrocution. Forensic Sci Int 16: 1

Marziano E, Lo Menzo G (1965) Aspetti microfluoroscopici del marchio elettrico. G Med Leg Infortun Tossicol 11: 389

Mazzucchelli B, Andreuzzi P (1966) Richerche istologiche sulle lesioni sperimentali da correnti ad alto voltaggio. Communicazione preliminare. Arch Soc Lobarda Med Leg 2: 49

Nevelös A, Rozsa Gy, Somogyi E, Soronyi P, Soronyi T (1971) Lesions of skeletal muscles following electrocution. Acta Med Leg Soc (Liege) 20: 203

Noeske K, Knothe W (1965) Pathologisch-anatomische Veränderungen im Bett von Schrittmacherelektroden. Thorac Cardiovasc Surg 13: 273

Pearse E (1961) Histochemistry. Churchill Ltd London

Pierucci G, Danesino P (1980) The macroscopic detection of metallization in the latent current mark. Z Rechtsmed 85: 97
Pioch W (1966) Histologisch-histochemische Untersuchungen zur Identifizierung von Strommarken. Dtsch Z Gerichtl Med 57: 165
Pioch W (1967) Zur gerichtsmedizinischen Untersuchung von Tötungsdelikten durch elektrischen Strom. Forschungsergebnisse der gerichtlichen Medizin. Festschr. z. 60. Geburtstag von Prof. Dr. H. Elbel. Schmidt-Römhild, Lübeck, p 31
Pioch W (1968) Zur gerichtsmedizinischen Untersuchung von Tötungsdelikten durch elektrischen Strom. Arch Kriminol 142: 143
Püschel K, Brinkmann B (1979) Zur Histomorphologie vitaler Muskelreaktionen nach Stromschädigung. Beitr Gerichtl Med 37: 141
Rozsa Gy, Somogyi E, Nevelós A, Varga T (1971) Kernveränderungen nach Stromeinwirkung. Acta Med Leg Soc (Liege) 20: 199
Sartorius H (1967) Nierenveränderungen nach Starkstromverletzungen. Therapiewoche 17: 839
Schäffner M (1965) Untersuchungen über Histologie und Metallisation nach elektrischen Einwirkungen auf die Haut. Dtsch Z Gerichtl Med 56: 269
Schmidt G (1963) Differenzierung von Strom- und Brandmarken. Contact
Schmidt G (1964) Identifizierung von Stromdurchtrittsstellen. Acta Med Leg Soc (Liege) 7: 51
Schmidt MB (1910) Über Starkstromverletzungen. Verh Dtsch Pathol Ges 14: 218
Schneider V, Hantsche H (1973) Über Untersuchungen an Strommarken mit Rasterelektronenmikroskop und Mikrosonde. Beitr Gerichtl Med 31: 192
Schrader G (1920) Experimentelle Untersuchungen zur Histopathologie elektrischer Hautschädigungen. Jena
Schridde H (1925) Der elektrische Stromtod. Pathologisch-anatomische Untersuchungen. Klin Wochenschr: 2142
Schwerd W, Lautenbach L (1960) Mord mit elektrischem Strom in der Badewanne. Arch Krim 126: 33
Sellier K (1966) Untersuchungen an Strommarken in Abhängigkeit von der Stromstärke und der Einwirkungsdauer. I. Metallnachweis und Temperaturmessung. Dtsch Z Gerichtl Med 57: 161
Sellier K (1975) Schäden und Tod durch Elektrizität. In: Mueller B (ed) Gerichtliche Medizin. Springer, Berlin Heidelberg New York: p 538
Somogyi E, Rozsa G, Sotonyi P (1965) Histochemische und fluoreszenzoptische Untersuchungen der Strommarke. Acta Morphol Acad Sci Hung 13: 311
Somogyi E, Sotonyi P, Rozsa G, Iranyi J, Ovorecz B, Iranyi K (1966a) Polarisationsoptische Untersuchungen der elektrischen Strommarke. Dtsch Z Gerichtl Med 57: 431
Somogyi Gy, Rozsa P, Sotonyi B, Orovecz J, Iranyi C (1966b) L'étude de la fluorescence et de la polarisation optique de la marque électrique. Acta Med Leg Soc (Liege) 19: 223
Spaar FW (1955) Hirnbefund nach Tod durch Blitzschlag. Virchows Arch 326: 732
Stichnoth E (1968) Zur Histologie der Strommarke. Beitr Gerichtl Med 24: 127
Tabbara W (1962) Présentation de pière microscopique: electrocution. Ann Med Leg 12: 340
Thomsen HK, Danielsen L, Nielsen O, Aalund O, Nielsen KG, Karlsmark T, Genefke IK (1981a) Early epidermal changes in heat- and electrically injured pig skin. I. A light microscopic study. Forensic Sci Int 17: 133
Thomsen HK, Danielsen L, Nielsen O, Aalund O, Nielsen KG, Karlsmark T, Genefke IK (1981b) Early epidermal changes in heat- and electrically injured pig skin. II. An electron microscopic study. Forensic Sci Int 17: 145
Timm F (1958) Zur Histochemie der Schwermetalle. Das Sulfit-Silberverfahren. Z Gerichtl Med 46: 706
Timm F (1968) Acta Histochem (Jena) 3: [Suppl 1]
Viterbo B, Pasetti M (1965) Modificazioni della musculatura scheletrica nella morte elettrocuzione. Med Leg (Genova) 13: 275
Voigt GE (1959) Untersuchungen mit der Sulfid-Silbermethode an menschlichen und tierischen Bauchspeicheldrüsen (unter besonderer Berücksichtigung des Diabetes mellitus und experimenteller Metallvergiftungen). Virch Arch 332: 295
Zollinger HO (1966) Niere und ableitende Harnwege. In: Doerr W, Uehlinger I (ed) Spezielle pathologische Anatomie, vol 3. Springer, Berlin Heidelberg New York

References to C VIII: Injuries Caused by Radiation and Ultrasound

Abbatt JD (1979) History of the use and toxicity of Thorotrast. Environ Res 18: 6

Becker F (1937) Kniegelenksarkom nach Röntgenbestrahlung. Dtsch Zschr Chir 248: 11

Berdjis CC (1971) Pathology of irradiation. Williams & Wilkens, Baltimore

Bergeder HD (1962) Grundlagen der biologischen Strahlenwirkung und Strahlenschäden. Ergeb Allg Pathol 42: 1

Bergeder HD, Braun H, Fasske E (1963) Strahlenpathologie der Zelle. Beiträge zur Cyto- und Histopathologie der Strahlenwirkung. Thieme, Stuttgart

Bergonié J, Tribondeau L (1906) Interpretation de quelques résultats de la radiotherapié et essai de fixation d'une technique rationelle. CR Acad Sci Paris 143: 983

Bianchi L (1961a) Experimentelle Untersuchungen über Gefäßveränderungen der Röntgenniere. Pathol Mikrobiol 24: 270

Bianchi L (1961b) Zur Morphologie und Funktion experimentell erzeugter Röntgennieren. Virch Arch [Pathol Anat] 334: 206

Brettschneider H (1952) Tierexperimentelle Beobachtungen über die Wirkung des Ultraschalls auf lebendes Gewebe. Ultraschall in Med 4: 45

Campanacci L, Patrese P, Romagnoli GF, Okolicsanyi L, Mendola R (1968) La nefropatia secondaria ad irradiazione. Folia Med (Napoli) 51: 905

Cottier H (1961) Strahlenbedingte Lebensverkürzung. Springer, Berlin Göttingen Heidelberg

Cottier H (1966) Histopathologie der Wirkung ionisierender Strahlen auf höhere Organismen (Tier und Mensch). In: Strahlenbiologie. Springer, Berlin Heidelberg New York (Handbuch der Medizinischen Radiologie, vol 2/2, p 35)

Cowden JW, Abell MR (1963) Some effects of ultrasonic radiation on normal tissues. Exp Molec Pathol 2: 367

Eger E, Gregl A (1965) Die Strahlenpneumonitis. Stuttgart, Hippokrates

Engelstad RB (1934) Über die Wirkung der Röntgenstrahlen auf die Lungen. Acta Radiolog 19 [Suppl] (Stockh.)

Fajardo LE (1977) Radiation-induced coronary artery disease. Chest 71: 563

Fliedner TM, Andrews GA, Cronkite EP, Bond VP (1964) Early and late cytologic effects of whole body irradiation on human marrow. Blood 23: 471

Franke H (1963) Die Strahlenempfindlichkeit des menschlichen Rückenmarks. Fortschr Med 81: 345

Fritz-Niggli H (1960) Allgemeine Strahlenbiologie. In: Roulet F (ed) Strahlung und Wetter. Springer, Berlin Heidelberg New York (Handbuch der allgemeinen Pathologie, vol X/1, p 1)

Fröscher W (1976) Die Strahlenschädigung des Rückenmarks. Fortschr Neurol Psychiatr 44: 94

Frýdl V (1962) Zusammenfassendes Referat über morphologische Veränderungen in der Leber durch Bestrahlung. Z Ges Inn Med 17: 624

Gehrmann G, Schäfer EL, Wunder M (1963) Klinische und radiologische Befunde bei Thorotrastschädigungen. Dtsch Med Wochenschr 88: 2050

Girgensohn H, Witzel D (1965) Rückenmarksschädigung durch Röntgenstrahlen von cervicalen und thoracalen Tumoren. Zentralbl Allg Pathol Pathol Anat 108: 121

Gössner W (1972) Grundlagen und allgemeine pathologische Anatomie der Strahlenschäden. Verhandl Dtsch Ges Pathol 56: 168

Günsel E (1953) Die Strahlenschäden am Erwachsenenknochen. Strahlentherapie 91: 595

Hennekeuser H-H, Citoler G, Niemczyk H, Gropp A (1970) Klinische, histologische und cytogenetische Befunde bei Patienten mit Thorotrastschaden. Klin Wochenschr 48: 895

Heyck H, Höpker W (1952) Hirnveränderungen bei der Ratte durch Ultraschall. Monatsschr Psychol Neurol 123: 42

Hieronymi G (1957) Kritische Untersuchungen sogenannter Thorotrasttumoren nebst Mitteilung zweier Fälle. Zentralbl Allg Pathol Pathol Anat 97: 513

Höpker W, Heyck H (1951) Ganglienzellschädigung nach kleinen Ultraschalldosen. Verhand Dtsch Ges Inn Med 57: 424

Itschev K, Dogramadjiew I, Dourmischev A (1979) Elektronenmikroskopische Untersuchungen der menschlichen Haut nach UV-Bestrahlung. Dermatol Monatsschr 165: 209

Jankowiak J, Majewski C, Kubiak E (1963) Histopathological changes in the adrenals of rabbits after direct action of ultrasound on the brain. Am J Physiol Med 42: 153

Jennings FL, Arden A (1962) Development of radiation pneumonitis. Time and dose factors. Arch Pathol Lab Med 74: 351
Klein H (1975) Körperschäden durch Strahlen. In: Mueller B (ed) Gerichtliche Medizin. Springer, Berlin Heidelberg New York, p 533
König W (1967) Die Wirkungsfaktoren einer Kernwaffendetonation auf den menschlichen Organismus und die Maßnahmen der medizinischen Hilfe. Z Aerztl Fortbild (Jena) 61: 453
Kosmider St, Jonek J (1963) Histochemische Untersuchungen über das Verhalten einiger Enzyme in der Lunge bei akuter Strahlenkrankheit sowie nach Lokal-Röntgenbestrahlung. Radiobiol Radiother (Berl) 4: 699
Kricke E (1961) Strahlenschäden der Arteria carotis interna nach Radiogold-Implantationen in die Hypophyse. Bruns Beitr Klin Chir 203: 311
Krompecher T (1971) Untersuchungen über die Cytochromoxidaseaktivität verschiedener Rattenorgane nach 200 RAD Ganzkörper-CO^{60}-Bestrahlung. Vortrag auf der 3. Tagung der Ges. f. gerichtl. Medizin der DDR, 1.10. 1971 in Berlin
Meissner J (1974) Aufgaben und Ergebnisse der Strahlenbiologie in ihren Beziehungen zu den Strahlenschutz- und Röntgenverordnungen. GIT
Melanotte BL, Follis RH (1961) Early effects of X-irradiation on cartilage and bone. Am J Pathol 39: 1
Mignard de VA, Patek PR, Bernick S (1965) Response of the liver to „target" irradiation. Am J Pathol 47: 339
Morgenroth K, Junge-Hülsing G, Hauss WH (1967) Über Veränderungen an Rattenherzen nach gezielter Röntgenbestrahlung. Strahlentherapie 133: 610
Oehlert W (1970) Pathologische Veränderungen in Organen und Geweben nach Applikation von Radioisotopen und Kontrastmitteln. Langenbeck Arch Chir 327: 229
Oehlert W, Wenig W (1975) Der latente Strahlenschaden der Leber, seine Manifestierung und seine Verstärkung durch zusätzliche Regenerationsreize. Zivilverteidigung 42
Opton AC (1969) Radiation injury. University of Chicago Press, Chicago
Peters G (1955) Schädigungen des Zentralnervensystems durch Ultraschall. In: Springer, Berlin Göttingen Heidelberg (Handbuch der spez. patholog. Anatomie und Histologie, p 363)
Rajewsky B (1956) Strahlendosis und Strahlenwirkung. Thieme, Stuttgart
Reed GB, Cox AJ (1966) The human liver after radiation injury. A form of veno-occlusive desease. Am J Pathol 48: 597
Rotter W (1951) Über Gewebsschäden durch Thorotrast. Unter besonderer Berücksichtigung der Gefäßveränderungen und aplastischen Knochenmarksreaktionen. Beitr Pathol Anat 111: 144
Scherer E, Stender HSt (1963) Strahlenpathologie der Zelle. Thieme, Stuttgart
Spath P (1963) Amyloide Lungenschrumpfung bei Röntgenbestrahlung. Frankf Z Pathol 72: 309
Staemmler M (1955) Thorotrastschaden. Zentralbl Allg Pathol Pathol Anat 93: 419
Steiner D, Brinkmann B (1974) Mitursächlichkeit eines Thorotrastschadens bei Tod durch stumpfe Gewalt. Z Rechtsmed 75: 213
Thalhammer O (1967) Pränatale Erkrankungen des Menschen. Thieme, Stuttgart
Thomas E, Forbus WD (1959) Irradiation injury to the aorta and the lung. Arch Pathol Lab Med 67: 256
Thurner J (1970) Iatrogene Pathologie. Urban & Schwarzenberg, München Berlin Wien
Vajardo LF, Steward JR, Cohn KE (1968) Morphology of radiation-induced heart disease. Arch Pathol Lab Med 86: 512
Villiers AJ, Gross P (1967) Radiation pneumonitis. X-ray induced lesions in hamsters and rats. Arch Environ Health 15: 650
Werthemann A (1930) Experimentelle Röntgenschädigung des Herzmuskels. Strahlentherapie 38: 702
Windholz (1933) Zur Histologie der Röntgenstrahlenwirkung. Zentralbl Allg Pathol 59: 190
Zeman W (1955) Elektrische Schädigungen und Veränderungen durch ionisierende Strahlen. In: Scholz W (ed) Erkrankungen des Zentralen Nervensystems III. Springer, Berlin (Handbuch der speziellen pathologischen Anatomie und Histologie, vol XIII/3, p 327)
Zollinger HU (1960) Radio-Histologie und Radio-Histopathologie. In: Roulet F (ed) Strahlung und Wetter. Springer, Berlin Göttingen Heidelberg (Handbuch der allgemeinen Pathologie, vol 10, part 1, p 127)

Zollinger HU (1966) Niere und ableitende Harnwege. In: Doerr W, Seifert G, Uehlinger E (eds) Spezielle pathologische Anatomie III. Springer, Berlin Heidelberg New York
Zülch KJ (1960) Über die Strahlensensibilität der Hirngeschwülste und die sogenannte Strahlenspätnekrose des Hirns. Dtsch Med Wochenschr 85: 293

References to C IX: Histological Findings in Starvation

Bade EG, Schumacher A (1964) Veränderungen der submikroskopischen Struktur der Leberzellen der Maus nach temporärer Ischämie. Frankfurt Z Pathol 74: 29
Baker RD (1964) Effect of starvation and glucose absorption in PAS-reactive granules in jejunal epithelium of mouse. Tex Rep Biol Med 22: 410
Baumann J, Jungmann H, Voigt KD (1966) Der Einfluß systematischer Nahrungskarenz und -zufuhr auf die 17-OH-Corticosteroidausscheidung von Normalpersonen. Klin Wochenschr 18: 1081
Becker V (1969) Pathomorphologie und Pathogenese der Malabsorption. Verh Dtsch Ges Pathol 53: 10
Feyrter F (1973) Über die zyanochrom-granuläre Entartung des braunen Fettgewebes des Menschen. Beitr Gerichtl Med 30: 97
Gerhartz H (1955) Das Verhalten der Schilddrüse unter dem Hunger. 2. Symposion der Deutschen Gesellschaft für Endokrinologie 1955, p 178
Gieseking R (1962) Die submikroskopischen Veränderungen der Skelettmuskelfaser bei Hungeratrophie. Frankf Z Pathol 71: 584
Harms K (1973) Das Malabsorptionssyndrom im Kindesalter. Med Klinik 68: 163
Houtrouw O (1973) Der Einfluß einer absoluten Nahrungskarenz auf die Aldosteron-Elektrolytausscheidung im Urin. Medizinische Dissertation Hamburg
Lamotte M, Bernier J-J, Oudéa P, Martin Et, Kleinknecht D (1965) Les dénutritions sévères. II. Etude anatomique du foie. Presse Med 73: 2189
Lange K, Giese W, Hörstebrock R (1962) Allgemeine Pathologie des exogenen, quantitativen Nahrungsmangels. In: Ernährung. Springer Berlin Göttingen Heidelberg (Handbuch der allgemeinen Pathologie, vol XI/1, pp 446, 552)
Lüdtke KCh (1973) Stoffwechseluntersuchungen bei Anorexia nervosa-Patientinnen vor, während und nach der Auffütterung. Teil III. Med Dissertation, Hamburg
Mueller B (1975) Gerichtliche Medizin, vol 1. Springer, Berlin Heidelberg New York, p 500
Napolitano L, Gagne HT (1963) Lipid-depleted white adipose cells; an electron microscope study. Anat Rec 147: 273
Otto H, Würstlein H (1964) Bioptische Untersuchungen zur Frage der Leberspätschäden nach Hungerdystrophie. Frankfurt Z Pathol 74: 4
Paradisi F (1965) Phase contrast microscope observations on the pancreas of fasting rats. Experientia (Basel) 21: 126
Reh H (1953) Die Fettzellgröße beim Menschen und ihre Abhängigkeit vom Ernährungszustand. Virchows Archiv 324: 234
Schlicht I (1955) Experimentelle Untersuchungen über den Ablauf der Leberverfettung bei Hunger und Sauerstoffmangel. Virchows Arch 326: 568
Stirling GA (1962) Renal pathology in malnourished infants. Arch Dis Child 37: 378
Svoboda D, Grady H, Higginson J (1966) The effects of chronic protein deficiency in rats. II. Biochemical and ultrastructural changes. Lab Invest 15: 731
Tarasitano F (1939) Erosioni emorragiche dello stomaco nella morte per il anizione acuta. Zacchia II. 3: 200
Tessmann D (1963) Fermenthistochemische Untersuchungen der Rattenleber unter den Bedingungen der akuten Inanition. Z Ges Exp Med 137: 464
Voigt KD, Apostolakis M (1969) Einfluß einer 20tägigen Nahrungskarenz auf Substrate des Kohlenhydrat- und Fettstoffwechsels und auf Enzymaktivitäten im Blut. Klin Wochenschr 47: 157
Voigt KD, Apostolakis M, Jungmann H (1967) Stoffwechsel- und Kreislaufstudien bei absoluter Nahrungskarenz. Klin Wochenschr 45: 924
Zaletaeva TA (1963) A study of destructive and reparative processes in the hepatic cells following starvation. Biull Eksp Biol Med 28: 112

References to C X: Histological Contribution to the Investigation of Gunshot Wounds

Francisco JT (1980) Histopathology of gunshot wounds. In: Perper, Wecht (eds) Microscopic diagnosis in forensic pathology. CC Thomas, Springfield Illinois
Henn R, Liebhardt E (1969) Zur Topik außerhalb des Schußkanals gelegener Hirnrindenblutungen. Arch Kriminol 143: 188
Hopkinson DAW (1964) The use of Giemsa stain to demonstrate histologically the extent of altered striated muscle around bullet wounds. J Pathol 87: 63
Hopkinson DAW, Watts JC (1963) Studies in experimental missile injuries of skeletal muscle. Proc Roy Soc Med 56: 461
Krauland W (1938) Die Basophilie des Bindegewebes als Zeichen des Einschusses und andere histologische Befunde an Schußwunden. Int Kongress gerichtl u soz Med Bonn/Rhine, 22.–24.9., p 125
Mueller B (1941) Gerichtlich-medizinische Studien an Bomben- und Granatsplitterverletzungen. Dtsch Z Ges Gerichtl Med 35: 173
Mueller B (1942) Untersuchungen über Schrägschüsse und über das Verhalten der Basophilie in der Umgebung von Schußöffnungen. Dtsch Z Ges Gerichtl Med 36: 53
Orsós F (1935) Die vitalen Reaktionen und ihre gerichtsmedizinische Bedeutung. Beitr Pathol Anat Allg Pathol 95: 163
Pollak St (1980) Zur Morphologie der Einschußwunden im Palmar- und Plantarbereich. Z Rechtsmed 86: 41
Rolfe HC, Curle D, Simmons D (1971) Eine histologische Technik für die forensische Ballistik. J Forensic Med 18: 47
Speeter D, Ohnsorge J (1973) Rasterelektronenmikroskopisch erfaßbare Schußzeichen am Knochen. Z Rechtsmed 73: 137
Venglinskaya EA, Svyatoshchik VL, Shchegel SM (1967) Immediate vascular reactions in the area of gun-shot wounds. Sud Med Ekspert 10: 20
Venglinskaya E, Svyatoshchik VL, Shchegel SM (1970) Zur Charakteristik reaktiver Veränderungen im Bereich einer Schußverletzung durch Einwirkung verschiedener Schußkomponenten. Sud Med Ekspert 13: 14

References to C XI: Histological Findings in Poisoning

Adebahr G (1954) Über Spättodesfälle nach Kohlenoxydvergiftung. Dtsch Z Gerichtl Med 43: 408
Adebahr G (1960) Nierenveränderungen bei der E 605-Vergiftung des Menschen. Arch Toxicol 18: 107
Adebahr G (1961) Die Niere bei Gehirnschäden infolge Barbiturat-Vergiftung und Schädeltrauma. Arch Toxicol 19: 169
Adebahr G (1963) Leberveränderungen bei der E 605-Vergiftung des Menschen. Beitr Gerichtl Med 22: 1
Adebahr G (1966) Veränderungen der Eizelle des Menschen bei E 605-Vergiftung. Dtsch Z Gerichtl Med 58: 248
Adebahr G (1970) Über lichtmikroskopisch sichtbare Spalten in der Zona pellucida der menschlichen Eizelle im Graafschen Follikel. Beitr Gerichtl Med 27: 86
Adebahr G (1971) Histochemische Befunde bei Barbituratvergiftung und Vergiftung mit E 605. Acta Histochemica [Suppl] 9: 493
Adebahr G (1976) Zur Pathologie der Organschäden nach diagnostischen und therapeutischen Eingriffen. Z Rechtsmed 78: 173
Adebahr G, Voigt GE (1963) Morphologische Veränderungen bei der akuten tödlichen Nicotinvergiftung. Dtsch Z Gerichtl Med 54: 304
Aenishänslin HW, Stalder GA, Bianchi L, Gudat F, Carmann H (1975) Hepatitis bei Drogensüchtigen, Verlaufskontrollen anhand bioptisch-histologischer Kriterien. Dtsch Med Wochenschr 100: 857
Aizawa S (1962) Beobachtete Veränderungen in Leberzellen und Nierentubuli bei akuter Tetrachlorkohlenstoff- und Diäthylenglycolvergiftung. Acta Pathol Jpn 12: 155

Al-Abadi H, Dumke K (1977) Donhuijsen K, Niedobitek F: Morphometrische Untersuchungen an Belegzellen des Rattenmagens unter chronischem Alkoholeinfluß. Z Gastroenterol 15: V

Alexander CS (1966) Idiopathische Herzhypertrophie. II. Elektronenmikroskopische Untersuchungen an Herzmuskelbiopsien bei alkoholischer Herzmuskelschädigung. Am J Med 41: 229

Alexander CS, Sekhri KK, Nagasawa HT (1977) Alcoholic cardiomyopathy in mice electron microscopic observations. J Mol Cell Cardiol 9: 247

Alterman K (1954) Untersuchungen über die Fibrose der Leber, hervorgerufen durch Tetrachlorkohlenstoff. I. Beziehung zwischen Leberzellschaden und Neubildung fibrösen Gewebes. Arch Pathol 57: 1

Altmann H-W (1973) In: Boekker W (ed) Gallenwege – Leber, 7. Bad Mergentheimer Stoffwechsel-Tagung. Thieme, Stuttgart

Altmann H-W (1980) Drug-induced liver reactions: A morphological approach. Curr Top Pathol 69: 69

Altmann H-W, Klinge C (1972) Drogenhepatopathie. – Morphologische Reaktionen menschlichen Lebergewebes auf Pharmaka. Verh Dtsch Ges Pathol 56: 194

Aragona F (1965) Das pathologisch-anatomische Kriterium bei der gerichtsmedizinischen Diagnose des Vergiftungstodes. Zacchia 40: 321

Asbeck F, Joist J, Löhrs U (1972) Lebervenenthrombose und Ovulationshemmer. Ein weiterer Fall von Budd-Chiari-Syndrom nach Einnahme eines oralen Kontrazeptivums. Med Klin 67: 82

Ashworth CT, Johnson CF, Wrightsman FJ (1965) Biochemische und morphologische Beziehungen der Eiweißsynthese der Rattenleber bei akuter Äthanolvergiftung. Am J Pathol 46: 757

Astolfi E, Donnewald H, Monserrat J, Calabrese A (1970) Die Lunge bei Vergiftungen durch organophosphorische Pesticide. Poumon Coeur 26: 1067

Asvadi S, Hayes JA (1978) Acute lung injury induced by cadmium aerosol. II. Free airway cell response during injury and repair. Am J Pathol 90: 89

Axelsson B, Piscator M (1966) Nierenschädigung nach längerer Cadmiumexposition. Experimentelle Untersuchungen. Arch Environm Health 12: 360

Bässler R (1961) Zur Pathogenese seltener Blutungen bei Leberzirrhosen mit Pseudolobulusnekrosen. Virch Arch [Pathol Anat] 334: 118

Balázs M, Várkonyi S, Pintér A (1977) Elektronenmikroskopische Untersuchung der alkoholischen Leberschädigung, insbesondere der Veränderungen der mesenchymalen Leberzellen. Morphol Igazsagugyi Orv Sz 17: 1

Balogh I, Sótonyi P (1977) Herzmuskelnekrosen bei akuter Kohlenmonoxidvergiftung. Morphol Igazsogugyi Orv Sz 17: 14

Balogh J, Rubányi G (1978) Elektronenmikroskopische Untersuchung des Herzmuskels nach Zyan-Vergiftung. Morphol Igazsagugyi Orv Sz 18: 10

Balzereit F, Arnold W (1965) Lungenödem nach Pentobarbitalvergiftungen. Nervenarzt 1: 42

Barckow D, Neuhaus G, Erdmann WD (1969) Zur Behandlung der schweren Parathion-(E-605)-Vergiftung mit dem Cholinesterase-Reaktivator Obidoxim (Toxogonin). Arch Toxicol 24: 133

Bartonićek VJ, Brun A (1979) Subacute and chronic trichloroethylene poisoning: a neuropathological study in rabbits. Acta Pharmacol 28: 359

Baumbach GL, Cancilla PA, Martin-Amat G, Tephly TR, McMartin KE, Makar AB, Hayreh MS (1977) Methylalcohol poisoning. IV. Alterations of the morphological findings of the retina and optic nerve. Arch Ophthalmol 95: 1859

Beckmann E-R, Püschel K (1982) Histologische Leberveränderungen bei Rauschgifttodesfällen. In: Kongreßbericht „XII. Kongreß der Internationalen Akademie für Gerichtliche und Soziale Medizin", vol II. Egermann, Wien

Bereznoy RV (1973) Morphological alterations in the rhomboid brain in fatal cases of acute alcoholic intoxication. Sud Med Ekspert 16: 15

Berghaus G (1978) Statistische Differenzierung zwischen Alkoholikern und Nichtalkoholikern anhand der Verfettung, des Fettsäuremusters und der Enzymaktivitäten der menschlichen Leber. Z Rechtsmed 82: 113

Blava C (1964) Eine bis jetzt einzigartige Schädigung des Ergastoplasmas der Leberepithelzellen. Lab Invest 13: 301

Böcker W, Seifert G (1972) Zur Pathologie der Alkohol-Pankreatitis. Dtsch Med Wochenschr 97: 803

Boelcke G, Gaaz J-W (1970) Zur Frage der Lebertoxicität von Nitrostigmin (E 605 forte) und Obidoxim (Toxogonin) an Hunden. Arch Toxicol 26: 93

Bonciu C, Dumitresco R, Petrovici M, Rotesco C (1962) Experimentelle Untersuchungen über die Giftwirkung des Atebrins. Arch Roum Pathol Exp Microbiol 21: 213

Borchard F, Grabensee B, Jax W, Huth F (1974) Morphologische Befunde bei Paraquatvergiftungen. Klin Wochenschr 52: 657

Brandt L, Walther G, Rothschenk H, von Lieven Th (1972) Enzymhistochemische Untersuchungen am Hoden der Ratte nach hyperbarer Sauerstoffvergiftung. Beitr Gerichtl Med 29: 312

Braunstein H, Stenger RJ (1966) Hyaline Körper in Tetrachlorkohlenstoff-geschädigten Leberzellen: Nucleosid-Diphosphatase-Aktivität. J Histochem Cytochem 14: 112

Bredemann W (1954) Zur Histopathologie der Thalliumvergiftung im Bereich des Nervensystems. Arch Psychiatr Nervenkr 192: 393

Brettel HF, Hiersch HH, Raudonat HW (1968) Beobachtungen bei einer mit Kobaltchelat behandelten percutanen Cyanidvergiftung. Hefte Unfallheilkd 94: 301

Broicher H, Heymer A, Hermanns O, Lelbach WK (1962) Chronischer Alkoholismus und Leber. Bioptische und klinische Befunde bei der alkoholischen Fettleber. Acta Hepatosplen 9: 37

Browning E (1965) Toxicity and metabolism of industrial solvents. Elsevier, Amsterdam London New York

Bruch J, Schlipköter H-W (1973) Veränderungen der Lungenalveolen bei der Maus nach chronischer Exposition mit Ozon in niedriger Konzentration. Virchows Arch [Pathol Anat] 358: 355

Bschor F, Keilbach H (1968) Die Bedeutung chronischer Organschäden für die tödliche Alkoholvergiftung. Dtsch Z Gerichtl Med 62: 183

Büsing CM (1978) Pathoanatomische Aspekte der Sauerstoff-Intoxikation (normobare Hypoxie). Beziehungen zur sog. Schock-Lunge. Fortschr Med 96: 673

Burck H-C, Portwich F (1964) Akute Niereninsuffizienz nach schwerer Kohlenmonoxyd-Intoxikation. Frankf Z Pathol 73: 520

Calderon JJ, Cualla U (1962) Ein interessanter Fall von Tod durch Fluorvergiftung. Rev Med Leg Colomb 17: 89, 145

Caroff J, Breton J, Hadengue A, Derobert L (1968) Histologische Aspekte der Leber bei der Phosphorvergiftung. Med Lég Dommage Corp 1: 178

Caulet T, Petit J, Adnet JJ, Diebold J (1972) Histoenzymologische Untersuchung der durch Tetrachlorkohlenstoff bei der Ratte ausgelösten Lebercirrhose. Ann Anat Pathol 17: 125

Cederberg A, Hellsten S, Miörner G (1965) Oxygen treatment and hyaline pulmonary membranes in adults. Acta Pathol Microbiol Scand 64: 450

Chomette G, Emerit J, Auriol M (1978) L'hépatocyte dans l'hépatite aigue alcoolique. Confrontation histoenzymologique et ultrastructurale. Virchows Arch [Pathol Anat] 380: 31

v. Clarmann M (1971) Grundzüge der klinischen Toxikologie. In: Kuemmerle HP, Garett ER, Spitzy KH (eds) Klinische Pharmakologie und Pharmakotherapie. Urban u. Schwarzenberg, München

Clausen E (1964) Histological changes in rabbit kidneys induced by phenacetin and acetylsalicylic acid. Lancet 11: 123

Cochran AJ, Watson AA (1969) Leberveränderungen bei einem Patienten nach Behandlung mit Cytostatica, ähnlich denjenigen bei akuter Phosphorvergiftung. Med Sci Law 9: 202

Colmant HJ (1968) Pathomorphologie des chronischen Alkoholismus. Internist 9: 256

Colmant HJ, Wever H (1963) Pränatale Kohlenoxydvergiftung mit „Organtod" des Zentralnervensystems. Arch Psychiatr Nervenkr 204: 271

Cucu F (1978) Carbon monoxide and its implications in atherosclerosis etiopathogeny. Med Interne 16: 229

Daalgard JB (1962) Postmortale Befunde bei Kohlenoxyd-Todesfällen. Acta Pathol Mircobiol Scand [Suppl] 154: 186, 189

Dammermann R, Gürtler K-F, Klöppel G, de Heer K (1979) Benigne Lebertumoren nach Einnahme oraler Kontrazeptiva. Inn Med 6: 115

De Bias DA, Banerjee N, Birkhead NC, Harrer WV, Kazal LA (1973) Carbon monoxide inhalation effects following myocardial infarction in monkeys. Arch Environ Health 27: 161

Dejung K (1963) Beitrag zur Histologie des Salyrganschadens an der Kaninchenniere. Z Ges Exp Med 137: 196

Dürr HK (1977) Alkoholschädigung des Pankreas. Internist 19: 123

Eisenburg J (1981) Leber und „Pille“. Part 2: Lebertumoren. Fortschr Med 99: 1527
Eisenmenger W, Henn R, Beckmann G (1974) Klinische und pathologisch-anatomische Befunde der Paraquat-Vergiftung. Beitr Gerichtl Med 32: 262
Eknoyan G, Gyärkey F, Dichoso C, Hyde SE, Gyärkey P, Suki WN, Martinez-Maldonado M (1973) Renal involvement in drug abuse. Arch Intern Med 132: 801
Factor SM (1976) Intramyocardial small-vessel disease in chronic alcoholism. Am Heart J 92: 561
Falk SA, Klein R, Haseman JK, Sanders GM, Talley FA, Lim DJ (1974) Acute methyl mercury intoxication and ototoxicity in guinea pigs. Arch Pathol 97: 297
Fasske E (1962) Akute Fluorvergiftung. Toxikologie des Fluors. Symposium Bern 15.–17. Oct. 1962. Schwabe, Basel Stuttgart
Fazekas I Gy (1964) Alkoholabbau und Nebennierenrinde. Acta Med Leg Soc (Liege) 17: 77
Fazekas IG (1957) Tödliche Pyramidonvergiftung bei einem Säugling mit besonderer Berücksichtigung der histologischen Veränderungen. Dtsch Z Gerichtl Med 46: 374
Fazekas IG (1971) Über die makroskopischen und mikroskopischen Veränderungen bei der Wofatox-Vergiftung (Methyl-Parathion). Z Rechtsmed 68: 189
Fazekas IG, Kosa F (1964) Drei Mordtaten mit Nicotin. Dtsch Z Gerichtl Med 55: 40
Fazekas IG, Kosa F (1970) Über histologische Veränderungen bei akuter Nikotinvergiftung. Zacchia 45: 200
Fazekas IG, Fazekas AGy, Bertok EF (1962) Über die histologische Veränderung der Nieren auf die Wirkung wiederholter großer Pyramidondosen. Zacchia 37: 1
Ferrans VJ, Hibbs RG, Weilbaecher DG, Black WC, Walsh JJ, Burch GE (1965) Alkoholische Kardiomyopathie. Eine histochemische Untersuchung. Am Heart J 69: 748
Finck P-A (1966) CO-Exposition. Literaturbericht und Beobachtungen an 567 Obduktionen. Military Med 131: 1513
Flax MH, Tisdale WA (1964) Elektronenmikroskopische Studie am Alkoholiker-Hyalin. Am J Pathol 44: 441
Fleischer J, Riedel H (1964) Histologische Organveränderungen beim Kaninchen nach Gaben von Prednison und Endoxan. Folia Haematol 82: 23
Force EE, Miller JW (1974) Liver disease in fatal narcotism. Role of chronic disease and alcohol consumption. Arch Pathol Lab Med 97: 166
Fouts JR, Rogers LA (1965) Morphologische Veränderungen der Leber bei Einwirkung von Phenyläthylbarbitursäure, Chlordan, Benzypren oder Methylcholanthren auf die enzymatische Aktivität der Mikrosomen. J Pharmacol Exp Ther 147: 112
Franke W, Kyrieleis Chr (1976) Gewerbliche Bleivergiftung als Todesursache. Med Welt 27: 233
Friedel H-P (1976) Die sogenannte Vinylchlorid-Krankheit in der Bundesrepublik Deutschland. Fortschr Med 94: 1416
Fritsch P, Schellander F, Konrad K (1971) Arsen und Epitheliome der Haut. Eine katamnestische Studie. Wien Klin Wochenschr 83: 7
Frommhold H (1964) Licht- und fluoreszenzmikroskopische Untersuchungen am Herzmuskel nach akut-tödlicher Kohlenoxydvergiftung. Med Dissertation, Hamburg
Fruscella FDER (1963 a) Die durch experimentelle Kadmiumvergiftung hervorgerufenen Schäden am Herzmuskel: histologische und ekgraphische Beiträge. Rass Med Industr 32: 559
Fruscella FDER (1963 b) Experimentelle Cadmiumpneumopathie: ein histologischer Beitrag. Rass Med Industr 32: 537
Galle P, Morel-Maroger L (1965) Nierenveränderungen bei klinischer und experimenteller Bleivergiftung. Nephron 2: 273
Gebbers J-O, Burkhardt A, Höltje WJ (1975) Morphologische Lungenveränderungen nach Bleomycin-Therapie. Verh Dtsch Ges Pathol 59: 561
Geipel A (1969) Versehentliche Einnahme von Marcumar mit Überdosierung. Münch Med Wochenschr 34: 1681
Geldmacher v. Mallinckrodt M (1975) Forensische Toxikologie. In: Mueller B (ed) Gerichtliche Medizin. Springer, Berlin Heidelberg New York
Geldmacher v. Mallinckrodt M, Zober A, Dumbach J, Geldmacher JH, Lautenbach L, Machbert G, Reinhardt G (1976) Todesfälle durch kombinierte Wirkung von Alkohol und Medikamenten. Z Rechtsmed 78: 97
Gerber A (1976) Rauschmitteltodesfälle. Arch Kriminol 157: 42
Gerlach D (1978) Histopathologische Befunde bei Rauschmittelkonsumenten. Z Rechtsmed 80: 299

Gerlach E, Lycko E, Ludwig B (1978) Untersuchungen über die Pathomorphologie von Organen nach Rauschmittelintoxikationen. Forsch.-Bericht d. Landes NRW, Westdeutscher Verlag

Gerstenbrand F, Mamoli B, Binder H (1976) Zur schwersten Verlaufsform der CO-Intoxikation. Wien Klin Wochenschr 88: 418

Gerstenbrand F, Hamdi T, Kothbauer P, Rustam H, Badri MA (1977) Apallisches Syndrom bei chronischer Quecksilbervergiftung. Eur Neurol 15: 249

Girard R, Malleim ML, Bertholon J, Couer P, Tolot F (1970) Die alkalische Phosphatase der Leukocyten bei Benzolexposition. Med Lav 61: 502

Giusti GV, Gentile V (1974) Hyaline membrane disease in adults after artificial ventilation: a histopathologic study. Forensic Sci Int 4: 207

Goertchen R (1973) Hirngefäßthrombosen nach hormonaler Kontrazeption. Dtsch Gesundheitswesen 28: 161

Grabensee B, Veltmann G, Mürtz R, Borchard F (1971) Vergiftung durch Paraquat. Dtsch Med Wochenschr 96: 498

Grabinski E (1975) Die Paraquatvergiftung. Toxikologische und histologische Untersuchungen zur Frage der Korrelation zwischen Giftkonzentration und morphologischem Organbefund. Dissertation Göttingen

Greendyke RM, Hodge HC (1964) Unfallbedingte Todesfälle durch Fluorwasserstoff. J Forensic Sci 9: 383

Grosgogeat Y, Roubelakis G (1965) Die experimentelle Wirkung von Nicotin auf die Aortenwand des Kaninchens. Eine lichtmikroskopische und elektronenmikroskopische Untersuchung. Pathol Biol 13: 1140

Gsell O (1974) Von der Phenacetinniere zur Analgetikanephropathie. Praxis 63: 1299

Hagedorn M, Böttcher D, Hasler K, Mittermayer Ch (1975) Pathogenetic aspects of bromocarbamide intoxication. Arch Dermatol Forsch 252: 111

Hallermann W, Pribilla O (1959) Tödliche Vergiftungen mit Phosphorwasserstoff. Arch Toxikol 17: 219

Hanson JW, Jones KL, Smith DW (1976) Fetal alcohol syndrome, experience with 41 patients. J Am Med Assoc 235: 1458

Hawkins HL (1978) Acute alcoholic hepatitis with gradual progression to cirrhosis. Gastroenterology 74: 276

Heber R, Helmig L (1976) Hand- und Unterarmgangrän nach versehentlicher intraarterieller Injektion von Phenothiazinen. Med Welt 27: 2026

Heilmann K, Linhart P, Weizel A (1970) Morphologische Aspekte des Leberschadens bei Rauschmittelsucht und -mißbrauch. Dtsch Med Wochenschr 96: 453

Heinemann HO (1977) Alcohol and the lung. A brief review. Am J Med 63: 81

Heusermann U, Stutte HJ (1977) Enzymhistochemische, histometrische und ultrastrukturelle Untersuchungen von Milzen bei der Vinylchlorid-Krankheit. Virchows Arch [Pathol Anat] 375: 303

Hibbs RG, Ferrans VJ, Black WC, Weilbaecher DG, Walsh JJ, Burch GE (1965) Alkoholische Kardiomyopathie. Eine elektronenmikroskopische Studie. Am Heart J 69: 766

Hoffmeister W (1957) Kortikoidtherapie, Wirkungen und Nebenwirkungen. Therapiewoche 17: 1899

Holczabek W (1953) Mors in tabula. Dtsch Z Gerichtl Med 42: 385

Horn J (1970) Isolierung und Untersuchung von Einschlußkörperchen in der Rattenniere nach chronischer Bleivergiftung. Virchows Arch [Cell Pathol] 6: 313

Huebner G (1965) Direkte Tetrachlorkohlenstoffwirkung auf die Membransysteme der Zelle. Rev Int Hepat 15: 455

Hübner K (1976) Morphologie der Arzneimittelschäden der Leber. Therapiewoche 26: 590

Hundsdörfer S, Röse I (1980) Zur Pathogenese der Hämatoxylinkörperchen. Beobachtungen an einem tierexperimentellen Modell. Z Erkr Atmungsorgane 154: 60

Ichida F (1970) Morphologische Befunde bei chronischer Alkoholintoxikation in Japan. Therapiewoche 20: 2351

Iff HW, Brewis RAL, Mallick NP, Mawer GE, McNorr W, Stern MA (1971) Paraquatvergiftungen. Schweiz Med Wochenschr 101: 84

Illchmann-Christ A (1952) Zur Pathologie der akuten Kampfer-(Cardiazol)-Vergiftung im Kleinkindesalter. Arch Toxicol 14: 196

Illchmann-Christ A (1954) Zur Pathologie der tödlichen Antabus-Alkoholreaktion. Dtsch Z Ges Gerichtl Med 43: 95

Illig L (1976) Purpura. – Einteilung, Klinik und Ätiopathogenese aus der Sicht des Dermatologen. Fortschr Med 94: 1379

Ito M, Shoji M, Kiribayashi K (1966) Morphologische Veränderungen am Myokard von Kaninchen nach experimenteller Alkoholvergiftung. Jpn J Stud Alcohol 1: 265

Iturriaga H, Insunza I, Ugarte G, Altschiller H (1966) Pathologie der Leber bei Alkoholikern. 1. Grundlegende morphologische Aspekte. Rev Med Chile 94: 399

Jaklinska A (1968) Über den Einfluß experimenteller Lebernekrosen auf den Verlauf der Alkoholausscheidung aus dem Blut von Kaninchen. Arch Med Sadowej 18: 73

Jansen HH (1967) Gefäßveränderungen bei Knocheninfarkten nach Cortison. Vortrag a. d. Tagung der Nord- u. Westdeutschen Pathologen v. 27.–29. 10. 67 in Lüneburg

Jansen HH (1977) Tödliche Arzneimittelnebenwirkungen aus pathologisch-anatomischer Sicht. Verh Dtsch Ges Inn Med 83: 1530

Janssen W (1962) Eitrige Myocarditis als ungewöhnliche Organmanifestation einer subacuten Tetrachlorkohlenstoffvergiftung. Dtsch Z Gerichtl Med 53: 72

Janssen W (1963) Zur Morphologie und Pathogenese des Corticosteroidschadens. Frankf Z Pathol 72: 462

Janssen W, Burger E (1968) Ungewöhnliche Art einer tödlichen Vergiftung durch Kaliumzyanid mit außergewöhnlichem Organbefund. Arch Kriminol 141: 99

Janssen W, Michot F (1960) Über die Pathomorphose der Periarteriitis nodosa nach Behandlung mit Corticosteroiden. Pathol Microbiol 4: 511

Jonek J (1964) Histochemische Untersuchungen über das Verhalten einiger Enzyme im Herzmuskel nach experimenteller Vergiftung mit Quecksilberdämpfen. Int Arch Gewerbepathol Gewerbehyg 21: 1

Jonek J, Kosmider S (1964) Verhalten der Atmungsfermente und der alkalischen Phosphatase in der Leber bei experimenteller Vergiftung mit Quecksilberdämpfen. Int Arch Gewerbepathol Gewerbehyg 20: 496

Jonek J, Pacholek A, Jez W (1964 a) Histochemische Untersuchungen über das Verhalten der Adenosintriphosphatase, 5-Nucleotidase, sauren Phosphatase, sauren Desoxyribonuclease II und der unspezifischen Esterasen in der Leber bei experimenteller Vergiftung mit Quecksilberdämpfen. Int Arch Gewerbepathol Gewerbehyg 20: 562

Jonek J, Waclawczyk H, Kosmider S, Cichon A (1964 b) Histochemische Untersuchungen einiger Enzyme in Nieren bei experimenteller Vergiftung mit Quecksilberdämpfen. Zentralbl Arbeitsmed Arbeitsschutz 14: 205

Kagawa M (1970) Histopathologische Leberuntersuchungen an unausgewählten Sektionsfällen. Überprüfung des Vorkommens von „Mallory-Körpern", Fett-Cirrhosen und „acidophilen Einschlüssen". Jpn J Leg Med 24: 427

Kaindl F (1971) Medikamentös bedingte pulmonale Hypertonie. Wien Klin Wochenschr 83: 373

Kapanci Y, Kaplan Y, Weibel ER (1967) Elektronenmikroskopische und morphometrische Studien zum Effekt des reinen Sauerstoffes auf die Lunge des Affen. Jahresversammlung d. Schweizerischen Pathologen, 17.–18. 11. 1967, Basel

Kaufmann G (1953) Tetrachlorkohlenstoff-Cirrhose und Restauration der Leber. Beitr Pathol Anat 113: 253

Kaufmann M, Müller A, Paweletz N, Haller U, Kubli F (1978) Fetale Schädigung bei einer Knollenblätterpilzvergiftung der Mutter in der Frühschwangerschaft. Geburtshilfe Frauenheilkd 38: 122

Kenyeres I, Balogh I, Somogyi E (1978) Angaben zur Pathogenese von Lungenveränderungen durch Inhalation eines organischen Lösungsmittels. Morphol Igazsagugyi Orv Sz 18: 23

Kessler G, Klöppel G, Schaarschmidt W (1975) Licht- und elektronenmikroskopische Untersuchungen der Rattenleber nach intraperitonealer Applikation von Halothan. Anaesth prax 11: 41

Kibler WB (1973) Skeletal muscle necrosis secondary to parathion. Toxicol Appl Pharmacol 25: 117

Kimbrough RD, Linder RE (1973) The ultrastructure of the paraquat lung lesion in the rat. Environ Res 6: 265

Klavis G, Schulz LCL (1966) Herzschäden bei der akuten Kohlenmonoxyd-Vergiftung. Arch Toxicol 21: 250

Klein H (1950) Zur pathologischen Histologie nach akuter Benzinvergiftung. Ein Beitrag zur primären toxischen Lipoidbildung im Gehirn. Dtsch Z Gerichtl Med 40: 76
Klima T, Ort M (1966) Akute corticale Nekrose der Nieren im Verlaufe der Corticoidtherapie. Monatsschr Kinderheilkd 114: 38
Klinge O (1973) Cytologische und histologische Aspekte toxisch induzierter Leberreaktionen. Curr Top Pathol 58: 91
Klinge O (1979) Arzneimittelbedingte Reaktionen der kindlichen Leber. Monatsschr Kinderheilkd 127: 115
Koch HK, Agostini B, Lesch R (1978) Die Topik der Leberzellnekrosen und -proliferation nach subletaler Phalloidinvergiftung junger und adulter Ratten. Verh Dtsch Ges Pathol 62: 265
Kodagoda N, Jayewardene RP, Attygalle D (1973) Poisoning with paraquat. Forensic Sci Int 2: 107
Kojima K (1973) Pancreatic lesions in alcoholism. Acta Med Biol 20: 111
Korb G (1962) Licht- und fluorescenzmikroskopische Befunde am Herzmuskel bei der akuten Leuchtgasvergiftung. Dtsch Z Gerichtl Med 52: 357
Korb G, David H (1962) Fluorescenzmikroskopische und elektronenoptische Untersuchungen am Herzmuskel der Ratte nach Leuchtgasvergiftungen. Dtsch Z Gerichtl Med 52: 549
Korenke HE, Pribilla O (1969) Suicid durch einmalige Inhalation von Tetrachlorkohlenstoff (CCl_4) mit Leukoencephalopathie. Arch Toxicol 25: 109
Krienke EG (1975) Knollenblätterpilz-Vergiftung. Dtsch Aerztebl 72: 2251
Krishnan N, Stenger RJ (1966) Auswirkungen des Hungerzustandes auf die leberschädigende Wirkung des Tetrachlorkohlenstoffes. Am J Pathol 49: 239
Krug H (1965) Die Hirnkonsistenz bei tödlicher Kohlenmonoxydvergiftung. Dtsch Z Ges Gerichtl Med 56: 74
Kühn H, Arnold W (1963) Über pathologische und chemische Befunde bei Kalypnon-Vergiftungen. Arch Toxicol 20: 148
Kühne D, Götze P (1978) Verschlüsse der A. cerebri posterior unter besonderer Berücksichtigung des Nikotinabusus und der hormonalen Antikonzeptiva. Eine klinische und angiographische Studie. Fortschr Neurol Psychiatr 46: 1
Kuhn H, Loogen F (1977) Die Wirkung von Alkohol auf das Herz einschließlich der Alkoholkardiomyopathie. Internist 19: 97
Kurstak C, Côte MG, Plaa GL (1973) Die Wirkung der Unterkühlung auf Tetrachlorkohlenstoff-induzierte Veränderungen der Ultrastruktur der Leber. Toxicol Appl Pharmacol 26: 14
Kuschinsky G, Lüllmann H (1972) Kurzes Lehrbuch der Pharmakologie, 5th edn. Thieme, Stuttgart
Lahl R (1973) Fettembolien nach experimenteller Tetrachlorkohlenstoffintoxikation. Z Gesamte Inn Med 28: 367
Lang E, Haupt EJ, Köhler JA, Schmidt J (1969) Cor pulmonale durch Appetitzügler? Münch Med Wochenschr 111: 405
Lange HP, Dippell J (1970) Über Schädigungen der Niere nach hochdosierter Cytostaticatherapie. Zentralbl Allg Pathol 113: 313
Langohr HD, Schumm F, Luithle HJ, Mayer K, Rentschler R (1977) Vergleichende biochemische und elektrophysiologische Untersuchungen in der Skelettmuskulatur bei Alkoholismus. Arch Psychiatr Nervenkr 223: 249
Lanzinger G, Ritz E, Franz HE, Kuhn HM, Klein H: Akute interstitielle Lungenfibrose bei Paraquat-Vergiftung. Klinisch-anatomische Beobachtung eines Falles mit tödlichem Ausgang. Münch Med Wochenschr 111: 944
Larson RE, Plaa GL, Crews LM (1964) Die Wirkung der Rückenmarksdurchtrennung auf die Toxicität von Tetrachlorkohlenstoff. Toxicol Appl Pharmacol 6: 154
Leithoff H, Leithoff J (1969) Organveränderungen als Leitsymptome bei der Ausmittelung von Giften. In: Graf E, Preuss FR (eds) Gadamers Lehrbuch der chemischen Toxikologie und Anleitung zur Ausmittelung der Gifte, vol I/1. Vandenhoeck u. Ruprecht, Göttingen
Lelbach WK (1972) Die alkoholische Fettleber. Münch Med Wochenschr 113: 1549
Lesch R (1968) Histologische und histoautoradiographische Befunde bei der experimentellen chronischen Bleivergiftung. Verh Dtsch Ges Pathol 542
Lesch R (1974) Das morphologische Bild der alkoholischen Fettleberhepatitis. Z Allgemeinmed 50: 927
Lesch R, Hoppe-Seyler P, Heißmeyer HH, Hoensch D, Jenss H, Wimmer B, Wenz W (1980) Orale Kontrazeptiva und gutartige tumoröse Veränderungen der Leber. Radiologe 20: 565

Letterer E (1957) Die pathologische Anatomie des Vergiftungstodes. In: Ponsold A (ed) Lehrbuch der gerichtlichen Medizin, 2nd edn. Thieme, Stuttgart
Leuschner U, Strohm WD, Czygan P, Ast E, Fröhling W, Stiehl A (1976) Elektronenmikroskopische Untersuchungen am Lebergewebe von Patienten mit Knollenblätterpilzvergiftung (Amanita phalloides). Z Gastroenterol 14: 767
Liebegott G (1967) Morphologische Befunde nach Anwendung von Kurznarkotika. Therapeutische Berichte 39: 25
Lieber CS (1975) Liver disease and alcohol: fatty liver, alcoholic hepatitis, cirrhosis and their interrelationships. Ann NY Acad Sci 252: 63
Liem CF (1970) Die chronische alkoholische Pankreatitis. Schweiz Med Wochenschr 100: 1473
Lindner H, du Bosque G, Dammermann, R, Klöppel G, Krause D (1975) Phenolisatin-induzierte Lebererkrankungen. Dtsch Med Wochenschr 49: 2530
Linke H (1971) Kumarinnekrosen, Pathogenese, Klinik und Therapie. Unter Berücksichtigung 6 eigener Fälle. Z Gesamte Inn Med 26: 271
Lisch H-J, Leiner G, Schwarzmüller B (1977) Letale Panmyelophthise nach 8jährigem Abusus von Appetitzüglern. Schweiz Med Wochenschr 107: 347
Liu HM, Maurer HS, Vongsvivut S, Conway JJ (1978) Methotrexate encephalopathy. A neuropathologic study. Hum Pathol 9: 635
Lo Menzo G (1966) Il comportamento dell'attività citocromossidasica e succinodeidrogenasica di taluni organi nell' avvelenamento acute da CO. Folia Medica 8: 607
Lorenz G (1978) Bioptische Leberveränderungen bei chronischem Alkoholismus. Z Gesamt Inn Med 33: 145
Ludwig H, Werthemann A (1962) Benzol-Myelopathien. Schweiz Med Wochenschr 92: 378
Lüchtrath H, Krüger R (1971) Arsen und Lebercirrhose in der Begutachtung heute. Int Arch Arbeitsmed 28: 330
Majewski F, Bierich JR, Löser H, Michaelis R, Leiber B, Bettecken F (1976) Zur Klinik und Pathogenese der Alkohol-Embryopathie, Bericht über 68 Fälle. Münch Med Wochenschr 118: 1635
Marek Z, Piejko M (1972) Circulatory failure in acute carbon monoxide poisoning. Forensic Sci Int 1: 419
Maresch W (1978) Der pathologisch-anatomische Befund bei Arsenikvergiftungen. Beitr Gerichtl Med 36: 41
Maresch W, Probst A (1962) Tödliche intravenöse Petroleuminjektion. Dtsch Z Gerichtl Med 52: 234
Mari E, Corsi Bargellini P, Pozone F (1967) Physikalisch-chemische und histologische Probleme der Thanatologie. Experimentelle Untersuchungen an Rattenlebern bei Phosphorvergiftung. G Med Leg Infortun Tossicol 13: 236
Meier W (1962) Experimentelle Untersuchungen zur Bedeutung der vacuoligen Umwandlung der Leber für die Diagnostik der Kohlenmonoxydvergiftung. Dtsch Z Gerichtl Med 52: 258
Metter D (1978) Pathologisch-anatomische Befunde bei Heroinvergiftung. Beitr Gerichtl Med 36: 433
Meyer J-E (1961) Hirnveränderungen vom Typ der intervallären CO-Vergiftung nach Stickoxydul-Narkose. Arch Psychiatr Nervenkr 202: 113
Milana V, Fichera G (1962) Experimentelle Untersuchungen über eventuelle schädliche Wirkungen durch das Einatmen von Polytetrafluoräthylen (PTFE)-Dämpfen. Folia Med (Napoli) 45: 1295
Miyabe I (1976) Studies on the fatty liver in acute dead bodies. Fatty acid composition in the alcoholic fatty liver. Jpn J Stud Alcohol 11: 31
Miyakawa T, Hattori E, Shikai I, Shimoi A, Nagatoshi K, Suzuki T (1977) Histopathological changes of chronic alcoholism. Folia Psychiatr Neurol Jpn 31: 253
Mölbert E, Huhn D, Büchner F (1964) Elektronenmikroskopische Untersuchungen am Tubulusepithel der Niere sublimatvergifteter Ratten. Beitr Pathol Anat 129: 222
Möllhoff G, Schmidt G (1976) Deaths resulting from drugs by abuse. Forensic Sci Int 7: 31
Moeschlin S (1972) Klinik und Therapie der Vergiftungen. 5 edn. Thieme, Stuttgart
Molz G (1971) Pneumopathien bei Neugeborenen nach langfristiger intratrachealer Druckbeatmung mit hochgespanntem Sauerstoff. Beitr Gerichtl Med 28: 66
Montalto B, Bartoloni Saint Omer F, Maurri M (1978) Pathologisch-anatomische Befunde bei 6 Vergiftungsfällen durch Betäubungsmittel. Minerva Med Leg 98: 79

Morgan JM, Hartley MW, Miller RE (1966) Nephropathie bei chronischer Bleivergiftung. Arch Intern Med 118: 17

Mosinger M, Fiorentini et Quicke H (1953) Zur Pathologie der experimentellen Kohlenoxydvergiftung. Sitzg, Luxembourg, 27.–29. 5. 1953, p 427

Müller PH (1965) Rezidivierende Lungenembolien mit sekundärer Thrombose der Pulmonalarterien bei Einnahme eines oralen Ovulationshemmers. Schweiz Med Wochenschr 95: 1367

Müller S, Wiesendanger V, Wegmann W, Scheitlin W, Moccetti T (1973) Akutes Nierenversagen durch Cephalothin? Schweiz Med Wochenschr 103: 889

Müller GL, Graham S (1955) Intrauteriner Fruchttod durch Kohlenmonoxydvergiftung. N Engl J Med 252: 1075

Nanikawa R, Hamaoka H, Awata Y (1960) Studies on the succinic dehydrogenase of cardiac muscle. Chemical and histochemical findings in carbon monoxide poisoning, death from cold, and hypoxygen respiration. Nagoya Med J 6: 27

Nasseri M, Kirstaedter H-J, Bücherl ES (1966) Experimentelle Untersuchungen über das Allgemeinverhalten und die morphologischen Veränderungen unter hohem Sauerstoffdruck. Virchows Arch [Pathol Anat] 341: 148

Neoral L, Dusek J, Smysl B (1977) Beitrag zur kausalen und formalen Pathogenese tödlicher Paraquatvergiftungen. Z Rechtsmed 80: 1

Nienhaus H, Poche R, Reimold E, (1963) Elektrolytverschiebungen, histologische Veränderungen der Organe und Ultrastruktur des Herzmuskels nach Belastung mit Cortisol, Aldosteron und primärem Natriumphosphat bei der Ratte. Virch Arch [Pathol Anat] 337: 245

Noeske K, Martens H (1972) Histologische und histometrische Untersuchungen am Benzolgeschädigten Rattenknochenmark. Virchows Arch [Pathol Anat] 355: 50

Okamura K (1976) A study on Mallory bodies. Isolation, ultrastructure and preliminary biochemical characterization of Mallory bodies from livers of alcoholic cirrhosis and malignant hepatoma. Acta Pathol Jpn 26: 649

Okonek S (1976) Vergiftungen durch Paraquat oder Deiquat. Med Welt 27: 1401

Okumura T (1969) Untersuchungen über Arzneimittelschock-Fälle bei Menschen (vorwiegend anhand histologischer Untersuchungen von Leber und Nebenniere). Jpn J Leg Med 23: 450

Paraf A, Coste Th, Gouffier Er (1971) Die Störungen der Hämatopoese bei schwerem Alkoholismus. Presse Med 79: 2219

Patscheider H, Hetzel H (1961) Histologische Befunde bei einem Fall akuter Vergiftung durch Äthylenglykol. Arch Toxicol 19: 143

Patscheider H, Dirnhofer R (1973) Über eine alimentäre, protrahiert verlaufende Cyanvergiftung. Z Rechtsmed 71: 315

Peiffer J (1963) Symmetrische Pallidum- und Nigranekrosen nach unbemerkt gebliebenem Zwischenfall bei Barbituratnarkose. Z Nervenheilkd 184: 586

Persson LI, Rosengren LE, Johansson BB, Hansson HA (1979) Blood-brain barrier dysfunction to peroxidase after air embolism, aggravated by acute ethanol intoxication. J Neurol Sci 42: 65

Pesendorfer F, Platthy G (1973) Gefäßwandschädigung und thromboembolische Gefäßverschlüsse nach Einnahme von Ovulationshemmern. Med Klin 68: 74

Petelenz T, Zajusz K, Dukat R, Misiewicz A, Zeleznik B (1972) Badania Doswiadczalne Dzilania Tlenku Wegla Na Ustroj. Archiwum Medycyny Sadowej i. Krymninilogii 12: 219

Peter H (1955) Organbefunde nach akuter Cadmiumvergiftung. Verh Dtsch Ges Pathol 225

Petersen P (1977) Alcoholic hyalin, microfilaments and microtubules in alcoholic hepatitis. Acta Pathol Microbiol Scand [A] 85: 384

Petri E (1930) Pathologische Anatomie und Histologie der Vergiftungen. In: Henke F, Lubarsch O (eds) Pathologische Anatomie und Histologie der Vergiftungen. Springer, Berlin (Handbuch der speziellen pathologischen Anatomie und Histologie, vol 10)

Pioch W (1960) Mordversuch und Mord durch Einspritzung von Luft, Benzin und Insulin. Dtsch Z Ges Gerichtl Med 49: 665

Podlesch I (1972) Sauerstoffüberdruckbehandlung. Probleme und Anwendung. Bericht über ein Colloquium am 13. u. 14. Nov. 1970 in Düsseldorf. Anaesthesiol Resusc 42

Poisson M (1969) Die muskulären Komplikationen des Alkoholismus. Rev Alcohol 15: 169

Pribilla O (1966) Tödliche Vergiftungen mit Salzen der Kieselfluorwasserstoffsäure. In: Gerchow J (ed) An den Grenzen von Medizin und Recht. Enke, Stuttgart

Pribilla W, Härtel G, Albrecht M (1966) Veränderungen des Knochenmarks bei chronischem Alkoholismus. Med Klin 61: 1031
Prick JJG, Sillievis-Smith WG, Müller L (1955) Thallium poisoning. Elsevier, Amsterdam Houston London New York
Próchnicka B, Marek Z (1973) Microscopical changes of myocardium in acute carbon monoxide poisoning. Arch Med Sadowej 23: 289
Prokop O (1950) Vacuolige Degeneration des Herzens bei der Methylalkoholvergiftung. Dtsch Z Gerichtl Med 40: 127
Püschel K (1982) Zum morphologischen Nachweis des intravenösen Drogenkonsums. In: Arnold W, Püschel, K (eds) Kongreßbericht Internationales Symposium: Fortschritte der forensischen Chemie. Verlag Dr. D Helm, Heppenheim
Püschel K, Mätzsch T (1981) Alkoholintoxikation im Kindesalter. Z Rechtsmed 86: 269
Püschel K, Seifert H (1979) Bedeutung des Alkohols in der Embryofetalperiode und beim Neugeborenen. Z Rechtsmed 83: 69
Püschel K, Schulz F, Naeve W, Arnold W (1980) Todesfälle nach nasaler Applikation von Heroin. Z Rechtsmed 84: 279
Radford DJ, Oliver MF (1973) Oral contraceptives and myocardial infarction. Br Med J 3: 428
Raestrup O (1926) Über cutane Schädigungen durch Zyankalium. Zentralbl Bakteriol [B] 3: 103
Raszeja S (1960) Histologische Untersuchungen der Leber bei Pilzvergiftung (Amanita phalloides). Dtsch Z Gerichtl Med 50: 417
Rauschke J (1963) Über Art, Entstehung und Spezifität der morphologischen Haarbefunde bei Thalliumvergiftung. Acta Med Leg Soc (Liege) 16: 103
Reichel W, Tönnis H, Scheler F (1973) Goodpasture-Syndrom nach Kohlenwasserstoff-Exposition. Umweltmedizin 111: 75
Reineke H (1977) Lungenveränderungen während Dauerbeatmung. Anaesthesiol Resusc 105
Reppart JT, Peters RL, Edmondson HA, Baker RF (1963) Elektronen- und Lichtmikroskopie der sklerosierenden hyalinen Nekrose der Leber. Die Entwicklung alkoholischer Hyalinkörper. Lab Invest 12: 1138
Reuter F (1938) Methoden der forensischen Beurteilung von Vergiftungen. In: Abderhalden E (ed) Handbuch der biologischen Arbeitsmethoden. Urban u. Schwarzenberg, Berlin Wien
Rewcastle NB, Humphrey JG (1965) Vacuoläre Myopathie. Eine klinische, histochemische und mikroskopische Studie. Arch Neurol 12: 570
Reynolds ES (1963) Leberparenchymschaden. I. Frühe Zellveränderungen nach Vergiftung mit Tetrachlorkohlenstoff. J Cell Biol 19: 139
Reynolds ES, Ree HJ, Moslen MG (1972) Leberparenchymschädigung. IX. Durch Phenobarbital verstärkte Denaturierung von endoplasmatischem Reticulum nach Gaben von Tetrachlorkohlenstoff. Lab Invest 26: 290
Riesner K, Janssen W (1978) Alkoholbedingte Kardiomyopathie und plötzlicher Herztod. Beitr Gerichtl Med 36: 351
Rizzi A (1962) Pathologisch-anatomische Studien bei akuter Colchicin-Vergiftung. Folia Med (Napoli) 45: 913
Robert A, Nezamis JE (1964) Die Histopathologie des Steroidulcus. Eine experimentelle Studie an Ratten. Arch Pathol Lab Med 77: 407
Roschlau G (1977) Die alkoholische Zirrhose aus bioptischer Sicht. Dtsch Gesundheitswes 32: 1211
Rouiller Ch, Colombey N, Haenni B, Perrelet A, de Torrente A (1965) Strukturveränderungen an der Wand der Lebersinusoide bei akuten experimentellen Intoxikationen. Rev Int Hépatol 15: 437
Rubin E (1979) Alcoholic myopathy in heart and skeletal muscle. N Engl J Med 301: 28
Rüdell E, Berg S, Pöhlmann K (1978) Das Verhalten der Lungen-Mastzellen bei der akuten Vergiftung mit Barbituraten und Bromureiden. Z Rechtsmed 82: 189
Ryvarden G (1973) Die „Alkoholische Fettleber" aus forensischer Sicht. Beitr Gerichtl Med 31: 267
Salamone L, Scorsone A (1961) Myocardinfarkt als Folge einer Blausäurevergiftung. Folia Med (Napoli) 44: 609
Salfelder K, Seelkopf C (1963) Über akute Phosphorvergiftungen beim Mensch mit Sektionsbefunden. Frankf Z Pathol 72: 357
Sattes H (1973) Schäden des Nervensystems durch Alkohol. Med Klin 68: 1493

Schaffner F, Felig P (1965) Veränderungen der Leberstruktur bei Ratten durch Einatmen reinen Sauerstoffs. J Cell Biol 27: 505
Schaffner F, Loebel A, Weiner HA, Barka T (1963) Veränderungen am Cytoplasma der Leberzelle bei „akuter Alkohol-Hepatitis". JAMA 183: 343
Schattenberg PJ, Totović V, Gedigk P, Marsteller HJ (1977) Die Ultrastruktur der Leberschädigung bei der chronischen Vinylchlorid-Intoxikation. Virchows Arch [Pathol Anat] 373: 233
Scheda W (1960) Über diffuse Hirnrindennekrose im Anschluß an akute Alkoholvergiftung. Psychiatr Neurol Med Psychol (Leipz) 12: 312
Schimassek H, Jeckel D (1978) Wirkung von Phalloidin auf Leberzellen: Bindung, Strukturveränderung und Elimination. Cytobiologie 17: 73
Schlipköter H-W, Bruch J (1973) Funktionelle und morphologische Veränderung bei Ozon-Expositionen. Zentrlbl Bakteriologie [B] 156: 486
Schmidtmann M (1934) Experimentelle Untersuchungen über die Wirkungen der Autoabgase. Verhand Dtsch Pathol Ges 134
Scholler KL (1968) Elektronenmikroskopische und autoradiographische Untersuchungen über die Wirkung von Halothan und Chloroform auf die Leberzellen. Univ flg, Aarhus
Schollmeyer W (1961) Die pathologische Histologie der Kalypnonvergiftung. Dtsch Z Gerichtl Med 52: 46
Schreiner GE, Maher JF (1965) Toxische Nephropathien. Am J Med 38: 409
Schweikert CH, Kapfhammer V (1965) Zur Frage der Hepatotoxicität des Halothans. Ein tierexperimenteller Beitrag unter besonderer Berücksichtigung der Hypoxydosen. Anaesthesist 14: 74
Seidel HJ (1978) Ätiologie der Leukämien. In: Begemann H (ed) Leukämie. Springer, Berlin Heidelberg New York (Handbuch der inneren Medizin, vol II/6, p 49)
Shanoff HM (1972) Alcoholic cardiomyopathy: an introductory review. Can Med Assoc J 106: 55
Simon H, Kemmer Chr, Müller M (1964) Über die Wirkung hoher Chlorochin- und Prednisongaben auf Fermente und Strukturen der Leberepithelzellen weißer Ratten. Frankf Z Pathol 74: 109
Slodkowska J, Szendzikowski S, Stetkiewicz J, Muszynski J (1980) The histological picture and mechanism of development of the liver changes in poisoning with Amanita phalloides. Pathol Pol 31: 55
Smith B (1964) Histological and histochemical changes in the muscles of rabbits given the corticosteroid triamcinolone. Neurology 114/9: 857
Smith HJ, Roche AHG, Jagusch MF, Herodson PB (1976) Cardiomyopathy associated with amphetamine administration. Am Heart J 91: 792
Somogyi E (1972) Clinical and medico-legal aspects of hyperbaric oxygenation. Z Rechtsmed 71: 79
Sorgo G (1976) Trichloräthylen-, Tetrachlorkohlenstoff- und Benzinintoxikation als ätiologischer Faktor bei der Entstehung der Arterio- bzw. Koronarsklerose. Arch Toxicol 35: 295
Sosnierz M, Szczurek Z, Knapek R, Kolodziejczyk A (1970) Morphologische Befunde bei Ratten in der Folge von subakuter und chronischer Intoxikation durch das phosphororganische Schädlingsbekämpfungsmittel „Naled", Arch Med Sadowej 20: 239
Stahl CJ, Fatteh AV, Dominguez AM (1969) Trichloroethane poisoning: Observations of the pathology and toxicology in six fatal cases. J Forensic Sci 14: 393
Stenger RJ (1966) Konzentrische lamelläre Strukturen in der Leberparenchymzelle der Ratte nach Tetrachlorkohlenstoffvergiftung. J Ultrastruct Res 14: 240
Stenger RJ (1966) Lebersinusoide bei Tetrachlorkohlenstoffinduzierter Cirrhose. Arch Pathol 81: 439
Stötzner H, Jaross W, Schnentke KU, Hanefeld M, Herrmann V, Fuchs R (1973) Morphologische Leberveränderungen bei chronischen Alkoholikern ohne internistische Erkrankungen und ihre Überprüfung auf eine diagnostische Verwertbarkeit. Zentralbl Allg Pathol 117: 274
Stoll BA, Andrews JT, Motteram R (1966) Leberschäden durch orale empfängnisverhütende Mittel. Br Med J 1: 960
Strassmann G, Sturner W, Helpern M (1969) Gehirnschädigungen, insbesondere Linsenkernerweichungen bei Heroinsüchtigen, nach Barbituratvergiftung, Spättod nach Erhängen und Herzstillstand in der Narkose. Beitr Gerichtl Med 25: 236
Strauss RH, Palmer KC, Hayes JA (1976) Acute lung injury induced by cadmium aerosol. I. Evolution of alveolar cell damage. Am J Pathol 84: 561
Szabó G (1940) Zwerchfellveränderungen bei langsamer Erstickung. Dtsch Z Gerichtl Med 33: 1

Szadkowski D (1976) Klinik und Pathologie der sogenannten Vinylchlorid-Krankheit. Fortschr Med 94: 1412
Täschner K-L (1973) Veränderungen am Glomus caroticum des Menschen bei E 605-Vergiftung. Z Rechtsmed 73: 71
Taylor NS (1965) Histochemische Untersuchung der Nephrotoxizität subletaler Quecksilberdosen bei Ratten. Am J Pathol 46: 1
Tessmann D (1964) Zur Frage des Prednisoneffektes bei akuter Leberschädigung (Tetrachlorkohlenstoff-Test an der Rattenleber). Z Gesamt Inn Med 19: 204
Thaler H (1979) Die Alkoholhepatitis. Ist sie die ausschließliche Ursache einer Alkoholzirrhose? Internist 20: 179
Thurner J (1970) Iatrogene Pathologie. Urban & Schwarzenberg, München Berlin Wien
Tilling W (1968) Paraquat-Intoxikation. Dtsch Med Wochenschr 93: 2439
Timm F (1958) Zur Histochemie der Schwermetalle. Das Sulfidsilberverfahren. Dtsch Z Ges Gerichtl Med 46: 706
Timm F (1961) Der histochemische Nachweis der Sublimatvergiftung. Beitr Gerichtl Med 21: 195
Timm F (1962) Zur Histochemie der chronischen Quecksilbervergiftung. Beitr Gerichtl Med 22: 321
Totović V (1964) Elektronenmikroskopische Befunde in der Niere bei chronischer Bleivergiftung der Ratte. Verh Dtsch Ges Pathol 193
Tovo S (1962) Tödliche Lebernekrose nach akuter Bariumpolysulfidvergiftung. Minerva Med-Leg 82: 347
Tsinronis A, Papacharalampous NX (1973) Schnelles Auftreten einer Leberzirrhose durch gleichzeitige Tetrachlorkohlenstoff- und Phenobarbitalverabreichung bei Ratten. Zentralbl Allg Pathol 117: 176
Uehlinger E (1964) Aseptische Knochennekrosen (Infarkte) nach Prednisonbehandlung. Schweiz Med Wochenschr 94: 1527
Ule G, Pribilla O (1962) Hirnveränderungen nach Cyankalivergiftung mit protrahiertem (intervallärem) klinischem Verlauf. Acta Neuropathol 1: 406
Umiker W, Pearce J (1953) Natur und Entstehung von Lungenschäden bei Tetrachlorkohlenstoffvergiftung. Arch Pathol Lab Med 55: 203
Veragut UP (1967) Gibt es eine alkoholische Kardiopathie? Praxis 56: 1202
Voigt GE (1971) Metallnachweis. Acta Histochemica 9: 489
Voit D, Dorndorf W (1971) Schlaganfälle nach Einnahme von Ovulationshemmern? Dtsch Med Wochenschr 96: 412
Waldbott GL (1963) Akute Fluoridvergiftung. Acta Med Scand [Suppl] 400, 174: 44
Walther G (1972) Über den Reaktionsverlauf der Sauerstoffvergiftung. Beitr Gerichtl Med 29: 21
Walther G, v. Lieven Th (1971) Histochemische Organveränderungen in Leber und Herzmuskel der Ratte nach Sauerstoff-Intoxikation. Beitr Gerichtl Med 28: 50
Weinig E (1957) Gerichtliche Vergiftungslehre. In: Ponsold A (ed) Lehrbuch der gerichtlichen Medizin. Thieme, Stuttgart
Weinig, Schmidt G (1966) Zur Verteilung des Thalliums im Organismus bei tödlichen Thalliumvergiftungen. Arch Toxicol 21: 199
White DJ (1977) Histochemical and histological effects of lead on the liver and kidney of the dog. Br J Exp Pathol 58: 101
Wiedeman MP, Tuma RF, Mayrovitz HN: In vivo microscopic observations of intra-arterial injections of barbiturates. J Surg Res 22: 97
Wilson DL, Rosen DA, Bencosme SA (1962) Steroidnephropathie beim Kaninchen. Diabetes 11: 402
Wink K (1978) Diagnose und Differentialdiagnose der alkoholischen Myokardiopathie. Internist Praxis 18, 369
Wohlfeil R, Schiffter R, Schliack H (1973) Schlaganfälle junger Frauen bei Einnahme von Ovulationshemmern. Fortschr Neurol Psychiatr 41: 166
Woźniak L, Kosicki M (1973) Acute toxicity of trichlorethylene. II. Evaluation of morphological changes in liver and kidney of white rat. Arch Med Sadowej 23: 105
Wunderer A, Schuch P (1963) Beitrag zur Frage der Periarteriitis nodosa als Therapiefolge nach Corticocosteroidbehandlung. Arch Kinderheilkd 169: 162

Yates JC, Yates RD (1964) Einige morphologische Wirkungen von Strychnin auf das Rückenmark: eine licht- und elektronenmikroskopische Studie. Anat Rec 150: 279

Zollinger HU (1953) Durch chronische Bleivergiftung erzeugte Nierenadenome und -carcinome bei Ratten und ihre Beziehungen zu den entsprechenden Neubildungen des Menschen. Virchows Arch [Pathol Anat] 323: 694

Zollinger HU (1966) Niere und ableitende Harnwege. Springer, Berlin Heidelberg New York

Zschiesche W (1962) Über Insulinsuicid aus morphologischer Sicht. Dtsch Z Gerichtl Med 53: 34

E. Subject Index

E

F

M

T

GPSR Compliance
The European Union's (EU) General Product Safety Regulation (GPSR) is a set of rules that requires consumer products to be safe and our obligations to ensure this.

If you have any concerns about our products, you can contact us on

ProductSafety@springernature.com

In case Publisher is established outside the EU, the EU authorized representative is:

Springer Nature Customer Service Center GmbH
Europaplatz 3
69115 Heidelberg, Germany

www.ingramcontent.com/pod-product-compliance
Ingram Content Group UK Ltd.
Pitfield, Milton Keynes, MK11 3LW, UK
UKHW051839180926
475695UK00004B/117

* 9 7 8 3 6 4 2 6 9 1 4 4 7 *